Point-of-Care Testing

Point-of-Care Testing

Performance Improvement and Evidence-Based Outcomes

edited by

James H. Nichols

Baystate Health System
Springfield, Massachusetts
and
Tufts University School of Medicine
Boston, Massachusetts

MARCEL DEKKER, INC. NEW YORK • BASEL

Library of Congress Cataloging-in-Publication Data
A catalog record for this book is available from the Library of Congress.

ISBN: 0-8247-0868-7

This book is printed on acid-free paper.

Headquarters
Marcel Dekker, Inc.
270 Madison Avenue, New York, NY 10016
tel: 212-696-9000; fax: 212-685-4540

Eastern Hemisphere Distribution
Marcel Dekker AG
Hutgasse 4, Postfach 812, CH-4001 Basel, Switzerland
tel: 41-61-260-6300; fax: 41-61-260-6333

World Wide Web
http://www.dekker.com

The publisher offers discounts on this book when ordered in bulk quantities. For more information, write to Special Sales/Professional Marketing at the headquarters address above.

Current printing (last digit):
10 9 8 7 6 5 4 3 2 1

PRINTED IN THE UNITED STATES OF AMERICA

Preface

Why? This is the question that many find themselves asking regarding the performance of laboratory testing at the site of patient care (point-of-care testing, POCT). While clinicians can argue the need for faster turnaround time of results, decreased sample requirements, and convenience to patient care, there is little in the peer-reviewed literature that actually demonstrates improved patient outcomes as a direct result of implementing POCT. POCT popularity is on the rise, and every day additional devices with wider menus and enhanced features are being introduced to the market. However, much of this testing is being adopted without critical investigation of its limitations or impact on patient care. Only after careful assessment have clinicians found the impact of overutilization. While some testing may be vital and important to patient care, other testing is unnecessary and duplicative of services already being delivered in an institution. In light of increasing healthcare pressure for financial and resource management, the amount of labor that is required to ensure quality testing under current regulatory guidelines requires those testing practices to be questioned.

Yet, laboratorians and POCT coordinators implement testing and take on the demands of supervising and managing the testing process, without questioning the need or benefit of moving the test onto the medical unit. Technologists often feel intimidated and claim that it is not within their purview to question the demands of a clinician. However, it is essential that the laboratorian develop the skills not only to question the need for implementing new technologies, but also to reassess the continued need for delivery of current, ongoing POCT.

Medical technologists, pathologists, and even physicians are hesitant to question the patient care practices of other clinicians, partially due to their lack of knowledge of the entire patient situation and partially because there is poor evidence to support their reason to question an ongoing practice. Many clinicians think that if the practice has always been done this way and no one has ever been harmed, why make waves? Surely there must be something else that needs more urgent attention.

Unfortunately, many of these misconceptions arise from the lack of appreciation for what is required to maintain the testing process in a quality manner. POCT certainly has the potential to provide a faster result, but whether that faster result translates into improved patient care is another question. POCT without quality assurance can generate misleading results, to the patient's detriment and increased overall cost of care. Additionally, POCT reagents are more expensive than core laboratory reagents on a unit basis, and labor costs are often higher because the test requires the focused attention of nursing and medical staff that are higher paid due to their patient contact responsibilities. Common sense dictates that such increased expenditures should be balanced by increased benefits to the system somewhere, whether directly to the patient or in staff convenience, scheduling, or time management.

POCT thus presents a dilemma that has only recently been realized: that a fast result may not necessarily be a better result. The risks to the patient have been appearing in the literature both as a result of failure to comply with regulatory requirements and due to a general lack of staff awareness for testing nuances. Clinicians are so used to getting ''quality'' results from a core laboratory that they translate that quality to POCT. As long as a device gives a result, that result is assumed to be correct and comparable to the core test with which the clinician is familiar. POCT, however, is a different methodology and can present accuracy and precision differences that may impact some patient populations. POCT is thus not universally interchangeable with the core laboratory test, and many of those situations are not recognized until the test is adopted into clinical practice.

The peer literature has falsely promoted this equivalence of core and POCT, as the bulk of POCT studies concern technical performance and laboratory correlations, not patient outcomes. As long as a similar result is obtained, POCT is assumed to generate the same or better outcomes than the core laboratory test because the result is available faster. Actual outcomes are rarely examined, and even more rarely followed up after implementation. Whether a faster result is really a better result thus defines the current dilemma facing laboratorians. While we may not be able to deliver a test any faster in a core laboratory given current technology limitations, POCT may not necessarily be the universal solution to clinical turnaround time, patient complaints, and other clinical problems. Integration is the key. POCT is worthless without also changing clinical management and preparing the staff to act on the result in a timely, clinically useful manner.

This book thus presents a critical look at the field of POCT and the literary evidence supporting its impact on patient outcome. The first half of the book explores the principles and theory of POCT, quality issues, evidence-based medicine, the role of performance improvement in the development of effective testing, practice guidelines, and critical pathways of care. The second half of the book focuses on individual tests and published literature to support improved patient outcomes from the use of POCT. I would hope that the reader would acquire an appreciation of the evidence-based perspective and foundation of available literature in order to address the appropriate questions of patient benefit and clinical utility to physicians demanding POCT. Moreover, laboratory staff should gain the confidence to address utilization issues on an equal basis with physicians, since physicians are as concerned about patient care as laboratorians but may not be aware or have thought about whether their patients are actually achieving the predicted benefits. This book should provide the foundation for developing evidence-based point-of-care and for building clinicians' understanding of the role of POCT in patient care.

To address a potential criticism, this book is neither anti-POCT nor pro-POCT. It is pro–clinically useful testing as based on available, published evidence. This evidence should consist of randomized controlled trials demonstrating patient benefit in a convincing number of patients. Demanding evidence in the form of well-designed trials is not unreasonable and is also aligned with the current trends of peer-reviewed publications. Many publishers have adopted the recent CONSORT (Consolidated Standards of Reporting Trials) guidelines, and are currently assessing the publication potential of submitted studies by comparison to these standards.

This is indeed the era of evidence-based medicine. As the laboratory, nursing, and clinical departments experience greater staffing shortages, there will be increased pressure to implement POCT to obtain a result while the patient is being seen. There will also be increased need to justify the resources required to maintain POCT. We should be prepared to answer questions about clinical necessity, analytical methodology, and how the result will alter patient management.

This book is thus a tool to the understanding of available evidence-based literature and, more importantly, what studies need to be conducted to optimize the utilization of POCT. I hope you enjoy this book and find it as interesting to read as it was for me to construct. Indeed, many of the contributors claimed to have learned a considerable amount in the process of writing their chapters. I hope that you will find as much insight in reflecting on your own POCT practices.

This book is dedicated to my family (Denise, Ashley and Jacqueline) for the time they have allowed me to complete this work and to my parents (Barbara and Isaac) for their support and inspiration. Credit is also due the medical staff and laboratory professionals who have brought me their numerous POCT issues over the years. Most importantly, I want to thank Linda Hadley for her administrative assistance and the POCT staff at Baystate Medical Center (Dr. Carol Rauch, Dr. Deb Morsi, Mark Provost, Claudia Chiapuzzi, and Cathy Bartholomew) and the Johns Hopkins Medical Institutions (Sandra Humbertson, Karen Dyer and Juanita Stem) for their advice in developing an evidence-based POCT philosophy and realization of that philosophy in practice.

James H. Nichols

Contents

Contributors

Erika B. Ammirati, R.A.C., M.T.(ASCP) President, Ammirati Regulatory Consulting, Los Altos, California, U.S.A.

Hassan M. E. Azzazy El-Badawy, Ph.D., S.C.(ASCP), DABCC, FAC-B Assistant Professor, Departments of Pathology and Medical Research & Technology, University of Maryland School of Medicine, Baltimore, Maryland, U.S.A.

Robert H. Christenson, Ph.D., DABCC, FACB Professor, Department of Pathology, University of Maryland School of Medicine, Baltimore, Maryland, U.S.A.

William Clarke, Ph.D. Department of Pathology, Johns Hopkins Medical Institutions, Baltimore, Maryland, U.S.A.

Catherine J. Cox, M.D. Director, Medical Affairs, Thermo BioStar, Inc., Boulder, Colorado, U.S.A.

Martin Fleisher, Ph.D. Chief, Clinical Chemistry Service, Department of Clinical Laboratories, Memorial Sloan-Kettering Cancer Center, New York, New York, U.S.A.

David G. Grenache, Ph.D. Department of Pathology and Immunology, Washington University School of Medicine, St. Louis, Missouri, U.S.A.

Ann M. Gronowski, Ph.D. Department of Pathology and Immunology and Department of Obstetrics and Gynecology, Washington University School of Medicine, St. Louis, Missouri, U.S.A.

Charlmain Johnson, M.S.N., R.N. Critical Pathway Facilitator, The Johns Hopkins Hospital, Baltimore, Maryland, U.S.A.

Jay B. Jones, Ph.D., DABCC, FACB Director of Chemistry & Regional Labs, Department of Laboratory Medicine, Geisinger Health System, Danville, Pennsylvania, U.S.A.

Gerald J. Kost, M.D., Ph.D., M.S. Director, Point-of-Care Testing Center for Teaching and Research (POCT · CTR^{sm}) and Professor, Medical Pathology, Faculty, Biomedical Engineering, University of California–Davis; and Director, Clinical Chemistry, University of California–Davis Health System, Davis, California, U.S.A.

Carolann Liszewski President and CEO, Quality Dynamics International, Bel Air, Maryland, U.S.A.

James H. Nichols, Ph.D., DABCC, FACB Medical Director, Clinical Chemistry, Baystate Health System, Springfield, and Associate Professor of Pathology, Tufts University School of Medicine, Boston, Massachusetts, U.S.A.

Gregory A. Nuttall, M.D. Department of Anesthesiology, Mayo Clinic and Foundation, Rochester, Minnesota, U.S.A.

Dorothy Nyberg, M.S., R.N.* Director, Case Management/Critical Pathway Program, The Johns Hopkins Hospital, Baltimore, Maryland, U.S.A.

Darryl Erik Palmer-Toy, M.D., Ph.D.† Department of Pathology, Johns Hopkins Medical Institutions, Baltimore, Maryland, U.S.A.

Paula J. Santrach, M.D. Co-Director, Hospital Clinical Laboratories, Department of Laboratory Medicine and Pathology, Mayo Clinic and Foundation, Rochester, Minnesota, U.S.A.

---

* *Current affiliation*: Director, Outcomes Management Program, Suburban Hospital Healthcare System, Bethesda, Maryland, U.S.A.

† *Current affiliation*: Department of Pathology, Massachusetts General Hospital, Boston, Massachusetts, U.S.A.

Ronald J. Schoengold, M.S. Director, Scientific Affairs, Beckman Coulter, Inc., Palo Alto, California, U.S.A.

Lori J. Sokoll, Ph.D. Assistant Professor, Department of Pathology, and Associate Director of Clinical Chemistry Division, Johns Hopkins Medical Institutions, Baltimore, Maryland, U.S.A.

Patrice L. Spath, B.A., RHIT Health care quality specialist; President, Brown-Spath and Associates, Forest Grove, Oregon, U.S.A

William E. Winter, M.D., DABCC, FCAP Departments of Pathology, Immunology and Laboratory Medicine, Pediatrics, and Molecular Genetics and Microbiology; Medical Director and Section Chief, Clinical Chemistry; and Director, Pathology Residency Program, University of Florida, Gainesville, Florida, U.S.A.

Alan H. B. Wu, Ph.D. Director, Clinical Chemistry, Department of Pathology and Laboratory Medicine, Hartford Hospital, Hartford, Connecticut, U.S.A.

Point-of-Care Testing

1
Point-of-Care Testing

James H. Nichols
Baystate Health System, Springfield, and Tufts University School of Medicine, Boston, Massachusetts, U.S.A.

THE VALUE OF POINT-OF-CARE TESTING

Definition

Point-of-care testing (POCT) is laboratory testing conducted close to the site of patient care. Point-of-care testing is also commonly described as ancillary, bedside, near-patient, satellite, remote, and decentralized testing, among other terms. Laboratorians and clinical staff often use these terms synonymously, but POCT can be delivered in many different ways. It is thus important to distinguish the particular scenario, or the manner in which the test is being conducted, when discussing POCT or reading the scientific literature, since each scenario may present unique operational aspects that could turn a beneficial test into a disadvantage to the patient. Understanding the complexity of the testing process is fundamental to determining the utility of a test in practice. This chapter explores the features of POCT delivery and the essentials of critically reviewing the scientific literature that serve as the basis of determining whether a specific test will improve patient outcomes.

Advantages

Point-of-care testing has become increasingly popular in the past two decades because it offers several advantages over core laboratory analysis (Table 1). Recent market surveys indicate that one in every four tests is currently being conducted outside of a traditional, central laboratory (1). With a 12% annual growth rate, over 40% of laboratory testing is predicted to be conducted at the point-of-

Table 1 Advantages and Disadvantages of Point-of-Care Testing

Advantages	Disadvantages
Portable	Quality of result
Rapid result	Clinically focused operators
Small sample volume	Inappropriate and over-utilization
Unprocessed samples	Regulatory compliance
Ease of use	Cost

care within the next decade. A wide range of analytes are now available to clinicians for POCT (Table 2).

Point-of-care testing is generally conducted on small, portable, handheld devices that can be easily carried onto a medical ward or out into the field. As opposed to traditional laboratory analysis in a central facility, POCT can be conducted on inpatient medical units, e.g., at the patient's bedside, in the patient's bathroom, or in a spare utility room on a nursing unit. The testing also can be performed in an outpatient clinic, physician's office laboratory (POL), and even the patient's home. Point-of-care testing is found in mobile transport vehicles, e.g., ambulances, fire engines, helicopters, and even cruise ships and the space shuttle. The variety of scenarios for POCT is unlimited given the portable nature of the instrumentation.

For POCT, the analytical time is short, on the order of minutes, allowing for a result often while the patient is still being examined. This decreases the therapeutic time (or the time to institute therapy) and offers the "potential" to improve patient outcome by reducing delays in wait time for laboratory results. When patient management is dependent on the test result, laboratory testing can be a significant bottleneck, resulting in longer wait times and poorer outcomes in particularly unstable patients. Point-of-care testing, providing a rapid result, can prevent such bottlenecks.

Clinician time may also be reduced, since physicians can obtain results while the patient and diagnostic issues are still fresh in their minds. If a sample needs to be collected and sent to a laboratory, the clinician is going to move on to other patients. Once test results are available, clinicians will need time to refamiliarize with the patient, their diagnosis, and where they left off in the treatment pathway. Thus, POCT has the potential to improve physician efficiency by enhancing result turnaround time and better fitting within clinical workflow.

The small volume of specimen required for POCT is also a benefit for patients with bleeding disorders, neonates, and others for whom collection of the standard sample volume could be an issue. Point-of-care testing utilizes unpro-

Table 2 Partial List of Variety of Analytes Available in POCT Format That Are Waived by the Clinical Laboratory Improvement Amendments of 1988

Alanine aminotransferase (ALT/SGPT)
Alcohol (saliva)
Amines
Amphetamines
Bladder tumor associated antigen
Cannabinoids (THC)
Catalase, urine
Cholesterol
Cocaine metabolite
Creatinine
Erythrocyte sedimentation rate (nonautomated)
Estrone 3-glucuronide
Ethanol (alcohol)
Fecal occult blood
Follicle stimulating hormone (FSH)
Fructosamine
Gastric occult blood
Glucose
Glucose monitoring devices (FDA cleared/home use)
Glucose, fluid (approved by FDA for prescription home use)
Glycosylated hemoglobin (Hgb Alc)
Human chorionic gonadotropin (HCG, urine)
HDL cholesterol
Influenza A/B
Ketone, blood and urine
Luteinizing Hormone (LH)
Methamphetamines
Microalbumin
Nicotine and/or metabolites
Opiates
Ovulation test (LH) by visual color comparison
pH
Phencyclidine (PCP)
Prothrombin time (PT)
Spun microhematocrit
Streptococcus, group A
Triglyceride
Urine dipstick or tablet analytes, nonautomated
Helicobacter pylori antibodies
Helicobacter pylori
Hematocrit
Hemoglobin by copper sulfate, nonautomated
Hemoglobin, single analyte instrument with self-control
Infectious mononucleosis antibodies (mono)
Vaginal pH

Source: Clara Sliva, Acting CLIA Coordinator, tests waived by FDA from January 31, 2000 to May 2, 2001; Centers for Disease Control (CDC) through March 2000 (*www.fda.gov/cdrh/clia/analyteswaived.html*).

cessed specimens, which further reduces the amount of specimen required for tests such as electrolytes, glucose, and enzymes that are traditionally conducted on serum or plasma in centralized laboratories, requiring larger volumes for centrifugation and the removal of erythrocytes. Elimination of sample processing is an additional feature of POCT that contributes to a faster result.

Point-of-care testing devices are simple to operate. The Food and Drug Administration (FDA) has approved many tests for home use. The technologies employed are simple enough that nontechnical people and those without formal laboratory training can perform the tests. There are also safeguards in many POCT devices that suppress the result if the test is not performed properly. The features of portability, rapid result, small sample volume, no sample processing, and ease of use have promoted the use of POCT in patient care.

Disadvantages

The Institute of Medicine and other survey reports have placed the number of deaths due to medical errors somewhere between 44,000 and 98,000 per year (2–5). Lucien Leape, Harvard Professor of Public Health, has claimed that medical errors are the "number one problem facing healthcare" today (4,5). Although many errors have been linked to pharmacy and medication administration, laboratory testing is not exempt. Errors continue to occur with laboratory testing despite the focus of laboratory professionals on quality and the enforcement of stricter federal and state regulations.

Managing the quality of POCT is a challenge due to the number of different devices and scenarios for delivery of testing. With the rapid rise in POCT popularity, quality has become a growing concern. A number of incidents involving POCT have appeared in the literature over the past several years. Self-monitoring (home use) blood glucose meters represent the largest number of complaints filed with the FDA for any medical device, with 16 deaths and over 3200 incidents of mismanagement (6,7). Poorly cleaned POCT devices can be reservoirs of nosocomial, antibiotic-resistant organisms on the nursing unit. *Enterobacter cloacae* infections on a neonatal intensive care unit have been linked to a blood gas analyzer (8) and the spread of *Serratia marcescens* and *Pseudomonas aeruginosa* have been traced to dirty urinometers (9,10).

These issues are not just typical of performance in the United States, and quality of POCT is a global concern. Through the use of blind proficiency samples, desktop cholesterol analyzers in the United Kingdom were noted to generate misleading results with 21% of samples more than 39 mg/dL (1 mmol/L) away from target. Such results would have misclassified over 16% of patients (11).

Misleading results have also been noted on proficiency surveys, comparative samples that are sent blinded to all laboratories performing testing in order to determine the accuracy of the testing process. Performance on proficiency surveys is thus indicative of POCT performance in patient samples. Higher failure rates have been noted in POLs when compared with hospitals with the same testing devices. Historically, the better performance has been linked to staff competency and having staff trained in laboratory science supervising the testing process (12). Such statistics have been highly criticized by the POCT industry that claims the simplicity of POCT devices poses no risk of performance problems. Physicians operating office laboratories have further complained that more stringent POCT requirements would limit access to medical care. Yet, the most recent inspections of POCT laboratories in 15 states have found

- Laboratories not following manufacturer's instructions
- Failure to identify incorrect results
- Testing outside of the laboratory certificate level
- Untrained staff
- Lack of quality controls
- Poor storage of reagents
- Poor record keeping

State inspectors in Colorado and Ohio noted 56 and 45% of POCT laboratories, respectively, were out of compliance with federal regulations in those states (13).

Staff training and clinical focus may be one source of quality problems. Clinical staff do not have formal laboratory education and tend to be patient centered. The performance of laboratory testing requires dedicated attention to detailed, stepwise analysis. When a patient is in trouble, clinicians and nurses are going to react in the aid of the patient. The laboratory test becomes a secondary concern. In the heat of patient care, staff may forget to precisely time the testing device, may not take note of specific sample collection details, or may not necessarily label each sample appropriately.

Nurses and clinical staff may also not fully appreciate the preanalytical variables that can interfere with the test result. They often assume that if the test gives a result, it must be the correct result. This leads staff to believe that POCT is equivalent and freely interchangeable with a central laboratory test. A glucose is a glucose test, a pregnancy is a pregnancy test, etc. Historical management pathways developed from the use of central laboratory tests now utilize POCT without necessarily accounting for differences in methodology or test limitations. However, POCT differs significantly in precision and accuracy from its central laboratory counterpart. It utilizes different chemistries in order to provide a faster result. Thus, POCT has technical characteristics that are unique from the central laboratory methods.

Patient population characteristics can also contribute to POCT and central laboratory differences. Hospital use of POCT stresses the technical performance of devices that are approved and marketed for home use applications. Home patients are ambulant, generally well, and utilize easily collected samples, such as urine, saliva, or capillary blood. Yet, hospitalized patients have a variety of acute and chronic illnesses, are confined to bed, and are on a number of medications. Use of the device in this patient population may be challenged by unusual samples, such as arterial and venous blood and blood drawn from intravenous lines. Hematocrits are higher (neonates) and lower (oncology, surgical, and trauma patients) than in the outpatient population. Critically ill patients may further be on oxygen therapy that can alter some test results (14). Point-of-care testing on inpatients is thus a very different scenario. Application of devices to patient populations that have not been validated though clinical trials may lead to result discrepancies that were not predicted from studies on home use patients.

This diversity in patient populations often leads to differences between the POCT result and the central laboratory result. When conflicts arise, staff does not know which result to believe. The POCT may be repeated, or an additional sample sent to the central laboratory. Rather than being a replacement for the central laboratory and improving patient outcomes, POCT in this case causes overutilization of testing and increased cost of care.

Training is thus a critical factor in obtaining quality test results and appropriate test utilization. In one U.S. location, unsupervised bedside glucose testing conducted by nonlaboratory staff differed by over 34% from the clinical laboratory at a mean concentration of 180 mg/dL and led to inappropriate categorization of hypoglycemic and normoglycemic patients. However, these same personnel, after implementation of a quality assurance program involving standardized operator training, quality control, and laboratory supervision, were able to reduce the coefficient of variation of bedside glucose from 17 to 8% and improve results to clinically acceptable levels (15). Institution of a standardized training program also improved the appropriate interpretation of Hemoccult slides from 60 to 91% (16). This level of performance continued even 9 mo after the training.

The need for competent staff in the performance of POCT has led to state and federal mandates for initial training, ongoing competency checks, routine quality control testing, documentation, and development of an overall quality assurance program for POCT. In the United States, the Clinical Laboratory Improvement Amendments of 1988 (CLIA '88) (17–20), Joint Commission on Accreditation of Health Care Organizations (JCAHO) (21,22), College of American Pathologists (CAP) (23), Commission on Physician's Office Laboratory Accreditation (COLA) (24), and various state agencies specifically address quality of POCT by requiring

1. Definition of how the test is utilized in clinical practice (for screening with follow-up central laboratory testing or definitive for management or diagnosis)
2. A list of operators and management supervising the testing process

3. Standardized training on the specific POCT device and documentation of ongoing competency evaluation
4. Written procedure manuals available to all operators defining how to perform the test, maintenance, calibration, and policies specific to the organization.
5. Routine performance of quality control checks to the manufacturer's specifications
6. Documentation of a result trail linking the specific device, its initial validation, ongoing quality control, and maintenance to the operator, and the operator's initial training and ongoing competency

Comparable regulations governing device performance are being developed by the European Union (Sweden, Germany, Spain, France, and the United Kingdom), New Zealand, Canada, and Australia. Recommendations have been developed by global standardization organizations: the National Committee for Clinical Laboratory Standards (NCCLS) (25) in the United States, International Standardization Organization (ISO) (26), Agence Française de Sécurité Sanitaire des Produits de Santé (previously Agence du Médicament) (27), the U.K. Medical Devices Agency and British Standards Institute (28), Canadian Standards Association (29), Instituto Mexicano del Suguro Social (30), the TNO Center for Medical Technology of the Netherlands (31), and the European Committee for Standardization. Consensus conferences have also developed and published guidelines for POCT device performance: the American Diabetes Association (ADA) (32,33), CAP, American Association of Bioanalysts (AAB), FDA (34), the German Working Group on Medical Laboratory Testing, and the U.K. Association of Clinical Biochemists (26).

These regulations have defined minimum criteria for obtaining quality results from POCT devices. Yet, institutions have a difficult time complying with these regulations. Clinical staff, due to their patient focus, fail to recognize the need for quality control and do not always document results and training in a consistent manner. Many do not feel it is necessary to be trained, since anyone can go to a pharmacy and buy the test. The root of the problem is that staff still tend to view POCT as a routine part of their medical evaluation and not a formal laboratory test. They were trained in medical and nursing school, and therefore they must be competent. This discrepancy in viewpoint indicates a failure to acknowledge the complexity of the testing process and the need for a quality assurance program to deliver acceptable test results.

Many have utilized screening tests for years, as their mentors trained them, without ever questioning the need for the test or whether the expected outcome is achieved. This point is emphasized in a study on urine dipsticks from Australia. A retrospective audit of routine dipstick testing performed at a large private hospital of 2294 medical records indicated that 12% of records had no result recorded, 9% of cases obtained abnormal (but expected) results, and 4% of results were abnormal and unexpected. A survey was sent to the physicians of those unexpected results. Only a third were aware of the abnormality and of those, none altered clinical treatment based on the results (35). Of note, 15 patients had further diagnostic testing or procedures conducted at increased cost without a change in patient outcome or treatment. In light of these data, one must question the value of routine dipstick screening to this institution.

Examples of such overutilization are common. When asked about such practices, clinical staff tend to reply that it has always been done this way or that it is hospital policy. Yet, few can actually cite the reasoning behind such policies.

Periodic re-examination of device clinical utility is thus justified in light of the tighter constraints on healthcare costs in recent years. In the previous urine dipstick example from Australia, the fundamental question is whether the use of dipsticks on all patients was worth the cost of managing the delivery of the test in a quality manner. None can doubt the value of urine dipstick testing in symptomatic patients and the importance of this test as a diagnostic tool in clinical assessment. Yet, while a single dipstick may appear innocuous in comparison with the total cost of overall care to a patient, the cumulative cost of thousands of dipsticks, the time spent in training hundreds of operators, competency assessment, performance and documentation of quality control, and laboratory supervision amounts to a significant effort. This total cost of rapid, POCT delivery needs to be balanced with a measurable patient outcome in order to justify the expense of such effort in comparison with obtaining the test from a central laboratory.

THE POCT DILEMMA

Point-of-care testing has the potential to enhance test result turnaround time and patient outcomes. Yet, it can also have no effect or actually be a detriment to patient care by leading to further diagnostic procedures and increased cost when applied inappropriately or overutilized. This is the POCT dilemma. Clinicians are under the impression that to improve patient care, they need a faster test result. Point-of-care testing is the means to that faster result. However, faster doesn't necessarily translate into better care until it is actually proven that a faster result alters treatment in such a way that the patient receives a better outcome. Clinical staff often infer that faster is better and are ready to make the leap-of-faith translation to improved outcomes without tangible demonstration of those outcomes because POCT is so convenient and readily available, and proving improved patient outcomes is challenging given the complexities of the testing process.

One of the best ways to establish the value of POCT is during the implementation of a new test. This situation allows the quantitative measurement of outcomes before and after access to a test. One recent study examining the impact of POCT evaluated patient wait times in a cardiovascular procedure area of an academic institution (36). Patients requiring coagulation (prothrombin time [PT] or activated partial thromboplastin time [aPTT]) or renal function (urea nitrogen, creatinine, sodium, or potassium) testing were prospectively studied over a 7-mo period. Patients without recent test results were requested to arrive 2 hr prior to scheduled procedure (interventional radiology, invasive cardiology, and electrophysiology procedures) to allow time for central laboratory testing in order to determine the type (standard or modified) of procedure that would be performed. Yet, many results were not available before the scheduled time, resulting in delays, open procedure rooms, rescheduling, staff overtime, and inefficiencies for the clinical staff.

The effect of implementing POCT was examined in four phases. In the initial phase, patient management and workflow were detailed. Fewer than 8% of patients requiring renal testing and 29% requiring coagulation testing had results back in time for their scheduled procedure. Mean wait times (arrival to procedure) were 188 ± 54 min for patients requiring renal testing and 171 ± 76 min for patients needing coagulation testing. In phase 2, POCT was implemented, but central results were still utilized for patient management. Timing studies indicated the potential for over 92% of patients to have POCT results available prior to scheduled procedure time. In phase 3, clinicians were allowed to treat patients based on the POCT results, but surprisingly, a significant change was not seen in the patient wait times. Only 23% of patients receiving coagulation POCT and 33% of patients with renal function POCT actually met scheduled procedure time. The prediction that faster results would lead to improvements in the percentage of patients prepared by the scheduled procedure time was not realized.

Overall workflow was then reexamined and changes made to better integrate the POCT into the overall patient care pathway. Once the optimized workflow was implemented in phase 4, significant improvement in wait time was achieved for both coagulation POCT (171 vs. 109 min) and renal function POCT (188 vs. 141 min) patients. Even with this improvement, though, only 42% of coagulation POCT and 22% of renal function POCT patients met their scheduled procedure time (36). Patient wait time was improved through the faster results of POCT, but the percentage of patients that met scheduled procedure time still did not attain the 92% predicted solely on the basis of POCT result turnaround time. The speed of POCT led to an overestimation of perceived benefit in this instance that was not achieved in reality even with optimized workflow changes.

This study highlights several important elements about POCT. Merely providing POCT does not guarantee improved patient outcomes. Point-of-care testing must be integrated into the entire patient care workflow in order to achieve some benefit. Many criteria must come together to achieve a final outcome. In this instance, the test results must be available, but there must also be a vacant procedure room; the patient must be prepared, have met with the clinician, and consented to the procedure; and clinical staff must be available before a procedure can begin. It is this coordination and the role that POCT plays in the overall workflow that ultimately determines the value of POCT.

Additionally, the prediction that faster test results will lead to improvement overestimates what can actually be achieved. The perception of "faster is better" obviously depends on how the staff is prepared to utilize the result. If a test result is available faster, but other factors are also important, the final outcome may not be changed. A test result is thus rarely the only bottleneck in the patient care pathway. If a test result is not immediately acknowledged and sits in the medical record, the benefit of a faster result is lost and there also may be no difference in outcome. Physicians must acknowledge the result before treatment can be instituted. Communication is thus an important factor that has been supported by other studies as well (37,38).

Communication further leads to unexpected benefits. Outcomes studies, such as the previous example, have demonstrated improved collaborations after study completion. The clinical staff can start to place faces and become familiar with the laboratory that promotes discussion of issues as they arise in the future. Improved interdepartmental relations are one patient benefit that is subjective, hard to quantitate, but fundamentally important to improving patient care.

OUTCOMES STUDIES

The previous study emphasized the difficulty in generalizing data from scientific literature. Point-of-care testing implemented in one institution may have beneficial outcomes, and the same POCT device in a different institution may have poor outcomes. The difference is in the degree of test integration into patient management and the level to which staff are attuned to acting on a test result at each institution. To obtain beneficial outcomes, the utilization of POCT must be optimized into patient workflow. Institutions and clinics that implement the technology solely because it is the latest device on the market or because their colleagues have bought it may not have thought out the entire management structure that needs to be in place to deliver quality results and obtain the outcomes desired. There are also an equal number of sites that implement POCT to solve a laboratory turnaround time problem or with the intent of improving patient care that never actually investigate whether the expected outcomes are ever achieved. One survey of U.S. hospitals noted that despite concerns over quality and cost of POCT, fewer than 7% of hospitals have conducted a cost comparison and

Table 3 Areas of Focus to Identify Patient Outcomes

Outcome measures
Efficacy
Appropriateness
Availability
Timeliness
Effectiveness
Continuity
Safety
Efficiency
Respect and caring
Service utilization

fewer than 2% of hospitals have evaluated the impact of POCT on outcomes (such as length of stay) (39).

Determining the benefit of POCT to patient care requires assessment of a specific outcome (Table 3). An outcome is something that is measurable as a consequence of some event. The JCAHO has further defined a number of possible areas of focus for general patient outcomes measures: efficacy, efficiency, patient safety, availability, appropriateness, timeliness, and continuity of care (40). Some of the outcomes may be defined quantitatively (minutes, dollars, test sensitivity and specificity) while others may be more subjective (qualitative surveys of patient satisfaction). Each outcome, however, is measured on a numerical scale for comparison before and after a clinical event, such as a change in practice.

For POCT, any parameter can be an outcome, provided that it can be measured numerically. The POCT outcomes can be clinical, social, or economic (Table 4). Other outcomes found in the POCT literature include therapeutic and decision time, time to procedure, volume of blood products transfused, nutritional and pharmacy orders, duplicate or repeat testing, and time in therapeutic range.

The Lack of POCT Outcomes Studies

Patient outcomes are complex and often involve a number of factors that can influence the final outcome. Laboratory testing is only one component of the care process. Radiology, pharmacy, available beds and procedure rooms, and adequate staff and facilities also impact the care decisions and management of a patient's treatment. In order to determine the laboratory's role, the entire process from the time the patient enters the health system until the patient is discharged needs to

Table 4 General Categories of Patient Outcomes and Examples of Specific Outcome Measures

Clinical
Turnaround time
Length of stay
Disease severity
Mortality or morbidity
Social
Patient satisfaction
Return to work
Pain
Suffering
Economic
Cost of care
Number of tests
Type of procedure

be defined—each decision, medication, and procedure documented; the interaction with clinical staff defined; and the impact of a laboratory test assessed. The complexity of the process and the subjective nature of assessing test impact are some of the factors that have limited the number of laboratory-focused outcomes studies, in general. For POCT, there are fewer, a mere handful, of randomized controlled outcomes studies in the peer-reviewed literature.

Why? Point-of-care testing is a fairly new technology that has only recently been added to the clinical repertoire of diagnostic tools. Conducting outcomes research takes some time to collect a sufficiently convincing volume of data. Until recently, there have also been few guidelines on the conduct of quality outcomes research or criteria for assessing the value of scientific literature as evidence for developing clinical practice recommendations. Consensus statements, such as CONSORT (Consolidated Standards of Reporting Trials) for the conduct of randomized controlled trials, are now available, and are starting to be adopted as criteria for grading the submission of manuscripts to the top scientific journals (41,42).

Point-of-care testing has also been historically viewed as a replacement for the core laboratory, so most studies have been comparative in nature rather than outcomes based. These studies have examined the correlation of a POCT method to a laboratory comparative method and calculation of the test's sensitivity and specificity. Few studies have focused on the effect on patient outcomes from obtaining a faster test result (i.e., choosing a point-of-care over a central laboratory test).

In light of the methodology differences, it is appropriate to consider POCT outcomes distinct from those of the central laboratory counterpart. The question, Does POCT lead to the same outcome as the central laboratory test in all patients and clinical situations? needs to be asked. Point-of-care testing cannot just be assumed to be the same laboratory test, only faster. As scientists, we need to ask, What is the effect of a faster result on patient outcome, and further, how does the outcome change if the point-of-care test is less accurate or precise than the central laboratory test?

Another factor complicating the conduct of POCT outcomes research is collection of data. Data collection from POCT devices is difficult, since half of the devices are manual, visually interpreted test strips and kits where the result may or may not get recorded into a patient's chart. The results may also not appear in a consistent manner in any given chart, complicating the data collection task.

The advent of computerized POCT instrumentation in the past few years has helped in the electronic collection and transmission of results for glucose, blood gases, electrolytes, and, most recently, coagulation tests. Unfortunately, devices from different manufacturers utilize proprietary communication protocols limiting the ability to synthesize data from different devices in the same database. An NCCLS standard for universal POCT device connectivity and communication has just been approved, but will take some months before implementation on devices currently on the market, and even longer for true data integration to occur. All of these factors have limited the ability to conduct POCT outcomes research. There is an immediate need for POCT outcomes research not only to justify the administrative cost of supporting the testing process, but also to establish the value of POCT in patient care.

Outcomes Research as Performance Improvement

Just getting started is the first hurdle in conducting outcomes studies. With such a complex process as modern medical care, the number of variables and factors to consider can be overwhelming. Most outcomes studies, though, are not comprehensive. In fact, many look at only one or two outcome measures and work toward defining the effects of various factors on those outcomes. Limiting the scope of the project is a good way to start an outcomes project.

In simplest terms, outcomes studies should be viewed as performance improvement. Most laboratorians are already familiar with the concept of total quality management and quality improvement. Problems in process that lead to laboratory errors are the first step. In order to determine how the problem occurred, staff must assess and outline the testing process from order through sample collection, analysis, and utilization of result in treatment. The trail that the sample follows is traced. Each step is evaluated for possible sources of error and areas for performance improvement are identified. This starts a cycle of continuous quality improvement with the following steps (Figure 1):

- Plan—find a problem or opportunity to improve
- Design—set goals and objectives
- Measure—identify quantitative measures and collect data
- Assess—statistically analyze the data
- Improve—review the results and determine selective areas for targeted improvement
- Communicate—inform and educate staff on the performance initiative
- Monitor improvement—provide regular performance feedback

This cycle then repeats by indicating further opportunities for improvement (43). Ultimately, this sets up an environment of progress surrounding the testing process. Outcomes are the measurable data to assess performance that drive the improvement process. Outcomes indicate if a problem exists, demonstrate the magnitude of the issue, and document when improvement occurs.

As performance improvement initiatives, the best sites for conducting outcomes studies are those areas that are at a higher risk for medical errors. High-volume nursing units with unstable, infectious, and multisystem failure patients, such as the intensive care units and operating rooms, are good areas to look for problems with POCT quality. These units are busy and the patients are critically

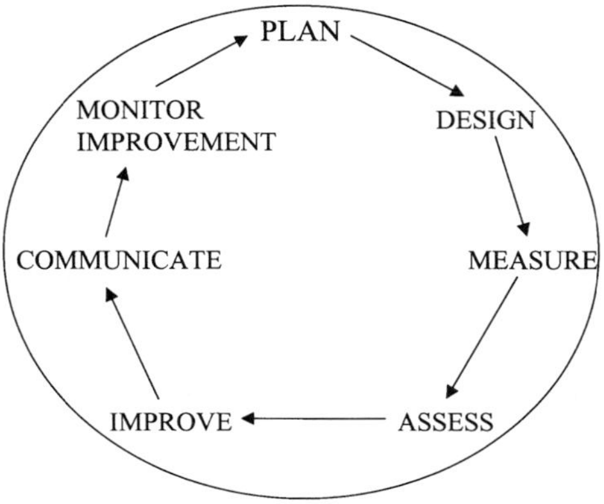

Figure 1 The continuous performance improvement cycle.

ill. These units place higher patient care demands on staff, and routine POCT quality assurance may get overlooked.

Sites shared by multiple departments also tend to have more issues, because these areas require extra effort in coordination. The basic responsibilities of quality control, documentation, and equipment maintenance tend not to get shared equally. Unless assigned, staff assume others have already conducted maintenance or performed controls, particularly when another department is involved. When compliance issues are noted, staff are less likely to take the time to clean up after those outside their nursing unit or department. Problems multiply in theses shared facilities, since no single department is willing to take responsibility for staff outside their purview.

In summary, there are few well-conducted outcomes studies involving POCT because of the recent introduction of the technology and the misconception that POCT is just a substitution for the core laboratory test and leads to comparable outcomes. There is also a hesitation to conduct outcomes studies because of the difficulty in design and construction of these studies to encompass all possible variables that may affect a terminal outcome such as length of stay. Viewing outcomes studies, however, as performance improvement is often a more manageable prospect. The ultimate goal of such outcomes studies is the development of practice guidelines regarding the use of POCT that define the patient population, settings, and criteria for choosing between the point-of-care and central laboratory tests that will optimize patient care.

The Pathway of Maturation for Laboratory Testing

The maturity of POCT is a consideration. Whether the technology is new or well characterized will determine if it is ready for clinical use or still at the level of basic research. Clinicians frequently request a laboratory test because they saw it in a medical journal. The clinician wants such tests because they are new. By offering the test, physicians have the illusion that they are providing better care, solely based on the novelty of the technology and its "potential" for improving outcomes. At which point, though, is a test ready for widespread versus selective clinical use? There is a path of development where research translates into clinical utility and may eventually change practice and ultimately become a practice guideline (Figure 2). Understanding the maturity of POCT along this path can help in assessing the evidence of scientific literature.

Few can doubt that POCT has the potential to deliver a faster result, but the fundamental issue is what a faster result means to patient care. Is POCT just a convenience or does it translate into improved patient outcomes? The rapid growth in POCT has led to the development of a wide range of tests. Every day, there seems to be a new test kit or device available, and sales representatives are placing increasing pressure on clinicians to purchase the latest products. So, how

"Potential"

"FDA Approval" "Outcomes" "Weight of Evidence"

Research → Clinical Utility → Consensus Recommendations → Standard of Practice

Figure 2 Development pathway for a laboratory test. What begins with research may indicate the potential for a test in clinical practice. With successful trials of the test in practice, the test may eventually gain clinical utility. In the United States, the FDA would need to review and approve the test for marketing prior to clinical use. With maturity, those tests that are particularly sensitive or selective may demonstrate significant patient outcomes and ultimately gain popularity through consensus recommendations or practice guidelines of professional organizations. With enough clinical experience and the weight of well-designed clinical studies, a test may eventually become a standard practice. While this is the preferred pathway for developing standards of evidence-based practice, some POCT has become a standard of practice because of convenience (a rapid result) without the weight of scientific evidence of improved patient outcome.

are clinicians to choose the most appropriate POCT for their particular patients? The clinician must critically appraise the scientific literature and weigh the evidence. The clinician must look beyond the "novelty effect" of a method and determine if the study design was sound or if it was biased toward the new device. Were there a sufficient number of subjects examined? Did the study population match patients found in real-world practice? Were appropriate controls utilized and did the results of the study support the author's conclusions? Only by evaluating the design of a study can the clinician determine whether any particular study provides sufficient evidence to implement a technology or change clinical practice. The laboratorian is uniquely trained in assessing technologies and weighing evidence. Thus, the pathologist and laboratory staff should assist clinicians in interpreting the scientific literature with respect to laboratory tests and POCT.

EVIDENCE-BASED MEDICINE

Evidence-based medicine (EBM) is defined as the conscientious, explicit, and judicious use of current best evidence in making decisions about the care of individual patients (44). Evidence-based medicine integrates systematic research in medical science with physician practice experience to optimize the best care for individual patients. In the past, EBM has been misunderstood to be "cookbook" medicine, but it is actually the opposite, since it seeks to determine the best care based on existing literature and professional experience for the particular situation of a given patient. Evidence-based medicine synthesizes the scientific literature, grading the design and weighting the conduct of each study to make recommendations or "practice guidelines." These guidelines do not dictate care, but indicate the general practice that leads to optimal patient outcomes and cost effectiveness in the average uncomplicated patient. Some patients fall exactly within the expectations of practice guidelines, while other cases are too complex. Evidence-based medicine is thus a tool for the physician to utilize in the process of decision making, offering support for one treatment over another in given situations.

Developing Evidence-Based Practice Guidelines

Criteria for reviewing medical and scientific literature have been under development for nearly 30 years. The first clinical-epidemiological approach to making practice recommendations was announced jointly by the Canadian Task Force on the Periodic Health Examination and the U.S. Preventive Services Task Force in 1979 (45–48). This approach was different from the traditional consensus development conference used by the U.S. National Institutes of Health, as consensus conferences were short (only a few days), involved expert speakers and a consensus panel of members, and culminated in a consensus opinion statement at the end of the conference. The evidence-based approach utilized by the joint task forces is a much longer process, in which the task force

- Defines criteria of effectiveness
- Reviews evidence
- Develops clinical practice recommendations
- Manages the committee analysis

A set of criteria for assessing the clinical effectiveness of preventive medicine or therapeutic interventions is first defined. These criteria rank the quality of evidence derived from the medical and scientific literature (Table 5). In reviewing

Table 5 Criteria for Ranking Quality of Medical and Scientific Evidence

	Rules of evidence
I:	Evidence obtained from at least one properly randomized controlled trial.
II-1:	Evidence obtained from well-designed controlled trials without randomization.
II-2:	Evidence obtained from well-designed cohort or case-control analytical studies, preferably from more than one center or research group.
II-3:	Evidence obtained from comparisons between times or places with or without the intervention. Dramatic results in uncontrolled experiments could also be included in this category.
III:	Opinions of respected authorities, based on clinical experience, descriptive studies, or reports of expert committees.

Source: Adapted from Ref. 46.

the literature, the task force balances the benefits from clinical interventions against the burden of suffering caused by the condition and the characteristics of early detection. Recommendations are then made for inclusion or exclusion of preventive practices in the periodic health examination, and each recommendation is graded based on the strength of the evidence to support the practice (Table 6). The graded recommendations acknowledge explicitly the degree of scientific certainty among different preventive services and assist clinicians in deciding whether or not to incorporate preventive activities in their own practices. Graded recommendations can also form the basis for insurance agency reimbursement determinations. This evidence-based process ultimately carries more weight in its recommendations when compared with a consensus conference since the task force process is optimized to ensure comprehensive inclusion of data, impartial weighting of the evidence, and documentation of the reasoning behind each recommendation. Most importantly, the task force functions so that no single expert or task force member can bias the recommendations.

The evidence-based approach utilized by the Canadian and U.S. task forces offers a foundation for examining scientific literature, in general, and this approach has been employed by other organizations (49–51). While the task force process is similar, different classification schemes for evidence have been proposed (Table 7). In all of the various classifications, conclusions from well-designed, randomized controlled trials of sufficient size carry the greatest weight, while nonrandomized, case-control, and observational studies offer less support. Consensus conferences and opinions of experts have the least strength as evidence. Multiple randomized trials conducted at different institutions with comparable conclusions add more weight to a recommendation than a single study or

Table 6 Strength of Recommendations for Clinical Practice Guidelines

	Task force classification of recommendations
A:	There is good evidence to support the recommendation that the condition be specifically considered in a periodic health examination.
B:	There is fair evidence to support the recommendation that the condition be specifically considered in a periodic health examination.
C:	There is poor evidence regarding the inclusion of the condition in a periodic health examination, but recommendations may be made on other grounds.
D:	There is fair evidence to support the recommendation that the condition be excluded from consideration in a periodic examination.
E:	There is good evidence to support the recommendation that the condition be excluded from consideration in a periodic health examination.

Source: Adapted from Ref. 46.

Table 7 Grades of Recommendations

	Grades of evidence
A1.	Randomized controlled trials (RCT), no heterogeneity in conclusions, confidence intervals (CI) all on one side of threshold number needed to treat (NNT) to avoid one unwanted outcome
A2.	RCTs, no heterogeneity, CIs overlap threshold NNT
B1.	RCTs, heterogeneity, CIs all on one side of threshold NNT
B2.	RCTs, heterogeneity, CIs overlap threshold NNT
C1.	Observational studies, CIs all on one side of threshold NNT
C2.	Observational studies, CIs overlap threshold NNT
	Grades of recommendations
Strongest	Based on A1 and B1 evidence
Intermediate	Based on A2 and B2 evidence
Weakest	Based on C1 and C2 evidence

Source: Adapted from Ref. 49.

multiple trials with disparate conclusions. Practice recommendations are thus graded so that the strongest recommendations are supported by the best evidence.

TRANSLATING LITERATURE INTO PRACTICE

Although the task force, evidence-based process was developed to help clinicians assess preventive health recommendations, these principles can also be applied to diagnostic testing and, more specifically, POCT. The process can synthesize the scientific literature to provide support for recommendations involving the appropriate clinical criteria for obtaining a laboratory test, the selection of appropriate test methodology, and even the impact of utilizing POCT on patient outcomes. Unfortunately, the scarcity of definitive POCT outcomes studies has hindered the incorporation of POCT into practice recommendations. To date, few practice guidelines have developed to the depth of including detailed recommendations for laboratory testing, let alone specifics regarding the criteria for selecting between POCT and core laboratory testing. Without a database of good, randomized controlled trials in POCT, laboratorians must determine the strength of research that is available. Application of the task force criteria can help laboratorians individually assess of the appropriateness of study design and determine the suitability of the research conclusions to real-world situations.

Assessing the design of a study requires an understanding of the causal

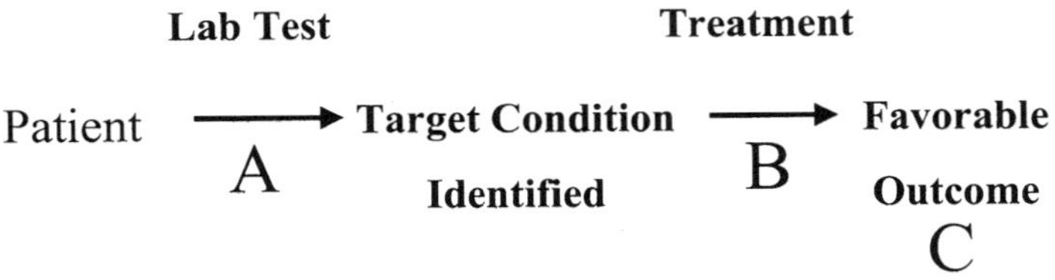

Figure 3 A simple causal pathway. If a laboratory test identifies a target condition (A → B), and treatment of the condition leads to a favorable outcome (B → C), then does the laboratory test generate a favorable outcome (A + B = C)? Only if proven through scientific study!

pathways set up by the study's authors. The validity of the causal assumptions will ultimately determine the applicability of the study to a real-world patient care scenario. A causal pathway defines a set of cause and effect relationships (Figure 3). In Figure 3, a patient obtains a laboratory test that defines the diagnosis of a target condition, the treatment of which leads to a favorable outcome.

Can POCT Substitute for Laboratory Testing?

The simple causal pathway in Figure 3 could be describing a fasting glucose test where a patient is diagnosed with diabetes and obtains treatment that leads to the lowering of blood sugar with concurrent prevention of long-term cardiovascular complications. In this instance, the fasting glucose level (A) leads to diagnosis and treatment (B) that improves patient outcome (C). This is a simple causal pathway. A (the laboratory test) + B (treatment) leads to C (the measurable, improved patient outcome). This example describes a common causal pathway to patient care that utilizes a fasting plasma glucose. What would happen, though, if whole blood POCT conducted on capillary blood were exchanged for the fasting plasma venous glucose? Would the same outcome be achieved (Figure 4)?

The same outcomes may not necessarily be achieved, because the methods are different. The precision and accuracy of blood glucose meters vary much more than core laboratory methods (52,53). In our laboratory, the core methodology is capable of obtaining total precision of less than 1.0% coefficient of variation (CV) in the range of 94–283 mg/dL, while our glucose meter has CVs of 5.3–18.6% in a comparable range of 49.0–283 mg/dL. Comparisons among various glucose meters on both CAP and AAB proficiency surveys indicate a wide range of results on the same sample (54,55). In one recent survey from the AAB, results varied from 134–285, 76.1–155.4, and 34–117 mg/dL on three separate samples (55). While manufacturers have complained that this variability is the result of the stabilized erythrocytes in such manipulated samples, similar differ-

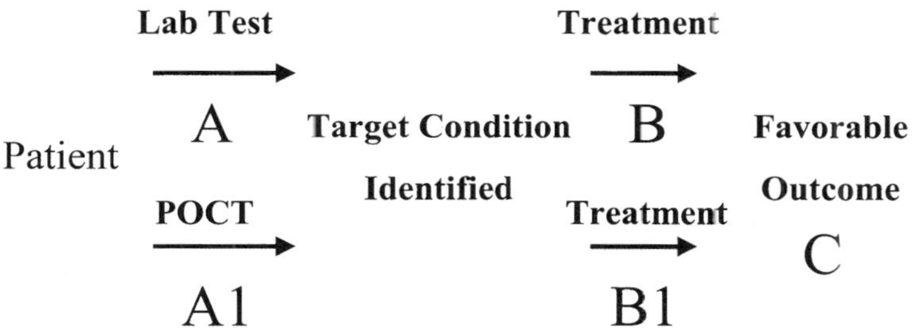

Figure 4 The effect of substituting POCT for a central laboratory test on patient outcome. A central laboratory test with proven patient outcome benefit (A + B = C) is replaced with POCT to provide a faster result. Does POCT also lead to the same outcome (C)? Not necessarily, because POCT takes a different pathway to the outcome from the original laboratory test. The POCT could generate better outcomes or worse outcomes because the pathway to the outcome has changed. The equivalence of patient outcome between POCT and central laboratory testing must be proven through separate investigation (A1 + B1 = A + B = C???).

ences have been obtained on fresh patient samples in several recent studies (52,53,56). Glucose meters apparently do not generate the same result on the same sample, despite the ADA recommendation that all glucose meters should strive for precision within 5% CV and accuracy within 5% of a comparative laboratory method (33).

Use of whole blood glucose meters as a substitute for plasma glucose from a core laboratory could generate significantly different results given the differences in accuracy and precision of the two methods. Whole blood is an unstable sample and glycolysis can occur in transit. Capillary blood samples may further be contaminated with tissue fluid if the fingerstick sample collection was not conducted properly. These features, together with the technical performance characteristics of glucose meters, have led to consensus recommendation for use of plasma venous glucose levels in the diagnosis of diabetes from professional societies.

Recommendations for use of the most accurate and precise method in diagnosis is further supported by a recent Monte Carlo simulation in which a mathematical model of glucose meters having defined imprecision and bias was utilized to generate 10,000–20,000 random “true and “measured” glucose results (57). A mathematical simulation was used in this study, since the actual collection of such a large number of samples would have been cost and labor prohibitive. The conclusions indicate that analytical errors, exceeding 10–15% total error, lead to twofold or greater insulin dosage errors more than 5% of the time. In order to guarantee acceptable insulin dosage more than 95% of the time, the total error of glucose meters would have to be less than 1–2% (57). Currently marketed meters are not yet capable of achieving this level of performance.

Substituting a whole blood glucose meter for central laboratory plasma glucose testing could, therefore, lead to different patient outcomes. Use of a glucose meter in the causal pathway of Figure 3 might lead to the same diagnosis, if the measured glucose were significantly higher or lower than the diagnostic cutoff for diabetes. However, if the meter result were close to the diagnostic cutoff (within the meter's variability), the meter could generate an alternate interpretation and be misleading. Given that total error is two standard deviations (imprecision) plus the bias (inaccuracy), meters within 20 or 25% of the diagnostic cutoff could generate discrepant results solely based on technical performance. This is before consideration of the added effects of operator errors in sample collection and analytical performance.

Such discrepancies have been noted in routine patient care, particularly in the neonatal hypoglycemic range around 40 mg/dL. Consider the ability of a glucose meter to identify hypoglycemia effectively when glucose meters may demonstrate variability as much as ±20 mg/dL by some standards (27). At this level of error, the user would not be able to discriminate a level of 20 from 60 mg/dL. Compare this performance with a laboratory method with a total error of <5%. Such a method would have the ability to discriminate between 38 and 42 mg/dL in 95% of the cases. The glucose meter is obviously more of an estimate of true glucose when compared against a method with better total error at this level. The risk for patient mismanagement and incorrect diagnosis has thus led to practice recommendations against the use of glucose meters in the diagnosis of diabetes. While POCT glucose meters may be useful as screening devices, their utility may break down when used in making diagnostic and finer management decisions. Thus, replacing glucose meters for plasma glucose in the causal pathway of Figure 3 does not necessarily lead to the same favorable outcome in all patient care applications where the core laboratory test may be utilized (see Figure 4).

Remember that in defining a causal pathway, a research study is indicating the cause and effect that led to the publication's conclusions. These conclusions are really only valid under the conditions stipulated in the study, and generalizations may not be applicable. In this example, some patients may be in a gray zone, or have questionable POCT results that may lead to further (repeat) testing or other diagnostic procedures rather than the preferred outcome. Substituting one method for another in the causal pathway changes the interrelationship of care and necessitates reexamination of the new cause and effect relationship on the patient outcome.

In the glucose example, the assumption that "faster is better" also isn't correct, since the tests are not equivalent. By substituting POCT for a fasting plasma glucose, a clinician is making a "leap of faith" based on the assumption that POCT is equivalent to the laboratory test in the clinical situations where the beneficial patient outcomes were proven (see Figure 4). However, this leap of faith may not be correct. Because of differences in accuracy and precision, the use of POCT (glucose meters in the previous example) is going to lead to different sensitivity (positivity in patients with diabetes) and specificity (negativity in the absence of diabetes, normal patients). If a rapid test is less sensitive than a core laboratory test, it will miss patients and compromise the effectiveness of the test by allowing some patients with disease to escape detection. On the other hand, if a test has low specificity, false positives will result in an increased number of patients being treated, unnecessarily increasing cost and risk of treatment side effects.

Patient Factors to Consider in Applying Research to Clinical Care

Other factors need to be considered as well in determining whether POCT research can be generalized to real-world, clinical applications (Table 8). The differences in technical performance of POCT may alter the clinician's treatment, which could then change patient outcomes. With POCT, compliance with required performance criteria, quality control, timing, sample collection, and application are also concerns that may cause different outcomes in actual use as compared with published research. Research studies are conducted with well-trained operators under conditions with motivated staff and patients. Yet, in routine practice, recent surveys of POCT sites have found significant quality problems associated with rapid diagnostics in about half of the inspected sites. Use of outdated reagents, performance by untrained operators, and failure to follow manufacturer's instructions can result in incorrect test results. What is the value of an incorrect test result in patient management? Does the incorrect result lead to additional testing, and what is the ultimate effect on patient outcomes? These questions support the need for investigating the impact of POCT on patient outcomes independent of results from a central laboratory method.

The study methodology should also be critically assessed to determine applicability to clinical practice. Research bias, whether unintentional or implied, is difficult to totally eliminate and requires a conscious effort within the study design to control. How were the sites, clinicians, and patients selected? Were they randomly selected, or was selection by need, or by preexisting POCT instrumentation? Was the comparative method a defined standard for the analyte in question, or were comparisons made to an existing laboratory methodology? Were comparisons made on the same sample or were two different samples collected that could contribute bias (e.g., capillary vs. venous samples)? Were all patients analyzed by the comparative method, and if not, how were patients randomized? Consider gas chromatography and mass spectrometry (GC/MS), an expensive but gold standard method for determining the presence of drugs of

Table 8 Some Considerations in Generalizing Scientific Research Literature into Specific Clinical Applications and Ensuring that the Same Study Outcomes will be Achieved in Practice

Study Design	
	Design Methods—randomized, controlled, or observational?
	Treatment—differences between control and study groups?
	Comparative method—performed on all tests or a select group of tests?
	Sampling—were comparative and study tests conducted on same or different samples?
	Blinding—random and adequate?
	Description—is study described in enough detail to reasonably repeat investigation?
	Hypothesis—clearly stated?
	Outcomes—practical and measurable in ongoing clinical practice?
Patient Population	
	Sample size—convincing number utilized?
	Follow-up—were patients followed for an adequate time period?
	Recruitment—randomized?
	Characteristics—same disease prevalence and severity as real-world patients?
Test Performance	
	Compliance—is similar management structure in place to guarantee quality of results?
	Performance—comparable to sensitivity and specificity of reported results in practice?
	Motivation—do staff have same motivation as staff performing test in study?
Study Conclusions	
	Appropriateness—do data support the conclusions?
	Convincing—do all sites and studies lead to same or different results?
	Statistics—are data statistically significant?
	Treatment—will conclusion change patient management in practice?

abuse. If a POCT drug study was conducted, were all of the samples analyzed by both the POCT and GC/MS methods, or were only the discrepant samples tested? Were the clinicians and study investigators blinded to the results of the comparative method until after the study was completed, or was the selection of comparative testing made on the basis of the POCT result (as in the drugs of abuse example)?

The patient population is an important determinant of whether study conclusions are applicable to specific patient care situations. Did the study patients match the intended patient population in terms of disease prevalence and severity? Is the patient population or clinician as motivated as the researchers during the conduct of the study? Were an adequate number of patients examined for the data to be convincing? Will the POCT results change patient management in the same manner as the study population? Is the clinical staff prepared to act on the POCT results in a timely manner?

These are some of the considerations in weighing the applicability of any specific study to actual patient care. The variety of possible effects on test utilization indicates the difficulty in extrapolating POCT and outcomes research to real-world implementations of new technology. Replacing of existing laboratory methods with POCT devices may generate a faster test result, but the effect on patient outcomes is still questionable. The research may demonstrate great value and beneficial outcomes, but poor management and utilization at a given site could yield opposite effects on actual patients. It is this variability in outcomes that necessitates both the critical review of the scientific literature before considering the implementation of new technology and a careful assessment during and after implementation to determine if expected outcomes were achieved.

OUTCOMES MANAGEMENT

With few randomized trials published in the POCT literature, how is the laboratorian to guide the appropriate use of POCT technologies? Staff need to be familiar enough with the scientific literature to be able to select methodologies based on the technical performance, patient need, and management practices of the medical unit. Implementations must seek to optimize test utilization in patient management and strive to eliminate those technologies that do not demonstrate a value-added benefit to patient care. Thus, institutions require a POCT staff to coordinate and manage patient outcomes. Most POCT staff are so involved with managing compliance problems on the medical unit that they do not have time to monitor test utilization. The POCT staff also tend to not question clinicians regarding the medical necessity of testing practices. Yet, until the clinicians appreciate the value of a quality laboratory test in patient care and the need for proactively developing quality systems surrounding POCT, progress on performance improvement is difficult. The laboratory staff can help the clinician understand the test sensitivity and specificity, the suitable situations for POCT, and the need for quality management. Laboratory staff collaboration with clinicians is the foundation for building improvements in POCT quality that will ultimately lead to better patient outcomes.

Patient outcomes management for POCT thus involves optimizing the use of laboratory testing to maximize patient benefit. Appropriate use and critical appraisal of the literature forms the basis for supporting this philosophy. As clinical issues are noted, areas for improvement are identified and the opportunity for assessing the steps involved in patient care and test utilization can be defined.

Scientific literature can indicate the technical performance and expected patient outcomes if such studies have been conducted. If not, decisions to implement POCT should involve the measurement of baseline outcomes and systematic assessment of treatment and management decisions to optimize patient outcomes.

Optimally, the field needs a foundation of sound randomized controlled trials in a large number of patients from which to develop practice guidelines for when and how to utilize POCT for optimal patient benefit. Unfortunately, there is a lack of POCT outcomes studies published in the peer literature. Even with the strongest of literature evidence, POCT may fail to immediately demonstrate an evident patient benefit in practice without optimization of patient care pathways. This is the role of outcomes management and the need for POCT staff involvement as POCT may further fail to benefit patients without ongoing outcomes assessment. Optimum patient benefit thus requires not only a fast result but also the management structure to support a quality result and the quick utilization of the result in patient care.

SUMMARY

Point-of-care testing is rapid diagnostic testing provided at the site of patient care. A fast result, however, doesn't guarantee improved patient outcomes. The relationship of POCT to patient outcomes must be proven through well-designed, randomized controlled trials in a convincing number of subjects. Unfortunately, the POCT scientific literature has few unbiased outcomes studies. Most of the literature evaluates POCT technical performance with respect to traditional, central laboratory testing. Patient outcomes are assumed based on comparability of the test results without proving that faster is really better for patients. With increasing fiscal and staffing constraints on nursing and laboratory staff, there is enhanced pressure to evaluate the actual value of delivering a faster result given the additional demands required for training, competency, and quality assurance documentation to deliver a quality test result at the point of care.

This book explores the foundation of scientific literature that is available and how that literature can be generalized to clinical practice. The book is divided into two halves. The first half outlines the fundamentals of device approval, laboratory regulations, hospital performance improvement and how performance improvement can lead to an understanding of clinical processes, and recommendations for clinical guidelines to change clinical practice. The second half of this book investigates specific examples of tests conducted at the point of care. The existing literature is reviewed and assessed from a patient outcomes perspective. Where such evidence doesn't exist, the authors have indicated the key considerations that need to be investigated. It is hoped that through such discussions, this text will spark research and interest in asking practice questions and the value of POCT to patient care.

REFERENCES

1. Stephans EJ. Developing open standards for point-of-care connectivity. IVD Tech 5:22–25, 1999.
2. Kohn LT, Corrigan JM, Donaldson MS, eds. To Err is Human—Building a Safer Health System. Committee on Quality of Healthcare in America, Institute of Medicine. Washington, D.C.: National Academy Press, 2000.
3. Thomas EJ, Studdert DM, Burstin HR, et al. Costs of medical injuries in Utah and Colorado. Inquiry 36:255–264, 1999.
4. Brennan TA, Leape LL, Laird NM, et al. Incidence of adverse events and negligence in hospitalized patients: Results of the Harvard Medical Practice Study I. N Engl J Med 324:370–376, 1991.
5. Leape LL, Brennan TA, Laird NM. The nature of adverse events in hospitalized patients: Results of the Harvard Medical Practice Study II. N Engl J Med 324:377–384, 1991.
6. Greyson J. Quality control in patient self-monitoring of blood glucose. Diabet Care 16:1306–1308, 1993.
7. Meadows S, Kubic M. Improving glucose monitoring for diabetics. FDA Consumer May:32–35, 1990.
8. Acolet D, Ahmet Z, Houang E, Hurley R, Kaufman ME. *Enterobacter cloacae* in a neonatal intensive care unit: Account of an outbreak and its relationship to use of third generation cephalosporins. J Hosp Infect 28:273–286, 1994.
9. Rutala WA, Kennedy VA, Loflin HB, Sarubbi FA. *Serratia marcescens* nosocomial infection of the urinary tract associated with urine measuring containers and urinometers. Am J Med 70:659–663, 1981.
10. Kocka FE, Roemisch E, Causey WA, O'Dell A. The urinometer as a reservoir of infectious organisms. Am J Clin Pathol 67:106–107, 1977.
11. Summerton AM, Summerton N. The use of desk-top cholesterol analysers in general practice. Pub Health 109:363–367, 1995.
12. Centers for Disease Control, Laboratory Practice Assessment Branch, Division of Laboratory Systems, Public Health Practice Program Office. Clinical laboratory performance on proficiency testing samples—United States, 1994. Morbid Mortal Wkly Rep 45:193–196, 1996.
13. Rehnquist J, Office of Inspector General. Enrollment and Certification Processes in the Clinical Laboratory Improvement Amendments Program. OEI-05-00-00251. Department of Health and Human Services, Washington, DC, 2001.
14. Tang Z, Louie RF, Payes M, Chang KCJ, Kost GJ. Oxygen effects on glucose measurements with a reference analyzer and three handheld meters. Diabetes Technol Ther 2:349–362, 2000.
15. Belsey R, Morrison JI, Whitlow KJ, Baer DM, Nelson S, Hardwick DF. Managing bedside glucose testing in the hospital. JAMA 12:1634–1638, 1987.

16. Fleisher M, Winawer SJ, Zauber AG, Smith C, Schwartz MK and the National Polyp Study Work Group. Accuracy of fecal occult blood test interpretation. Ann Intern Med 114:875–876, 1991.
17. Department of Health and Human Services, Health Care Finance Administration. Clinical laboratory improvement amendments of 1988, Final Rule. Fed Regist 7001–7288, Feb 28, 1992.
18. Department of Health and Human Services, Health Care Finance Administration. Medicare, Medicaid and CLIA programs: CLIA program fee collection: Correction and final rule. Fed Regist 5211–5237, Jan 19, 1993.
19. Department of Health and Human Services, Health Care Finance Administration. CLIA program: Categorization of tests and personnel modifications. Fed Regist 20035–20051, Apr 24 1995.
20. Department of Health and Human Services, Health Care Finance Administration. CLIA program: Categorization of waived tests. Fed Regist 47534–47543, Sept 13, 1995.
21. Joint Commission on Accreditation of Healthcare Organizations. 2002–2003 Comprehensive Accreditation Manual for Pathology and Clinical Laboratory Services. JCAHO, Oakbrook Terrace, IL, 2001.
22. Joint Commission on Accreditation of Healthcare Organizations. Comprehensive Accreditation Manual for Hospitals. JCAHO, Oakbrook Terrace, IL, 2001.
23. College of American Pathologists Laboratory Accreditation Program. Inspection Checklist: Point-of-Care Testing. CAP, Northfield, IL, 2001.
24. Commission on Office Laboratory Accreditation. Laboratory Accreditation Manual. COLA, Columbia, MD, 2000.
25. National Committee for Clinical Laboratory Standards. Ancillary (Bedside) Blood Glucose Testing in Acute and Chronic Care Facilities; Approved Guideline. NCCLS C30-A. NCCLS, Wayne, PA, 1994.
26. International Standardization Organization. Determination of Performance Criteria for In Vitro Blood Glucose Monitoring Systems for Management of Human Diabetes Mellitus. Draft International Standard ISO/DIS 15197. ISO, Geneva, Switzerland, 2000.
27. Agence Française de Sécurité Sanitaire des Produits de Santé (previously Agence du Médicament). Evaluation Protocol for Self Blood Glucose Monitoring Devices. AFSPS, Paris, France, 1998.
28. United Kingdom Medical Devices Agency. MDA Evaluation Reports. MDA, London, UK. For a complete list see *www.medical-devices.gov.uk/catalogu.pdf*
29. Canadian Standards Association. Performance Specifications for Portable Whole Blood Glucose Monitor Systems for Use in Diabetes Management. CSA Z316.4-94. CSA, 1994.
30. Insituto Mexicano del Seguro Social. Reactive Strip Assessment Protocol for Determination of Glucose in Blood. IMSS, Mexico City, Mexico, 1998.
31. TNO Center for Medical Technology. Quality guideline for non-implantable portable blood glucose monitors for self monitoring. TNO-CMT/90.021 E. 1991.
32. American Diabetes Association. Self monitoring of blood glucose. Diabetes Care 17:81–86, 1994.

33. American Diabetes Association. Consensus statement on self-monitoring of blood glucose. Diabetes Care 9(suppl):S62–S66, 1996.
34. U.S. Food and Drug Administration, Division of Clinical Laboratory Devices. Review Criteria for Assessment of Portable Invasive Blood Glucose Monitoring In Vitro Diagnostic Devices Which Use Glucose Oxidase, Dehydrogenase or Hexokinase Methodology. USFDA, Rockville, MD, 1998.
35. Del Mar C, Badger P. The place of routine urine testing on admission to hospital. Med J Aust 151:151–153, 1989.
36. Nichols JH, Kickler TS, Dyer KL, Humbertson SK, Cooper PC, Maughan WL, Oechsle DG. Clinical outcomes of point-of-care testing in the interventional radiology and invasive cardiology setting. Clin Chem 46:543–550, 2000.
37. Saxena S, Wong ET. Does the emergency department need a dedicated stat laboratory? Continuous quality improvement as a management tool for the clinical laboratory. Am J Clin Pathol 100:606–610, 1993.
38. Parvin CA, Lo SF, Deuser SM, Weaver LG, Lewis LM, Scott MG. Impact of point-of-care testing on patients' length of stay in a large emergency department. Clin Chem 42(5):711–717, 1996.
39. Bickford G. Decentralized testing in the 1990s: A survey of United States hospitals. Clinics Lab Med 14:623–645, 1994.
40. Joint Commission on Accreditation of Healthcare Organizations. Using Performance Measurement to Improve Outcomes in Behavioral Healthcare. JCAHO, Oakbrook Terrace, IL, 1998.
41. Moher D, Schulz KF, Altman DG, for the CONSORT Group. The CONSORT statement: Revised recommendations for improving the quality of reports of parallel-group randomised trials. Lancet 357:1191–1194, 2001.
42. Altman DG, Schulz KF, Moher D, Egger M, Davidoff F, Elbourne D, Gøtzsche PC, Lang T, for the CONSORT Group. The revised CONSORT statement for reporting randomized trials: Explanation and elaboration. Ann Intern Med 134:663–694, 2001.
43. Joint Commission on Accreditation of Healthcare Organizations. Using Performance Improvement Tools in Healthcare Settings. JCAHO, Oakbrook Terrace, IL, 1996.
44. Sackett DL, Rosenberg WMC, Gray JAM, Haynes RB, Richardson WS. Evidence based medicine: What it is and what it isn't. Br Med J 312:71–72, 1996.
45. Canadian Task Force on the Periodic Health Examination. The periodic health examination. Can Med Assoc J 121:1193–1254, 1979.
46. Woolf SH, Battista RN, Anderson GM, Logan AG, Wang E, and the Canadian Task Force on the Periodic Health Examination. Assessing the clinical effectiveness of preventive maneuvers: Analytic principles and systematic methods in reviewing evidence and developing clinical practice recommendations. J Clin Epidemiol 43:891–905, 1990.
47. Battista RN, Fletcher SW. Making recommendations on preventive practices: Methodological issues. Am J Prevent Med 4:53–76, 1988.
48. Goldbloom R, Battista RN. The periodic health examination: 2. 1987 update. Can Med Assoc J 138:617–626, 1988.
49. Guyatt GH, Sackett DL, Cinclair JC, Hayward R, Cook DJ, Cook RJ, for the Evidence-Based Medicine Working Group. Users' guide to the medical literature. IX. A method for grading health care recommendations. JAMA 274:1800–1804, 1995.

50. Cook DJ, Guyatt GH, Laupacis A, Sackett DL. Rules of evidence and clinical recommendations on the use of antithrombotic agents. Chest 102(suppl):305S–311S, 1992.
51. Jaeschke R, Guyatt D, Sackett DL, for the Evidence-Based Medicine Working Group. Users' guides to the medical literature. III. How to use an article about a diagnostic test. A. Are the results of the study valid? JAMA 271:389–391, 1994.
52. Nichols JH, Howard C, Loman K, Miller C, Nyberg D, Chan DW. Laboratory and bedside evaluation of portable glucose meters. Am J Clin Pathol 103:244–251, 1995.
53. Chance JJ, Li DJ, Jones KA, Dyer KL, Nichols JH. Technical evaluation of five glucose meters with data management capabilities. Am J Clin Pathol 111:547–556, 1999.
54. College of American Pathologists. EXCEL Proficiency Survey. CAP, Northfield, IL, 2001.
55. American Association of Bioanalysts. Whole Blood Glucose Proficiency Testing Service. AAB, Brownsville, TX, 2001.
56. Chen ET, Nichols J, Duh S, Hortin G, Fonzalez L. A study of the factors that affect the performance of blood glucose monitoring devices. Clin Chem 47(suppl):A189, 2001.
57. Boyd JC, Bruns DR. Quality specifications for glucose meters: Assessment by simulation modeling of errors in insulin dose. Clin Chem 47:209–214, 2001.

2
The Device Approval Process

Erika B. Ammirati
Ammirati Regulatory Consulting, Los Altos, California, U.S.A.

FOOD AND DRUG ADMINISTRATION PROCESSES FOR DEVICE QUALIFICATION

In vitro diagnostics (IVDs), (see Table 1 for list of chapter abbreviations and definitions) are regulated as medical devices by the U.S. Food and Drug Administration (FDA). This means IVD manufacturers must satisfy specific FDA requirements, and obtain FDA's approval, before a product can be legally marketed in the United States. In vitro diagnostics represent a unique subset of medical devices, and therefore their safety and effectiveness are supported by unique types of data. Further, IVDs specifically designed for point-of-care environments are subject to additional regulatory oversight beyond what is required for IVDs designed for traditional environments, i.e., the hospital or reference laboratory. This chapter begins with a review of the regulatory requirements for traditional IVDs, and continues with a description of specific requirements for point-of-care IVDs. The chapter then presents a discussion of the time and costs involved with bringing a point-of-care IVD to market, followed by the necessary elements for keeping an IVD on the market (quality and compliance issues).

FDA's Premarket Notification Process

Manufacturers desiring to bring an IVD through the FDA must, most often, prepare and file the necessary documentation via one of two regulatory routes. Recently, new FDA regulation has provided a third option that exempts certain low-risk IVDs from this type of documentation, but all point-of-care IVDs have been

Table 1 List of Abbreviations and Definitions

Abrreviation	Name	Definition (if applicable)
510(k)	510(k) or premarket notification	Name of regulatory document that must be filed with the FDA by the manufacturer for most laboratory products
CDC	Centers for Disease Control and Prevention	
DMR	Device master record	Manufacturer's official log for a product that includes all manufacturing information
FDA	Food and Drug Administration	
FD&C	Food, Drug and Cosmetic Act	Name of the law that regulates food, drugs, devices, and cosmetics
IRB	Institutional review board	Committee designed to protect human subjects who are enrolled in clinical studies
IVD	In vitro diagnostic	
NCCLS	National Committee for Clinical Laboratory Standards	
%CV	Percent coefficient of variation	Statistical term to express imprecision of an assay system
PMA	Premarket approval	Name of regulatory document that must be filed with the FDA by the manufacturer for selected laboratory products
QSR	Quality System Regulation	Name of the federal regulation (law) that covers device manufacturers to ensure medical devices will be safe and effective, and otherwise in compliance with the FD&C
SOP	Standard operating procedure	

classified as "reserved" devices, and therefore the exemption cannot apply (1). All reserved devices must undergo conventional FDA review.

The first regulatory route is a premarket notification, or clearance, and this document has been given the jargon name of "510(k)." The 510(k) is named after the section in the Food Drug and Cosmetic Act where this regulatory path is described (2). The second regulatory route is the premarket approval process, and this document is abbreviated as "PMA." The 510(k) is the more streamlined and straightforward submission, and this pathway applies to most IVDs as well as other medical devices. In vitro diagnostic PMAs are reserved for those tests that are considered novel in terms of the analyte being measured or the measurement technology, or for those tests where the consequences of the clinical interpretation are of the highest risk. For example, tests that diagnose cancer are regulated as PMAs. Since most point-of-care IVDs are regulated as 510(k)s, this chapter will limit itself to that regulatory route.

The manufacturer's primary objective in preparing the 510(k) document is the demonstration of substantial equivalence between the new IVD and a similar product already being marketed domestically (the "predicate device"). In other words, the manufacturer must show that the new device and the predicate device have physical and performance characteristics in common. Substantial equivalence is a relative term for many medical devices, but in the realm of IVDs, substantial equivalence is almost exclusively defined by a test's intended use, its physical/technological characteristics, its analytical performance characteristics, and its clinical performance characteristics. Each of these elements of substantial equivalence is described below.

Intended Use

An IVD's intended use encompasses the "who, what, where, and why" of the assay or test system. The intended use describes which analyte is measured, and in which particular matrix (e.g., calcium in serum or urine, or cholesterol in fingerstick whole blood); it also defines whether the test will be used for screening, monitoring, or diagnostic purposes. The intended use describes the environment where the test will be used (e.g., traditional laboratory, emergency room or doctor's office), and also describes the relationship between levels of the analyte and a medical condition or risk factor. For example, elevated levels of cholesterol are associated with coronary risk, and elevated levels of the MB isoenzyme of creatine kinase (CK-MB) are diagnostic of coronary infarction. This last relationship is often referred to as the clinical utility of a test, or the test's indications for use.

The intended use is an extremely important factor when determining substantial equivalence, and the FDA carefully reviews 510(k) applications to ensure that the labeling for the new IVD does not claim uses or indications that exceed those described by the predicate device. In order for a new IVD to be substantially equivalent to its predicate, the two intended uses must closely relate to one another, but do not need to match identically.

Technological Characteristics

Another element for demonstrating substantial equivalence between the two IVDs is the comparison of the physical and technological characteristics. Examples of various IVD formats include 96-well plate enzyme immunoassays, classical, stoichiometric "wet-chemistry" assays, high-throughput chemistry analyzers, and biosensor-based systems. Most point-of-care devices consist of unitary, disposable units, or easy-to-operate "permanent" instruments with single-use, disposable cartridges, cassettes, or test strips for each patient sample.

Other test system characteristics include the sample type(s) of choice, and the procedural steps. An IVD may be designed for only one matrix, or it may be designed for multiple matrices; it may require a high level of technical expertise and manual dexterity, or it may have "walk-away" attributes where there are essentially no procedural steps after sample addition. This last category is often seen with point-of-care devices.

In contrast to the intended use discussion described above, it is not mandatory that a new IVD be of the same format as its predicate device or share the same technological characteristics. In fact, one of the most common reasons for developing a new IVD is to modernize a test from a more labor-intensive format to that of a less labor-intensive format. This is quite often the case for many point-of-care devices in which internal and external components have been unitized, miniaturized, and procedurally simplified. In terms of substantial equivalence, the FDA requires that the manufacturer describe why the changes in test formats do not raise new issues of safety and effectiveness. For example, if the transformation of an assay from a desktop analyzer to a point-of-care unitary device does not put additional risk burdens on the operator (safety) and the results obtained from the point-of-care device are comparable to the predicate device (effectiveness), it can be claimed that no new issues of safety and effectiveness have been raised, and a substantially equivalent determination can be made.

Analytical Performance Characteristics

An IVD's analytical performance characteristics include the standard laboratory measurements of analytical sensitivity, analytical specificity, linearity, and spike recovery. Other analytical measurements may be added, depending on the test system. The analytical performance characteristics are almost always generated in-house in the manufacturer's laboratory, and this is in contrast to how the clinical performance characteristics of accuracy and precision are evaluated. Accuracy and precision are best supported by field studies (or clinical trials) conducted outside of the manufacturer's laboratory in actual clinical settings (see next section).

A manufacturer must demonstrate that the analytical performance of the new IVD is comparable to that described in the labeling (package insert) of the predicate IVD. A brief discussion of the experimental objectives and designs for the major analytical components (sensitivity, specificity, linearity, and recovery) follows.

Analytical Sensitivity. The analytical sensitivity of an assay is defined as the lowest level of the analyte that can be measured with reasonable precision. This is also referred to as an assay's limit of detection. There are various means for establishing analytical sensitivity, and a common method is to assay the test system's buffer matrix or "zero calibrator" in 20–30 replicates. From these measurements, a mean value and the standard deviation are calculated. The value of two standard deviations is added to the mean value of the signal, and this becomes the lowest limit of detection, or the lowest level that can be distinguished from zero.

Analytical Specificity. The analytical specificity of an assay is defined by two sets of requirements. The first requirement is the system's ability to measure a distinct entity and not compounds that are closely related to the analyte of interest. For example, if the IVD is intended to measure levels of luteinizing hormone (LH), the level of crossreactivity with beta human chorionic gonadotropin (hCG), which shares a common alpha subunit with LH, must be identified and included in the labeling. Another example of two closely related compounds is thyroxine (T_4) and triiodothyronine (T_3) in thyroid testing.

The second specificity requirement is the evaluation of interfering substances. Interfering substances are those constituents in the blood (or other matrix) that may cause falsely positive or falsely negative results in qualitative systems, or may cause falsely depressed or falsely elevated results in quantitative systems. Although there is an infinite list of substances that could be tested for interference, it is the manufacturer's responsibility to test a reasonable number of candidate substances. These substances generally fall into one of three categories: elevated levels of biological compounds (e.g., bilirubin, hemoglobin, and lipids), elevated levels of over-the-counter medications, and elevated levels of prescription drugs that are associated with the analyte being measured.

Since many IVD systems utilize color, or a color change, as the measurement endpoint, substances that impart color changes to the testing matrix need to be evaluated. Elevated levels of bilirubin, hemoglobin, and lipids are routinely included in specificity testing because high levels of these substances can cause subtle color changes of yellow, red (or green), and milky white, respectively. The second category of candidate testing substances are over-the-counter medications. Many patients self-prescribe high doses of analgesics or vitamins, and the effects of these products need to be tested. The third category of potentially interfering substances is prescription medications. Here the manufacturer should try to include the testing of those medications that bear a relationship to the analyte being identified or measured. For example, a test for cholesterol should include in its interference testing some form of lipid-lowering drugs; patients or consumers who have a need to monitor their cholesterol levels often have this class of pharmaceutical prescribed to them. Similarly, a manufacturer of an IVD for the monitoring of bone metabolism would include high levels of calcium in its interference testing because calcium supplements are widely recommended and prescribed.

Interference testing may be accomplished in a number of ways, and a common method is described as follows. Elevated levels of the various potentially interfering substances are added to two pools with known quantities of the analyte (controls). The pools are generally "positive" and "negative" for the particular analyte when evaluating qualitative systems, and are "low level" and "high level" for the particular analyte when evaluating quantitative systems.

All samples are tested as routine "unknowns," and the difference between the "true results" (controls) and the "on-test results" (samples with interfering substances) are compared. If the differences between the two results are within the imprecision of the assay, then the substance is considered to be noninterfering. If the differences are large, then those substances are considered to be potentially interfering, and are disclosed as such in the limitations section of the product labeling (package insert). The National Committee for Clinical Laboratory Standards (NCCLS) EP-7 document (3) describes numerous candidate substances, target levels for interfering concentrations, and guidelines for statistical evaluation.

Linearity. Linearity measures the ability of an assay to "read" predictably throughout the reportable range. It also can be an indication of the presence (or absence) of matrix effects from clinical samples. Some systems are susceptible to quantitative biases at the high or low ends of the measurement ranges, and linearity experiments are designed to identify these errors. Like specificity testing, the linearity of an assay can also be determined by various testing routes. One well-accepted method is described in the NCCLS EP-6 document (4) and a brief description of that method follows.

Two levels of neat samples are identified—one at (or near) the lower limit of the measurement range, and the other at (or near) the upper limit. From these two extreme samples, three intermediate samples are prepared—at the midpoint between the "high" and "low" samples, at an intermediate low point, and at an intermediate high point. The "formulations" of the five levels are presented in Table 2.

Once all samples have been prepared, they are analyzed by the new IVD system. The quantitations of samples 1 and 5 at the extremes of the range are used to calculate the expected quantitations of the three intermediate levels. Sometimes an independent reference method is used to assay samples 1 and 5 in order to achieve the highest level of accuracy. Sample 3 is expected to lie midway between samples 1 and 5, sample 2 is expected to be midway between samples 1 and 3, and sample 4 is expected to be midway between samples 3 and 5. The observed values (y) are plotted against the expected values (x), and the data are, at a minimum, visually examined for linearity. In addition, there are

Table 2 Formulations of Samples for Linearity Testing

Sample	Level	Preparation
1	Lower limit of range ("low")	Neat[a]
2	Intermediate low	3 Parts sample 1 and 1 part sample 5
3	Midpoint	Equal parts of samples 1 and 5
4	Intermediate high	1 Part sample 1 and 3 parts sample 5
5	Upper limit of range ("high")	Neat

[a] Undiluted, unchanged.

various statistical tests that can be used to confirm linearity. The IVD's claimed dynamic range has to be consistent with those limits established by the linearity experiments.

Spike Recovery. Spike recovery is somewhat analogous to linearity. Both measurements are an indication of systematic biases or matrix effects, but the measurement techniques are different. While linearity begins with known levels of the analyte and studies the dilutional effects, spike recovery begins with a "zero" or very low levels of the analyte in a base pool, and known amounts of the analyte are added and tested.

To perform spike recovery, generally four or five samples with varying levels of the analyte are tested. Five "negative" pools (samples) are prepared, and known amounts of increasingly concentrated analyte are added to each sample. All samples are assayed as unknowns, and the observed measurements are compared with the expected measurements based on the amount of analyte added. The percent recovery of each sample is the mathematical calculation of (observed) − (expected)/(expected) × 100. A general guideline is that each level should be within 10% of the expected measurement, with biases being nonsystematic—meaning that differences should be both positive (>100% recovery) and negative (<100% recovery).

Clinical Performance Characteristics

The clinical performance characteristics are the next benchmark for the determination of substantial equivalence between the new IVD and the predicate IVD. The clinical characteristics are often considered the "heart and soul" of the premarket notification, because here is where precision and accuracy data are presented, and thereby the question "does the test work right," gets answered.

Precision and accuracy can be established in-house by the manufacturer's laboratories, but over the past 10 yr the FDA has placed an increasingly larger focus on these studies (termed clinical trials, field studies, or method comparisons) being conducted in their eventual settings. This means manufacturers will recruit hospital laboratories for the evaluation of traditional IVDs, and emergency rooms, doctor's offices, and even consumers for the evaluation of point-of-care IVDs. The reason for this is to provide the most realistic view of the IVD's precision and accuracy, and thereby allow the eventual end user to have an accurate expectation of system performance.

Precision. Precision reflects the IVDs ability to provide reproducible results. The manufacturer's challenge is to optimize the IVD system so that aliquots of the same sample demonstrate very similar results each time a sample is tested. Precision data are generally expressed as within-day reproducibility, and between-day reproducibility. The conventional within-run terminology is not appropriate for point-of-care technology because each analysis is, in practice, a separate "run." Precision may also be evaluated interlaboratory with the one lot of product, or may be evaluated with multiple lots of product at one or more facilities.

Precision is always evaluated at more than one level within the measurement range because precision generally varies depending on concentration. For qualitative systems, precision is usually evaluated with a negative sample, a positive sample, and a low positive sample that has been titered near the cutoff value. For quantitative systems, precision is usually evaluated at two to four levels, depending on the breadth of the measurement range. An IVD with a wider range of reportable results will require more precision samples than an IVD with a narrower reportable range. Further, precision samples for quantitative tests should be targeted at or near medical decision points (5). This way the manufacturer can demonstrate precision statistics at those levels associated with clinical diagnoses.

Precision may be evaluated and analyzed in several ways, but it always requires repeat testing of a multilevel precision panel over several runs. The NCCLS EP-5 document (5) describes a well-accepted protocol for precision testing that requires the sampling of two runs per day over 20 days with each run consisting of two aliquots of test material for each concentration. However, as stated previously, point-of-care testing should not be affected by day-to-day variations since each test is a separate run. Therefore, rather than conducting a study over 20 days to generate 80 values (2 runs $\times$ 20 days $\times$ 2 aliquots), it is more practical to generate a comparable number of results over fewer days. Regardless of the precision testing design, the raw data from this testing are used to calculate means, standard deviations, and percent coefficients of variation (%CVs). The "bottom line" for precision testing is expressed as %CVs, and acceptable %CVs for IVDs can range from 2–15%, depending on the specific technology. IVDs that are heavily technique dependent, or with multiple internal steps, are expected to reflect greater assay-to-assay variation than the simpler IVDs.

Accuracy. Accuracy is the IVD's ability to report the "right answer." The right answer is defined by the result obtained by an existing IVD (the predicate device) or by a recognized reference method when split, aliquoted samples from the same individual are tested by both methods. Good accuracy is largely achieved by close calibration of the new IVD against its predicate device. Accuracy must also be defined and supported for multiple matrices, as appropriate. If product labeling specifies that multiple matrices may be used, e.g., whole blood, plasma, and serum, all claims must be validated.

For IVD clinical trials, the field site performs the analyses using the new IVD, and comparative testing with the existing IVD may be performed either by the field site or by the manufacturer. There is more latitude with the testing of the predicate method because this method is a legally marketed device, and the performance characteristics have already been established. In either case, it is imperative that all testing be performed in a blinded fashion where the operator has no knowledge of the comparative result or the clinical status of the patient from whom the sample was collected.

Accuracy may be evaluated and expressed in a variety of ways, and the NCCLS recommends that accuracy be expressed as the percent biases throughout the reportable range. In their EP-9 document (6), it is stated that the manufacturer must collect and analyze comparative data from a minimum of 40 split patient samples, and these samples must cover most of the reportable range. Manufacturers generally include 100–200 samples in their comparative testing in order to obtain more representative data and to fully characterize the effects from different operators and other environmental factors. Also, if samples are being collected and tested prospectively by the participating field site (i.e., stored, banked samples are not being used), it is likely that more than 40 samples will be necessary due to the natural tendency of results to cluster around the middle or "normal" range. In the event that the majority of the measurement range is still not covered by patient samples, it is allowable to supplement the data set with contrived samples that have been specifically prepared at the high and/or low ends of the IVD's dynamic range. These samples are prepared by the manufacturer and then sent to the field site for blinded comparative testing.

Once the assays have been performed by the field site and the results have been sent to the manufacturer, it is the manufacturer's responsibility to summarize and analyze the data. For qualitative tests, data are analyzed as the percentages of true positive/true negative results, and false positive/false negative results. The results from the new method are compared with those results obtained with the predicate method. For quantitative tests, the data are most often analyzed by linear regression statistics (e.g., least squares, or Deming), in which the reference, predicate, or "true" results comprise the x-axis, and the new IVD results comprise the y-axis. There are numerous software packages available for performing these analyses, complete with graphics and calculations of the slope, y-intercept, correlation coefficient, and 95% confidence intervals.

After the linear regression equation is determined, percent biases throughout the new IVD's dynamic range are calculated. The manufacturer has the discretion to choose appropriate levels for bias estimation, but usually the chosen levels include clinical decision points. A good example is provided by cholesterol, for which the National Cholesterol Education Program (NCEP) has determined that the levels of 200 and 240 mg/dL are the cutpoints between "desirable" (<200 mg/dL) and "borderline high" (200–240 mg/dL), and "borderline high" and "high" (>240 mg/dL), respectively. The manufacturer will likely calculate the biases at 150 (arbitrary low concentration), 200, 240 (the two cutpoints), and 300 mg/dL (arbitrary high concentration). This way, data are provided for high and low levels, and at the two medical decision points. Results between or beyond the four levels may be interpolated from the calculated data. An example of calculated percent biases from a hypothetical study is presented below.

In our example, the linear regression equation for a 152-sample data set is: $y = 1.02x - 12$. From this equation, the percent biases are estimated at the four quantitation levels described above. The data are presented in Table 3. It is demonstrated from these data that percent biases ranged from −2% at the high end, to −6% at the low end, and the range of clinical units from 6–9 mg/dL lower than the true result.

Another statistical tool for expressing accuracy is the measurement of clinical sensitivity and specificity. Clinical sensitivity and specificity differ from their analytical counterparts and have separate definitions. The clinical sensitivity of an assay is its ability to identify true positives for a given disease or condition, and the clinical specificity is the ability of an assay to identify truly negative clinical conditions. Clinical sensitivity and specificity are used less commonly than regression statistics for determining IVD accuracy, but they can be valuable tools. Examples of appropriate situations are the evaluations of microbiology systems in which an assay is compared with routine culture results, and also for

Table 3 Estimated Percent Biases from Cholesterol Example (all units mg/dL)

"True" result	Estimated result	Difference in clinical units	Percent bias
150	141	9	−6%
200	192	8	−4%
240	233	7	−3%
300	294	6	−2%

tumor marker assays that monitor disease progression. Here assay results are compared with clinical symptoms and other diagnostic tools, e.g., x-rays, magnetic resonance technology.

Using the example of a new IVD immunoassay for Group A streptococcus (Strep A), suppose a clinical study were conducted with 100 throat swab samples in which there were 50 positive samples and 50 negative samples as determined by routine culture on blood agar plates. The new IVD was evaluated with a second throat swab from the same individuals, and this method identified 52 positive samples and 48 negative samples. The new IVD would therefore demonstrate a clinical sensitivity of 100% (all true positive samples were correctly identified), and a clinical specificity of 96% (two false positive results). This type of accuracy data is most often presented as 2 × 2 contingency tables as shown in Table 4.

Clinical sensitivity and specificity are also useful measures for determining the accuracy of tumor marker assays for monitoring disease progression. If an assay claims that disease is likely to be present above a certain threshold level, and that below this level there should be no evidence of disease, then the clinical sensitivity from a particular study would be the percentage of cases in which the threshold value was reached or exceeded in the presence of disease progression (as determined by appropriate clinical markers), and the clinical specificity would be the percentage of cases in which the results were below the threshold and there was no evidence of disease. A false positive result would occur when the

Table 4 Hypothetical 2 × 2 Accuracy Data

	Culture positive	Culture negative	Total
IVD positive	50	2	52
IVD negative	0	48	48

Formulae for computing sensitivity and specificity, and positive and negative predictive values:

Sensitivity = True positives/(true positives + false negatives)

Specificity = True negatives/(true negatives + false positives)

Positive predictive value = True positives/(true positives + false positives)

Negative predictive value = True negatives/(true negatives + false negatives)

From the hypothetical example:

IVD sensitivity = 50/50 + 0 = 50/50 = 100%

IVD specificity = 50/50 + 2 = 50/52 = 96%

IVD positive predictive value = 50/50 + 2 = 50/52 = 96%

IVD negative predictive value = 50/50 + 0 = 50/50 = 100%

assay result was above the threshold but disease progression was not evident, while a false negative result would occur, conversely, when the assay result was not elevated but there was evidence of disease progression.

It is these various performance characteristics (analytical and clinical) that are provided in the product's package labeling. All labeling is carefully reviewed by the FDA as part of the 510(k) process. With this disclosure of the data, the end user (customer) has an expectation of how the IVD should perform in their particular setting. It is understood that another set of experiments with the same IVD would not produce the exact same statistics, but it would be expected that overall performance would be similar. Further discussion of the FDA's labeling requirements is provided below.

Labeling Requirements

Manufacturers are required to provide draft package inserts and manuals (as appropriate) as part of the 510(K) submission. The contents of the package inserts are well defined within the Code of Federal Regulations (21 CFR. 809.10), and inserts are reviewed for consistency among product lines and between product lines. Some of the labeling requirements are purely administrative (company's name and address), and some requirements are highly technical. There are 15 required elements for IVD package inserts:

- Proprietary and established test name
- Intended use(s)
- Summary and explanation of why the test is useful (discussion of disease, etc.)
- Principle of the test procedure
- Information on the reagents
- Information on the instrumentation
- Information on sample collection and preparation
- Test procedures
- Test results (calculations, etc.)
- Limitations
- Expected values
- Performance characteristics (both analytical and clinical)
- Bibliography
- Name and place of business
- Date and revision number (if applicable) of the latest version of the package insert

In summary, the 510(k) is a composite of an IVD's description (including the intended use), its performance characteristics (both analytical and clinical), and its labeling. The manufacturer's goal is to demonstrate, via scientific evidence, substantial equivalence between the new IVD and the predicate IVD, and thereby show the safety and effectiveness of the new IVD.

CLIA'88 and Test Categorization

Clinical Laboratory Improvement Amendments of 1988 (CLIA'88) is a federal law that regulates laboratories. As such, manufacturers are not directly affected by CLIA'88, but CLIA'88 has a tremendous impact on manufacturers because it is the laboratories (defined broadly to include clinics and doctors' offices) that purchase the IVD products. Although CLIA'88 could be discussed from the viewpoint of the laboratories, this discussion is limited to the industry view.

CLIA'88 regulates laboratories by monitoring their compliance to five standards:

Personnel requirements
Proficiency testing
Quality control
Quality assurance
Patient test management

All laboratories in the United States (inclusive of traditional and nontraditional sites) must comply with these five standards, but CLIA'88 makes some distinctions among laboratories regarding the level of rigor required to meet the standards. Those distinctions are described below.

There are three classifications of laboratories: waived, moderately complex, and highly complex. The decision of which classification is applied to each laboratory is dependent upon the tests performed by each laboratory. All laboratory tests have similarly been categorized as waived, moderately complex, or highly complex, and a laboratory is classified according to its highest "ranking" test. That is to say, if a laboratory performs all moderately complex tests except for one highly complex test, then the laboratory is highly complex. The CLIA test categorization was originally performed by the Centers for Disease Control and Prevention (CDC), but this responsibility was transferred to the FDA in February, 2000.

The regulatory differences between moderately complex tests and highly complex tests are minimal. Highly complex tests can only be performed by personnel with a higher level of education and training (personnel standards), but the differences in the four remaining CLIA'88 standards are invisible or much subtler. In contrast, there are enormous differences between the requirements for waived tests and nonwaived tests. Waived tests are, as would be surmised by the name, waived from all five standards. Functionally, waived laboratories are free to hire personnel with any level of education and training, need only follow the manufacturer's recommendations for quality control testing (normally this is specified as two levels of controls for each day patient results are reported), and do not need to participate in a proficiency testing program. The other two standards (quality assurance and patient test management) deal with global quality issues and are not specific to IVD testing.

With this administrative structure, manufacturers see the advantage of commercializing waived tests. Waived tests have a much lower regulatory burden for market entry because these products may be used with less governmental oversight. This is especially beneficial to many point-of-care sites that do not have the advantages of large staffs and other elements of a traditional laboratory's infrastructure. Clearly, a doctor's office using point-of-care IVDs has different staffing and administrative concerns than a critical care unit within a hospital using the same IVD. The critical care unit is most likely operating under the main laboratory's CLIA license, and is not impacted by a test's CLIA categorization. In contrast, the doctor's office, as a stand-alone unit, may be reluctant to perform IVD testing of nonwaived tests due to the financial and administrative constraints.

As was stated above, the FDA now has the responsibility of categorizing IVDs for complexity. If no special request is made, a new IVD will generally be assigned the CLIA test categorization of its predicate, assuming the predicate is moderately or highly complex. The request for waived status always requires special considerations.

An IVD may become waived by one of three routes: (1) the test system may be one of the original eight products that became waived by congressional regulation (see below), (2) the IVD may be "down-classified" from moderate complexity or high complexity by petition, or (3) an IVD may be waived by virtue of being cleared for home use by the FDA. (Home use IVDs are automatically CLIA waived.) The original eight waived (by regulation) tests are

- Dipstick/tablet urinalysis (nonautomated)
- Ovulation test kit (visual color comparison)
- Urine pregnancy test (visual color comparison)
- Erythrocyte sedimentation rate (nonautomated)
- Hemoglobin (copper sulfate)
- Fecal occult blood
- Spun hematocrit
- Blood glucose (FDA-cleared home use device)

If a manufacturer wishes to obtain FDA clearance and market these assays (and not all these tests could be formatted as test kits), nothing more is required for waived status. Similarly, home use IVDs do not require additional efforts for waived status.

The most common route for a manufacturer to obtain waived status is through the petition process. As of this writing, final guidelines for the petition process have not yet been agreed upon, but an FDA Draft Guidance issued March, 2001 indicates that petitions will need to include the following elements:

- Conformance of the IVD to established waived criteria (see below)
- Demonstration, through hazard analysis studies, of an insignificant risk of an erroneous result
- Lay-user field studies for accuracy (qualitative tests), or accuracy and precision (quantitative tests)

The FDA has proposed the following test system criteria for waived IVDs:

- Is a fully automated instrument, unitized, or self-contained test
- Uses direct unprocessed specimens (only whole blood- and urine-based assays may be waived)
- Requires only basic, non-technique-dependent specimen manipulation
- Requires only basic, non-technique-dependent reagent manipulation
- Has no operator intervention during analysis
- Requires no technical or specialized training with respect to troubleshooting (interpreting error codes does not constitute troubleshooting)
- Requires no electronic or mechanical maintenance
- Produces a direct readout or result that requires no calibration, interpretation, or calculations
- Contains instructions for use written at no higher than a seventh-grade reading level

Clearly many point-of-care IVDs are well suited for waived status based on these criteria. This is especially true of IVDs targeted to the doctor's offices.

The second criterion to fulfill a waived petition is the demonstration of insignificant risk of an erroneous result. This has been interpreted to mean that failure alert mechanisms should be integrated into waived devices, thereby producing no result in the event a test system malfunctions. The guidance document suggests that failure alert mechanisms be addressed as a two-tiered approach: the first step would be the identification of potential test system failures via a comprehensive hazard analysis, and the second step would be the conducting of stress (or flex) studies that characterize the operational limits of the test system.

The third criterion to fulfill a waived petition is the demonstration of field performance. Qualitative tests are challenged with accuracy studies, while quantitative tests are challenged with accuracy and precision studies. For accuracy studies, it has been suggested that 300 lay users each test one blinded sample solely by following the written instructions. These results would then be compared with results obtained from trained users who have tested separate aliquots of the same samples. For precision studies, it has been suggested that 20 lay users at each of three separate site locations perform testing with three samples, each sample containing varying concentrations (low, middle, and high) of the analyte(s) of interest. As with the accuracy studies, results obtained by the lay populations would be compared with results obtained by the trained populations.

FOOD AND DRUG ADMINISTRATION REGULATORY PROCESSES UNIQUE TO POINT-OF-CARE IN VITRO DIAGNOSTICS

The previous section reviewed the FDA's general requirements for bringing traditional IVDs to market. This section identifies those issues that manufacturers must consider when designing the clinical trials and preparing the 510(k) for point-of-care IVDs. The issues center on the clinical trial design and the study's personnel requirements.

Clinical Trial Design

Testing Sites

As was already discussed, the FDA places an emphasis on clinical trials being conducted in the IVD's eventual setting. For the point-of-care IVD, this means studies may need to be conducted in doctor's offices, emergency rooms, and critical care units, as appropriate. The FDA's general policy is that these studies need to be conducted at a minimum of three sites, and preferably at three sites that are geographically located in different parts of the country (7). This is to ensure that regional demographical factors regarding patients and laboratory personnel have been sufficiently addressed.

Rate of Subject Recruitment

Two important aspects of any study's clinical design are the rate of patient recruitment and the possible constraints of sample processing. Since it is less likely that samples can be batch tested for point-of-care technology, a point-of-care study often requires more time for completion than its traditional IVD counterpart. Samples may need to be analyzed "one at a time," with continual replacement of the system's disposable components. Also, if an IVD is targeted for the doctor's office, the office staff may need to specifically recruit certain subjects, or wait for "foot traffic" to enter the office. To assist with this issue, the FDA often allows a percentage of the clinical samples to be banked instead of freshly collected. The manufacturer may collect and store serum, plasma, or urine samples, and then deliver the samples to the testing site. These samples may be tested in batches over a few days, while several more days or weeks may be required to prospectively collect fresh samples.

Sample Matrices

Another aspect of point-of-care clinical design is the stability and volume of the sample matrix. Whole blood assays are very convenient from the standpoint of not requiring clotting time and/or centrifugation, but whole blood is not a stable matrix and therefore arrangements must be made to obtain adequate sample for the comparative method. Further, fingerstick whole blood samples will almost always be of insufficient volume for comparative testing.

In order to work around the matrix issue, many studies require that a second, more stable sample be collected in addition to the sample for the point-of-care IVD. For example, a study designed for a new fingerstick whole blood hCG test will need a separate sample for analysis with the predicate IVD. This is because the predicate IVD will most likely be a conventional system that uses venous serum or plasma. In this case, the testing site must be able and willing to obtain a venous draw in addition to the fingerstick sample.

Personnel Requirements

Point-of-care testing is quite often performed by nonlaboratory personnel who have not received extensive education and training. Because of this, the FDA requires that the individuals who are performing the testing are representative of the eventual end user. In the case of doctor's offices, the testers are likely to be medical assistants and office staff; in the case of emergency rooms and critical care units, the testers are likely to be nurses and paramedical personnel. The FDA frequently asks that the 510(k) include the resumes of the personnel who performed the testing for the new point-of-care IVD.

COSTS AND TIME REQUIRED FOR MARKET INTRODUCTION

There is a tremendous amount of variation in the amount of time and financial resources that are required to bring a point-of-care IVD to market. A general rule is that the more novel the analyte or the technology, the longer and more costly the route. This section provides general details on the major components of the product development phase, the clinical trial phase, and the regulatory interaction phase.

Product Development Phase

The product development phase is arbitrarily being defined here as the time from when a product is an idea, to the time it enters clinical trials. This can easily require 1–2 yr, depending on the "newness" of the technology. Clearly a manufacturer develops in-house expertise over time concerning a particular test platform, and sequential products reap the benefit of institutional knowledge from their predecessor products. Still, every new IVD brings with it a new set of challenges.

To begin the process, a product in the research stage must be shown to be viable from the marketing point of view, i.e., it is believed someone will wish to buy it. A feasibility effort begins to determine if the test system can perform to predetermined minimum specifications. These specifications should be established by all functional departments within the company (Research and Development, Clinical/Regulatory, Operations, and Marketing), and there should be consensus among the departments regarding the outcome of the feasibility testing. Feasibility should also take into account the eventual "manufacturability" of the final product, even if feasibility lots were "handmade" on a small scale.

After feasibility has been shown, true development begins with numerous iterative versions of prepilot and pilot lots. Experimentation with various materials and processes is undertaken so that performance is optimized. Modern IVDs (point-of-care and traditional) often include sophisticated software and hardware systems, thereby adding new levels of complexity that were not a part of conventional "wet chemistry" technology.

After there is a high level of confidence with the pilot lots, the IVD is ready for clinical trials. These clinical trials will produce the performance characteristics that will support the 510(k) and will define the product from the marketing point of view (data provided in package insert). Due to the tremendous cost and time associated with the trials, it is best to not begin clinical trials before a product is fully characterized and has been shown to meet preliminary specifications. It is estimated that development costs to this point range from $10–20 million for the first product on a newly developed platform, and then $2–3 million are needed for additional assays and applications.

Clinical Trials Phase

Successful clinical trials will show that a point-of-care IVD is substantially equivalent to a predicate IVD. This will be done mostly by the demonstration of accuracy and precision in the hands of the eventual end user. Before this can begin, there are many administrative tasks that need to be completed. These preparatory tasks may require 3–6 mo, and are briefly described below.

- Writing the study protocol (inclusive of identifying the predicate device, establishing appropriate inclusion/exclusion criteria for subjects and samples, and developing case report forms and data summary sheets, as appropriate)

- Identifying a minimum of three clinical sites
- Qualifying the clinical sites
- Negotiating budgets with the clinical sites
- Obtaining institutional review board (IRB) approval for the testing of human subjects
- Training the clinical sites with the new IVD procedure, processing steps, and administrative steps
- Coordinating the shipment of samples and supplies to the clinical sites
- Training the clinical sites with the comparative methods, as needed
- Coordinating the shipment of samples and data back to the manufacturer

Once the trials have begun, monitoring is necessary to ensure the protocol is being followed and data are being recorded correctly. Monitoring of IVD trials is far less complex and time consuming than the monitoring of pharmaceutical trials due to the shorter duration (usually measured in weeks rather than years) and the in-vitro component of the study objectives. Samples are being withdrawn and tested, rather than the subject being required to ingest a pharmacological compound.

The costs for point-of-care IVD clinical trials can range from $30,000–60,000 above the company's general overhead. There are potential expenses for IRB approvals, compensation to the investigational site, compensation to the recruited subjects, purchasing of reagents and instrumentation for the comparative method, shipping costs, copying costs, and travel costs to the three clinical sites.

Regulatory Interactions Phase

Once the clinical sites have completed the testing, the data are summarized and analyzed by the manufacturer. This may require a few weeks to many months, depending on the complexity of the data. The data are then prepared in a logical format and the balance of the 510(k) is written. There is no mandatory format for the 510(k), but, along with the performance sections for analytical performance and clinical performance, the document includes sections for the product description, a comparative chart showing the similarities and differences between the new IVD and the predicate IVD, an overview of the manufacturing processes, and a software validation section, if needed. The preparation of the 510(k) may need a few weeks to a few months, depending on the scope of the data and in-house resources.

When the 510(k) is complete, it is submitted to a specific branch within a specific division at the FDA. The FDA is organized in such a way that like products are reviewed together. There is no charge to the manufacturer for the FDA's review, although there is continual discussion of user fees for all devices. The submission is logged into the FDA's system and the "clock" begins. The FDA makes a good effort to complete its initial review within 60 days, and there is almost always a round of questions that is asked of the manufacturer for additional information. The manufacturer must supply the information, or come to agreement with the FDA that the information is already present in the document, or that the request is not feasible or appropriate. If the FDA believes the additional information cannot be obtained within 30 days, the FDA retains the right to withdraw the document from their system. The manufacturer would then need to resubmit the 510(k) at a later date with the added information.

If the request for additional information is such that it can be, and is, submitted within 30 days of its request, then a new FDA cycle begins. The FDA generally tries to complete this review within the next 30 days, but the time limits are nonstatutory and the FDA may exceed this target. Usually there are one or two additional minor rounds of questions, and labeling issues are discussed in great detail at this point. Once the FDA is satisfied that all policy, statutory, and scientific requirements have been met, a substantially equivalent determination is granted. Only then can the IVD be legally marketed. The time frame for this can be 3 mo to 2 yr, with the majority of point-of-care IVDs needing 6–9 mo for clearance. The FDA believes a higher level of scrutiny is required of point-of-care IVDs in order to protect the public's health. This is largely due to the nontraditional environments where the tests are used.

QUALITY SYSTEMS AND COMPLIANCE ISSUES

Once an IVD has been cleared by the FDA, a manufacturer's focus shifts to compliance issues to ensure the product stays on the market and in good regulatory stead. This is largely accomplished through compliance to FDA's Quality System Regulation (QSR). The QSR is an "umbrella" regulation that was designed to ensure consistent product quality for all devices. The regulation was written in general terms to fit a wide array of devices and technologies, so an IVD manufacturer must identify which aspects of the regulation apply to their products, and design the company's quality system accordingly. The QSR mostly identifies the goals for product quality, but also provides some specifics on how to accomplish those goals.

Under the QSR, manufacturers are responsible for ensuring that all purchased goods and services meet established criteria so that the devices meet specifications and perform as expected. The QSR includes provisions for virtually every aspect of a device's design, manufacturing process, and finished acceptance testing. A list of those major provisions appear in Table 5.

Clearly a comprehensive discussion of all QSR provisions is beyond the

Table 5 QSR Provisions

Management responsibilities
Buildings and physical space
Internal audit procedures
Personnel requirements and training
Design controls
Document controls
Purchasing controls
Materials identification and traceability
Production and process controls
Inspection, measuring and test equipment
Process validation
Acceptance activities (receiving, in-process, finished device)
Nonconforming product
Corrective and preventative action
Labeling and packaging control
Product handling, storage, distribution, and installation
Records and records retention
Complaint files
Servicing

scope of this section. However, an abbreviated presentation of manufacturing responsibilities for product lot acceptance activities is provided. The acceptance activities have been categorized by the QSR as receiving, in-process, and finished device activities.

Receiving Activities

Since a product can only be as good as its starting material, it is important that the manufacturing process begins with qualified components, reagents, and other materials. The QSR states that incoming product must be inspected, tested, or otherwise verified as conforming to specified requirements, and that product acceptance or rejection must be documented [21 CFR 820.80(b)]. Before this can be done, however, the manufacturer must decide what specific characteristics of the components will determine their acceptability, and must create specific acceptance criteria (via inspection or testing) that will confirm component/reagent acceptability. The tested characteristics may include appearance, dimensions, and performance. For an IVD manufacturer, receiving criteria may be the purity of an antigen or chemical, the affinity of an antibody, or the reliability of hardware components.

In-Process Activities

In-process activities refers to those controls that are imposed during the manufacturing process. Manufacturers are given discretion to decide when it is appropriate to establish and maintain acceptance procedures for in-process product [21 CFR 820.80(c)]. In-process testing is valuable because it can prevent further loss of time and materials when it is clear a lot of product will fail to meet its final release criteria. As an IVD example, the optical density of an enzyme conjugate may be obtained "off the line" before it is lyophilized to a dried pellet. If the reagent does not meet its targeted range of acceptable values, the manufacturer has the options of "reworking" the conjugate (if this is possible), placing the product in quarantine for further evaluation, or discarding the lot. All recourses must be documented.

Final Acceptance Activities

Final acceptance procedures must be established and maintained so that each production run, lot, or batch of finished devices meets acceptance criteria identified in the device master record (DMR) [21 CFR 820.80(d)]. (The DMR is the "official log" for a product, and it contains the device specifications; production process specifications; quality assurance procedures and specifications; and installation, maintenance, and servicing procedures and methods.) Acceptance criteria should include all parameters that the device must meet to perform its intended use. Manufacturers have the discretion to choose a combination of methods for finished device inspection and/or testing. The inspection/testing methods should ensure that the finished run, lot, or batch meets specified requirements.

For an IVD manufacturer, final product testing usually includes the evaluation of accuracy and precision. Accuracy may be confirmed by means of testing a well-characterized accuracy panel with each lot. The panel typically consists of 3–10 samples that span the assay's dynamic range. The standard operating procedure (SOP) for this testing specifies how close the quantitations need to be to the "right answers." Accuracy may be expressed as the percent differences between the two sets of data (established panel results and the on-test lot) or by linear regression statistics. These specifications define the accuracy pass/fail for the lot.

Final acceptance testing for precision is conducted in much of the same manner. A two- to-four-level precision panel may be assayed with the new lot in multiple runs. From this testing, means, standard deviations, and percent coefficients of variation are calculated, and the precision testing SOP provides the limits for the amount of allowable variation. These specifications define the precision pass/fail for the lot. The objective of this combined final acceptance testing is to confirm that each lot of product meets the product's claim for accuracy and precision.

Until the new lots of devices have satisfied the final acceptance procedures and have been released, they must be held in quarantine or controlled by some other means. Finished devices may not be released until the manufacturer completes activities required in the DMR, reviews associated data and documentation, and a designated individual signs, authorizes, and the dates the release.

Compliance Implications: Warning Letter, Seizure, Injunction, and Prosecution

The FDA maintains oversight of manufacturers and the devices they produce by two primary mechanisms—by performing on-site inspections and by monitoring device problems as identified through product recalls (see below). The Food, Drug and Cosmetic Act (FD&C) allows inspections for purposes of enforcement, and it permits the FDA to inspect all documents specified in the QSR. Therefore, a company may get cited for a violation of any of the provisions discussed in the previous QSR section.

The FDA may routinely inspect a manufacturer as often as every 2 yr, although realistically the frequency is much less. Routine inspections will include review of the 510(k) status for each of the company's devices, and will also focus on complaint handling, changes manufacturers have made in design and production processes, and a review of records showing in-process or finished device testing failures. This information provides the FDA inspectors with an overview of the company's quality system. An FDA inspector has access to all company records except those dealing with financial matters, customer lists, and personnel issues beyond training and education.

If the FDA inspector finds a serious violation of the QSR, meaning (1) finished devices are unsafe or ineffective or (2) conditions exist whereby there is a reasonable probability that unsafe or ineffective devices will be produced, a warning letter may be issued detailing the observation(s) and identifying the provision(s) of the QSR that was violated. The manufacturer must provide a written response to the warning letter within a defined amount of time, and the response must include the steps that will be taken to correct the violation (corrective action) and the estimated amount of time that will be needed. A comprehensive follow-up inspection will reinspect the condition(s) that led to the original citing, plus the balance of the QSR requirements will be reviewed and inspected. The manufacturer may be allowed to continue production of the device while the quality issues are being resolved, depending on the nature of the product and the violation.

If the FDA inspector finds less serious QSR violations or deviations where it is believed there is only a minimal probability that nonconforming product will result if the deviations are not corrected, then a Notice of Inspectional Observations (Form 483) will be issued. The notice will advise the company of the deviations, and the company should respond to the "483" promptly and thoroughly. Responses should present the manufacturer's views of the facts and their interpretations of the relevant QSR requirements. If the violations alleged in the 483 are more serious, the manufacturer should consider submitting to the FDA a proposal for voluntary corrective action.

The FDA's goal in enforcing the QSR is to bring manufacturers into a "state of control" by eliciting voluntary, cooperative efforts. When voluntary cooperation is insufficient, the FDA may initiate further regulatory or judicial action. In the event there is inadequate response to a warning letter, or if initial observations appear to harm public health, the FDA may escalate enforcement activities through seizure, injunction, and prosecution.

Seizure of a product is generally limited to devices that are misbranded or adulterated, and not for violations of the QSR. This is an extreme measure whereby the government can gain control of an allegedly violative product based merely on a complaint (8). In these extreme cases, seizures are often accompanied by injunction orders. An injunction is a remedy against a person, including individuals or corporations, that orders the person to do or not to do something. Typically, injunction orders under FD&C prohibit the conduct of business "unless and until" certain actions are taken and approved by the FDA. The FDA usually pursues injunctions only for the following circumstances:

- When adequate warning to a defendant has been given
- When the FDA believes violations of the FD&C are clear
- When the defendant refuses to discontinue the allegedly violative conduct voluntarily
- When a seizure does not appear to adequately protect public health

The FDA is also more apt to seek injunctions rather than seizures against violations of the QSR because injunctions effectively close a business until the QSR is in place. Injunctions are more applicable when the violation is systemic rather than applying to only one product. Injunctive orders are also the FDA's remedy of choice when a violation presents a health risk.

As a final resort, persons who violate the FD&C may be subject to criminal prosecution and penalties, including imprisonment and/or monetary penalties. The amount of punishment is determined by the type of violation, namely a misdemeanor or a felony. Because felonies are knowing violations of the FD&C, they are subject to greater punishment than misdemeanors. The FDA has used criminal authority sparingly, but these are viable options for the agency.

Product Recalls

Most product recalls are initiated by the manufacturer when it is realized the device does not meet specifications. The FDA also has the authority to impose mandatory recalls when a device "presents an unreasonable risk of substantial harm to the public health," [Section 518(a) of the FD&C], but these recalls are less common.

Product recalls are categorized into one of three classifications: class I, II, or III. The significance of these classifications relates to the extent of the recall and the effectiveness checks that will be required to consider the recall closed in the FDA's view. Additionally, a correct recall classification is important because it represents the FDA's evaluation of the hazard a device presents to the public and, therefore, has potential significance to a product liability suit against the recalling firm.

A class I recall represents a situation in which there is "a reasonable probability that using a violative product will cause serious adverse health consequences or death." This is the most significant recall classification and would require the greatest recall depth, the greatest extension of the recall into the product distribution chain, and the greatest degree of follow-up to ensure the effectiveness of the recall, i.e., proof that any remaining product was returned to the company or destroyed. An example of a class I recall would be for a faulty surgical irrigation device that could result in an air embolism during surgery. Additionally, a class I recall may include public notification, which is reserved for urgent public health situations.

A class II recall is one in which "a violative product will cause temporary or medically reversible adverse health consequences," and the probability of serious effects is remote. Examples of class II recalls include defective latex gloves, printers not being compatible with alarm driver boards on ventilators, needle tips that may separate from the sheath during a surgical operation, possible inaccurate noninvasive blood pressure measurement devices, and cracked components that may compromise the sterility barrier.

A class III recall describes a violative product that is unlikely to cause adverse health consequences. Class III recalls commonly result from labeling errors and mix-ups. Examples of class III recalls include incorrect barcoding, incorrect packaging, control solutions not meeting their target values, and incorrect chemical formulations.

Recalls of IVD products, due to their nature of working outside the body and providing information instead of physical changes to the body, are always class II or III, and mainly class III. In vitro diagnostics can be recalled whenever any portion of the system cannot perform as intended. This includes situations when reagents lose stability or become contaminated, when instruments do not function properly, and when control solutions are mislabeled or erroneously quantitated.

CONCLUSIONS AND BEST APPROACHES FOR THE FUTURE

The regulatory considerations of bringing an IVD to market include interactions with the FDA. The FDA is responsible for:

- Granting market clearance via the decision that the product is safe and effective for its intended use
- Determining test categorization under CLIA'88 requirements
- Providing the regulatory oversight for quality issues to ensure the product continues to meet its performance claims.

Getting an IVD on the market requires the presentation of scientific data supporting analytical and clinical performance characteristics. Getting a point-of-care IVD on the market requires an increased regulatory burden to ensure the product will be used appropriately in the nontraditional laboratory environments.

Table 6 Internet Contacts for Regulatory and Related Organizations

Organization	Internet address
Food and Drug Administration	www.fda.gov
FDA Center for Devices and Radiological Health	www.fda.gov/cdrh/index.html
Code of Federal Regulations	www.access.gpo.gov/nara/cfr/cfr-table-search-html
Centers for Medicare and Medicaid Services (formerly Health Care Financing Administration)	www.hcfa.gov
Centers for Disease Control and Prevention	www.cdc.gov
Biotechnology Industry Association	www.bio.org
Food and Drug Law Institute	www.fdli.org
AdvaMed, Advanced Medical Technology Association (formerly Health Industry Manufacturers Association)	*www.advamed.com* or www.himanet.com
Regulatory Affairs Professionals Society	www.raps.org

Before point-of-care clinical trials are designed, it is very important to open a dialogue with FDA so that the agency's concerns and questions can be voiced. This is best done by contacting the specific branch that regulates the type of IVD, e.g., Clinical Chemistry, Hematology, Microbiology, etc., and speaking with the Branch Chief or a member of the review staff. While FDA regulations are slow to change, FDA policy can change rather quickly, so it is critical that manufacturers be aware of the most current regulatory attitudes towards point-of-care testing. Similarly, if a manufacturer is interested in obtaining waived status for an IVD, it is important to open a dialogue early with the FDA (before the field studies are conducted) so that subtle changes in the requirements can be addressed. Table 6 lists Internet addresses for the FDA and other agencies/organizations.

Keeping an IVD on the market requires compliance with the QSR and other statutory measures. The FDA keeps surveillance over IVD manufacturers by on-site inspections and by monitoring product recalls. In order to ensure that the QSR and other requirements are being met, it is critical that individuals within the company keep updated on the changes in laws and policy. The FDA has a considerable arsenal of regulatory and judicial remedies for those instances when violative product can affect public health.

REFERENCES

1. Federal Register Notice. Fed Regist 5387, Feb 2, 1998.
2. Federal Food, Drug, and Cosmetic Act. 21 USC §301 et seq.
3. National Committee on Clinical Laboratory Standards. Interference Testing in Clinical Chemistry: Proposed Guideline (EP7-P). Vol 6, No. 13. NCCLS, Villanova, PA, 1986.
4. National Committee on Clinical Laboratory Standards. Evaluation of the Linearity of Quantitative Analytical Methods: Proposed Guideline (EP6-P). Vol 6, No. 18. NCCLS, Villanova, PA, 1986.
5. National Committee on Clinical Laboratory Standards. Evaluation of Precision Performance of Clinical Chemistry Devices (EP5-T2). Vol 12, No. 4. NCCLS, Villanova, PA, 1992.
6. National Committee on Clinical Laboratory Standards. Method Comparison and Bias Estimation Using Patient Samples: Approved Guideline (EP9-A). Vol 6, No. 13. NCCLS, Villanova, PA, 1995.
7. U.S. Food and Drug Administration. FDA Guidance Document, Center for Devices and Radiological Health: Review Criteria for Assessment of Cholesterol In Vitro Diagnostic Devices Using Enzymatic Methodology for Clinical Laboratories, Physician's Office Laboratories, and Home Use. USFDA, Washington, DC, 1997.
8. Guide to Medical Device Regulation. Vol 1. Thompson Publishing Group, Washington, DC, 1993.

3

Information Management of Point-of-Care Testing: Strategies for Improving Outcomes

Jay B. Jones
Geisinger Health System
Danville, Pennsylvania, U.S.A.

INTRODUCTION

Management of point-of-care testing (POCT) information should be approached as a subject integrated in the mainstream flow of laboratory data and information to the laboratory information system (LIS) and electronic medical record (EMR). Aspects of POCT information management may be singled out for discrete discussion but even then should be kept in the context of integrated medical informatics (1,2). A basic strategy for improving outcomes in the health care enterprise is to build a holistic approach to medical informatics—beginning at the point of care.

Since laboratory POCT information is typically derived near the patient and the patient's provider, it is innately more integrated with medical informatics than is the more remote and centralized hospital clinical laboratory. Ideally, the *entire* laboratory should remain integrated via its departmental LIS to the broad activities of its healthcare enterprise (2). This broad perspective of laboratory informatics integration has been termed "the distributed laboratory."

Several aspects of POCT information management from this broad perspective need to be singled out for discussion. Detailed discussion of key aspects of POCT informatics is presented following a few introductory concepts.

Impact of New Information Management Technology on POCT

Point-of-care testing and particularly its connectivity to healthcare information systems is being greatly enabled and expanded by existing hardware and software technology. This trend will continue to expand at an accelerating pace as even newer communication hardware, connectivity standards (e.g., the National Committee for Clinical Laboratory Standards' NCCLS POCT1-A standards) (3), and personal computer (PC) technology improve and become increasingly affordable (4). Communication hardware technology (e.g., wide area network architecture) is a vital link between decentralized POCT and more centralized information systems, and as it becomes more ubiquitous (5) will facilitate aggregation and archiving of POCT information. Enhanced functionality of this communication network technology includes increasing bandwidth and speed of data transfer, more intelligent routers and interface engines, and more diffuse wide area network coverage. Information connectivity nodes on wide area networks will almost surely become the predominant model as POCT work station PCs precondition data for verification to the legal patient record. This PC connectivity hardware continues to become more powerful with processing speeds well above a gigahertz and terabyte local mass storage archival becoming feasible. The cost of much of this connectivity hardware continues to decrease on a per unit basis as increased connectivity is demanded, especially in large healthcare enterprises (2,6). The cost of expanded connectivity will likely be partially offset by the lower cost per unit installation but, as with all new technology, will be a rate-limiting factor for POCT connectivity implementation.

On the not too distant horizon is also broad application of wireless technology. Except for a few prototypical installations, this technology will probably not be broadly applied for a few more years. Options for wireless connectivity include (6)

1. Long range systems, such as wireless mobile, as is found with current paging and phone systems.
2. Wireless local area network found in the IEEE802.11B standards.
3. Personal LAN, such as found in the Bluetooth specifications.
4. More local solutions, such as those found in infrared wireless applications (IRDA).

Unless standardization occurs a priori, it is quite likely that there will be several flavors of wireless POCT connectivity initially implemented. Current specifications for device connectivity as listed in the NCCLS POCT1-A standard do not preclude use of wireless technology for POCT device access to its point of connection. On the other hand, NCCLS POCT1-A stops short of specifying wireless connectivity (3).

Wireless solutions may impact the decentralized POCT laboratory sooner than other healthcare sectors. The laboratory may hence be faced with the "first application on the block" scenario (i.e., similar to installing cable television in a new block of houses). It is likely that the attractiveness of wireless solutions will enlarge before the laboratory can readily afford its broad application. The laboratory may be the first to cost justify conversion to wireless technology and the first to be challenged by introducing a precedent-setting technology. One can only hope that broad application of wireless technology becomes more prevalent in the consumer market to help drive down cost prior to implementation in the healthcare enterprise. Perhaps wireless personal digital assistants (PDAs) or graphic tablets will prove a forerunner for wireless POCT device connectivity. It will be quite interesting to observe the evolution of powerful new wireless technology such as Bluetooth in this consumer market. Short-range real-time voice and data communication may occur point to point at low expense with speeds approaching 2.4 gigahertz/720 kilobytes per second using this specification. The range of this relatively local communication is approximately 50 m.

It is likely, however, that wired ethernet will remain the predominant medium for moving data from POCT access points to archival for the next few years. Use of POCT devices will continue to expand and connectivity will become the norm as close proximity IRDA standards continue as the norm for device connectivity. Low-cost point-to-point connectivity with respectable transfer speed can be accomplished with this "here and now" technology. Communication protocols using IRDA such as tiny exist in the NCCLS POCT1-A standard.

Advancement of technology will also greatly impact the POCT device. Miniaturization of electronic hardware, lower mass production cost, and increased affordability of components will encourage broader use of POCT devices. Miniaturized analytical components, such as those found in microfluidic, microarray, and molecular pathology technology, is evolving toward point-of-care applicability. Increasing sophistication in the POCT market will evolve concurrent with increased sophistication of POCT connectivity. Emergent acute infectious disease POCT is but one of many such new POCT applications.

Emergence of the Electronic Medical Record

Concurrent with the evolution of POCT connectivity is integration of POCT into the more global electronic medical record (EMR). Just as decentralized POCT is emerging, an "electronic cultural change" is occurring for the provider who has *always* practiced at the point of care. This "electronic cultural change" is impacting physicians largely by how they order and review tests by the EMR (6–9). The physician or provider interface to the EMR is increasingly a PC screen view in an examining room or physician's office at the point of care. Hence, POCT devices and data input/retrieval devices exist increasingly side by side in the clinic. It is important to realize that the provider customer of the laboratory interacts with "lab" at these PC hardware devices. This user interface to the EMR is the key point of delivery for the laboratory's product—information. The physician or provider of today and certainly tomorrow will be confronted with increasing quantities of information on a more real-time basis. The provider interface to the EMR will become almost as important as the provider interface to the patient. Information retrieval at the time and place that it can most positively impact decision making is a key process that medical care enterprises must design into their future (10,11). Point-of-care laboratory testing must also integrate into the mainstream of this rapid EMR information flow.

A patient's own EMR will become an important personal possession (12). This personal possession will also become more accessible to its owner. Point-of-care test results as well as most laboratory results will likely be broadly viewed by patients in the not too distant future. Access of a given patient's EMR will be shared among multiple healthcare providers in multiple healthcare systems as well as with the individual patient. A newly installed example of this information sharing exists in the Geisinger Health System through the use of an EMR product called "MyChart." This component of the Geisinger EMR allows patients to view laboratory results via the Internet from the home. This genre of information availability and sharing creates a new paradigm for information archival and security (13). The new paradigm will include sharing of information not just *from* the EMR but also *to* the EMR. One should envision the future of POCT to include connectivity from a home "appliance" (14) to a patient's personal EMR. Communication technology has long existed for prescribed home monitoring devices, such as Holter monitors, and the laboratory should prepare for similar connectivity.

It is important for the laboratory to realize that test migration from traditional core laboratory operations to POCT is a continuum rather than a one-step process. Laboratory testing will diffuse to increasing numbers of locations and to an increasing number of caregivers who will need to input POCT to the EMR. A key driver the laboratory must face squarely is that nearly *all* testing in the future will be integrated into the EMR. As such, laboratorians must view the "lab" not as merely a geographical location but rather as an information management service. As the laboratory distributes information to more testing locations, its management will become an increasing responsibility and burden. Since the amount of information in the electronic medical record that originates from the laboratory is estimated between 30 and 50% of the whole, laboratorians are faced with a very large challenge in their role as information managers.

Maintaining Integration of the "Distributed Laboratory"

Information management of POCT data is part of a much larger endeavor that includes all portions of the clinical laboratory and interfaced information systems

(6,15,56). Optimally, POCT should be integrated into the LIS to serve as the primary laboratory data source for the EMR. A good term for site neutral integration of test data in an enlarging clinical laboratory enterprise is "distributed laboratory." One must not envision POCT as a separate and distinct laboratory enterprise consisting of separate rules, quality control programs, purchasing, supply distribution, and data archiving, but rather as part of one "distributed laboratory." In maintaining the functional integrity of the clinical laboratory, point-of-care data management must be interleaved with total laboratory information management. All testing results from the clinical laboratory, whether derived from a POCT device or a central core laboratory instrument, must be presented to the EMR with a means of indicating where and how the laboratory test was done. If connectivity of a given POCT device is to be established to the LIS, it must employ test codes with standardized reference ranges and other relevant data to interleaf with central laboratory tests in the EMR (16). One may state that once a POCT result is verified via a POCT workstation to the LIS that the test becomes part of the mainstream of information flow. This mainstream includes flow of information through all additional information systems interfaced to the LIS (e.g., admission/discharge/transfer [A/D/T] information systems, billing information systems, decision support systems, as well as the EMR) (17).

This holistic approach to POCT information integration requires a broad scope of planning to seamlessly implement into the LIS and EMR. The end product of POCT—information—needs to be integrated into a useful provider EMR screen view. Traceability and specificity of clinical laboratory testing information (e.g., the POCT scientific record) may be archived at intermediate steps of information flow (i.e., POCT workstation and LIS); however, POCT and central laboratory test information needs to be universally retrievable from the EMR.

Combined and integrated archival of POCT and central laboratory testing (16) is also important for supporting disease management programs. For example, diabetes disease management in an integrated delivery system may benefit from initial population screen testing for random blood glucose performed on a "CLIA waived" glucose meter. Additional confirmatory testing for fasting plasma glucose in a gray-topped tube should be performed with a reference method such as hexose kinase in the central laboratory. Follow-up monitoring may include central laboratory hemoglobin A1c testing by HPLC or a point-of-care hemoglobin A1c device. To determine incipient nephropathy, a urine dipstick microalbumin test may be performed. If initial microalbumin in urine is positive upon screening, more accurate quantitative testing of urine microalbumin with a 24-hr collected specimen may be indicated. All of these tests must be verified in the LIS and logically archived to the EMR so the provider can determine which tests were done for screening purposes and which tests were done for confirmatory purposes. As evidence-based medicine (EBM) becomes the norm and these laboratory data elements are archived in a clinical repository to be searched for disease correlation, all standardized methods must be interpretable by LIS test code. A longitudinal record must be maintained in order to follow patient outcomes as various types of tests—centralized laboratory or POCT—are accumulated. Therefore, it is important for the laboratory to construct the LIS database with identifiable and standardized test methods that may be correlated. This interpretable complete laboratory database will form the basis of outcomes analyses, derivation of clinical pathways, and evidence-based medicine (EBM). This laboratory database may be termed a *data warehouse* (18), not to be confused with the more global *clinical repository.*

As the laboratory data warehouse and clinical repository in the electronic record are populated by POCT and central laboratory tests, the clinical laboratory will need to assist their colleagues in applying these data to EBM. The laboratory will have an expanding role in assisting the construct of EBM around useful parametric laboratory tests in data warehouses and clinical repositories. It is only with an understanding of the technical aspects of laboratory testing that verifiable outcomes measures may be formed across the continuum of care.

Expanding the Clinical Laboratory's Role in the Healthcare Enterprise

With the expansion of POCT information management, the laboratory is offered an expanding role in integrating laboratory testing into disease management and developing the EMR (6,19,55). Because there is a growing need to deliver laboratory information to the provider at the point of care, the laboratory has the opportunity to participate closer to where medicine is practiced. Laboratorians must understand that POCT information integration is but an entrance into a broader participation in reforming the "front end" of healthcare informatics. Understanding the dynamics of information flow from (1) when the patient is registered into the healthcare system as an encounter, to (2) where the patient is treated, to (3) where laboratory testing is performed, to (4) how laboratory results are reviewed in the clinical decision-making process are all tantamount to understanding the total integrated informatics process. System analyzing this total informatics process allows the laboratory to better understand how its product—information—fits into the entire process and the true value of a POCT. As previously mentioned, it is also important that once this information flows through the POCT workstation and the LIS to the EMR, that aggregated information can be formed into clinical pathways to support EBM. It will also be important that laboratorians be viewed as important team members in effecting improved outcomes by installing laboratory information in real time at key medical decision-making points.

POCT in vitro diagnostic (IVD) companies in general view the laboratory as an important entrance location for introducing their products to the market (20). Vendors understand that laboratorians will manage not only compliance as

CLIA regulations are maintained, but also will be instrumental in integrating connectivity to information systems in the healthcare enterprise. For this reason, laboratorians should collaborate with industry to enhance their role as change agents for the future of healthcare. Laboratorians must do more than simply provide POCT results. Laboratorians must become "informaticians" to help extract valuable information from test results. Part of this role as an "informatician" includes knowing some of the "nuts and bolts" of information systems implementation.

Since many clinical pathways embedded in EBM will be based on parametric laboratory values, laboratorians will have increasing influence upon outcomes management. As POCT migrates and distributes itself across the healthcare continuum, laboratorians will work more closely with their customers—providers and patients. Understanding laboratory medicine not just from a diagnostic standpoint but also from its integration into decision making (10) will empower the laboratorian to create increased value and quality to their product—information. Point-of-care testing, at one time viewed as an encroachment upon laboratory authority, has the potential of becoming the new vanguard of laboratory medicine.

LOCATION OF THE "USER VIEW" FOR POINT-OF-CARE TESTING

Clearly, the user's interaction with POCT, be it device operator, provider, laboratory, or consumer, will become increasingly important for managing test information (21). As healthcare becomes even more "paperless," user *screen views* via desktop, portable, graphic tablet, or palmtop devices will become primary tools of POCT information transfer. The "front end" of the laboratory will become vital for interacting with the full range of laboratory customers. Since the laboratory's product—information—will increasingly be delivered by this screen view, its design will determine the laboratory's success in providing clinical information. To begin an understanding of the user view and how it relates to the overall clinical laboratory testing process, one must analyze where screen views are (or will be) located.

Device User View

Currently, much of the information from POCT is provided real time directly from the device's screen view to its operator. Most clinical decision making from POCT is made based upon the dynamics of information flow from this "user" screen view. The operator is not the device's "user" per se but must transfer information to the "user" of this information. One cannot presuppose that a user screen view on the POCT device is the optimal way to integrate POCT into clinical decision making. As convenient as this user screen view is, there are numerous situations that require better informatics. At this point, it is important to differentiate device operator user from provider information user. The importance of the provider user view will be expanded upon in later sections.

Most information archived for review by primary or secondary provider users is verified by the device operator to the LIS. Most current POCT devices capable of data transfer to a LIS contain all result and demographical fields that are required for a legal reportable clinical laboratory test. In the future, these fields will likely be expanded to include accessory information that is available at the point of care to conveniently treat the patient. Expansion of the user view of a POCT device to a broader informatics screen view, especially for data input, may occur rapidly in the next few years. Point-of-care testing devices will be stressed to provide this expanded screen view. The importance of a strategically placed POCT device for data capture and input cannot be ignored.

Operator View

Current POCT devices have user views designed for convenient operation at the bedside. Most first-generation POCT devices tend to focus on emergent care (e.g., blood gas analysis), with user views designed for rapid display (22). In most cases, these POCT devices are operated by the provider or near the provider on a real-time basis. Controlling factors such as double entry of patient and/or operator identification (ID) are largely avoided because of provider need to get information rapidly. Features that would "lock out" an operator—for example, if quality control checks were not performed within a given time frame—are also largely suppressed.

With the advent of LIS connectivity, operator input information passes a second line of defense for verification, namely the POCT workstation. At the POCT workstation level, a result verifier, usually a laboratory POCT coordinator, can intercept improper patient and/or operator ID. If demographical information for a POCT is incorrect, or "excepted," it is corrected prior to verification to the LIS. Essential data must be input to the POCT device by the operator in order to produce a legal test result. Table 1 shows obligatory information elements that must be entered into the device via the user screen view to produce a legal result.

It will be increasingly important to design device operator views in the future to capture as high a rate of accurate information input as possible. User views that are overly convenient and easy to bypass should be discouraged to avoid possible medical errors. Operator convenience as well as accuracy may be accomplished with automated input such as bar code scanners and touch screens already found in several POCT devices. Bar code scanning capability is convenient not just for entry of patient ID via bar coded wristbands, but also for determining operator ID via bar coded badges and nameplates. Additionally, bar

Table 1 Obligatory Order Entry Data Elements for POCT

Patient identification	
1.*	Patient location
2.*	Patient encounter number
3.*	Patient provider identification
4.	Patient clinical parameters, if pertinent
5.	Operator identification
6.	Device name
7.	Device serial number
8.	Device error message or null
9.	Test name
10.	Test lot number
11.	Date of test
12.	Time of test

* Information assigned by A/D/T or billing system(s).

coded comments on carried cards (e.g., entering insulin dose) or perhaps voice input may evolve to facilitate input.

Equilibrium must be achieved between operator convenience and burdensome exception correction at the workstation level. One should not overly burden the operator with laborious lockout and verification protocols for every field input when current technology may build verification or "intelligence" into the POCT system (23). With bidirectionality of data transfer between device and workstation, the opportunity will eventually appear for echoing back information from the workstation to the operator on a real-time basis. Information from the workstation may eventually provide the "intelligence" for correction of improperly input fields (e.g., "try again" messaging). The NCCLS POCT1-A connectivity standards support this bidirectional real-time information flow. When and if this functionality becomes the norm, there will be autocorrection or at least intervention on a real-time basis between the information in the POCT workstation and the operator as the operator performs the test. For example, if a medical record number is entered as patient ID and that patient is not live in the system, an operator warning or prompt for rechecking of patient ID can occur. Such hardware "intelligence" built into the overall system may very well reduce transcription or keystroke errors.

Since the POCT workstation is simply a reflection of data input by the operator, it becomes a source of concern when archived. This archived information is now "discoverable" from a medicolegal standpoint. This "discoverable" information needs to have documented review and verification at the point-of-care workstation level. Hence the verifying laboratory shares the responsibility for correction of inaccurate test information. Point-of-care coordinators are currently plagued by recurring operator input errors at the POCT workstation level with exception rates (i.e., those results that must be corrected before verification) typically between 5 and 30%. Intervention with operators for training and remediation is commonly the most time intensive activity of today's point-of-care coordinator.

Patient Self-Testing View

The device user view must be specifically (re)designed for the consumer patient as POCT devices or "appliances" are employed for home testing. The responsibility for verifying correct information to a patient's own medical record will remain a shared responsibility between the patient entering their own information and the healthcare provider archiving it (24). Simplified large numerical displays predictably will need to be features of self-testing "appliances" (e.g., home prothrombin time testing). Again, intelligence built into the POCT workstation (or as specified in the NCCLS POCT1-A specification, the "observation reporter") will need to discover improper information input by the patient. Algorithms for early error detection must be designed to operate jointly between the device and the observation reporter. Simplified prompts will also need to be employed in consumer devices to alert self-testing patients of device malfunction or improper data entry.

Since an aging population will likely require this sort of self-testing device in the future, caregivers in the home or other care facility will increasingly perform the actual testing. The device user view designed for the consumer would likely be the most appropriate user view to employ for this genre of testing. The regulatory and medicolegal burden will continue to be borne largely by the healthcare provider, specialty service, or clinical laboratory that prescribes or issues the self-testing device to the consumer patient. This is a burden that laboratorians must face in order to remain involved in laboratory testing that will become part of the distributed laboratory of the future.

Ordering Healthcare Provider View

In the simplest scenario for ordering a POCT, a healthcare provider simply asks an operator to perform the test. The operator then typically performs electronic order entry while operating the POCT device. Upon test completion, the operator verbally transmits the results, passes a printed tape, or shows the device screen to the provider. This simple scenario requires proximity and real-time presence of operator and provider. This scenario is diminishing in frequency, however.

Providers infrequently perform their own POCT or are present to view the POCT result in real time. More frequently, point-of-care tests are ordered and results are viewed on electronic devices (or screen views) remote from the POCT device itself.

For example, in the Geisinger Health System (Danville, PA) the EMR EpicCare system provides the view where most POCT tests (and *all* distributed laboratory tests) are ordered and results viewed in outpatient clinics. Thus a pending order (a "hole") is created that is filled in one of two ways. Most manual point-of-care tests are resulted directly into EpicCare. Automated (i.e., instrumented) tests are reordered in the LIS and upon resulting fed to EpicCare to "fill the hole" in the test order. To the ordering provider, a virtual interface appears in EpicCare but a direct electronic orders interface does not currently exist between EpicCare and the LIS. In essence, EpicCare creates a work list for POCT that is printed locally. The instrumented POCT is performed, and order entry/results transmittal done concurrently to the LIS. Once verified to the LIS, "unsolicited" results are returned to EpicCare. Under development is an electronic version of this orders interface by which EpicCare POCT orders will pass to the LIS that will synchronize with test results coming from the POCT device. This is referred to as a "solicited" orders interface. A major unresolved problem in developing such an orders interface is how to get the LIS to handle solicited and unsolicited POCT orders concurrently.

There is a growing need in healthcare to synchronize the healthcare provider screen view with the test ordered and performed on the POCT device. The major question to resolve involves synchrony of an orders alert. The orders alert may come from the EMR (e.g., the EpicCare system in the case of the Geisinger Health System), the LIS, or perhaps, in the future, the device itself. In any case, there is a need to focus on synchronizing the "front end" provider order with the initiation of the POCT. Although it is currently the norm for operators to simply walk up to a POCT device and perform the test, one must not become complacent that all POCT orders will remain in this manual mode.

The ordering healthcare provider's graphical user interface (GUI, pronounced "goo-ey") will be a very broad multidepartmental desktop in the EMR (25). This EMR desktop GUI view will include clickable multidepartmental tabs to retrieve information from pharmacy, radiology, and appointments, as well as clinical laboratory. For that reason, the laboratory must understand it is sharing this EMR desktop view in a standardized format with multiple other departments with multiple data types and formats. Retrieval of information from the EMR must be quick, convenient, and accurate. Laboratory information must be seamlessly integrated interdepartmentally and intradepartmentally. The informatics of this interlaced distributed laboratory requires concise use of test identifiers that allow similar test results from the central laboratory and POC to be differentiated yet viewed together.

Different providers should also be allowed the flexibility in their EMR desktop to set preferences or synonyms for laboratory test identifiers (21). In the

EpicCare EMR this is accomplished with "SmartSets." Cross-reference tables must be built to map user POCT identifiers from the EMR to the LIS. This front end flexibility that funnels user convenience and preferences to a concise laboratory descriptor is a great advantage to the laboratory. A provider may call the test that they are ordering a "glucometer," an "accucheck," a "one touch," or a "fingerstick sugar" that will funnel to a single LIS test code. Information-overloaded providers often remember (and sometimes cannot forget) vendor-specific names for tests they performed on a previous generation POCT device. Rather than force immediate change in terminology, the laboratory is probably wise to educate providers in proper test terminology and evolve gradual change. The laboratory should not force terms on providers that may be concise to the laboratory but confusing to the laboratory customer.

The Laboratory View

Since the laboratory is legally responsible for providing a complete record of each testing event, the laboratory view for POCT must be the "source of truth" for technical management of all POCT results. Traceability of all POCT results to testing conditions existing when the test was done needs to be part of the laboratory's responsibility and screen view. Items listed in Table 2 are elements of this source-of-truth scientific or quality assurance (QA) record (26). Many outside of the laboratory have little appreciation for how much obligatory information is part of this QA or scientific record. Since most of these information elements do not typically pass to a LIS or EMR, the POCT workstation is the most appropriate location for archival. This workstation screen view is extensively used for correcting operator input errors as previously described. Archiving of all POCT information derived from operator and device must be retrievable in toto for the laboratory to technically manage and verify results to the legal medical record.

For the laboratory to bear the legal responsibility of technically managing POCT in a single source-of-truth system, it is imperative that POCT results are verified to a LIS. The LIS of the future may consist of a separate departmental system, a module within an EMR (27), or an "outside" application service provider (ASP) system or systems (28). The location of LIS hardware and how it integrates to the EMR is not as important to the laboratory as the laboratory's direct involvement in systems managing it. The laboratory must systems manage the LIS in order to verify POCT (and all laboratory) results. Besides device-generated patient results, all of the aforementioned scientific or QA record must reside in the LIS or the POCT workstation. Both LIS and POCT workstation (in whatever hardware configuration) should be owned and the legal responsibility of the clinical laboratory. The POCT workstation may be viewed as a clinical laboratory device or workstation just as PCs are configured in the main laboratory as workstation managers for other instruments. For example, a PC that controls

Table 2 Source-of-Truth Information in the Scientific or QA Record

Those data listed in Table 1 plus:

1. Reagent lot numbers
2. Quality control/calibrator lot numbers
3. Reagent/quality control calibrator expiration dates
4. Product recall or alert records
5. POCT device location (e.g., TCP/IP address)
6. POCT device error messages
7. POCT device reference ranges
8. POCT device reportable ranges
9. Operator competency checks
10. Operator lock out criteria
11. Accuracy of time/date (e.g., daylight savings time changes)
12. Quality control records (results, frequency, performed by)
13. Proficiency testing results
14. Patient identification changes
15. Operator identification changes
16. Operator input textual comments
17. Laboratory input textual comments
18. Calibration verification records
19. Test validation records
20. POCT result cancellation/change traceability
21. Input error traceability (e.g., wrong patient identification input event)

and aggregates information from chromatographic devices in a toxicology laboratory is very much akin to the PC workstation that controls and aggregates information from POCT devices.

With such tight control of information management, the laboratory may assume responsibility for aggregating information from multiple POCT devices and prevent misinformation from entering the EMR. With appropriate control from the POCT workstation to multiple devices, the laboratory may also exercise some control over not only operator input but also provider test utilization. An equilibrium exists between user convenience and control of user input. The dynamics of establishing this equilibrium over thousands of operators and providers is one of the most difficult operational responsibilities of the current laboratory and will become an increasing focus of activity for the distributed laboratory of the future.

Internet Strategies

The front end of the distributed laboratory will continue to evolve toward Internet access (29,30). Within the Geisinger System, the Internet has been applied as a browseable front end to both patients and referring providers via MyChart and EpicLink (Figure 1). Although current Internet access is enabled only for result review (including POCT), eventual order entry and self-testing result input via the Internet is envisioned. The market demand for convenient laboratory result review has been rapid and intense. It is important to pro-act to this market demand by examining the full scope of activities that Internet access will enable (31,32).

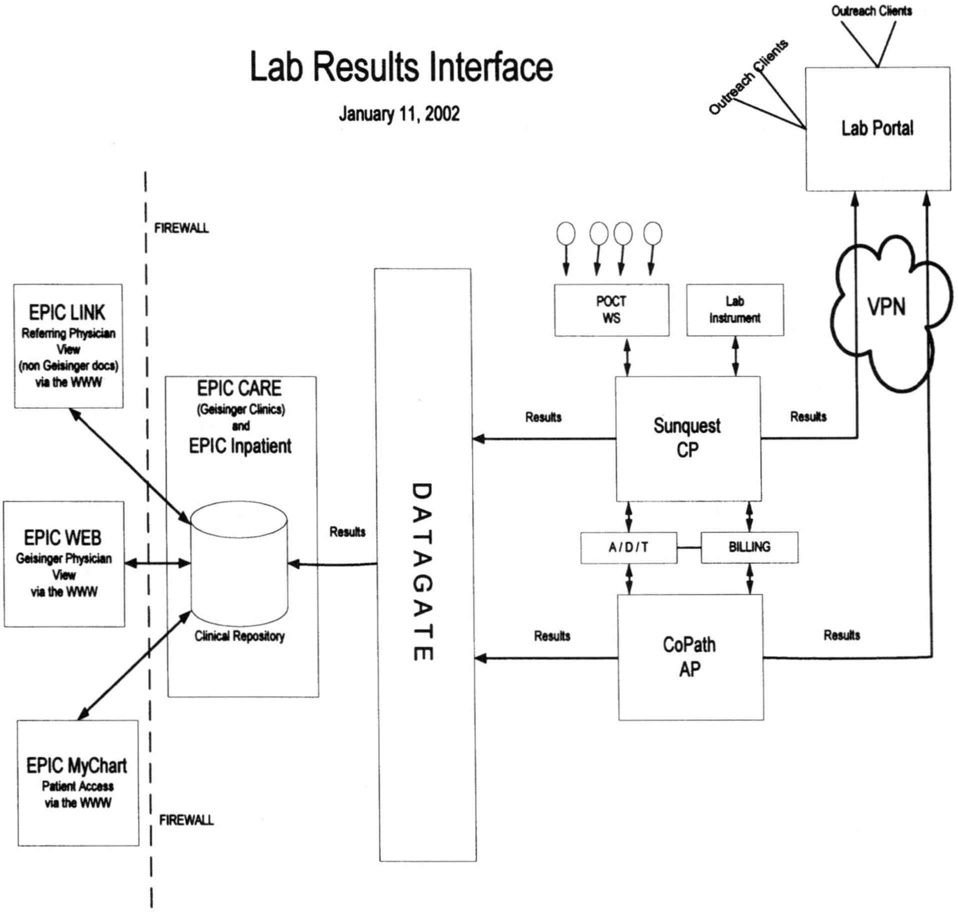

Figure 1 Integration of laboratory information systems and electronic medical record in the Geisinger Health System.

Since the Internet by its very nature is very branched and hyperlinked, one must look at all routes of access and input via a Web browser. It would be naive to think that a single browseable front end could be created for all applications and customers in a healthcare enterprise. Hence, one must look at all portals of entry into the LIS and EMR and judge how they may be browsed and hyperlinked (33,34).

The reverse side of convenient laboratory access via the Internet is (in)security of this access (12). One must plan firewall protection between *intra*net and *Inter*net sources of information. This firewall must protect from unauthorized access via open TCP/IP address portals to the enterprise's network. Some access to information may be authorized via intranet connectivity to salaried providers within a healthcare enterprise that should not be authorized for the provider community at large.

Information disseminated by intranet may be much more detailed and sensitive than that allowed via Internet connectivity. Hence, intranet information must be secured via firewall and access security (e.g., user identification by "what they know, what they have, who they are"). A dilemma exists as to "where the tween shall meet," i.e., where may the Internet appropriately hyperlink to the intranet? In most cases, such hyperlinking will be disallowed because it creates a "back door" to sensitive information. Hence parallel Internet and intranet portals will likely need to be segregated with only subsections hyperlinked with each other. Since almost all POCT devices do not send results via HIPAA-compliant encrypted messaging, it would be unwise to allow such connectivity outside of an enterprise's intranet firewall.

Figure 1 shows various Internet routes for access across the firewall to laboratory information in the Geisinger system. There are currently two such access routes that presently do not hyperlink. "Lab Portal" for test order entry and result reporting to for profit outreach customers is entirely separate from EpicCare, MyChart, EpicLink, and EpicWeb used for information retrieval by Geisinger patients, referral providers, and salaried providers, respectively. Future hyperlinking is being carefully considered.

A major information management consideration is whether or not all routes of results inquiry point to a single, legal, source-of-truth laboratory record (35). This ultimate source of truth resides in the full scientific QA record contained in the LIS and or LIS workstations. The EMR may be a summarized results repository but it only reflects the veracity of the LIS. The LIS with its associated POCT workstation represents the full data repository that feeds the EMR. In the future, it will become important to consider this full scientific and QA record as a source of truth when and if POCT laboratory results are entered via the Internet. Likewise, it will be important to judge the potential of conflicting information if central laboratory and point-of-care tests are ordered on the same patient and then viewed by the same patient. The laboratory may be in the position of having to explain and interpret differences between screening and confirmatory test methods to not only provider customers but also patient customers. The bottom line is that the laboratory must become expert at information management and verify its LIS as the source of truth for laboratory results no matter how they are accessed or where they are transferred.

In summary, the user views for POCT and central laboratory testing will become merged and expand via the Internet to customers within the traditional healthcare setting and to patients and providers in the community at large (6,32). The laboratory, and especially those laboratorians that are coordinating POCT, will help establish the distributed laboratory as it provides valuable information via new informatics tools. Laboratorians must broaden their view and prepare for this greatly expanded role.

LOCATION OF DATA AND INFORMATION TO BE MANAGED

Front End Feeder Systems

Information that becomes part of the source-of-truth legal POCT result aggregates from multiple sources and locations. The POCT result generation is an assembly process in terms of aggregating multiple data elements from front end feeder systems apart from both the LIS and POCT workstation in a time-dependent sequence. Such front end feeder systems are shown in Figure 1. After POCT results are verified in the LIS, they pass across a multiple departmental interface engine, termed "Datagate," to the EpicCare EMR. Once in EpicCare, results may be viewed quite universally by the aforementioned screen views.

Of prime importance for creating a POCT result are patient demographics for location and time of the POC test. These two information elements commonly come from an A/D/T system. For a valid laboratory order to occur, the patient must in some form be "admitted to the system." Frequently, this admission is tracked as an "encounter." This encounter is date and time specific as well as location specific. Since most A/D/T systems are a component of a financial system, this encounter frequently may also be referred to as a "billing number." Laboratory tests and other reimbursable charges in a healthcare system are posted via that encounter number to the patient's bill. Hence the A/D/T becomes an important source of truth for these patient demographics that are passed to the LIS (and EMR) when a laboratory test is ordered. Since an A/D/T system is almost assuredly a feeder system to the LIS for central laboratory testing, it is logical that it also would be for POCT. In fact, since POCT is more quickly performed as a patient moves between departments in a medical center, tracking patient location in real time in the A/D/T system becomes quite important. Time synchronization with patient location is a key consideration when planning POCT connectivity in a dynamic medical center with multiple outpatient and inpatient

POCT services. The common means of tracking patient demographics is the A/D/T system rather than the LIS or the EMR. The A/D/T function in the future may be merged into a single EMR system (as in many cases, hospital information systems [HISs], have already seamlessly merged). In implementing POCT connectivity, one cannot overemphasize the importance of integrating these front end systems.

In large integrated systems or multiple entity healthcare enterprises, there may be multiple A/D/T systems for identifying patients and locations (56). This presents a growing problem as healthcare systems merge and try to standardize efficient operations. Cross-referencing systems for merging separate patient identifiers to a single unique identifier that may be tracked in multiple healthcare entities is in a state of development. The so-called "master patient index" (MPI) is of growing importance for tracking patients seen at separate entities with separate patient identifiers at each. All of this complexity needs to be resolved if POCT connectivity is to be dispersed across the entire enterprise. This front end complexity must also be resolved in order to report POCT to a merged EMR. The MPI must be responsible for providing identity to a patient and hence routing to the proper EMR(s). Any potential mismatches of information may result in an exception in the A/D/T or other clinical system and prevent posting of a laboratory result. Of even greater consequence would be a potential misposting of one patient's test result to another patient. In dispersing POCT, one must have an intimate knowledge of the A/D/T system to prevent this type of mismatch error. Mismatch error may be created not just for patient identity but also provider identity and location identity. Again, this requires the laboratorian to aggregate POCT data through the LIS and to have a global understanding of front end feeder systems.

POCT Device

After POCT is performed, results are electronically stored within the device (36). These device-displayed results are typically acted upon in real time, especially in emergent situations. For more routine applications, device-stored results must remain robustly secured and unchanged as they await uploading to the POCT workstation and LIS. Editing of results is not in the operator domain (22,36).

Current-generation POCT devices are almost always batch rather than real-time uploaded to the POCT workstation (37). Until such time that POCT results are broadcast to the workstation on a real-time basis (i.e., wireless transmission), results must remain secure in the device or a device accessory at the point of care. Time of batch uploading is variable, typically occurring hourly to daily. Stored POCT results contain most pertinent demographics and test results and may be recalled from the device itself. Therefore, the POCT device to some degree may be used as an inquiry device.

However, results inquiry is most typically performed via the LIS or EMR. For this reason, batch uploading and verification from the device itself is commonly performed several times daily. Hence the scheduling of wired transmission from device to LIS and EMR is part of the data management responsibility of the laboratory. Explicitly stated, the POCT coordinator largely controls, and hence must decide, the overall timing of information flow through the various information systems. Security of this test information is also partly the responsibility of the laboratory or POCT coordinator. Although, current HIPAA (Health Insurance Portability and Accountability Act) regulations do not preclude placement of point-of-care devices in patient areas, it is logical that these devices be in secure treatment areas. Recent statements by HIPAA implementation study groups indicate that paper medical records may remain by the bedside. Therefore, one may feel some relief that rational restrictions will likely evolve for placement and use of POCT devices.

If POCT devices are prescribed by healthcare systems to patients for self-testing, data management issues will surely arise (38). Proper data input has already been discussed. Management of this information including transmission of test results typically over modem and Internet connection to the healthcare system will need to be supported and monitored. Encryption of now readable message content will need to be developed by POCT device vendors as well as receiver decrypting software in POCT workstations. In the case of coagulation testing, it is likely that the responsibility for proper data management and instruction of the user will be a partnership between the laboratory and pharmacy. If the archiving of test information from coagulation testing is to occur in the LIS, it may be that pharmacists or other designated providers be given editing and verification rights to the LIS. This is an example of how the laboratory must partner with other healthcare providers not just for performing POCT but also for data managing orders and results.

POCT Data Workstation Informatics Issues

Several issues arising from POCT data transfer from device to workstation and from workstation to LIS have already been discussed. Actual information management issues that arise at the workstation level are severalfold. A key consideration is not only how data transfers with complete source-of-truth information, but also how that data is modified, corrected, and archived within the workstation (1,39). If, for example, patient identification is not correctly entered into the POCT device and subsequently uploaded to the POCT workstation, the POCT coordinator will need to detect this misidentification and correct it. A record of this corrective action (old and new result and when and by whom the correction was made) should be part of the data archived in the workstation. After correction, the POCT coordinator may also follow-up with the appropriate operator at the point of care to remediate the error if severe or frequent.

For example, if a trauma patient in the Emergency Room prior to identification is input simply as a string of six 1s for blood gas analysis, results will be uploaded to the workstation that clearly need to be corrected. The POCT coordinator will need to establish subsequent identity by medical record number of this patient 111111 and change it in the POCT workstation. This example assumes that patient 111111 was not an active encounter in the A/D/T system and was identified as an exception. In order to assure that proper results go to the properly identified patient, it is sound practice to look at other tests performed to make sure there is no mismatch of results. Reestablishing time and location of testing may also help to verify identity of this patient. Clearly, policy should be implemented for such unidentified patients, using a system of unique identifiers.

In a similar but yet unacceptable scenario, an operator may enter six 1s for patient identity simply to shortcut lookup of the patient's medical record number. In this case, the POCT coordinator may need to launch more aggressive remedial action toward the operator not performing their duty. In this case, the POCT workstation may assist in documenting that an operator misidentified a patient (or more severely, falsified a medical record) on which the POCT was performed. This documentation may assist aggressive remedial action and be used as evidence for disciplinary action. The POCT data manager may thus be used in organizing operator training and documenting competency. This archived record needs to be maintained for QA purposes and also show due diligence in correcting medical errors prior to verification to the LIS (and hence the EMR). Table 3 shows several activities ensuing from archived data in the POCT workstation.

Laboratory Information System Informatics Issues

A very important location for information verification and archival is the LIS. As already mentioned, the LIS is a data repository that should be regarded as the source of truth for the laboratory testing record (40). This laboratory testing record includes not only all pertinent demographics and test results, but also the scientific and QA record required to establish most test conditions retrospectively. Hence, in many regards, the POCT workstation is part of the LIS. The systems management of the LIS and all associated workstations is the primary responsibility of the clinical laboratory (41). All preanalytical and postanalytical specifics of a test result need to remain under the purview of the clinical laboratory. Decisions regarding specimen suitability, analytical veracity, and test reporting to EMR and billing systems should be highly structured and controlled by the clinical laboratory. In the realm of POCT, all of this systems management of information is likewise required.

Table 3 POCT Workstation Information Management Activities

1. Tracing frequency of patient misidentification input errors by operator
2. Tracing frequency of operator misidentification input errors by operator
3. Tracing frequency of connectivity failure by location (e.g., network node troubleshooting)
4. Tracing frequency of "exceptions" (i.e., those POCT that do not autoverify)
5. Maintaining a roster of operators by service
6. Certifying operators after initial training
7. Validating operators with ongoing training (i.e., competency testing)
8. Tracing frequency of retesting POCT within protocol (e.g., retesting hypoglycemia)
9. Monitoring volume of testing by types and location
10. Monitoring volume of testing by time
11. Reconciling number of tests reported versus number of reagent strips consumed (i.e., inventory control)
12. Monitoring use of reagent lot numbers
13. Monitoring quality control compliance
14. Monitoring proficiency testing compliance

Selection of discriminatory LIS test neumonics needs to be under tight structure and control of the clinical laboratory (40). With the several hundred different procedures typically reported via the LIS to the EMR, it is important that the laboratory select and utilize these identifiers for their targeted purpose. For example, it is not uncommon for 20 different test identifiers to exist in a LIS for the test "glucose." These test codes are used specifically with given specimen types (e.g., cerebrospinal fluid, whole blood, plasma, urine), with given methods (e.g., substrate selective electrode, hexose kinase, test strip), as members of specified batteries (e.g., glucose tolerance tests), and under different clinical situations. The laboratory needs to manage test code information, as well as results with associated reference ranges, and critical limits for these different LIS test codes. Point-of-care test code assignment in the LIS is very important in order to discriminate methods that will be reported to a common source in the LIS and EMR. Many EMRs, including EpicCare do not have table-driven test code identifiers to allow such specificity and hence should not be used as source-of-truth laboratory data repositories. Simply stated, a glucose is not always just a glucose.

Assignment of specific CPT codes to bill specific LIS test codes is also typically under the purview of the clinical laboratory (42). Assignment of specific CPT codes to a glucose test in the above example is also a rather daunting task if one considers that levels of CLIA licensure require different CPT codes for the same test. For example, a rapid strep screen test would require different CPT codes in claims processing if submitted from a "waived" verses a "moderate complexity" CLIA-certified laboratory. In addition, in some healthcare organizations, tracking revenue back to a specific testing location may be accomplished by assigning specific LIS test codes to designate and map revenue to a given location. Hence "one size fits all" is not a practical model for managing POCT informatics. It is up to each laboratory to use different features and levels of their particular LIS to accomplish information management specific to their organization (35).

It is the experience of the author in evolving a 70-site distributed laboratory structure that standardized LIS test codes employing standardized POCT methods has reduced complexity to manageable proportions. Use of LIS test codes to map revenue back to performing locations has not been employed and hence the number of LIS test codes has been minimized. Under such a controlled structure, information management has been greatly facilitated.

One must remember these data will populate a large data repository in the LIS and optimally also post to a clinical repository in the EMR. The fewer the test codes and the more standardized the test results evolve in these repositories, the more capable a health care system will find itself in performing outcomes research. Laboratory results, including both those derived from the core laboratory and at point-of-care will be used in forming the parametric foundation of EBM. In a large integrated delivery system, the overhead of maintaining the LIS is also reduced if a simplified LIS test code menu is evolved. Standardized conventions for naming tests and test results, such as those of LOINC (Logical Observations Identifiers Names and Codes) developed within the Regenstrief Institute (www.regenstrief.org/loinc/) and SNOMED (Systematized Nomenclature of Medicine) developed within the College of American Pathologists (www.snomed.com/), will prove of great benefit as the laboratory distributes itself to more locations and more testing methods (7,43).

Another aspect of information management in the LIS involves the degree of information changeability. In the POCT workstation, some demographical errors may be corrected by an authorized laboratorian prior to verification to the LIS. Once verified in the LIS, a result may be changed only if "tagged" with all pertinent information, including previous result, testing conditions, who changed the result, when it was changed, and any other pertinent comments. As a table-driven source of truth the LIS has functioned to "tag" and track all of these changes—producing a time-tested medicolegal system. Such is not the case with several newly developed EMR systems, which in essence have evolved from document distribution systems. It is important that the table-driven and table-maintained LIS architecture be used for tracking laboratory results as the source of truth. Electronic medical record systems that have legacy LIS modules incorporated into them are more likely to perform as well structured table-driven systems. Those LISs that are interfaced to separate EMRs must remain as separate source-of-truth feeder systems. The EMR in the latter case is more of a result reporting system than a source-of-truth data repository.

Electronic Medical Record Informatics Issues

There is a host of electronic medical record to LIS integration issues that have already been stated. Principles that hold true for the LIS and EMR at large hold true for integrated POCT information. There is some urgency in planning POCT integration to the EMR. The dynamics of rapid change will increase the risk that POCT results will be integrated by various user departments not to the LIS but rather directly to the EMR (1,2). This may well create an "informatics short circuit" in terms of developing source-of-truth laboratory information. Since the EMR typically is not a table-driven information system, there is risk of evolving an incomplete scientific and QA laboratory record.

Many IVD vendors are approaching the market with their POCT devices and tests to support disease management. With this approach, IVD vendors are frequently selling directly to physician customers within a given specialty (e.g., diabetologist, endocrinologist, cardiologist, etc.). If not represented in these marketing approaches, there is increasing probability that the laboratory will be disintermediated in the process (38). Physician specialists who do not collaborate with the clinical laboratory in their own system may likewise find themselves disintermediated from information flow in their organization. Hence there is a three-way partnership that must be solidified when properly integrating POCT into the healthcare enterprise. This three-way collaborative triangle should include one leg where collaboration between vendor and laboratory is strengthened by technical and data assessment. A second leg of collaboration between IVD vendor and physician is strengthened via clinical consultation and application of IVD technology. The third leg between the laboratory and the physician is of increasing importance as the laboratory assists in constructing clinical pathways and supporting EBM in the EMR. Therefore, in this three-way partnership no one partner should be disintermediated.

As illustrated in Figure 1, the aggregation of data in the EMR and more specifically its clinical repository should be via source of truth feeder (or embedded) systems. It is likely that traditional LISs will become affiliated or embedded in the ERM systems of the future. Such LISs as Cerner and more recently Sunquest are on this track of having the LIS be a module seamlessly integrated into the EMR. Once the EMR receives a result that has been verified by the feeder system, it should be unchangeable. Only after changed in the feeder system, should a corrected result be received by the EMR.

The EMR may well be the apparatus for reformatting unchangeable data elements into graphic displays to assist physicians and providers in interpreting the clinical relevance of the result. Since the EMR display is what greatly influences the clinical decision-making process by the previously discussed user view, it must be carefully designed. Since most LIS systems, especially legacy LIS systems, have very limited ability to generate graphic reports, they should not be the focus for generating interpretive reports. Since interfaces between the LIS and EMR are limited largely to data streams and message context that is textual, it is unlikely that graphic information may be passed across an interface. Graphic and interpretive reports for LIS may be generated from LIS data warehouses, but these most typically will pass to accessory information system as bit-mapped (i.e., image file) objects. These bit-mapped objects may be disseminated to the EMR via various optical management systems. Discrepant information systems (i.e., information systems "outside" of a given medical enterprise) may pass data and laboratory reports to a specific EMR, but these are typically accomplished by scanning paper records and storing the scanned objects in that EMR. By this means collaboration with "outside" sources of laboratory data and interpretive reports will not touch the clinical repository or data warehouse.

One of the most important reasons for aggregating departmental systems including the LIS into the EMR is to enable storage of data from multiple departments in a single location (i.e., the clinical repository). The clinical repository will contain laboratory, pharmacy, radiology, cardiology, and a host of departmental systems records in a single relational database. Association of these records may be made via query of the clinical repository database. Such queries may be made for ad hoc reports or for routine reports that will be of great assistance for interpreting transdepartmental information. It can be confidently predicted that most significant clinical outcomes studies, clinical pathways, and EBM will result from data mining such broad and deep clinical repositories.

Another important reason for structuring a multidepartmental approach to the EMR is to generate medical error alerts (44). Such medical error alerts should be issued on a real-time basis in the future so that if conditions from various departments show that a dangerous risk is imminent to a patient, a warning will be broadcast via the EMR. For example, if Coumadin is about to be dosed at a dangerous level to a patient with an already elevated POCT prothrombin time, an alert should be issued to the physician or pharmacist. This type of medical error should be broadcast a priori and embedded in a clinical alert that supersedes all other information in the provider's user screen view.

ARCHIVING POINT-OF-CARE TESTING INFORMATION

POCT Workstation

Archiving of POCT information occurs at three levels (i.e., POCT workstation, LIS, and EMR) besides the testing device itself and should be viewed as contrib-

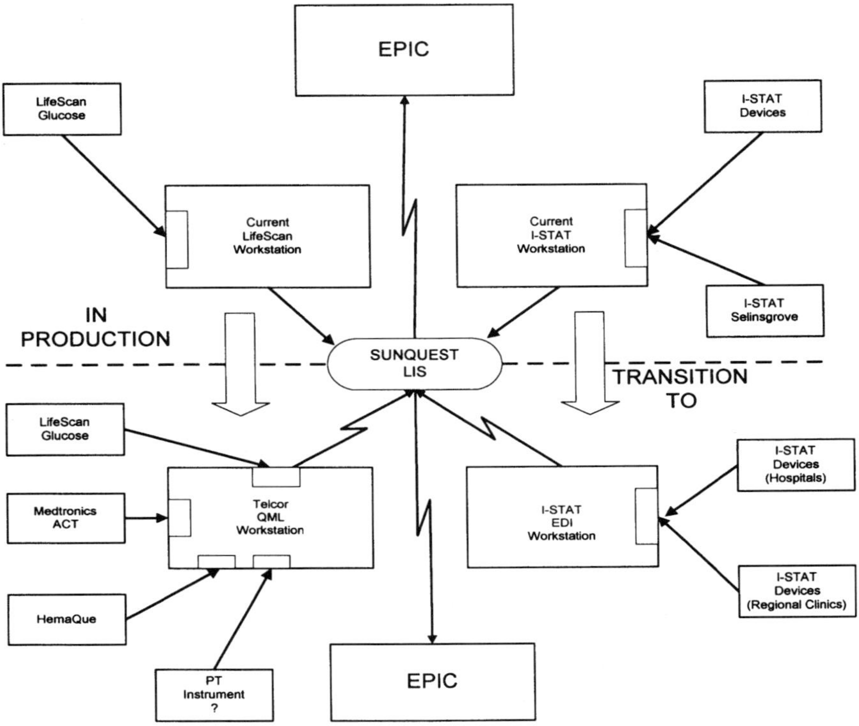

Figure 2 Point-of-care testing work station integration in the Geisinger Health System.

uting to the total legal record of a testing event. Figure 2 illustrates the current POCT workstation configuration at the Geisinger Medical Center (Danville, PA). Current components of POCT devices, POCT workstations, LIS, and EMR are listed by vendor but demonstrate a prototypical model for POCT integration used by several vendors. Figure 2 also illustrates the evolutionary nature of POCT workstation integration as two installed PC workstations remain in production and two upgraded workstations are parallel tested for implementation. Clearly, POCT workstation installation should not be viewed with oversimplified "plug and play" expectations. Some implementation assumptions for upgrading POCT connectivity are listed in Table 4.

Much of the scientific and QA record resides in the POCT workstation and should be regarded as the source-of-truth archival device for most of this information. It is important that data management principles be applied to the POCT workstation just as they are to the LIS and EMR. Regular backup and

Table 4 Some Implementation Assumptions for Upgrading POCT Workstation Connectivity

1. Archived results must be ported to the new POCT platform.
2. Workstation should have all demographics (operator ID, location codes, etc.) mirrored and ported from old POCT platform.
3. New POCT workstation should be tested on "test side" of LIS if one exists.
4. New POCT workstation should be synchronized with proper LIS software version.
5. POCT device TCP/IP addresses should be autodetected on network rather than fixed.
6. When possible, visit other site installations of identical POCT device/POCT work station/LIS.
7. Device connectivity should be parallel tested with existing network or modem lines.
8. Authorized laboratory POCT personnel should be trained and practiced on new POCT platform.
9. Operator involvement should be minimized and installation made transparent to them.
10. Use case scenarios should be tested before moving to new POCT platform.
11. Remote installation of POCT platform software and its configuration by software such as "PC Anywhere" should be monitored for network security.
12. "Open" POCT networks (i.e., those not behind a firewall) pose a security and HIPAA challenge.

storage of backup records should be systematized as they are in other laboratory areas. Since many hard drives are now capable of storing several years of data, some may be tempted simply to have all data reside on the hard drive. One must remember that hard drives are not infallible and even with free space on the hard drive a secondary backup should be maintained and stored in a separate location.

Most POCT workstations operate with versions of Microsoft Windows and integrate with other MS applications that make several PC workstations interoperable. For example, as operator performance is archived in a laboratory's POCT workstation, rosters of certified and validated operators may be shared with a nursing education department. This type of efficient data-sharing tool may encourage symbiotic collaborations and ease the POCT data management burden on the laboratory. Data files from imbedded databases in POCT application software may be queried and sent to other PCs via e-mail attachment (see Table 3).

In archiving numerous data to the POCT workstation, one must look at its basic archiving structure. Nonproprietary databases should be used if possible to create interoperability with other departmental applications. For example, Microsoft Access databases may be convenient for querying and sharing information with sister departments. Alternatively, file conversion from more proprietary databases systems, such as Cybase, SQL, and other application software, may require conversion of files via comma delimited, space delimited, or tab delimited format. Basic premises to follow are that archived information should be stable, traceable, and accessible. Preferably, users should be able to conduct their own sorts, queries, and reports from these POCT workstation databases.

Alterations to any datum element to the POCT workstation should be traceable to the new datum, the replaced datum, who changed the datum, and when the change was made. This data traceability should be part of the archived record. In general, device-generated test results should not be changed because they may have been acted upon. Other demographical data, such as patient ID and operator ID, may require changing because of keystroke errors. Once a POCT result is verified to the LIS, further changes in the POCT workstation should not be allowed. Verified numerical results from the actual test once verified in the LIS should only be changed in the LIS. One must plan for just what changes are enabled at the various levels of information transfer and recognize that the LIS is the source of truth for the end test result.

Since most LISs do not track data, such as lot numbers of reagent, frequency of operator input errors, device error messages, or serial numbers of POCT devices, these data should be archived at the POCT workstation level in the scientific and QA record. Few LISs can provide the functionality of tracking quality control performance at multiplexed and networked POCT device locations with operator identification in the thousands. For this reason, the quality control as well as scientific and QA record are usually in the realm of the POCT workstation rather than the LIS.

Laboratory Information System

Archiving of POCT information at the secondary level of the LIS should be virtually identical to that for all laboratory testing. Only in rare cases should POCT data be altered in the LIS, and traceability of all changes needs to part of the archived record.

It cannot be overemphasized that the LIS is the cornerstone for source-of-truth laboratory information archiving in the healthcare enterprise. Recently, several LIS vendors have developed what is widely described as data repositories or data warehouses. These LIS archival systems should produce a very rich source of information, including that from POCT devices, for data mining. User-friendly access to these data warehouses should be developed so that individual users may develop their own queries and perform laboratory data mining at their own PC.

This personalized database query or "data mining" of laboratory information may also be subarchived in one's own PC and referred to as a "data mart." This rich source-of-truth laboratory archive may be used in such studies as reference interval determination, workflow analyses, turnaround time studies, preanalytical and postanalytical QA, production and staffing scheduling, and utilization analysis to name a few. It must be recognized that the data warehouse is focused upon clinical laboratory analyses as opposed to more general clinical outcomes analyses, which is within the realm of the clinical repository (45).

EMR Clinical Repository

The third level of archiving for POCT information is that of the EMR and its associated clinical repository. Just as some data are parsed during information transfer from the POCT workstation to LIS, nonessential technical data are also parsed during transfer from the LIS to the EMR. Data must be archived in feeder information systems and each level of archiving requires maintenance. One must recognize that as we acquire more data, we process more data, and must archive more data. As various feeder systems send parsed data to the EMR for the acted upon result, it leaves an electronic trail that must be maintained by the laboratory. Most provider customers do not care about this electronic trail of data, but regulator customers do. The laboratory must send a "pedigreed" result to the EMR and bear the burden of its backup and traceability.

One of the largest informatics challenges that the laboratory faces is assuring that POCT information reaches the EMR by a quality means. As previously stressed, it is important that POCT information loop through the LIS as a source-of-truth feeder system to populate the EMR. There is great risk that POCT results may in some circumstances "short circuit" the LIS and be input directly to the EMR. In many EMR systems that are not table driven, this would be akin to placing laboratory results in the EMR as a nursing note. If nontabular results are placed in the EMR by such means, one may envision that a urinalyses result may be entered as "U/A neg." Another example might be envisioned of POC glucose entered as a textural result in the EMR without associated reference ranges based on specimen type. Such results could exist in the serial EMR interspersed with laboratory results as an unassociated glucose without appropriate interpretability. Such POCT results are simply not properly archived. Therefore, it is of critical importance whenever practicable that clinical laboratory data including POCT be archived in the EMR from a well-managed source-of-truth feeder system, such as the LIS.

Similarly, if outcomes research and EBM are to be based upon archived results from the EMR, they must be interpretable (46). All results that come from a source-of-truth feeder system, such as a LIS, will be interpretable if the distributed laboratory has a well-defined method test code file in the LIS. Hence, all the different types of glucose tests fed to the EMR would be clearly differentiated as to method, specimen, and application type. Likewise, it is important in constructing a clinical repository that all laboratory information be well defined and direct interfaces to "outside" LIS systems be avoided. The model the Geisinger Health System uses includes a single LIS to populate laboratory data to the EpicCare clinical repository. Laboratory results from other "outside" hospitals' LISs are scanned into the EpicCare system for bit-mapped screen view but the numerical results are not archived in the clinical repository database. Hence, providers using the EpicCare screen view have access to results, but only those results from the Geisinger LIS are used to support outcomes research.

The clinical repository and/or the laboratory data repository may be used to provide data to outside agencies for QA purposes (42). For example, hemoglobin A1c and lipid values from the Geisinger patient population are extracted and sent as a comma delimited file to information systems in the sister entity, the Geisinger Health Plan, which in turn uses these data to report quality perimeters to HEDIS. Reporting these population data to agencies such as HEDIS requires a degree of method standardization and well-managed archiving to comply with quality data standards. If POCT is used for HEDIS compliance (e.g., hemoglobin A1c or low density lipoprotein [LDL] cholesterol testing) these data should also be included in an archive that can produce an interpretable HEDIS report.

In summary, archiving of data is one of the more important activities that the laboratory must plan for in the future in healthcare. A well-planned "soup to nuts" strategy should be employed in producing quality data for such an archive. The laboratory must plan the continuum from selection of standard methods, to maintaining a stable method standard, to capturing all laboratory data in a repository. All laboratory test data must be archived and traceable from POCT device, to POCT work station, to LIS, to EMR. In the future, it is not an exaggeration to say that the quality of a health care organization will be judged by the quality of its archived data and how those data are converted to valuable information.

Cultural Change of Going Paperless

The conversion of the human interface in medicine from one of *paper* to provider to one of *screen view* to provider is very dynamic and at times difficult (6,47). One must not underestimate the impact of POCT with connectivity looping back to a human screen view. The immediate gratification of seeing a POCT result on a device's LCD (liquid crystal display) is one such loop, but as already mentioned, the EMR will increasingly be the provider's screen view. Removing a written paper order and a written paper result removes much potential for error and makes the process innately more efficient as one goes to a completely electronic process. However, the reworking of such an information loop requires much process and operational reengineering of individuals. To those newly initiated to an electronic process, removing paper removes some perceived QA as "nothing is written down." To others, information is more complete as legible data must be electronically input to complete the process. All of this change of operations and fundamental data input creates what can mildly be called a "cultural change." As one Geisinger clinician said, as the Geisinger Health System implemented the EpicCare EMR, "our world is being turned upside down."

One basic characteristic of a handheld POCT device is that it is essentially paperless. An order is generated upon the key pad or touch screen of the device itself. Necessary demographics are included in this input process and the test result is displayed on the same screen on a real-time basis—also paperless. Hence the laboratory may see itself as ushering in "the paperless revolution" via POCT devices. The laboratorian knows the device itself is simply the first step in information transfer through various information management systems to the EMR and this paperless revolution will occur at many levels in the integrated enterprise. The laboratory must assert that the gratification of an initial screen display result on the POCT device is no more adequate than writing a result on a scrap of paper and putting it in one's pocket. Providers may, however, receive information from POCT devices or EMR screen views as the old "paper trail" of a classic laboratory test dissolves into the "electronic archive" of the emerging era. The legal testing process is not complete until the verified result is archived in the proper format in the proper source of truth.

One of the greatest challenges for POCT information management is getting operators to perform quality data input (36). In a paperless healthcare system, quality keystroking will determine the quality of the data input and obviate any need to correct data prior to archiving. A basic cultural change for the POCT operator is compliance to requirements for quality keystroking.

Integration of various information systems to aggregate a legal laboratory test result (i.e., A/D/T, billing, and other clinical information systems) with proper sequence and timing will greatly impact multitudes of personnel in multiple operations (42). Not the least of these personnel will be clinical providers. This process reengineering is what prompted the one clinician to say, "our world is being turned upside down." One may envision a clinician performing a routine physical examination on a patient while ordering all required laboratory tests with ICD-9 coding and adhering to clinical pathways—all while sharing their attention between patient and CRT. All of the compulsive rules that various departments impose upon the test-ordering process funnel to this clinician who tries to engage the patient with a caring, attentive, pleasant attitude. The front end of data capture funnels directly through the human provider who is encountering the patient in a very complex and information-overloaded process. Providers in the information (or information overloaded) age will continue to be of prime importance to the healthcare enterprise. It will be up to the laboratory and other departments to help increase their efficiency and decrease their burden.

All data input needs to integrate across the healthcare enterprise and hence individual departments will increasingly influence the timeliness and data requirements of others. In our electronically interlinked enterprise we must maintain a

Table 5 The Four "Wares" of Information Technology

Hardware
Software
Warmware
Beware!

broad view and perform duties that do not initially appear to be part of our focused specialty. The upheaval of change in converting to a paperless healthcare system is very human intensive (30,47). Much training is required of clinicians, nurses, and clerical assistants to perform to systems requirements. For that reason it is important to include a new "ware" to the classical "wares" of the information technology world. Table 5 lists four "wares."

One must not take "warmware" whimsically. The human interface is as important in designing an integrated EMR as any of the other listed "wares." If all three—hardware, software, warmware—attributes are not designed into the EMR, be wary (i.e., beware) of the outcome.

Because of POCT, the laboratory is rapidly drawn into issues of this cultural upheaval. With our interpersonal skills, we must partner with clinical colleagues as their world is turned upside down. How the laboratory operationalizes POCT will depend to a great extent on how information management integration is configured in the arena of the healthcare provider. The laboratory is but a small part of this integrated change upheaval. The laboratory must not impose inflexible requirements that put an undue burden on providers. Rather, it needs to systems analyze what the wins are for their customers and help manage change. During this period of change the laboratory—especially those involved in POCT integration—has ample opportunity to partner with other professional groups that are similarly stressed with change. Change frequently creates new partnerships and breaks old ones. The following section outlines opportunities for laboratory transition into new roles.

USING POCT INFORMATION MANAGEMENT TO FORM STRATEGIC PARTNERSHIPS IN THE HEALTHCARE ENTERPRISE

A key component of any long-term laboratory strategy should be to partner with other providers and activities in its healthcare organization (6). A key strategic partnership to focus upon initially is disease management. As these strategic partnerships evolve, diverse groups of providers in the healthcare enterprise become natural allies. A core mission of healthcare is to diagnose and treat diseases. This core mission in many healthcare organizations is being organized around selected disease management. Meeting the needs of disease management in terms of point-of-care involvement for the laboratory draws one into designing joint operational systems across the entire healthcare enterprise. Point-of-care testing provides the laboratory a key entry way into the mainstream of clinical and business planning for a healthcare organization. Data management and systems development are pivotal areas of planning for which the laboratory needs increased involvement.

Disease Management

The laboratory is already greatly relied upon by specific disease management programs. At the same time, specific disease management activities are finding an increasing number of POCT devices and tests to meet their needs. Hence, an opportunity is created for the laboratory to technically manage testing and organize information for disease management activities in the healthcare enterprise.

An opportunity for greater laboratory involvement in diabetes disease management planning already exists in POCT and central laboratory information management. Few if any healthcare enterprises lack the ubiquitous glucose meter for performing POCT whole blood glucose analysis. The laboratory must not restrict itself to looking at glucose meter device connectivity as the sole information goal of the laboratory. Laboratories must think beyond connectivity of glucose meters to global diabetes disease management. There are currently three key parametric tests the laboratory needs to integrate across the entire healthcare continuum to support diabetes disease management—glucose, hemoglobin A1c, and urine microalbumin testing. Most if not all enterprise-wide diabetes disease management systems use these tests as a cornerstone in outcome measurement.

Integrating and supporting just these three tests for diabetes disease management is a large task if one considers all aspects of integration, methodology, and informatics. For example, the laboratory may maintain reference methods for a host of existing or potential POCT values. In the Geisinger enterprise, a patient collected by venipuncture for plasma glucose testing by a hexokinase method may concurrently self-test with their meter and have both results entered into the LIS for comparison. This is a means of quality checking the accuracy of the glucose meter and the patient's self-testing technique. These side-by-side results are reported to the physician and after review, to the patient via MyChart. Paired results with a calculated percentage difference are archived in SunQuest by meter type for device comparison.

Similarly, microalbumin may be screen tested on a variety of single-use urine strip tests to be followed by more quantitative urine microalbumin testing in the main laboratory. An initial screening test entered into the LIS may be correlated to urine microalbumin-creatinine ratios from a 24-hr or random urine collection. Efficacy of self-testing or screen testing for microalbuminuria may thus be judged by a quantitative central laboratory test.

Another example of useful integrated laboratory information management for test correlation may be found with hemoglobin A1c testing. Initial POCT or self-tested hemoglobin A1c may be compared to reference methodology and confirmatory testing of hemoglobin A1c by HPLC.

One may see similar usefulness in correlating information from a variety of laboratory tests across the medical continuum from POCT screening to confirmation, in other disease management activities. Numerous examples exist to illustrate how POCT and centralized testing need to be information managed to establish a basis for EBM and disease management; for instance, infectious disease testing, cardiovascular risk assessment, and coagulation testing (48).

All of these examples require the laboratory to define a primary reference methodology and to have a means of comparing results from a common information system. Evidence-based medicine algorithms that include screening methodologies should be based upon this sort of information management and outcomes analysis. Quality measurements for outcomes should be submitted to agencies such as the National Committee for Quality Assurance (NCQA) (e.g., the HEDIS data) with a reference methodology or at least a basis for comparison with peer organizations.

Interdepartmental Evolution of the Electronic Medical Record

As previously outlined, POCT exists at the front end of the healthcare enterprise. This location is heavily impacted by implementation of the EMR. The laboratory should be a valuable participant as the EMR is planned and rolled out. Partnering with radiology, cardiology, endocrinology, emergency, operating room, and a host of other departments is a prerequisite for establishing an efficient EMR. Since the laboratory is one of the more experienced departments, often having implemented several generations of LISs, it may help other departments understand proper information management. Since many departments—especially physician provider departments—are geared toward textural input (progress notes, discharge summaries, etc.), the laboratory needs to stress the importance of parametric values being entered and maintained in table-based information systems (8). Laboratory and other parametric values must not be input into the EMR merely as a textual string. Most information technology professionals understand the importance of table-based information systems and are a natural ally of the laboratory if rapid decisions are made rolling out an EMR.

Just as the laboratory serves a support role in analyzing specimens with requested tests, the laboratory must support providers at the point of care with information management. Assuring proper demographical identify during testing encounters is part of the information management responsibility of the laboratory. The laboratory must step up as an active participant in designing information management screens to meet regulatory requirements. By partnering with providers, the laboratory can help design screen views with a minimum of clutter and maximum of efficiency.

Home Visiting Nursing

Home visiting nurses will likely assume a greater role for POCT for their customers in the home setting (14,21,24,34). The laboratory may assist these professionals and benefit the entire healthcare enterprise by selecting system-compatible methodology for POCT. Just as POCT devices may connect at the bedside in the hospital, they may connect at the bedside in the patient home (e.g., via modem). Alternatively, test result upload may occur in the home visiting nurse office or clinic. This remote connectivity should be verified to the LIS just as is done in outpatient settings in the hospital. Depending upon the location of the home visiting nurse activity, a CLIA license may be maintained by the hospital laboratory or the home visiting nurse at multiple points in an integrated delivery system. In any of these cases, the laboratory should bear substantial responsibility for supporting the CLIA license.

The appropriate validation of the POCT devices, quality control information management, proficiency testing, and operator training should be standardized and under the purview of the distributed laboratory leadership structure (2). Although at first thought this may represent a large challenge and burden, the continued existence of the laboratory will depend upon de novo formation of such strategic partnerships. As the laboratory distributes itself closer to its customers, it must provide its service and prove its value through an increasing number of operator intermediaries. These operator intermediaries are those strategic partners that the laboratory coalesces over time.

Quality Assurance and Error Reduction

As the laboratory aggregates data across its distributed areas, these data become available for QA and may enable error reduction (26). As previously mentioned, different portions of the QA and scientific record exist in the POCT workstation, LIS, and the EMR. The laboratory may pay a key role in gleaning information from these data. Hence, strategic partnerships may be formed between the laboratory and different QA or process improvement (PI) entities in the health care enterprise. In doing so, the laboratory empowers itself by suggesting or mandating institutional policy.

For example, if patient misidentification is seen as a documented QA problem, the laboratory may suggest or even mandate the use of patient bar coded wristbands to reduce error rate. If data show improperly performing POCT operators, the data may be called to the attention of an operator's supervisor to launch remedial action.

Point-of-care testing coordinators should view laboratory information management as its most valuable infrastructural part and use it to improve specific QA/PI outcomes.

Information Technology Department, Wide Area Network, and Wireless Technology

One of the most important strategic partnerships and a source of key support for growth and development of the laboratory's future is the information technology (IT) department (50). Many clinical laboratories depend on IT support from outside of their departmental structure. Hence, the laboratory must form a mutually beneficial partnership with IT. As with any strategic partnership, two-way synergy is important. Laboratories must not "demand" IT support but "require" and "specify" it. Information technology support comes most strongly from well-defined specifications. As laboratorians develop the skill to design more integrated information systems and become conversant in IT jargon, they will become natural partners to successful implementation of point-of-care information systems. In developing this partnership, the laboratory must respect the role of the IT department and not "demand" specific hardware solutions or try to usurp the system role of the IT department. Likewise, the IT department must respect the laboratory's knowledge of its own application and operation. Mutual sharing must occur to make both partners partial experts in the other's domain. In this way, both departments develop and increase their informatics skills and success rates.

Emerging technology, such as that found in wide area networks and wireless communication, is merely a tool to an end. In other words, this linking technology is only as good as the applications it links (51). In defining and specifying application for laboratory connectivity, the IT-laboratory partnership may find one of its first wireless prototypes in POCT. As these communication tools are installed, the laboratory may well be viewed by IT as prototypical for full institutional use.

A degree of patience and reasonableness must prevail and current technology must be maximized before next step technology is "demanded." One should go back to the previously stated "wares" and realize that capability of hardware and software does not determine a successful IT implementation as much as the savvy and maturity of a user department. The laboratory-IT partnership should monitor an appropriate level of enthusiasm for future application tools as they reach the healthcare market. Streaming video and sound application software should not be purchased just because users consider them cool tools. When such streaming video and sound documents are distributed via Internet to wireless graphic tablets, the future laboratorian-IT partnership should look back to the evolutionary steps of its implementation (52). Clearly these advanced systems will not evolve without mature and realistic strategic planning.

The best working relationship between laboratory and IT may well be one where a partnership exists internal to the laboratory. Information technology personnel on assignment and permanently located in the laboratory may best evolve this strategic partnership.

Community Health and the Electronic Record

Many laboratories already perform POCT in a "health fair" format. As such, POCT information should not just be disseminated to the single patient being screen tested, but should also be returned to the healthcare enterprise for accumulation into a population record. This type of information may be managed to determine prevalence of positive results in a screened population. The dynamics of reporting a positive screening result to a patient's provider may be an informatics problem. There have been many instances where well-conducted "health fairs" have failed because providers have not been consulted prior to receiving their patient's positive result.

Advanced integrated delivery systems are beginning to establish not just an individual patient's EMR but also a community population electronic health record (EHR) (6,8,9,43). Examples of health record implementations exist in several communities. Systems in Helena, MT, Indianapolis, IN, and Birmingham, AL show how community supported health endeavors may be successful. The community-based EHR is in its infancy. Governmental agencies such as the Centers for Disease Control and Prevention (CDC) are interested in surveillance of chronic and acute disease states at a national level. A recent metadata registry project has been launched by ANSI/HISB (American National Standards Institute/Healthcare Informatics Standards Board) to examine how data may be compared from various EHR systems in the future.

Point-of-care testing, as it distributes to the home visiting nurse and patient self-testing in the home, may be envisioned as community based. One should see the healthcare enterprise as existing not only in the hospital or doctor's office, but also in the community. Point-of-care testing may be the first part of the laboratory enterprise that directly reaches the community. In fact, governmental agencies are envisioning patient self-testing POCT via "home appliances" as a matter of national security. Just as societal needs must be met by future wheat crop availability, in a few years baby boomers must have access to appropriate levels of healthcare technology. As a society, and as laboratory futurists, we must link POCT informatics technology to the EMR and EHR.

Group Purchasing

There is a natural alliance between laboratories that standardize methodologies for the purpose of simplifying information management and material management departments in the health care enterprise. Material management departments are constantly looking for group purchasing opportunities. Discounting on volume, dealing with fewer vendors, and producing fewer purchase orders are goals of most material management departments. These goals can best be reached after laboratory method standardization.

Several POCT vendors are partnering with distributors who have systems for electronic ordering and purchasing of their products. Other independent material managements systems for supply tracking exist. For example, in the Geisinger Health System much purchasing from designated vendors (i.e., "premier partners") is provided by the Lawson information system (www.lawson.com). Hence, the laboratory may electronically enter a purchase order for a POCT diagnostic kit and the order will be placed via the Lawson System. The Lawson System is programmed with designated POCT product numbers with appropriate distribution systems to track delivery as well contracted discounted system pricing. These systems track POCT consumable distribution and provide information not just to material management but also to the laboratory and/or POC location. Hence, the laboratory may monitor usage and possible wastage of product by given POC location.

Cost per test of a given POCT is commonly more expensive than a similar test performed in a centralized laboratory when judged on a reagent expense basis. The value of timeliness and the immediate intervention of diagnostic or treatment procedure by the provider must also factor into relative cost. The "bang for the buck" of POCT is most frequently enjoyed by the clinical service rather than the laboratory since the benefit of POCT is mostly external to the laboratory. The clinical value of embedding decision making into a clinical pathway (e.g., algorithms built into provider screen views) and hence into EBM must also be factored into cost-benefit analysis. It is likely that financial analysis of POCT delivery to providers and patients will become more broadly viewed as integrated systems develop. The laboratory must not allow material management decision support systems to dictate product use based on simple cost per test product comparisons. Again, the laboratory with its operational and clinical expertise must be a partner to the making of such financial decisions. The laboratory may well advocate that POCT has clinical value and that to take the test to the central laboratory with lower cost per test "is penny wise but pound foolish."

Data Mining

As previously mentioned, POCT data will exist in a number of locations, namely in the POCT device, POCT workstation, LIS, EMR, laboratory data warehouse, and the EMR clinical repository. The laboratory data repository and EMR clinical repository will be the most frequently used locations to conduct database sorts and queries for data mining. The laboratory must be an active participant in distributing these data from the primary source-of-truth LIS or its associated data repository. The clinical laboratory with its rich source of parametric data will be a primary resource for the overall healthcare data mining endeavor (49,53). The role of the laboratorian will likely change to some degree from that of a specimen analyst to a data analyst.

For the laboratorian to be an active participant in the data-mining process, new skills must be developed. Understanding information management and its capabilities for extracting information from data is a skill that may be learned from a number of sources. Statistics and research design courses, specific statistics software training, research project participation with statisticians, long-distance Internet learning, or simple self-teaching may all improve these skills. Application of test results to a population of patients is a natural outgrowth of understanding the application of test results of a single patient. With this clinical background and newly acquired data-mining expertise, the laboratorian may bring a key skill set to their organization for converting massive amounts of data into valuable information.

A partnership for data mining and conversion of laboratory test results to information and knowledge must include participants from several areas of expertise. Financial experts with their decision support systems (DSS) (54), clinicians with disease management objectives, administrators with operational goals, risk management with needs for security, as well as IT who must support hardware and software are the laboratory's partners in this endeavor. These various partners will compete for data to support their pre-existing notion of how the healthcare enterprise should be focused and managed. There will be alliances within this power structure as it struggles to balance between financial and clinical objectives. Much of the balance of decision making will likely be determined by parametric laboratory data and outcomes analysis. For this reason, the laboratory must be present to interpret not only its individual elements but also how those data elements are mined to produce information. This process basically represents the means for development and evolution of clinical pathways into EBM.

Since the basic nature of laboratory data is parametric (i.e., measurable and statistically governed) it will be used with great veracity to support decisions and outcomes analysis. One may see a basic paradigm of *data* being mined to produce *information*, and this information being interpreted to produce *knowledge*. Figure 3 shows a basic pyramid that supports evolution and conversion of data to infor-

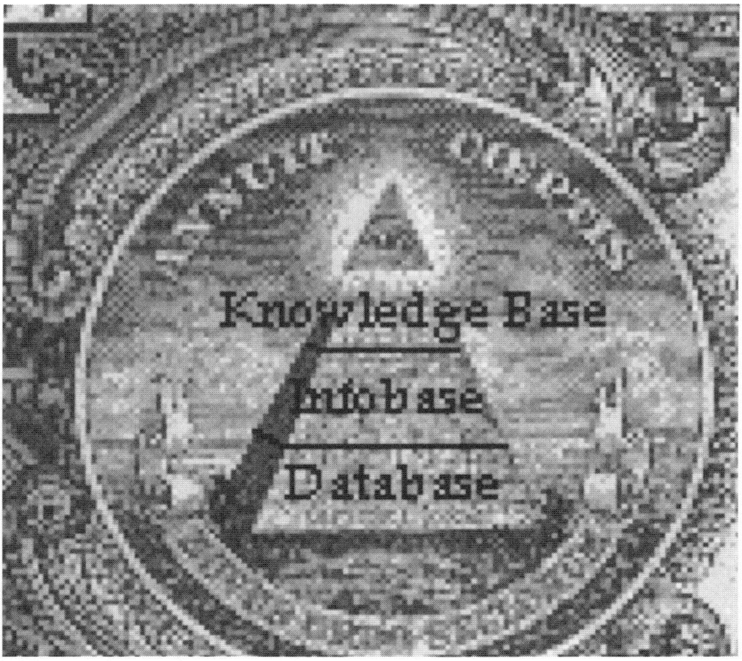

Figure 3 Sound data management forms a foundation supporting outcome studies.

mation, and information to knowledge. A knowledge base can only be supported upon a sound foundation of quality parametric information (i.e., the "infobase") and data (i.e., the database). Point-of-care testing will provide some of the parametric foundation of outcome based research, and this assumption alone should prove an impetus for archiving POCT results in the same databases as those used for central laboratory testing.

CONCLUSION

Point-of-care testing connectivity and archiving must be viewed as but a small niche in a much greater scheme of information management. As POCT becomes a greater portion of the laboratory's product—information—its integration into the "mainstream" of information management in the healthcare enterprise at large becomes increasingly important. The EMR, with its associated clinical repository, will increasingly represent this "mainstream." The EMR will also present the challenge of broadening information management issues as home testing and Internet integration issues appear.

A foresighted integrative approach must be taken when designing laboratory information systems—from POCT device connectivity to data mining of the clinical repository. Laboratory effort put into an integrative systems approach should pay dividends when broad outcomes studies and EBM become the cornerstones of healthcare.

REFERENCES

1. Jones JB. The importance of integrating POCT data into an organizational database. Advance for Administrators of the Laboratory, Sept 8, 1999.
2. Jones JB. In: G Kost, ed. Point-of-Care Testing in Physicians' Offices, Primary Care Networks, and Managed Care Point-of-Care Testing: Principles, Management and Clinical Practice. Lippincott/Williams & Wilkins, New York, 2002.
3. Dubois JA, Dunka L, Allred T, Callaghan J, Cooper T, Cross S, Hawker C, Jones J, Knafel AJ, Nichols J, Perry J, Schluter P. Point-of-Care Connectivity: Approved Standard (POCT1-A). Vol. 21. No. 8. National Committee for Clinical Laboratory Standards, Wayne, PA, 2001.
4. Lewis M. The New New Thing: A Silicon Valley Story. Norton, New York, 1999.
5. Starr P. Smart technology, stunted policy: Developing health information networks. Health Aff May/June:91, 1997.
6. Jones J, Steindel S, Chou D. Connecting the laboratory to the electronic medical record: Issues and opportunities [CD ROM]. Nat Acad Clin Biochem Symposium. AACC Press, Washington, DC, 2000.
7. Dexter PR, Perkins S, Overhage JM, Maharry K, Kohler RB, McDonald CJ. A computerized reminder system to increase the use of preventative care for hospitalized patients. N Engl J Med 345:991–993, 2001.
8. Shea S, McMouchel W, Bahamonde L. A meta-analysis of 16 randomized controlled trials to evaluate computer-based clinical reminder systems for preventative care in the ambulatory setting. J Am Med Inform Assoc 3:399–409, 1996.
9. Hunt DL, Hayes RB, Hanna SE, Smith K. Effects of computer-based clinical decision support systems on physician performance and patient outcomes: A systematic review. JAMA 280:1339–1346, 1998.
10. McDonald CJ. Protocol-based computer reminders, the quality of care and the non-perfectibility of man. N Engl J Med 295:1351–1355, 1976.
11. Tierney WM, Miller ME, Overhage JM, McDonald CJ. Physician inpatient order writing on microcomputer workstations: Effects on resource utilization. JAMA 269: 379–383, 1993.
12. Burkhartsmeier G. HIPAA and the clinical laboratory. Health Mgt Tech Nov:26–28, 2001.
13. Goldsmith J. How will the Internet change our health system? Health Aff Jan/Feb: 148–156, 2000.

14. Peddicord H. Extending disease management: A home monitoring system for vital signs. Am Clin Lab Nov/Dec:22, 2000.
15. Taylor M, Nichols JH, Saltz J. POCT connectivity: Opening the door to a laboratory without walls. Am Clin Lab 19:12–13, 2000.
16. Stem JE, Humbertson SK, Silverman BC, Nichols JH. Harmonization of point-of-care results. Diagn Endocrin Metab 18:375–378, 2000.
17. Kassirer JP. The next transformation in the delivery of health care. N Engl J Med Jan:52–53, 1995.
18. Taylor M, Saltz J, Nichols JH. Design of an integrated clinical data warehouse. JALA 5:54–59, 2000.
19. Bissell MG, Petersen JR. Automated Integration of Clinical Laboratories: A Reference. AACC Press, Washington, DC, 1998.
20. Miller T. The Health Care Industry in Transition: The Online Mandate to Change. Cyber Dialog Inc, Intel Corp, July, 1998.
21. Schou J. Information where it's needed: Function-rich and diverse applications make point-of-care data access a healthcare reality. Health Mgt Tech Oct:48–51, 2001.
22. Jacobs E, Vadasdi E, Sarkozi L, Colman N. Analytical evaluation of I-Stat portable clinical analyzer and use by nonlaboratory health-care professionals. Clin Chem 39: 1069–1074, 1993.
23. Hurst J, Nickel K, Hilborne LH. Are physician office laboratory results of comparable quality to those produced in other laboratory settings? JAMA Feb 11:468–471, 1998.
24. Lehman C. Home health care: The next frontier for clinical laboratory services? Clin Lab News Aug:8–10, 2001.
25. Teich JM, Merchia PR, Schmiz JL, Kuperman GJ, Spur CD, Bates DW. Effects of computerized physician order entry on prescribing practices. Arch Intern Med 160: 2741–2747, 2000.
26. Nichols JH, Poe SS. Quality assurance, practical management, and outcomes of point-of-care testing: laboratory perspectives. Clin Lab Manag Rev 13:341–350, 1999.
27. Skjei E. Disappearing acts—Coping with LIS mergers. CAP Today 15:1–66, 2001.
28. Blick KE. Lab computer system: Will your lab be a winner or a loser in the next millenium? Clin Lab News 25:22, 1996.
29. Freudenheim M. Six health plans are developing online venture. New York Times 30 Mar, 2000.
30. Larkin M. E-health continues to make headway. Lancet 358:517, 2001.
31. Kassirer JP. Patients, physicians and the Internet. Health Aff Nov/Dec:115–123, 2000.
32. Cochrane JD. Delivering patient care on the Internet. Health Sys Exec Sept:1–12, 2001.
33. Dark RL, ed. Eight "must have" features for web lab test reports. The Dark Report 10:5–7, 2001.
34. Stewart RL. Home care info. Is the future now? The Remington Report (special issue) 4–6, 2000.
35. Francis K. Laboratory information systems: A novel approach for defining your laboratory. Clin Lab News Nov:12–13, 2001.

36. Price CP, Hicks JM. Point-of-Care Testing. AACC Press, Washington, DC, 1999.
37. Bailey TM, Topham TM, Wantz S, Grant M, Cox C, Jones D, Zerbe T, Spears T. Laboratory process improvement through point-of-care testing. J Qual Improve 7: 363–380, 1997.
38. Jones JB. A Zen approach to ordering/reporting lab tests. Advance for Administrators of the Laboratory, June 2001.
39. Jones JB. Emerging applications of point-of-care connectivity are offering accuracy, expediency, and convenience for POCT data management. Advance for Administrators of the Laboratory, April 2001.
40. Cowan DF, Gray RZ, Campbell B. Validation of the laboratory information system. Arch Pathol Lab Med 122:239, 1998.
41. Blick KE. Selecting a laboratory information system. Clin Lab News 22:44, 1996.
42. Paquin MD. Integration of the back office with the EMR. Health Mgt Tech Sept: 68–69, 2001.
43. McDonald CJ, Overhage JM, Tierney WM. The Regenstrief Medical Record System: A quarter century experience. Int J Med Inf 54:225–253, 1999.
44. Overhage JM, Tierney WM, Zhou XH, McDonald CJ. A randomized trial of "corollary orders" to prevent errors of omission. J Am Med Inform Assoc 4:364–375, 1997.
45. Warner Jr H. Mining the gems: Strategies to help CIOs effectively use clinical databases while avoiding the data warehouse money pit. Health Mgt Tech Oct:30–32, 2001.
46. Seliger R. Laying the foundation: Characterizing and conceptualizing an integrated healthcare information system is a critical step in building one. Health Mgt Tech Oct:22–24, 2001.
47. Starr P. The Social Transformation of American Medicine. Basic Books, New York, 1982.
48. Geerts WH, Heit JA, Clagett GP. Prevention of venous thromboembolism. Chest 119(suppl):132S–175S, 2001.
49. Zeger SL, Liang KY. Longitudinal data analysis for discrete and continuous outcomes. Biometrics 42:121–130, 1995.
50. Hagland M. IT and point-of-care. Health Mgt Tech Oct:10–14,69–70, 1998.
51. Bennehum D. The hot new medium is...Email. Wired Apr:104, 1998.
52. Klienke JD. Release 0.0 Info. Tech. in the real world. Health Aff Nov/Dec:23, 1998.
53. Rogoski RR. Integration crossroads. Health Mgt Tech Oct:14–20, 2001.
54. Workman RD, Lewis MJ, Bradford TH. Enhancing the financial performance of a health system laboratory network using an information system. Am J Clin Pathol 114:9–15, 2000.
55. Britton BP, Rains D. Negotiating the PPS maze: Can tele-homecare help? The Remington Report 8:8–10, 2000.
56. Jones JB. Penn State Geisinger Building "Distributed Lab" Around POCT. The Dark Report 6:9–15, 1999.

4

Understanding and Preventing Medical Errors in Point-of-Care Testing (and the Use of FAST-QC)

Gerald J. Kost (with technical contributions by Brian D. Evans)
University of California–Davis, and University of California–Davis Health System, Davis, California, U.S.A.

GOAL AND OBJECTIVES

The fundamental goal of this chapter is to improve the performance, safety, and quality of point-of-care testing (POCT) by assuring reliable clinical practice. The objectives of the chapter are:

- To highlight recent guidelines on medical errors issued by the Institute of Medicine (IOM) and the National Committee for Clinical Laboratory Standards (NCCLS)
- To understand why a systems approach to error prevention is most efficient and efficacious
- To categorize potential preanalytical, analytical, and postanalytical errors in POCT
- To introduce a multidimensional pattern recognition technique: Fingerprinting-Analysis Systems-Testing Quality Control (FAST-QC™)
- To summarize practical security, validation, performance, and emergency systems for preventing errors in POCT
- To briefly assess the role of connectivity and safeguards in error reduction

Hopefully, at the conclusion of this chapter the reader will agree that POCT instruments need to provide more software and hardware options that operators can use to prevent medical errors in POCT and to foster its continued growth, safety, and success.

BACKGROUND

Multidimensional Challenges

Point-of-care testing is testing at or near the site of patient care (1,2). Although exact preanalytical, analytical, and postanalytical error rates are not known, bedside diagnostic testing outside the clinical laboratory may contribute to serious medical errors (1–3). Point-of-care testing is expanding rapidly and has a growth rate of 12–15% per annum, one several times larger than that of the central laboratory (4). As more testing shifts to the bedside (5,6) and is performed by increasing numbers of physicians, nurses, and nurse practitioners, there must be adequate safeguards to prevent medical errors and reduce risk. Errors in laboratory testing often are preanalytical and can contribute to inappropriate care or modification of therapy (7,8). Reduction of preanalytical errors represents a potential advantage of POCT. However, POCT may be prone to serious disadvantages (2,9), such as

- Inadequate automated and parallel quality control (QC)
- Insufficient validation of trained and certified operators
- Lack of algorithms to assess the competency of operators
- Little or no security of patient test results and QC data
- Limited connectivity (bidirectional communication between computerized information systems and remote devices) with the electronic medical record

The use of unauthorized POCT results in diagnosis and treatment does not comply with practice standards, accreditation requirements, or the security, confidentiality, authentication, integrity, and auditing requirements of the Health Insurance Portability and Accountability Act (HIPAA) (10). Thus, POCT faces multidimensional challenges for improved performance and error reduction.

New Guidelines from the Institute of Medicine and the National Committee for Clinical Laboratory Standards

The Committee on Quality of Health Care in America of the IOM recently published two extensive sets of guidelines intended to reduce patient deaths caused by medical errors (11,12). The first set of IOM guidelines recommended that national leadership focus on raising expectations, improving safety standards, and implementing safer practices at the delivery level within healthcare systems, and additionally, that the Food and Drug Administration (FDA) increase attention to the safe use of drugs and devices. Other recommendations included communicating and disseminating methods to prevent, identify, and analyze errors; integrating competency certification and recertification into the delivery of professional services; requiring error reporting systems in hospital and ambulatory care settings; and enhancing patient safety through standardizing and simplifying equipment, supplies, and processes. The second set of guidelines will be discussed in Chapter 8. Identification of error modes, prediction of error expression, training and design for self-detection, and interdiction before transformation into harmful accidents fundamentally protect patients, while new NCCLS guidelines for infectious diseases (13) help protect clinical laboratory staff and POCT operators.

Systems Improvement Approach to Error Reduction

Point-of-care testing instruments should be designed with respect for human limitations. Additionally, timely discovery and recognition of errors will improve patient safety. A systems approach to error prevention like that presented in this chapter generally is recognized as productive and is favored over approaches focusing on repeated discipline of personnel and punitive measures. Recognized methods of error reduction include (11–15)

- Avoiding reliance on memory and vigilance
- Error proofing devices
- Designing procedures to make errors visible
- Structuring critical tasks with constraints and "forcing functions" (required actions)
- Standardizing processes and data displays
- Simplifying key steps
- Automating complex routines
- Improving information access
- Facilitating decision making
- Training by means of problem simulation to develop skills in failure mode analysis

Connectivity of POCT devices is essential to the successful implementation of systems for reducing and tracking errors. Mitigating harm from known errors also will improve patient welfare (12). This philosophy of designing systems improvements to prevent medical errors in POCT is the rationale for the methods proposed in this chapter.

National Concern, Local Responsibility

The frequency of serious medical errors caused by POCT is not known (16) and generally, medical error rates may be overestimated or underestimated (17,18). However, rapid growth of this modality of diagnostic testing in the United States and other countries warrants investment in error detection and prevention, even if only a fraction of the sentinel events or errors actually lead to significant harm, since test menus and test volumes are increasing progressively. Legislation inspired by the two recent sets of IOM guidelines will fund research to identify sources of medical errors and mechanisms for reducing preventable injuries and deaths, including those attributable to diagnostic testing. This legislation, which will require providers to measurably reduce errors, affirms the IOM goal of cutting the medical error rate by 50%. These initiatives reflect the high level of national concern about prevention and reduction of medical errors. Therefore, it is incumbent upon manufacturers to implement safety features. In turn, users must assure the safe practice of POCT in all health system settings without exception!

THE QUALITY CYCLE AND TOTAL QUALITY PRINCIPLE FOR POINT-OF-CARE TESTING

There are several studies in the literature that address the accuracy and precision of POCT and cover a wide array of instruments, formats, and settings (19). Experimental designs and operational factors, such as operator competency and professional experience, represent large factors in determining the outcomes of these studies, which may or may not reflect the actual "real-world" performance of POCT. Clinicians have mixed feelings about their tolerances for errors. For example, once the diagnosis of diabetes is known and the patient is relatively stable, speed and convenience may take precedence over accuracy and precision in routine handheld glucose monitoring. In fact, some clinicians feel that accuracy must be individualized for each test and its application, and that precision may be sacrificed for lower cost, increased availability, and faster turnaround time (20). On the other hand, quantitative systematic concepts of POCT error tolerances have emerged in formal studies, such as simulation modeling (21), patient-derived quality specifications (22), and multicenter evaluations (23,24). This type of evidence-based research is more effective than professional opinion in motivating users, industry, accreditation agencies, and the FDA to improve the quality of POCT.

At this point in the evolution of POCT, the debate about accuracy and precision, especially for handheld instruments, is being forced into the marketplace where improved overall performance generates sales that reward investment in higher quality, in effect producing an appropriate *quality cycle*: The more accurate and precise a POC device is, the greater its competitive edge, the broader its medical applications, and the safer its operation. Therefore, users should set high standards in order to foster the appropriate ethic of this quality cycle among manufacturers. Based on the accepted concept of site neutrality for diagnostic testing, which derives from the Clinical Laboratory Improvement Amendments of 1988, the *total quality principle* for POCT (25,26) means empowering professionals who proactively integrate QC, quality monitors, proficiency testing, and performance improvement into one patient-focused package that meets customer needs *irrespective of where the diagnostic testing is performed.* Inaccuracy and imprecision, therefore, are viewed more as symptomatic of revolutionary new technologies, rather than as necessary or permanent attributes of POCT. The quality cycle and the total quality principle call for *perpetual improvement* in POCT and its practice.

PRINCIPLES FOR PREVENTING ERRORS

Table 1 lists potential preanalytical, analytical, and postanalytical sources of errors in POCT. The table applies broadly to transportable, portable, and handheld instrument formats and to in vitro, ex vivo, and in vivo testing modalities, and was compiled from several sources including common deficiencies found during accreditation inspections by the College of American Pathologists (CAP) and the Joint Commission on Accreditation of Healthcare Organizations (JCAHO). Data currently available do not allow prioritization of the sources of errors. The heterogeneous assortment of POCT devices available complicates systematic analysis because different methods and instruments have unique strengths and weaknesses. Therefore, key principles of error prevention are

- Adopt consistent methods.
- Use relatively few different types of instruments.
- Focus efforts on reduction of anticipated defects in those methods and instruments.
- Educate, certify, and validate POCT operators.

The error prevention systems presented below provide methods that implement these important principles. Strong leadership by the POC director and the coordinator is needed to assure that these principles are followed throughout the entire healthcare system for uniform and safe practice of POCT.

The learning organization (27) identifies causes, learns from mistakes, and adjusts its culture. Point-of-care testing program design, professional integrity, and performance monitors represent crucial factors in preventing adverse events. The most important programmatic principles include

Table 1 Potential Sources of Errors in POCT

A. Preanalytical
- Patient identity, record number, time, or date incorrect or missing
- Specimen collection protocol not known, followed, or timed, or improper collection site
- Wrong specimen source (i.e., capillary, venous, or arterial; in vitro, ex vivo, or in vivo)
- Inconsistent or incorrect specimen handling, application, dosing, or volume
- Absent or wrong anticoagulant (if required)
- Inappropriate sample icing, instability, delay, dilution, contaminants, or storage
- Hemolysis, erythrocyte settling, poor mixing, microclots, or degradation (e.g., metabolism)
- Incorrect, mishandled, expired, unlabeled or unstable test strips, cartridges, cassettes, or reagents
- Indwelling sensor artifacts (e.g., $\downarrow pO_2$, $\uparrow pCO_2$, $\downarrow$pH, $\downarrow\uparrow$temperature, or clotting around probe)
- Leukocytosis (>50,000/μL), thrombocytosis (>600,000/μL), or anemia. (hgb <7.5 g/dL)
- Clinical contraindications (e.g., digit capillary in shock or poor peripheral perfusion)
- Direct or indirect effects of transfused blood products or additives

B. Analytical
- Physical perturbations (e.g., temperature, altitude, vibration, or humidity)
- Extrinsic or intrinsic sample or aspiration anomalies (e.g., bubbles, viscosity, or thrombi)
- Confounding variables (e.g., pO_2, pCO_2, pH, hematocrit, or osmolality) high, low, or changed
- Matrix effects (e.g., proteins, lipids, dyes, cryoglobulins, or radiocontrast agents)
- Native interferents (e.g., heterophile antibodies or autoimmune biproducts)
- Interfering diluents, contaminants, preservatives, or drugs (pharmacologic or substance abuse)
- Clotting/anticlotting activators (e.g., Coumadin, heparin, hirudin, or thrombolytic)
- Method not calibrated, calibration protocol not followed, or calibration code wrong
- Ex vivo blood cycling, calibration, or measurement problems
- Calibration interval expired (e.g., in vivo sensor calibrated periodically to in vitro measurement)
- Linear or reportable range exceeded, nonlinearity, drift, or sensor aging
- Licensed (vendor-specified) range violated (e.g., newborn glucose limits or hematocrit)
- Fundamental method or instrument inaccuracy, imprecision, or inconsistency
- Lack of quality control (QC), proficiency testing (PT), or performance monitors
- QC or PT not done by the correct person or no follow-up of problems (critical for accreditation)
- QC reagents unstable, volatile, expired, undated, contaminated, or mislabeled

Table 1 Continued

QC inappropriate for the clinical decision thresholds (e.g., cTnI low control too high)
Test performed despite QC out of range or without periodic linearity check
Operator not educated, experienced, qualified, certified, or validated in testing or maintenance
Lack of recognition of instrument defect, malfunction, failure, or abnormality
Unstable power source (e.g., surges) or power interruption (e.g., blackout)
C. Postanalytical
Critical values omitted, not recognized, or not alerted
Incomplete test cluster from selection, deletion, or suppression error
Results not communicated to the physician, or communication lost, misplaced, or delayed
Instrument or data station memory, power, or battery failure
Transcription mistake, wrong units, no reference interval, or garbled data on printout
Software delays, errors, bugs, or failures
No results documentation or transfer of data to the electronic medical record
Test results or quality monitors not reviewed per statutes or accreditation requirements
Lack of bidirectional exchange of demographics, test results, quality data, or errors

- Detection and description of COT sentinel events
- Assessment of their significance
- Prioritized investigation including, if warranted, root cause analysis to determine the true source of the accident, incident, error, near miss, deviation, or variance
- Description, classification, and systematic archiving, tracking, and following up
- Heuristic grouping, such as trend plotting, pattern analysis, and cluster formation
- Standardized and computerized process, reporting, and corrective actions
- Loop closure through collaborative changes in attitude, behavior, or paradigms
- Risk management including legal counsel, liability reduction, economic projection, and loss write-off

Since medical malpractice can accumulate staggering losses, implementation of the principles above requires skillful collaboration and cooperation at all levels in the health system, as well as, when required, careful interaction with state and federal agencies, such as the FDA, which recently extended its reporting requirements for clinical laboratory accidents and errors.

FINGERPRINT-ANALYSIS SYSTEMS-TESTING QUALITY CONTROL

Fingerprint-Analysis Systems-Testing Quality Control (28) allows simultaneous analysis of multichannel test results. In this technique, data points from each channel of a whole blood analyzer are presented simultaneously on a single graphic display. Then, the graphic is examined by the human eye or a computer algorithm for patterns, that is, "fingerprints" that reveal system errors and mainte-

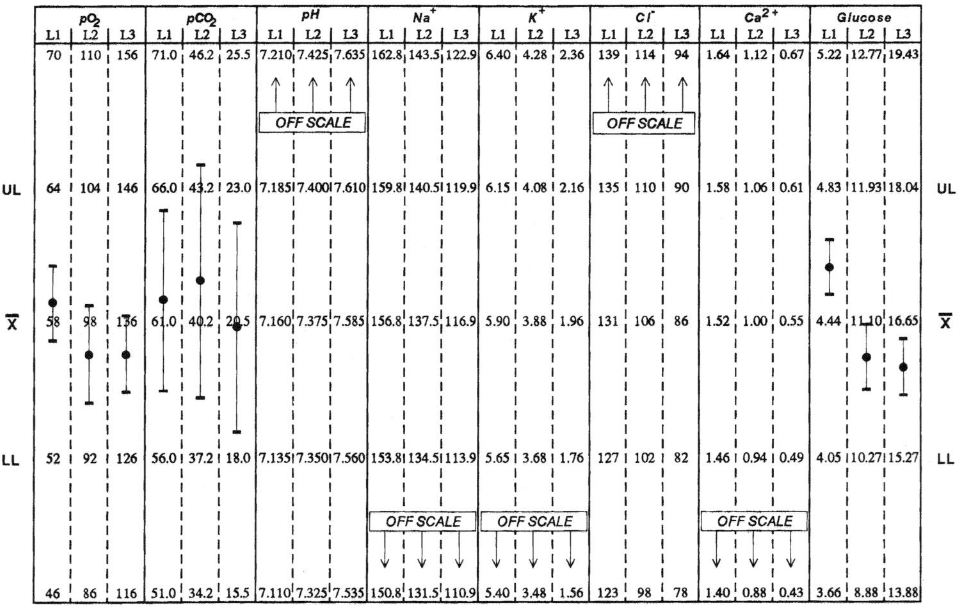

Figure 1 FAST-QC detects a reference electrode problem. The fingerprint pattern reveals the dependence of the pH, Na^+, K^+, Cl^-, and Ca^{++} channels on the common reference electrode and the direction of their deviations off scale. Changes from normal operation were statistically significant ($p \ll 0.01$, Student's t-test). The points are control level means $\pm$SD ($n = 20$). The center numeric value is the expected mean for each of three control levels (L1, L2, and L3) for each of the eight analytes. UL is the upper control limit; LL is the lower control limit.

nance problems. The objective of this section is to illustrate briefly the usefulness of FAST-QC for the evaluation of the quality of performance of biosensor-based whole blood analyzers using control materials. Fingerprints were produced during normal operating conditions and simulated instrument failures. The fingerprints taken during normal conditions should be statistically and visually different from those taken during periods of mechanical or electrochemical failures, and vice versa. A second objective of this section is to demonstrate how FAST-QC reveals interactions among multiple channels. FAST-QC is a performance map (6,25) technique for quality improvement that also can be used to visualize patient data, critical limits, and diagnostic patterns.

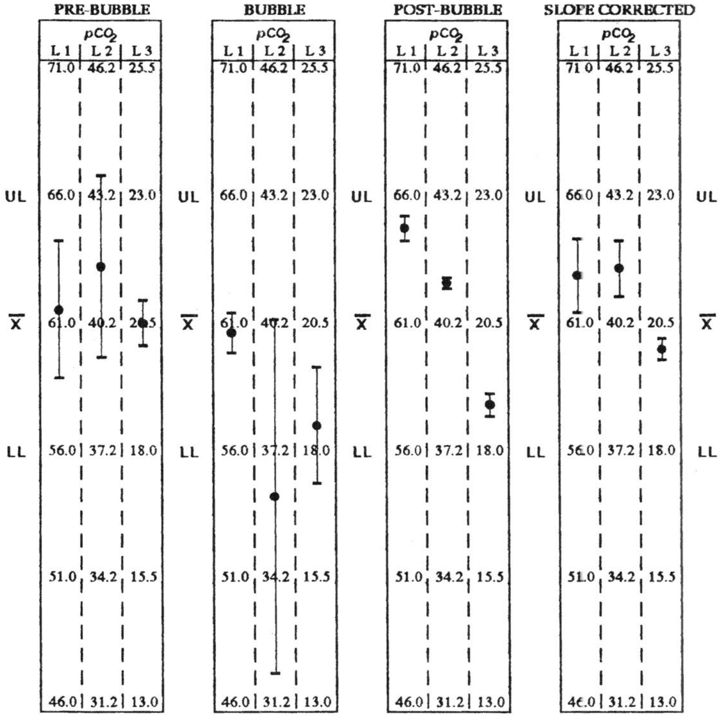

Figure 2 Effects of a biosensor bubble on FAST-QC. The frames show pCO_2 control measurements before, during, and after the presence of a bubble. With the interference of the bubble, measurements were both inaccurate and imprecise. Postbubble, the points revealed a proportional calibration error. Slope correction (right) restored the original quality of the measurements. Group means differed significantly ($p < 0.01$, analysis of variance). Plots show mean $\pm$SD ($n = 6$).

Figure 1 demonstrates a FAST-QC pattern produced by disruption of the integrity of the reference electrode. Figure 2 illustrates the effects of measurement errors caused by introducing a bubble into the pCO_2 electrode measurement process. Figure 3 shows the effects of temperature perturbations on blood gas and pH measurements. FAST-QC can be displayed serially over time in three-dimensional topologies, and draws on the unique human ability of quickly recognizing patterns, even in the two-dimensional displays shown in Figures 1 through 3. Future studies are needed to determine the usefulness of FAST-QC for detection and elimination of errors in POCT under varied clinical conditions. Ultimately, POCT error reduction will benefit from nanofabricated designs with internal ("wet") QC performed in parallel to or in sequence with patient testing, even on unit-use disposables; immediate graphic display of patterns, such as FAST-QC, for both QC and patient test data; and rapid computer-facilitated detection, inter-

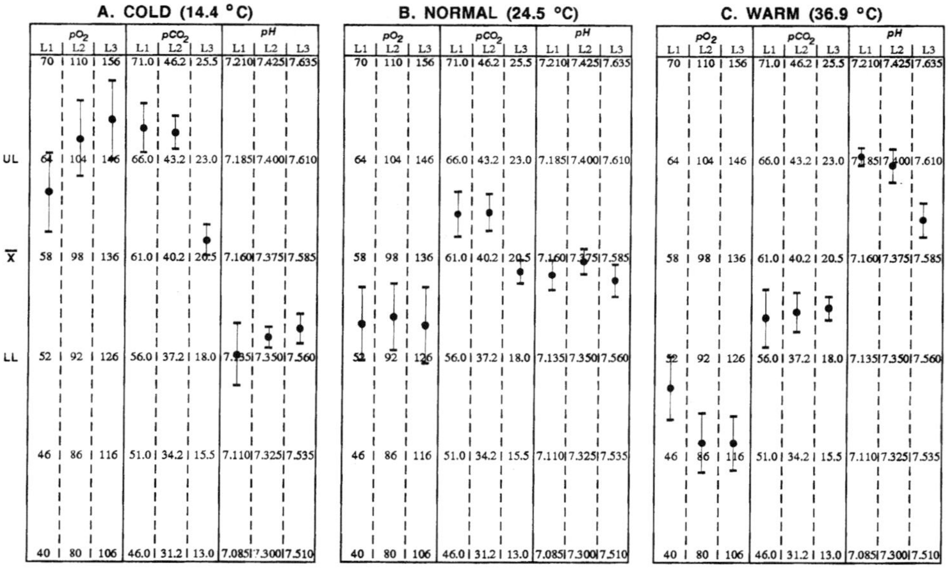

Figure 3 FAST-QC pattern for temperature perturbations. The three frames compare blood gas and pH measurements during serial temperature changes in control solutions using a 26-min, five-step cycle consisting of (1) room temperature (RT); (2) cold (A); (3) RT (B); (4) warm (C); and (5) RT. Temperature fluctuations, similar to what might happen with inappropriately prepared whole blood samples, drove the results out of control. The instrument measurement temperature was 37°C in each case. Differences were statistically significant ($p < 0.01$, Tukey multiple comparison test). Plots show mean $\pm$SD ($n = 20$).

pretation, and rectification of problems. In addition, electronic ("dry") QC can be performed concurrently with or prior to patient testing.

SYSTEMS FOR ERROR REDUCTION

This section summarizes systems for error prevention with POCT devices (Table 2). These systems are based on results of a U.S. national survey of experts, followed by progressive improvements through serial critiques by POCT professionals at several presentations. Please consult Ref. 29 for details. The systems can be implemented with instrument software and hardware. The fundamental error prevention functions include security, validation, and performance, three elements that must be managed efficiently and professionally by a collaborative team of laboratorians and clinicians who establish and enforce program rules in conjunction with the POCT director and coordinator. For example, a portable

Table 2 Systems for POCT Error Prevention

A. Fundamental functions
  1. Security
     Operator is required to enter personal identification number (PIN) and password.
  2. Validation
     Operator with valid credentials can review and/or download (transfer) test results, and perform patient testing, quality control (QC), and proficiency testing (PT).
  3. Performance
     QC is required at timed intervals (e.g., day of use, each shift, or defined period) or when use of the device triggers a QC check.
     QC check is demanded if range exceeded, result rejected, or error detected.

B. Emergency override
   Emergency personnel must be trained and certified periodically in point-of-care testing.
   Hospital defines conditions for emergency access to testing, which is flagged and tracked, following mandatory entry of operator's PIN.
   Password or special emergency code (e.g., in a "break box") also may be required.
   During emergencies, operator is warned, initiates testing, and is accountable for recovery actions.
   For instruments with override capability and those used during disasters, QC is performed in advance as part of daily workflow to assure that each instrument is prepared for critical patient testing.

POCT device for use in critical care could require the operator to enter a personal identification number (PIN) and password to gain access to instrument function (see Table 2, A1). Next, the system must have a method (e.g., list, database, or connectivity) for validating that operator prior to patient testing (see Table 2, A2). Finally, there must be an instrument-based, well-defined protocol for QC, which the operator must complete upon request (see Table 2, A3).

In contrast, a consumer meter for self-monitoring of blood glucose could use only PIN-gated access and remind the user to perform a QC check each new day of testing. However, except for patient training in self-monitoring (e.g., glucose or prothrombin time) prior to discharge, the use of "open" access consumer meters or nonsecured POCT instruments that anyone can operate invites errors and is not recommended in hospital settings. Protection features, access levels, and QC interrupts can be used in conjunction with tracking, monitoring, and auditing of the rate of nonvalidated operator use and other compliance metrics to identify errors by function, correct them promptly, and reduce occurrence rates. On simple instruments, QC results can be "pass/fail" to avoid the abuse of QC routines being used for patient testing.

Users cannot bypass the security, validation, and performance systems, except in emergencies (see Table 2, B). Following emergencies, the same users are held accountable within 24 hr for actions by tracking their PIN- and/or password-gated entry to instrument use. All such operators should be trained on site-specific instruments made available for emergencies and disasters, and these operators should be trained in effective recovery from crises (12). Emergency override allows testing in critical situations when not testing could harm patients and expose the hospital to excess liability. Emergency override is problematic (especially for blood gases) because of potential errors in clinical decisions based on erroneous test results, management difficulties controlling emergency access, and resulting inconsistent testing practices. A viable option is to send emergency specimens to the core laboratory by courier or to call laboratory personnel to perform testing on site.

However, during a rapidly evolving disaster, communications may be interrupted or sites of emergency care may be physically inaccessible, necessitating testing by available clinical personnel. Therefore, the operation of the emergency override system is conditional to diminish the drawbacks of override through requirements for

- Formal planning of staff who will have access
- Training and certifying of these individuals
- Documenting written attestations that PINs and passwords will not be shared
- Performing QC in advance as part of daily workflow so that emergency-designated instruments are perpetually ready

With this conservative approach, security features will not obstruct medically needed, rapid response testing during emergencies and disasters.

Diagnostic testing continues to shift from the clinical laboratory to the point of care as devices become smaller, smarter, and faster (5,6,14,25,26,30–32). It is the responsibility of industry to provide systems that are safe for the intended application, such as the operating room, intensive care unit, clinical specialty ward, outpatient care center, or patient's home. To fulfill IOM and NCCLS guidelines, HIPAA regulations (10), and other sound advice (13,15,33), manufacturers should proactively incorporate into instruments the consensus security, validation, performance, and emergency systems presented here, so that users will have the tools necessary to improve the safety of POCT and to test objectively manufacturers' claims of accurate and precise performance. The FDA, which works through manufacturers' claims, could require nonvalidated operator lockout, noncertified operator lockout, and error reduction options, such as lockout when QC is not performed or data are not transferred (Table 3), and software-based safeguards (29) on instruments when licensing new devices and tests for POCT. Availability of these options would allow POCT coordinators to track and analyze error-to-injury translation sequences.

Human factor problems, especially when cumulative opportunities for errors exist, are more likely to occur with technologically complicated instruments,

Table 3 Lockout Features for POCT Error Reduction and Their Significance

Acronym	Lockout	Significance
NVO	Nonvalidated operator	Protects system from unauthorized and inappropriate use
NCO	Noncertified operator	Prevents testing if the operator lacks education, experience, or current skills appropriate for the setting, as required by the collaborative agreement of the POCT director, POCT coordinator, and clinical team
NQC	No quality control performed	Prevents testing if the quality control protocol for the instrument is not followed or quality control is not performed in a timely fashion
NDT	No data transferred	Assures the integrity of the medical electronic record and facilitates several other functions, such as monitoring of patient data, checking quality control compliance, and tracking medical errors

complex procedures, and poorly trained operators. Instrument access is a critical control point. Therefore, only certified and validated operators should be allowed to perform POCT, and security standards should be comparable to those used for access to other hospital systems, such as computerized medical records. Use of a PIN plus password (alphanumeric) combination is preferred because of the potential for sharing, which creates problems tracking the origin of test results, determining if results were produced by competent users, and correcting deficiencies.

Competency is the ability to perform all phases of POCT correctly. Competency can be documented through certifications that assure individual operators meet training and experience standards. Competency is deemed crucial by JCAHO (34,35), CAP, and other accreditation agencies. Each health system must define its own goals for operator training, certification, and recertification and its own criteria for operator validation. Training and certification alone probably will not prevent errors. Resolution must occur through periodic human contact and communication. For example, monthly e-mail notification of QC compliance and success rates improves operator performance (32). Real-time QC interrupts should be designed carefully to match clinical needs, fulfill manufacturers' specifications, and integrate accreditation requirements (e.g., no patient results if QC is out of the control range).

ESSENTIAL CONNECTIVITY

Connectivity is critical to the prevention, detection, and tracking of medical errors in POCT. Error management cannot be implemented easily without bidirectional connectivity. Table 4 lists user connectivity specifications summarized from proceedings of the Connectivity Industry Consortium (CIC), a nonprofit corporation launched October 20, 1999 (36). Connectivity standards (published by the NCCLS as document POCT 1-A) facilitate secure data transmissions and help organize patient information (37). For example, bidirectional communication can help synchronize time and date functions, provide interpretive information with test results, and send alerts to POCT operators (e.g., hematocrit out of range during glucose meter testing).

Important user requirements encompass confidentiality, security, legality, compatibility, interoperability, timeliness, and convenience of processes, data, communications, and software. The CIC members believe that connectivity should not increase therapeutic turnaround time (TTAT), the time from test order to patient treatment (1,2), for POCT results. Fast TTAT is associated with improved patient care (38). Connectivity will improve the efficiency and efficacy of the error prevention systems, facilitate use of safeguards through shared instrument software, help track and store error episodes in clinical information systems

Table 4 User Requirements and Priorities for Connectivity[a,b]

A. Transmission, confidentiality, and security
   1. *Transmit bidirectionally between point-of-care devices, coordinators, and data bases*
   2. *Use existing communication infrastructures (e.g., LAN/WAN, intranet, Internet, & WWW)*
   3. *Conserve IP (Internet protocol) addresses and use existing ones where possible*
   4. *Guarantee confidentiality and security (encrypt as necessary)*

B. Accreditation, legality, and regulation
   1. *Satisfy regulatory agency guidelines (e.g., JCAHO, CAP, COLA, and individual states)*
   2. *Facilitate test ordering and resulting at the point of care and via computerized systems*
   3. Enhance performance, quality compliance, and QC/QA training

C. Software and hardware compatibility and interoperability
   1. *Standardize device connections ("plug and play") and minimize space needed*
   2. *Ensure compatibility and interoperability with commercial software*
   3. Strive for compatibility with U.S. and foreign information systems

D. Timeliness, convenience, and information content
   1. *Minimize therapeutic turnaround time (≤1–2 min pre-/postanalytic reception/transmission)*
   2. *Design an intuitive, functionally simple standard that is easy to use and operate*
   3. Qualify and archive results with relevant descriptors (e.g., patient test, QC, or critical value)

E. Downloading, uploading, access, flexibility, and integration
   1. Download point-of-care testing data automatically, seamlessly, and on demand
   2. Interface directly to LIS, HIS, CIS, and/or CDR, and avoid intermediates (e.g., laptops)
   3. Allow user-defined, multilevel access to test menus/results, QC/QA setup, and order entry
   4. Let operators configure data model, optimize density/content, and customize uses
   5. Integrate informatics fully and automate information processes (e.g., automated e-mail alerts)

F. Future requirements
   1. Real-time verification of operator/patient IDs and communication of test results
   2. Wireless operation with locator capability, site annotation, and regional communication
   3. Compatibility/communication with personal digital assistants and other devices
   4. Intelligent processing and interpretation of information using expert systems
   5. Efficient data retrieving, mining, sharing, analyzing, trending, and managing
   6. Information consolidation and condensation for outcomes optimization

[a] Top 10 connectivity priorities are in *italics*.

[b] Abbreviations: JCAHO, Joint Commission on Accreditation of Healthcare Organizations; CAP, College of American Pathologists; COLA, Commission on Laboratory Accreditation; LIS, laboratory information system; HIS, hospital information system; CIS, clinical information system; CDR, clinical data repository; ID, identification; LAN, local area network; PC, personal computer; QA, quality assurance; QC, quality control; WAN, wide area network; WWW, world-wide web.

for identification of serious accidents, and allow POCT informatics to merge with computerized hospital systems and clinical data repositories (39).

SAFEGUARDS

Safeguards (29) can be implemented through instrument system software and connectivity. The most important safeguards include

- Identifying the patient
- Integrating critical limits (40–43)
- Assuring the integrity of specimens, formats, test results, and statistical process control

Some safeguards, such as verifying the sequence and timing of patient test results, QC, and proficiency testing for JCAHO accreditation inspections, require a combination of "smart" instruments, data archiving, and collaborative management of the hospital-based POCT program to complete the "quality loop" (34,35). Fulfillment of other requirements, such as alerting interference from confounding variables (44) and drugs (45), requires bidirectional connectivity with hospital computerized databases. Root-cause analyses show that serious adverse events frequently are attributed to drug accidents (11,12). If a drug regimen interferes with test methods, physicians making rapid bedside decisions should be informed of possible analytical errors by means of a viewable comment shown when analyte results are displayed on the POCT device.

CONCLUSIONS AND RECOMMENDATIONS

Existing options (Table 5), especially on portable and handheld instruments, offer no, few, or inconsistent features that do not adequately assure operator competency or the integrity of test results. Often, these features can be bypassed by operating instruments in an open access mode. Provision of adequate safety options will help decrease the costs of detecting and reducing medical errors. Health system providers, government agencies, accreditation organizations, and commercial corporations should collaborate to provide consensus security, validation, performance, emergency, safeguard, and connectivity solutions (36,37,39) in order to identify and prevent errors, improve the performance of POCT, preserve fast TTAT, and help improve medical and economic outcomes (46).

Point-of-care testing has become the standard of practice in critical emergencies because of the immediate availability of critical results and fast TTAT (1–3). The goals of POCT are to provide rapid response and to improve patient outcomes (1,2), not to increase the frequency of medical errors. In the U.S. na-

Table 5 Current Status of Six Key Error Reduction Functions on POCT Devices

System	Status
Security	Several commonly used POCT instruments run only in open access mode.
	Protection varies from none to PINs and/or passwords on handhelds and portables.
	Even when protection features are available, an option for open access is typical.
Validation	Nonvalidated operator lockout is not common on portables and handhelds.
	Some devices offer basic and intermediate access levels via computer data stations.
	Downloading and uploading of valid operator lists typically are cumbersome.
Performance	QC lockout is available on a few portable and handheld POCT devices.
	Nurses and physicians are reluctant to implement QC lockout at the bedside.
	Most practical approach would be automated QC concurrent with patient testing.
Emergency	Methods of emergency override at the point of care are not proven.
	Override is dangerous if it allows potentially inaccurate testing.
	Experts feel that emergency operators should be trained, certified, and validated.
Safeguards	Lockout of expired QC materials and incorrect code keys is a common strength.
	Lack of positive patient identification is a weakness of portables and handhelds.
	Emerging algorithmic software offers some user-definable safeguards.
Connectivity	Transportables, some portables, and handhelds with computer data stations have basic connectivity.
	Bidirectional communication generally is not available for portable and handheld POCT devices.
	Handheld devices use proprietary docking stations, which are not interchangeable and waste space at the bedside or nursing station.

tional survey (29), 100% of experts recommended the practice of validating trained and certified operators before they use hospital-based instruments for POCT. Leadership must assure at least this minimum level of safety and should proactively support use of the consensus error prevention systems and lockout features. Additionally, collaborative hospital teams (11,12) and a culture of safety

(47) are necessary to make safety a primary concern and responsibility among hybrid staff (5,6) participating in a POCT program.

ACKNOWLEDGMENTS

The author is indebted to the many generous students and colleagues who contributed to this work. FAST-QC experimental results were based on the Honor Thesis of Brian D. Evans (28) and were developed with the advice of Robert L. Coleman and Paul W. McDonald. The author sincerely thanks each of the participants who contributed to the U.S. national survey and development of systems for preventing medical errors in POCT (29). Table and figure concepts are used with the permission of Knowledge Optimization®, Davis, CA. Tables 4 and 5 reproduced with the permission of the Archives of Pathology and Laboratory Medicine.

REFERENCES

1. Kost GJ. Guidelines for point-of-care testing: Improving patient outcomes. Pathol Patterns, Am J Clin Pathol 104(suppl):S111–S127, 1995.
2. Kost GJ, Ehrmeyer SS, Chernow B, et al. The laboratory-clinical interface: Point-of-care testing. Chest 115:1140–1154, 1999.
3. Kilgore ML, Steindel SJ, Smith JA. Continuous quality improvement for point-of-care testing using background monitoring of duplicate specimens. Arch Pathol Lab Med 123:824–828, 1999.
4. Stephans EJ. Hospital point-of-care survey report (Enterprise Analysis Corporation). Presented at the Connectivity Industry Consortium Meeting, October 20, 1999, Redwood City, CA.
5. Kost GJ. The hybrid laboratory: Shifting the focus to the point of care. Med Lab Observer 24:17–28, 1992.
6. Kost GJ. Point-of-care testing ⇒ The hybrid laboratory ⇒ Knowledge optimization. In: Kost GJ, ed., Handbook of Clinical Automation, Robotics, and Optimization. Wiley, New York, 1996, pp 757–838.
7. Plebani M, Carraro P. Mistakes in a stat laboratory: Types and frequency. Clin Chem 43:1348–1351, 1997.
8. Witte DL, VanNess SA, Angstadt DS, Pennell BJ. Errors, mistakes, blunders, outliers, or unacceptable results: How many? Clin Chem 43:1352–1356, 1997.
9. Jenny RW, Jackson-Tarentino KY. Causes of unsatisfactory performance in proficiency testing. Clin Chem 46:89–99, 2000.
10. Ballam H. HIPAA, security and electronic signature: A closer look. J AHIMA 70: 26–30, 1999.
11. Kohn LT, Corrigan JM, Donaldson MS, eds. Committee on Quality of Health Care

in America, Institute of Medicine. To Err is Human: Building a Safer Health System. National Academy Press, Washington, DC, 2000.
12. Richardson WL, Berwick DM, Bisgard JC, et al. Crossing the Quality Chasm: A New Health System for the 21st Century. National Academy Press, Washington, DC, 2001.
13. National Committee for Clinical Laboratory Standards. Protection of Laboratory Workers from Occupationally Acquired Infections. NCCLS M29-A2. NCCLS, Wayne, PA, 2002.
14. Kost GJ. Optimizing point-of-care testing in clinical systems management. Clin Lab Manage Rev 12:353–363, 1998.
15. Leape LL. Error in medicine. JAMA 272:1851–1857, 1994.
16. Witte DL, Van Ness SA. Frequency of unacceptable results in point-of-care testing [editorial]. Arch Pathol Lab Med 123:761, 1999.
17. McDonald CJ, Weiner M, Hui SL. Deaths due to medical errors are exaggerated in Institute of Medicine report. JAMA 284:93–95, 2000.
18. Leape LL. Institute of Medicine medical error figures are not exaggerated. JAMA 284:95–97, 2000.
19. Tang Z, Louie RF, Kost GJ. Principles and performance of point-of-care instruments. In: Kost GJ, ed. Principles and Practice of Point-of-Care Testing. Lippincott/Williams & Wilkins, Philadelphia, 2002.
20. Watts NB. Reproducibility (precision) in alternate site testing. Arch Pathol Lab Med 119:914–917, 1995.
21. Boyd JC, Bruns DE. Quality specifications for glucose meters: Assessment by simulation modeling of errors in insulin dose. Clin Chem 47:209–214, 2001.
22. Skeie S, Thue G, Sandberg S. Patient-derived quality specifications for instruments used in self-monitoring of blood glucose. Clin Chem 47:67–73, 2001.
23. Kost GJ, Vu HT, Lee JH, et al. Multicenter study of oxygen-insensitive handheld glucose point-of-care testing in critical care/hospital/ambulatory patients in the United States and Canada. Crit Care Med 26:581–590, 1998.
24. Kost GJ, Vu HT, Inn M, et al. Multicenter study of whole-blood creatinine, total carbon dioxide content, and chemistry profiling for laboratory and point-of-care testing in critical care in the United States. Crit Care Med 28:2379–2389, 2000.
25. Kost GJ. Point-of-care testing in intensive care. In: Tobin MJ, ed. Principles and Practice of Intensive Care Monitoring. McGraw-Hill, New York, 1998, pp 1267–1296.
26. Kost GJ. Point-of-care testing. In: Meyers RA, ed. Encyclopedia of Analytical Chemistry: Instrumentation and Applications. Wiley, England, 2000, pp 1603–1625.
27. Senge PM. The Fifth Discipline: The Art and Practice of the Learning Organization. Currency Doubleday, New York, 1990.
28. Evans BD. Pattern recognition "fingerprinting" for continuous quality improvement of point-of-care whole blood testing. Honor thesis, University of California, Davis, CA.
29. Kost GJ. Preventing medical errors in point-of-care testing: Security, validation, performance, safeguards, and connectivity. Arch Pathol Lab Med 125:1307–1315, 2001.
30. Kost GJ, Hague C. In vitro, ex vivo, and in vivo biosensor systems. In: Kost GJ,

ed. Handbook of Clinical Automation, Robotics, and Optimization. Wiley, New York, 1996, pp 648–753.
31. Kost GJ. Planning and implementing point-of-care testing systems. In: Tobin MJ, ed. Principles and Practice of Intensive Care Monitoring. McGraw-Hill, New York, 1998, pp 1297–1328.
32. Louie RF, Tang Z, Shelby DG, Kost GJ. Point-of-care testing: Millennium technology for critical care. Lab Med 31:402–408, 2000.
33. Witte DL, Astion ML. Panel discussion: How to monitor and minimize variation and mistakes. Clin Chem 43:880–885, 1997.
34. Joint Commission on Accreditation of Healthcare Organizations. Quality Point of Care Testing: A Joint Commission Handbook. JCAHO, Oakbrook Terrace, IL, 1999, p 94.
35. Joint Commission on Accreditation of Healthcare Organizations. How to Meet the Most Frequently Cited Laboratory Standards. JCAHO, Oakbrook Terrace, IL, 2001.
36. Nichols J, ed. User Needs (Provider Review Committee). Version 2.0, CIC web site, www.poccic.org, 2000; Provider Review Committee Survey, www.poccic.org, 2000; and AACC Milestone Status, San Francisco—July 2000; and Standards Documents. Agilent Technologies, www.poccic.org, 2001.
37. National Committee for Clinical Laboratory Standards. Point-of-Care Connectivity. NCCLS POCT 1-A (formerly AUTO 6-P), NCCLS, Wayne, PA, 2001.
38. Kilgore ML, Steindel SJ, Smith JA. Evaluating stat testing options in an academic health center: Therapeutic turnaround time and staff satisfaction. Clin Chem 44: 1597–1603, 1998.
39. Kost GJ. Connectivity: The millennium challenge for point-of-care testing [editorial]. Arch Pathol Lab Med 124:1108–1110, 2000.
40. Kost GJ. Critical limits for urgent clinician notification at U.S. medical centers. JAMA 263:704–707, 1990.
41. Kost GJ. Critical limits for emergency clinician notification at United States children's hospitals. Pediatrics 88:597–603, 1991.
42. Kost GJ. Using critical limits to improve patient outcome. Med Lab Observer 25: 22–27, 1993.
43. Kost, GJ. Designing critical limit systems for knowledge optimization. Arch Pathol Lab Med 120:616–618, 1996.
44. Louie RF, Tang Z, Sutton DV, Lee JH, Kost GJ. Point-of-care testing: Effects of critical care variables, influence of reference instruments, and a modular glucose meter design. Arch Pathol Lab Med 124:257–266, 2000.
45. Tang Z, Du X, Louie RF, Kost GJ. Effects of drugs on glucose measurements with handheld glucose meters and a portable glucose analyzer. Am J Clin Pathol 113: 75–86, 2000.
46. Kern DA, Bennett ST. Quality improvement in the information age. Med Lab Observer 31:24–28, 1999.
47. Sirota RL. The Institute of Medicine's report on medical error: Implications for pathology. Arch Pathol Lab Med 124:1674–1678, 2000.

5
Performance Improvement

Carolann Liszewski
Quality Dynamics International, Bel Air, Maryland, U.S.A.

INTRODUCTION

Performance improvement in point-of-care testing has taken many forms. Consumerism and a plethora of new technical advancements that have fostered laboratory testing of patients at the point of care have been the catalyst in improving availability of test results. This is certainly seen as an improvement from the consumer point of view. In hospitals and medical practices, point-of-care testing has served as the commonality between medical professionals. It has helped non-laboratorians appreciate the laboratorian's job as well as highlighted for the laboratorian the realization that the laboratory result is a piece of the total healthcare puzzle, thus fostering an improvement in cooperation and understanding among healthcare providers. Does increased availability and increased communication mean improved performance?

The measurement of performance improvement involves a systematic plan. Models of improvement need to be designed. Measurement criteria need to be developed. Data need to be collected and assessed to discover improvement opportunities. This chapter describes the natural progression of performance improvement from quality control and quality assurance and provides the tools needed to design quality systems, which include identification of opportunities for both process and performance improvement that could be used for any testing process regardless of where it is performed.

PATIENT CARE RESPONSIBILITIES

In the traditional patient care model, the patient was serviced by two separate entities, the clinician and the laboratory scientist, working conjointly. The clinician assisted the patient through establishing diagnosis and directing management. The laboratory scientist assisted the patient through working with the clinician to provide appropriate in vitro laboratory tests and procedures. The clinician's responsibility extended to understanding the test that was requested and requesting the test that best met the clinician's goals. The laboratory scientist's responsibility was to perform tests appropriate to the question being asked and assure the best quality result.

CHANGING ENVIRONMENT

Significant changes in various areas related to the delivery of patient care have occurred. Among these are the financial constraints brought about by managed care and heightened consumer awareness. Guarantors' expectations are that medical services are coordinated and efficient and that care is delivered in a cost-effective manner. Managed care systems require that documentation is complete and timely and that there is an identified system for solving problems and fulfilling requirements. Consumers are seeking the "one-stop" shop that will allow for accessibility to a broad range of healthcare options and assure the continuity of care, seamless referrals, and timely communications between primary care and tertiary care providers.

The medical field has seen improvement in the availability of laboratory tests. Some are now sold in pharmacies. Patients can now get laboratory test results in the privacy of their own home. People perform testing with no training in the laboratory. Patients can use the test results to self-manage their illnesses.

THE RESPONSE

The technology industry has responded with developments in simplified instrumentation and packaged reagents. Manufacturers continue to produce smaller and smaller instruments so testing is portable. It can be done in any place at any time. Regulators have also heard the consumers' mandate and have lessened regulatory requirements for certain types of laboratory testing. All of this has led to the growth of the "super clinician" who takes on both of the roles described above.

THE CHALLENGES

The goal is to achieve the desired outcomes of increased patient satisfaction and improved clinical outcomes while reducing costs. In this market-driven environment, there are growing demands for accountability. Assuring quality of care is paramount. Quality of care is defined by the Joint Commission for Accreditation of Healthcare Organizations (JCAHO) as, "the degree to which health services for individuals and populations increase the likelihood of desired health outcomes and are consistent with current professional knowledge" (1). The American Association of Family Practitioners recommends that "quality care should produce optimal health outcomes in the most effective manner and result in high patient satisfaction" (2). The assurance of quality affects every resource used by the clinician in the delivery of patient care. These resources can fall in the following categories: men, materials, machines, and methods. Quality assurance systems need to be developed which consider all of these elements.

QUALITY CONTROL

Quality control is the piece of the quality assurance puzzle that deals with process and product control. In the point-of-care laboratory testing arena, the process is the actual testing of the sample and the product is the laboratory result. Most manufactures will include quality control material to be run just as a patient sample. This type of material controls the performance of the entire analytical process and assures that the reagents are working properly. These controls need to be appropriately chosen to mimic a patient's result at a certain concentration where the result would trigger changes in patient management. Some instruments require an additional control material that is used to verify that the instrument is functioning correctly. This type of control monitors the electronic functions of the instrument. Both of these types of controls serve a different purpose and need to be used in tandem to assure the accuracy of the test result. Both of these types of controls are considered "internal controls" as they give information on how the test system, which comprises the instrumentation and the reagents, is working. Additionally, "external" controls should be used. These are controls that give information on how the test system that you use compares with similar test systems used in other settings by other users. Standardized proficiency testing programs and/or specimen exchange programs are used as external controls. Both internal and external quality control material and the information gathered from their usage can be used to assure that other resources (men, materials, machines, and methods) are functioning properly.

The use of traditional laboratory quality control in the point-of-care setting has been highly debated. The National Committee for Clinical Laboratory Standards (NCCLS) has developed a guideline for point-of-care in vitro diagnostic testing (3), which recommends daily usage of quality control material both for single use devices as well as multiple use point-of-care devices. The College of American Pathologists (CAP) position is that any test improperly performed can lead to patient injury. The CAP guidelines designate the "internal" quality control material as either procedural controls or instrument controls and sets the criteria for when instrument only controls are appropriate for assuring the quality of the complete system. The NCCLS guideline for unit-use devices recommends that the testing site must understand the sources of error based on the device, the operator, and the setting (4). Quality control systems need to be uniquely tailored to the methodology so that frequency of control usage increases when monitors indicate deterioration in analytical performance and decreases when performance improves.

QUALITY ASSURANCE SYSTEM

These quality control tools and information are integral parts of the quality assurance system and give information regarding methodology, but used alone cannot provide all the information necessary to assure an accurate test result. Human resource also is a key factor. The federal government, in the Clinical Laboratory Improvement Amendments of 1988 (CLIA'88), guidelines (5) has set standards for testing personnel who are performing various levels of laboratory testing. The levels are well defined and categorized according to the perceived level of risk to the patient of an inaccurate result. Individual state licensing regulations may also apply. As expressed previously, accrediting agencies such as the College of American Pathologists believe that any test improperly performed can lead to patient injury. The key components needed in this part of the quality assurance system are job descriptions defining responsibility and accountability. The development of criteria for establishing and re-evaluating competency needs to be tied to the responsibilities defined in the job description as well as the tasks to be performed. In the point-of-care setting, initial verification of the task-specific training is often accomplished by the manufacturer. The responsibility for continued verification of competency and competency of new staff remains the responsibility of the point-of-care testing area and falls upon its designated director. This can be accomplished by using the tools in the quality assurance system, such as both internal and external quality control, instrument function records, records documenting testing process, result verification, and result reporting. Continuing education is a requirement for continued and updated competency of testing personnel. This requirement may be particularly difficult for smaller self-contained areas that provide point-of-care testing. When the documentation gathered as part of the quality assurance system detects opportunities for improvement, the point-of-care testing area progresses from quality assurance to performance improvement.

Management of material resource involves purchasing, standardization, traceability, and trackability of reagents and equipment. Documentation that the point-of-care testing area can replicate calibration and standardization of the assay as proclaimed by the manufacturer is needed before the patient testing is performed. Quality management of machines requires systems that assure maintenance, calibration, verification of accuracy, precision, specificity and sensitivity as needed to serve the patient population. Environmental control of machines is also very important. Some equipment and reagents work well only within certain temperature ranges. In the point-of-care setting, all of these requirements may initially be accomplished by the manufacturer. It is important to note that the testing systems require continuous monitoring in order to assure an accurate test result.

The quality system must include a documentation system that describes all policies, work processes, and procedures. Policies explain "what to do," processes explain "how it happens," and procedures explain "how to do it" (6). The system tracks the patient and the patient's specimen from test request through interpretation of test result. It tracks monitors set up by the quality system that document conformity to the criteria for proper management of the specimen. Examples of these monitors are the internal process controls and the instrument function checks. Inherent in each component of a quality assurance system are the criteria used to detect nonconformity in the system and the corrective actions used to limit the risk of repeating the nonconformity. Therefore, establishing a document control system that requires review of all documents at a preset frequency is key to the quality assurance system. The document control system enables the point-of-care testing area to discover potential opportunities for performance improvement.

The National Committee for Clinical Laboratory Standards (7) addresses the issues noted as well as describes additional essential components in the areas of organization, internal assessment, service, satisfaction, and process improvement. The NCCLS standard includes the following quality system essentials:

- Organization [4.1–4.3]
- Personnel [4.18]
- Equipment [4.11]
- Purchasing and inventory [4.6, 4.7]
- Process control [4.4, 4.8–4.10, 4.12, 4.15, 4.20]
- Documents and records [4.5, 4.16]
- Occurrence management [4.13]
- Internal assessment [4.17]
- Process improvement [4.14]
- Service and satisfaction [4.19]

PERFORMANCE IMPROVEMENT EXPLAINED?

As described, performance improvement is a natural outgrowth of quality systems. There are various terms given to management systems that detect opportunities for improvement and the resulting improvement systems that occur. The NCCLS guideline uses "process improvement" as opposed to performance improvement, which is a term used by the Joint Commission for Accreditation of Healthcare Organizations. The JCAHO defines "performance improvement" as, "the continuous study and adaptation of a healthcare organization's or network's functions and processes to increase the probability of achieving desired outcomes and to better meet the needs of individuals and other users of services" (8). It is further described as the third part of a system of performance measurement, assessment, and improvement. The NCCLS wording is aligned with the International Standards of Operation (ISO 9004-2000) guidelines, which were explained in the *ISO 9004-2000 and Healthcare* document. "This standard promotes the adoption of the process approach when developing, implementing, and improving the effectiveness and efficiency of a quality management system" (9).

"Total quality management" was developed from the work of Deming as a management system that planned management by teams to achieve improvement. "Continuous quality improvement" (CQI) is the term used to refer to the system of implementation and management of improvement. Continuous quality improvement is both an organizational philosophy as well as a systematic process. The philosophy is that members of an organization, including its leadership, are committed to strategic planning and teamwork that will result in ongoing quality improvement and satisfy customer needs. The process is a systematic total management approach that facilitates continuous quality improvement (10). The American Academy of Family Physicians defines quality management in patient care as "a systematic process by which quality of patient care is continually evaluated and improved to assure that optimal patient care outcomes are achieved, and that patient care is consistent with current professional knowledge" (11).

PERFORMANCE IMPROVEMENT: IDENTIFYING OPPORTUNITIES

Despite differences in terminology, systems of improvement naturally follow from information gathered by the tools used in the quality assurance system. An important aspect of the CQI philosophy is that improvement opportunities are inherent in all processes and do not necessarily need to be identified by problems. In this manner, CQI can be used to enhance outcomes for patient care.

DIMENSIONS OF PERFORMANCE

The Joint Commission for Accreditation of Healthcare Organizations defines two basic dimensions of performance. These are "doing the right thing" and "doing the right thing well" (12). Improvement opportunities can be found by assessing how well the point-of-care testing area performs in these areas. "Doing the right thing" involves the effectiveness and appropriateness of the laboratory services.

Does the testing accomplish the desired patient outcome?
Is the testing relevant to the patient's needs?

To assess whether the testing area is "doing the right thing well," certain operational processes need to be reviewed:

Is testing provided to the patient at the most beneficial time?
Is there a system in place, which assures that the testing is performed to produce the best result?
Is the testing provided as part of the continuum of care and coordinated with other providers and services?
Is the safety of the patient and all providers of service assured?
Are resources used effectively to produce the best outcome of care?
Are the patient's needs and expectations respected?

Answers to these questions can be found in many sources. The first approach discussed suggests gathering information from all interested parties. The second approach looks to examining workflow process. The best approach for a particular testing area might be a combination of both, the people approach and the process approach.

STAKEHOLDERS

Identification of stakeholders can involve two distinct populations: those involved in defining the opportunity and those involved in responding. Each entity performing point-of-care testing will have its interested parties, such as patients, clinicians, scientists, testing personnel, suppliers, guarantors, and owners/investors. Feedback from these stakeholders can provide valuable information on potential improvements.

Patients judge the quality of the laboratory services by the following:

- Accessibility of the phlebotomy area
- Skill, attitude, and appearance of healthcare provider who performs the fingerstick or draws the blood
- How long they wait for the provider to review their result
- Information that they receive from the healthcare provider regarding the laboratory result
- Their perceived value of the lab result in managing their health
- The bill that they receive
- Overall appearance of the environment.

As expressed previously, the clinician and the laboratory scientist have the opportunity to take separate but complimentary roles. Clinicians are focused on the patient's clinical presentation and seek the best outcome; therefore, clinical relevance of the testing performed is important. The laboratory scientist is focused on the technical aspects of the testing and has a pulse on the latest developments in the laboratory testing field. They can advise on the best methodology/equipment that will provide the clinician with accurate information regarding the health status of the patient. Combining the feedback from these stakeholders, the point-of-care testing area will be able to identify opportunities to provide the patient with better information. Testing personnel can advise on workflow process, documentation systems, equipment, work satisfaction, and personal development. Suppliers can advise on product safety, product liability, delivery, price, and life cycle costs. Owners/investors can advise on financial impact, environmental impact, and impact of services on society/community. The key is to determine if the services satisfy the needs and expectations of all the stakeholders. Where there are gaps, there are identified areas for improvement. Improvement opportunities can also be detected by analyzing workflow processes.

PATH OF WORKFLOW: TRADITIONAL LABORATORY TESTING

Patient assessment → Test request → Specimen collection
→ Specimen transport → Specimen receipt → Testing/review
→ Laboratory interpretations → Results reporting
→ Post test specimen management → Information management LIS
→ Clinician interpretation → Treatment decision

In this traditional laboratory testing model, workflow includes processes in several venues: the point of patient contact as well as the laboratory setting and back to the clinician's office.

PATH OF WORKFLOW: POINT-OF-CARE TESTING

Test requested (physician) → Supplies gathered (nurse)
→ Sample drawn (nurse) → Test run (nurse/technician)
→ Results reviewed (nurse/physician)
→ Treatment decision made (physician)

In the point-of-care testing model, the steps are decreased because every process is performed in the same venue. When testing performed at the point of care needs to be validated by the laboratory, both sets of processes would be combined.

The quality system essentials (QSEs) (i.e., organization, personnel, equipment, purchasing/inventory, process control, documents/records, occurrence management, internal assessment, process improvement, and service and satisfaction) as described in the NCCLS document (13) apply to all operations in the path of workflow. These QSEs are the tools that can be used to identify opportunities for performance and process improvement. Some basic examples of improvement opportunities and how they relate to the QSEs are discussed in the following section. All of the processes involved have been divided into three distinct phases depending on when they occur: preanalytical, analytical, and postanalytical. Although these phases are distinct, it should be noted that each area is dependent on interactions with the other phases as part of a continuum.

IMPROVEMENT OPPORTUNITIES: PREANALYTICAL PHASE

Preanalytical functions include everything that happens before the actual testing. This can also refer to every process that occurs in order to assure that the best specimen is procured. Potential opportunities exist in patient education. Outreach activities that include point-of-care laboratory testing as part of health screenings or literature outlining steps for monitoring of certain conditions can improve customer satisfaction (QSE: service and satisfaction). The process of specimen collection lends itself to improvement opportunities (QSE: process control). Assuring that the person procuring the specimen is provided with the appropriate updated information regarding technique and educated in both technical and customer service provides the opportunity of expanding the roles of healthcare providers (QSEs: documents, personnel, organization). Working with vendors to assure that supplies are available (QSEs: purchasing/inventory, equipment) and are used before their expiration date (QSE: internal assessment) will improve the experience for the patient. Assuring that systems are in place to properly identify both the patient and the blood will also reduce the potential of subjecting the patient to another blood draw or finger stick (QSEs: documents, occurrence management). The opportunity to have access to information regarding the best test for the best information to achieve the best patient outcome limits the risk of misdiagnosis and the need for return visits.

IMPROVEMENT OPPORTUNITIES: ANALYTICAL PHASE

Analytical functions refer to all processes that involve the actual testing of the specimen. They also include the processes that lead to the generation of the laboratory result. In ISO terminology, laboratory testing is considered a service industry, which provides a product. The product provided by the laboratory testing is information in the form of a test result. The key is to set performance standards for analytical testing delineated in job descriptions. Using quality system competency review, gaps in skill and knowledge can be identified. Training programs and continuing education opportunities can be designed from this information (QSEs: organization, personnel). Evaluation programs such as the POCTE program under the American Society of Clinical Pathologists (ASCP) can assist in providing materials. Opportunities to obtain continuing education for testing personnel may exist in the local medical community. Continuing education can be achieved without sacrificing staffing time as staff could view public television programs that are related and/or read articles found in trade and professional journals.

Careful planning of workflow process can save time and effort. It can also minimize risk in that it promotes a standardized process that assures integrity of the patient's specimen throughout the process. Disorganized work space could lead to errors in specimen identification, mistakes in technical process and promote the reporting of inaccurate results (QSEs: process control, documents/records, occurrence management). Environments need to be designed to achieve staff and patient safety and effective infection control (QSE: personnel). Opportunities to select equipment that will work effectively in the particular environment of temperature control and workflow process will prevent the need for unnecessary delay in obtaining accurate patient results due to equipment malfunction (QSEs: purchasing/inventory, process control, occurrence management, internal assessment, service and satisfaction). As has been discussed previously, opportunities for collaboration of the clinician with the laboratory scientist will allow for optimization of test methodologies. Assistance is available from the scientists employed by the vendors from which the assays and reagents are purchased. They can provide information regarding verification of calibration and standardization and keep the point-of-care testing area aware of changes in operational characteristics. The point-of-care testing area can provide feedback on actual test performance and information on clinical correlations. There is increased opportunity within the point-of-care setting to optimize usage of quality control to effectively monitor the patient-specific population (QSEs: equipment, process control, occurrence management, documents). The most visible improvement recognized by clinicians and patients is reduction of turnaround time. The opportunity for this improvement is inherent in all of the phases. As shown by the workflow model, in the point-of-care testing setting, the number of preanalytical and postanalytical processes have been decreased whereas, the processes in the analytical phase remain the same. Therefore, the best opportunity for improving turnaround time in the point-of-care testing setting is in the analytical phase (QSE: service and satisfaction).

IMPROVEMENT OPPORTUNITIES: POSTANALYTICAL PHASE

Postanalytical functions include how the result is documented in the patient record, communicated to the clinician, verified and interpreted by the clinician, and utilized in the management of patient care. When the laboratory result is received, the clinician will need to be assured that the result belongs to the patient identified. In the point-of-care setting, there is a unique opportunity to design reporting systems that will document the patient's test result as part of a permanent record and include identifying information by which that result can be traced back through the path of workflow. This is important to assist the clinician in the verification process. The identifier could be alpha or numeric but should be assigned at time of specimen procurement and used in all documentation involving the specimen. The information given to the clinician in the reporting format regarding expected normal values that have been optimized to the served patient population can be helpful in assisting in the interpretation. The format should highlight critical or panic values that require immediate attention from the clinician (QSEs: documents/records, internal assessment, service and satisfaction). All of these opportunities assist in assuring that the patient will be able to receive the appropriate information regarding health status (QSE: service and satisfaction).

PERFORMANCE IMPROVEMENT PLANS

Once an improvement opportunity is identified, the next step is development of the opportunity as a performance improvement initiative. Several performance improvement plans will be discussed. The particular testing area needs to decide what plan works best for their operation. A key consideration for each testing area is to attempt to coordinate their improvement initiatives with the improvement initiatives of the organization of which it is a part. Success of performance improvement relies on the support of the leadership of the organization. Without that support, the information needed to develop the initiative and achieve the improvement could be very difficult to attain. The best initiatives cross disciplines and involve various groups of people.

The philosophy of early promoters of total quality management and continuous quality improvement such as Deming and Shewhart espoused systems that involved only four steps, which were connected in a continuous circle. The steps in Deming's cycle were: plan, do, act, and study. Shewhart's four steps differed slightly in that his cycle placed the evaluation step before the action step: plan, do, check, act. Others, including the JCAHO, have developed templates, which expand on these basic steps in an attempt to guide users in developing their own performance improvement matrix. The Hospital Corporation of America (HCA) uses the acronym FOCUS to help those using the system to remember the key components (14):

F—Find an opportunity.
O—Organize a team.

C—Clarify the process.
U—Understand causes for variation.
S—Select the process.

Other systems use FADE:

F—Focus.
A—Analyze the process.
D—Develop the plan for improvement.
E—Execute.

The JCAHO has streamlined its original 10-step plan to seven steps emphasizing how all of the steps are incorporated in the cyclic process. The JCAHO seven steps to process improvement are

Plan—Find a problem or opportunity to improve.
Design—Set goals and objectives.
Measure—Identify indicators and collect data.
Assess—Analyze data.
Improve—Try out the improvement.
Communicate—Inform and educate people on the results.
Monitor improvement—Provide regular performance feedback.

THE PLAN

The planning step answers the question "Where do we start?" Improvement opportunities may need to be prioritized. The American Academy of Family Physicians recommends that the following criteria be used to evaluate improvement opportunities (15):

There should be reasonable belief that the initiative will improve patient outcomes.
There needs to be a substantial potential for improvement.
There should be a significant gap between optimal and current practice.
The improvement should have the potential of making a substantial impact on a significant number of patients.
The initiative can be measured by scientifically valid methods.
The initiative can be accomplished within a realistic time frame.

The Health Care Financing Administration (HCFA) uses three guiding principles when selecting its performance improvement initiatives (16):

The initiative needs to be consumer and purchaser driven.
Collection tools needed to collect data should be in the public domain.

> The content and collection of data and the resulting performance initiative should be standardized.

It is important at this step to define the opportunity, evaluate its frequency of occurrence, and determine the population who could be affected. Since leadership support and team involvement are key to the success of the initiative, selecting improvement opportunities that align with the mission and strategic plan of the parent organization is important. It is beneficial to gather information regarding the initiative's impact on overall institutional factors, such as cost, quality, service, and satisfaction, as part of the initiative selection process.

Once the initiative has been selected, it is important to form a team of all those who will work on the initiative. The team should be small but should include those who work closely with the processes to be improved. Involvement of these stakeholders in the plan will increase their commitment to the resultant improvement. It is important to involve persons who have the authority to make a change. With the team in place, the opportunity can be fine-tuned.

THE DESIGN

In this stage of the development of the initiative, goals for improvement can be formalized. A goal is defined as a first-level planning element that delineates how to accomplish a specific strategy. Objectives are second-level planning elements that delineate how to accomplish a specific goal (17). As specific objectives are developed depending on information gathered from the team, meetings of the team should focus on the part that each individual will play, allowing for more detailed work or tasks to be done by individual members and/or smaller groups. Tasks are defined as third-level planning elements that delineate how to accomplish a specific objective (18). Each meeting should have an agenda and minutes should be documented. Factors that will limit success of the initiative need to be realized. Timelines can be established for data collection as resources and data sources are identified. If an improvement initiative is too complex, and includes multiple factors, it is better to choose a measure that will address a specific area, rather than the entire initiative.

DEVELOPMENT OF THE MEASURE

The next step involves developing specific performance indicators to measure. The JCAHO defines an indicator as a measure used to determine, over time, an organization's performance of functions, processes, and outcomes. There are two categories of improvement opportunities: symptomatic and asymptomatic. Symptomatic opportunities are those that are evidenced by pre-established surveillance indicators and may have set thresholds. An example of a symptomatic opportunity is one identified as part of the CAP Laboratory Improvement Q-Probes Program that uses benchmarking data to establish thresholds. Asymptomatic opportunities are those that are not clearly evidenced by pre-established indicators. Indicators can be based on rate of occurrence, a step in a process, or a patient care outcome. Measures are based on change in process either from a frequency aspect, such as it occurs more/less frequently, or an improvement aspect, such as better quality or increased patient satisfaction. Measures need to be designed to monitor success in reaching the goal. A measure should clearly identify what improvement opportunity it addresses. Concentrating on the most likely changes that could occur and/or the most likely causes for the problem being reviewed will help define specific measures and identify the data elements needed.

Certain thresholds should be established. A threshold is the target point for the improvement initiative. Thresholds can be established by use of benchmarking data obtained from reference studies. The benchmark is the point of reference or standard by which performance can be measured. Most thresholds are set to achieve between 90% and 95% of the goal. This accounts for human error and also allows the opportunity for continued improvement after the threshold is reached.

One measurement system that is growing in popularity and promoted by the American Society for Quality (ASQ) is Six Sigma. This system is a high-performance data-driven approach to analyzing root causes of problems. The premise of this system is that some processes are capable of being improved to be defect-free. Defects are considered as anything that results in customer dissatisfaction. In this system, the threshold for achieving success increases to 99.99966%. Efforts to incorporate Six Sigma have been successful in the manufacturing arena but have not yet been widely applied to the healthcare arena. This information is included only to give the reader a glimpse of possible future goals for performance improvement.

COLLECTION OF DATA

After the measures are defined and the thresholds established, data will need to be collected. Defining the purpose of the initiative also determines what information and data need to be collected. There are two fundamental kinds of studies: qualitative and quantitative. Qualitative studies entail direct observation and interviews. Qualitative data are narrative and descriptive. Quantitative studies use techniques to understand relationships among the variables of interest. Quantitative data are objective and measurable. A finite period of time should be determined for collection of data. Time frames should be short enough to allow for repeated collection to allow for analysis of trending over time. Data collection should involve as many people and sources as needed.

There are several standardized methods for data collection. Checklists can be used and designed to allow for interpretation of data directly from the form. Questionnaires can be designed when input is needed from a large group of people. This type of collection tool works better when collecting perceptions not facts. Interviews and other discussion formats are useful for collecting data on a one-to-one basis. Data can also be collected by direct observation of the process. The tools take more time and energy and require sharp interpersonal skills. No matter what tools are used, certain errors could be inherent. The measure may not have been designed to adequately address the specific question. Samples selected may not be adequate either in number or in composition. The timing of the collection may not be optimal and additional factors, such as process changes, that were not considered by the measure could cause potential errors in the database.

ASSESSMENT OF DATA

Data can be displayed in many formats. It is key to select the format or combination of formats that best demonstrate answers to the question: What does this tell us? Graphs and charts used to organize the data in different ways can assist people in understanding the results and making conclusions. Run charts are used to analyze and illustrate an outcome or process over a period of time. They can depict shifts and trends in the process. Bar charts are used to compare data from one group with the same data from another group or the same data over a period of time. Histograms are used to show variation in a set of data. Scatter diagrams display relationships between two variables (19). Analyzed data is information and applied information is knowledge. Using the knowledge gained from the analysis of the initiative will lead to improvement.

When the initiative has resulted from a serious problem that needs to be corrected, a root-cause analysis should be performed. Root-cause analysis is not a single tool but an approach using several tools including the ones already discussed. The process flow diagram is useful in detailing how the targeted process operates. Process analysis looks for useless actions, redundancy, and frequent or common obstacles in the process. As already discussed, this tool can help identify improvement opportunities as well as highlight problem areas. The cause–effect diagram is another tool used as part of a root cause analysis. This tool takes into account factors that cause certain results. The factors considered in this type of analysis coincide with the resources discussed previously: men, methods, machines, and materials. Another tool called Pareto analysis is commonly used to identify the proportional contribution of different causative factors to a particular outcome. Pareto analysis is based on the theory that 80% of the effects result from 20% of the causes (20).

IMPROVEMENT

It needs to be determined what the improvement is and how it will be implemented. Reviewing objectives and the data will tell whether the problem or opportunity has been successfully addressed by the tested indicator and to what extent improvement will occur. Initial efforts may not be successful. Re-evaluating the reason for failure and changing the indicator can subsequently result in improved outcomes. When the analysis of the data provides a solution, it is good practice to design a pilot to test out the improvement before it is completely implemented. The pilot should be limited to a subset of the representative group that will be affected by the improvement and to those performance measures that will determine whether the improvement will be successful.

COMMUNICATION

Communication is key to implementation of the pilot study as well as the improvement. The improvement will mostly likely involve change or redesign of process. Leadership must be involved from the beginning of the project in order to send the message to the entire staff that the improvement is important and the resulting process changes will be supported. Initially, both time and resources will be needed to assess the impact of the improvement. Top management needs to be aware of the impact of changes on employees. Change management teams often report that top management tends to focus on the business issues and neglect the employee side. Employees can become fearful and confused without adequate information and guidance. The following change management guidelines should be utilized:

- Educate your employees about the reasons for change.
- Demonstrate to your employees that you have a stake in them.
- Describe the phases of the change and what employees can expect.
- Answer questions many employees are unwilling to ask.
- Give employees the tools to deal with change both personally and professionally.
- Reinforce why the change is happening; explain the business reasons and the priority for the business.
- Share the change with all levels in the organization.

Provide answers to “What does this change mean to me?” and “What is expected of me?”
Listen to resistance and respond to feedback from the organization.
Create a positive network of conversation about the project with peers and project stakeholders.
Actively participate in implementation planning; stay involved with the project; monitor progress and remove obstacles.
Ensure that adequate resources are available or adjust the implementation plan to fit available resources.
Engage middle managers in transition planning; define their role for the transition and set clear expectations.

CHALLENGES

There are many challenges to developing a continuous quality improvement system that incorporates quality assurance monitors, performance improvement indicators, and corresponding action response plans. The point-of-care testing setting adds its own set of challenges. Physician buy-in is essential but difficult as there can be an environment of resistance to change. Overburdened work schedules and decreasing resources add to the burden of considering to implement a CQI program. Those areas that develop indicators may have difficulty with patient participation. Patient autonomy exists in the outpatient setting, patients might decline care or only partially comply with the process of care. These factors could lead to inaccurate and misleading data and the subsequent lack of benchmarking information.

The following are offered as some “rules for success”:

Undo the past.
Find a champion.
Get leadership commitment.
Involve everyone.
Overcome resistance.
Learn from failure.
Have persistence and patience.

MONITORING IMPROVEMENT

After a continuous quality improvement system is designed and implemented, it is important to develop an internal auditing system that can monitor all of the aspects of the quality system and the success of performance improvement initiatives. The system should be standardized so that it can apply to any laboratory testing area and should include all of the resources of the laboratory testing area. As expressed in the NCCLS guideline, all quality system essentials (QSEs) need to be addressed. As improvements are implemented and found to be successful, these processes become part of the standard operating procedure. The cycle continues to identify additional improvement opportunities and each opportunity is developed using the same steps.

Improvements are continuously re-evaluated as part of this cyclic process. It is helpful to include in the criteria for internal audit, not only the QSE guidelines discussed above but also all guidelines from regulatory and other accrediting bodies as the internal audit can assure success during the external audit conducted by any one of these agencies. Development of a standardized checklist assists in educating all interested parties in what is required by the guidelines and in the training of internal auditors. For obvious reasons, it is best if these auditors are not part of the everyday point-of-care testing process. For this reason, many testing areas solicit the assistance of an outside consultant to perform these internal audits. Whatever technique is used, the ultimate goal of these internal audits needs to be consultative and educational. The golden rule for an auditor should be "Don't cite anything unless you can suggest an appropriate corrective action" (R. I. Bosman, personal communication, 1979). If the monitoring system lives up to this rule, it will add to the success of the continuous quality improvement system.

REFERENCES

1. Joint Commission for Accreditation of Healthcare Organization. Comprehensive Accreditation Manual for Pathology and Clinical Laboratory Services. JCAHO, Oakbrook Terrace, IL, 2002, p GL-10.
2. *HTTP://www.aafp.org/quality/main.html* (accessed 3/02).
3. National Committee for Clinical Laboratory Standards. In vitro Diagnostic Testing; Approved Guideline. NCCLS AST-A. NCCLS, Wayne, PA, 1999.
4. National Committee for Clinical Laboratory Standards. Quality Management for Unit Use Testing. NCCLS EP18. NCCLS, Wayne, PA, 2000.
5. Department of Health and Human Services, Health Care Finance Administration. Clinical Laboratory Improvement Amendments of 1988, final rule. 42CFR 493 Subpart M, Personnel for Moderate and High Complexity Testing. Fed Regist Feb 28:7172–7183, 1992.
6. National Committee for Clinical Laboratory Standards. A Quality System Model for Healthcare. NCCLS, Wayne, PA, 1999, p 14.
7. National Committee for Clinical Laboratory Standards. A Quality System Model for Healthcare. NCCLS, Wayne, PA, 1999, p GP-26.
8. Joint Commission for Accreditation of Healthcare Organizations. Comprehensive

Accreditation Manual for Pathology and Clinical Laboratory Services. JCAHO, Oakbrook Terrace, IL, 2002, p GL-9.
9. International Organization for Standardization. ISO 9004-2000 and Healthcare, Quality Management Systems—Guidelines for Process Improvements in Healthcare Organizations. ISO, Geneva, Switzerland, 2001.
10. National Committee for Clinical Laboratory Standards. Continuous Quality Improvement: Essential Management Approaches and Their Use in Proficiency Testing. NCCLS GP-22. NCCLS, Wayne, PA, 1998.
11. *HTTP://www.aafp.org/quality/main.html* (accessed 3/02).
12. Joint Commission for Accreditation of Healthcare Organizations. Comprehensive Accreditation Manual for Pathology and Clinical Laboratory Services. JCAHO, Oakbrook Terrace, IL, 2002, p PI-3.
13. National Committee for Clinical Laboratory Standards. A Quality System Model for Healthcare. NCCLS, Wayne, PA, 1999, p GP-26.
14. National Committee for Clinical Laboratory Standards. Continuous Quality Improvement: Essential Management Approaches and Their Use in Proficiency Testing. NCCLS GP-22. NCCLS, Wayne, PA, 1998.
15. *HTTP://www.aafp.org/quality/projects/criteria/index.html* (accessed 3/02).
16. *HTTP://www.hcfa.gov/quality/10a.htm* (accessed 3/02).
17. National Committee for Clinical Laboratory Standards. Continuous Quality Improvement: Essential Management Approaches and Their Use in Proficiency Testing. NCCLS GP-22. NCCLS, Wayne, PA, 1998.
18. National Committee for Clinical Laboratory Standards. Continuous Quality Improvement: Essential Management Approaches and Their Use in Proficiency Testing. NCCLS GP-22. NCCLS, Wayne, PA, 1998.
19. Maryland Healthcare Education Institute. Quality Improvement: Methods and Tools, Skills Training for Team Leaders. MHEI, Elkridge, MD, 1995.
20. Joint Commission on Accreditation of Healthcare Organizations. Designing and Implementing and Outcomes-Based Performance Improvement Project. JCAHO, Oakbrook Terrace, IL, 1998, pp 435–445.

6

Patient Care Pathways

Dorothy Nyberg and Charlmain Johnson
The Johns Hopkins Hospital, Baltimore, Maryland, U.S.A.

INTRODUCTION

Increased competition in the healthcare industry over the past decade has placed tremendous pressure on healthcare organizations to reduce costs while maintaining or improving the quality of care. In response to these pressures, many healthcare organizations have adopted strategies to reduce unexplained variation in medical care, decrease resource utilization, and measure the outcomes of care in an attempt to identify opportunities for improvement. Case management and critical pathways are strategies that have been implemented in many hospitals to meet these challenges (1–3). Case management is a care delivery model that focuses on the delivery of high-quality care and achievement of positive patient outcomes within a designated time frame by effectively and efficiently using resources during a patient's episode of illness. A critical pathway, a tool used in case management, is a guideline that highlights key processes of care that must occur in a timely and predictable manner to achieve an appropriate length of stay and desired patient outcomes. The purpose of this chapter is to describe the development, implementation, and evaluation of critical pathways in healthcare and their role in performance improvement and evidence-based outcomes.

CRITICAL PATHWAYS

Background

The critical pathway method originated in the 1950s in the construction and engineering fields as a technique to identify the key sequence of events in a process, the beginning and end times, and the expected time frames for each activity. The purpose of this technique is to identify opportunities to improve efficiency and eliminate redundancies, to manage the time-limiting steps in the process, and to understand and coordinate the roles of multiple personnel involved in the process (1,4). Critical pathways have subsequently been used as project management tools in many different business sectors for years. In healthcare, concepts related to critical pathways were discussed and researched in the early 1970s but the fee-for-service reimbursement system did not provide incentives to hospitals and healthcare providers to implement these techniques. However, in the early 1980s, prospective payment and competitive bidding were introduced as features of hospital reimbursement systems to control escalating healthcare costs. These changes stimulated renewed interest in critical pathways and other related topics such as clinical practice guidelines and algorithms. Other factors driving this renewed interest included the increasing evidence of unexplained variation in clinical care and outcomes, a greater emphasis on the involvement of other healthcare professionals in the patient care decision-making process, the rising costs of malpractice, and a focus on outcomes management (4).

Critical pathways are based on the premise that the care of a patient with a specific condition or procedure requires many interdependent services to be provided for the patient during hospitalization. If these are not appropriately planned, coordinated, and communicated, the quality of the care decreases, delays occur, additional resources are required, and costs increase (5). It is theorized that the adaptation of critical pathways to healthcare, particularly inpatient care, can facilitate the efficient delivery of quality patient care resulting in reduced costs and improved patient safety, quality, and outcomes (6).

Definitions

The term, critical pathway, is often used interchangeably with many different terms, including clinical pathways, care paths, clinical protocols, clinical practice guidelines, and algorithms. Although the concepts of these terms differ, they are all based on the basic principle of standardizing care that is consistent with available scientific evidence and presenting that information in a format that can be easily understood by the clinicians providing care in the clinical setting. The conceptual differences in these terms are described in the following paragraphs and summarized in Figure 1.

Critical or clinical pathways are patient care management plans that display in graphic format the optimal sequencing and timing of interventions by physicians, nurses, and other staff involved in the delivery of care to the patient for a particular diagnosis or procedure. The critical pathway is developed by a multidisciplinary team of clinicians and designed to minimize delays and resource utilization, facilitate the coordination of care among the various disciplines, and maximize the quality of care (4). In healthcare, critical pathways highlight key processes of care that may include the following categories: assessments, con-

Critical Pathway	Evidence based multidisciplinary plans of care for a diagnosis or procedure; defines the optimal timing and sequencing of clinical processes; improves outcomes of care through improved coordination and communication; standardizes clinical practices.
Clinical Practice Guideline	Systematically developed statements based on scientific evidence that guide patient management decisions for specific clinical conditions; purpose is to decrease variation in clinical practices
Clinical Protocol	Decreases practice variation by prescribing treatment interventions for a specific clinical problem that may apply across diagnoses or procedures
Clinical Algorithm	Step-by-step approach involving conditional logic to analyze and solve a defined clinical problem given a particular clinical characteristic; useful to manage high-risk subgroups within a cohort of patients

Figure 1 Differentiation of terms for practice standardization.

sults, tests, treatments, diet, medications, discharge planning, patient teaching, and interventions that should occur within the designated length of stay for a diagnosis or procedure related group. Desired patient outcomes to be achieved are defined for each day or phase of care and at discharge. A clinical pathway or care path may differ from a critical pathway by incorporating more comprehensively all the clinical activities in the treatment regimen whereas a critical pathway identifies the minimal but critical clinical activities required to meet the expected outcomes within the designated time parameters. An example of a critical pathway for normal pressure hydrocephalus is presented in Figure 2.

Clinical practice guidelines are systematically developed statements based on current scientific knowledge and expert clinical judgment regarding the best ways to prevent, diagnose, treat, or manage diseases and disorders (7). Guidelines are developed by professional medical organizations and specialty societies at the national level as a resource to practitioners in making patient management decisions related to specific clinical circumstances. Guidelines address the appropriateness of care by delineating the indications for tests or treatments for a particular clinical condition (8). Critical pathways should be derived from clinical practice guidelines, which may define both the clinical processes and outcomes of care to be included on the pathway. Critical pathways are one of the tools whereby clinical practice guidelines can be adapted at the local level for implementation in a clinical setting and communicated to the clinicians at the bedside. Pathways are implemented after a clinical decision has been made to treat the patient or perform the procedure and focus on the efficiency and quality of the care provided. Critical pathways differ from clinical practice guidelines by their multidis-

JOHNS HOPKINS HOSPITAL

DEPARTMENT OF NEUROSCIENCES

NORMAL PRESSURE HYDROCEPHALUS (NPH) PATHWAY **(Target LOS: 7 days)**

NOTE: This pathway is a guideline for routine care. It requires daily updates/changes to meet unique individual patient care needs.

	GOALS	OUTCOMES
CLINIC (MD)	1. Previous MD notes, records, and consults reviewed by MD.	1. _____Met ____ Not met_____
	2. History and Physical complete (MD).	2. _____Met ____ Not met_____
	3. Patient questionnaire completed.	3. _____Met ____ Not met_____
	4. Gait videography completed.	4. _____Met ____ Not met_____
	5. Patient's meds reviewed.	5. _____Met ____ Not met_____
	6. Pre-procedure teaching completed: ➢ Risk/Benefits of: Intracranial pressure. Shunt.	6. _____Met ____ Not met_____
	7. Appropriate consults initiated and forms faxed.	7. ____SW ____OT ____PT ____PM& R _____NEUROCOGNITIVE (Argye Hillis)
MONITORING PHASE **(DAY 1)**	8. Admission orders signed by MD within one hour upon arrival to floor.	8. _____Met ____ Not met_____
	9. Consent signed and in chart (MD).	9. _____Met ____ Not met_____
	10. Neuro exam at baseline or improved.	10. _____Met ____ Not met_____
	11. Mini Mental State Exam obtained on admission	11. _____Met (_____/30) ____ Not met_____
	12. Protocols initiated.	12. _____ Elective ICP monitoring _____Mechanical restraint _____Fall
	13. Transducer and lumbar drainage system set up by RN.	13. _____Yes ____ No_____
	14. IV Saline lock inserted.	14. _____Met ____ Not met_____
	15. First dose of antibiotic given on call for insertion of lumbar catheter.	15. _____Yes ____ No_____
	16. Patient teaching complete: ➢ Hospital environment. ➢ Sleep aid. ➢ Restraints. ➢ When to call RN for assistance.	16. _____Met ____ Not met_____
	17. Need for labs evaluated.	17. _____Met ____ Not met_____
	18. Able to sleep at night.	18. _____Yes ____ No_____
	19. 30 ft walk & 180 degree turn completed (MD).	19. _____Met ____ Not met_____
	20. Lumbar dressing dry and intact.	20. _____Met ____ Not met_____
	21. Lumbar catheter intact.	21. _____Met ____ Not met_____
	22. Appropriate consults initiated.	22. _____SW _____PT _____OT
	23. Ambulating with assist twice daily.	23. _____Met once _____Met twice ____ Not met_____
	24. SW assessment completed.	24. _____Met ____ Not met_____
	25. Pain level.	25. Pain level_____/10 (<3/10) Pain level_____/10 (>3/10)_____
MONITORING PHASE **(DAY 2)**	26. Neuro exam unchanged from previous day or improved.	26. _____Met ____ Not met_____
	27. Protocols continued.	27. _____ Elective ICP monitoring _____Mechanical restraint _____Fall
	28. Able to sleep at night.	28. _____Yes ____ No_____
	29. 30 ft. walk & 180 degree turn completed (MD).	29. _____Met ____ Not met_____
	30. Lumbar dressing dry and intact.	30. _____Met ____ Not met_____
	31. Lumbar catheter intact.	31. _____Met ____ Not met_____
	32. Ambulating with assistance twice daily.	32. _____Met once _____Met twice ____ Not met_____
	33. Pain level.	33. Pain level_____/10 (<3/10) Pain level_____/10 (>3/10)_____
	34. Afebrile (<38.3C).	34. _____Met _____Not met_____

(a)

ciplinary approach to development and scope of implementation. Other distinguishing features of critical pathways are the format and comprehensiveness of their design that streamlines documentation and allows them to be used as a part of the patient medical record, often replacing other documentation entirely.

In contrast to critical pathways and clinical practice guidelines, clinical protocols prescribe treatment interventions for a specific clinical problem that may occur in patients across many different diagnostic or procedural groups. Examples of clinical protocols include the management of the patient with acute pain or the management of patients receiving sedation for diagnostic and/or invasive procedures. Like critical pathways, protocols are often based on clinical practice guidelines and may be used to decrease treatment variation (2). However, clinical protocols often focus on guideline compliance rather than the identification of the rate-limiting steps in the process of patient care delivery. They may be included as a component of a critical pathway. Protocols may or may not include a continuous monitoring and data evaluation component, which is an important feature of critical pathways.

Clinical algorithms differ from critical pathways by providing the clinician with a step-by-step approach to analyzing and solving a defined clinical problem given a particular circumstance or characteristic, such as a laboratory test result or presenting symptom. Clinical algorithms involve conditional logic, for example if/then statements, presented in a structured flowchart or decision tree that clearly guides the clinicians in making decisions about the actions to be taken for that circumstance. Algorithms are useful in the management of high-risk subgroups within the cohort of patients; however, they do not address the rate-limiting steps in the patient care process (7,9). A clinical algorithm may also be included as a component of a critical pathway. An example of a clinical algorithm guiding the selection of a treatment plan and the appropriate pathway for post allogeneic bone marrow transplant patients with liver dysfunction is presented in Figure 3.

Variance Analysis

Variance and variance analysis are key concepts in the critical pathway method. In industry, any variation in the production process is suboptimal. By defining,

---

Figure 2 (a–c) Example of a critical pathway for normal pressure hydrocephalus. Definitions: MD, medical doctor; SW, social worker; OT, occupational therapist; PT, physical therapist; PM&R, physical medicine and rehabilitation; NUS, neurosurgery; UA, urinalysis; D/C'd, discontinued; S&S, signs and symptoms; CSF, cerebrospinal fluid. (Reprinted with permission of Michael Williams, MD, Johns Hopkins Hospital, Baltimore, MD.)

JOHNS HOPKINS HOSPITAL

DEPARTMENT OF NEUROSCIENCES
NORMAL PRESSURE HYDROCEPHALUS (NPH) PATHWAY (Target LOS: 7 days)

NOTE: This pathway is a guideline for routine care. It requires daily updates/changes to meet unique individual patient care needs.

	GOALS	OUTCOMES
CSF DRAINAGE TRIAL **(DAY 3)**	35. Neuro exam unchanged from previous day or improved.	35. ____Met ____ Not met________
	36. Protocols continued.	36. ____ Elective ICP monitoring ____Mechanical restraint ____Fall
	37. 30 ft walk & 180 degree turn completed (MD).	37. ____Met ____ Not met________
	38. Lumbar dressing dry and intact.	38. ____Met ____ Not met________
	39. Lumbar catheter intact.	39. ____Met ____ Not met________
	40. Ambulating with assistance three times daily.	40. ____Met once ____Met twice ____Met three times ____ Not met
	41. Pain level.	41. Pain level ____/10 (<3/10) Pain level ____/10 (>3/10) ________
	42. Afebrile (<38.3C).	42. ____Met ____ Not Met________
	43. Consults completed.	43. ____PT/OT (by morning) ____PM & R (by evening, if appropriate).
CSF DRAINAGE TRIAL **(DAY 4)**	44. Neuro exam unchanged from previous day or improved.	44. ____Met ____ Not met________
	45. Protocols continued.	45. ____ Elective ICP monitoring ____Mechanical restraint ____Fall
	46. 30 ft walk & 180 degree turn completed (MD).	46. ____Met ____ Not met________
	47. Lumbar dressing dry and intact.	47. ____Met ____ Not met________
	48. Lumbar catheter intact.	48. ____Met ____ Not met________
	49. Ambulating with assistance three times daily.	49. ____Met once ____Met twice ____Met three times ____ Not met
	50. Pain level.	50. Pain level ____/10 (<3/10) Pain level ____/10 (>3/10) ________
	51. Afebrile (<38.3C).	51. ____Met ____ Not met________
	52. Appropriate candidate for surgery (MD).	52. ____Yes ____ No________
	If Yes, appropriate consults and tests obtained.	If Yes, (select appropriate consults) ____Anesthetist ____Neurocognitive ____NUS ____PM & R ____Chest X ray ____UA
CSF DRAINAGE TRIAL **(DAY 5)**	53. Neuro exam unchanged from previous day or improved.	53. ____Met ____ Not met________
	54. 30 ft walk & 180 degree turn completed (MD).	54. ____Met ____ Not met________
	55. Lumbar dressing dry and intact.	55. ____Met ____ Not met________
	56. Lumbar catheter intact.	56. ____Met ____ Not met________
	57. Lumbar catheter assessed for removal (MD).	57. ____Met ____ Not met________
	58. Ambulating with assistance three times daily.	58. ____Met once ____Met twice ____Met three times ____ Not met
	59. Pain level.	59. Pain level ____/10 (<3/10) Pain level ____/10 (>3/10) ________
	60. Afebrile (<38.3C).	60. ____Met ____ Not met________
	61. Appropriate candidate for surgery (MD).	61. ____Yes ____ No________
	If Yes, appropriate consults and tests obtained.	If Yes (select appropriate consults) ____Anesthetist ____Neurocognitive ____NUS ____PM & R ____Chest X ray ____UA

(b)

Figure 2 Continued

JOHNS HOPKINS HOSPITAL

DEPARTMENT OF NEUROSCIENCES

NORMAL PRESSURE HYDROCEPHALUS (NPH) PATHWAY **(Target LOS: 7 days)**

NOTE: This pathway is a guideline for routine care. It requires daily updates/changes to meet unique individual patient care needs.

	GOALS	OUTCOMES
CSF DRAINAGE TRIAL	62. Neuro exam unchanged from previous day or improved.	62. _____Met ____ Not met____________
	63. 30 ft walk & 180 degree turn completed (MD).	63. _____Met ____ Not met____________
	64. Lumbar catheter removed (MD).	64. _____Met ____ Not met____________
	65. One additional antibiotic dose administered after lumbar drain D/C'd.	65. _____Met ____ Not met____________
(DAY 6)	66. Ambulating with assistance three times daily.	66. _____Met ____ Not met____________
	67. Pain level.	67. Pain level ______/10 (<3/10) Pain level _____/10 (>3/10) __________
	68. Afebrile (<38.3C).	68. _____Met ____ Not met____________
	69. Appropriate candidate for surgery (MD).	69. _____Yes ____ No____________
	If Yes, appropriate consults and tests obtained.	If Yes (select consults) _____Anesthetist _____Neurocognitive _____NUS _____PM & R _____ Chest X ray _____UA
DISCHARGE DAY	70. Neuro exam unchanged from previous day or improved.	70. _____Met ____ Not met____________
	71. Mini mental State Exam obtained at discharge.	71. _____Met (_____/30) ____ Not met____________
	72. 30 ft walk & 180 degree turn completed (MD).	72. _____Met ____ Not met____________
	73. Ambulating with assistance three times daily.	73. _____Met ____ Not met____________
	74. Pain level.	74. Pain level ______/10 (<3/10) Pain level _____/10 (>3/10) __________
	75. Afebrile (<38.3C).	75. _____Met ____ Not met____________
	76. Appropriate candidate for surgery (MD).	76. _____Yes ____ No____________
	If Yes, appropriate consults initiated.	If Yes (select consults) _____Anesthetist _____Neurocognitive _____NUS _____PM & R _____ Chest X ray _____ UA _____SW (for subactue facility upon discharge).
	77. Chest X-ray and UA completed if returning for surgery (MD).	77. _____Met ____ Not met____________
	78. Discharge teaching complete: ➢ S & S of meningitis. ➢ S & S of low CSF pressure.	78. _____Met ____ Not met____________
	79. If applicable, surgery date obtained.	79. _____Surgery necessary (_____/_____/_____) Date _____Surgery not needed

(c)

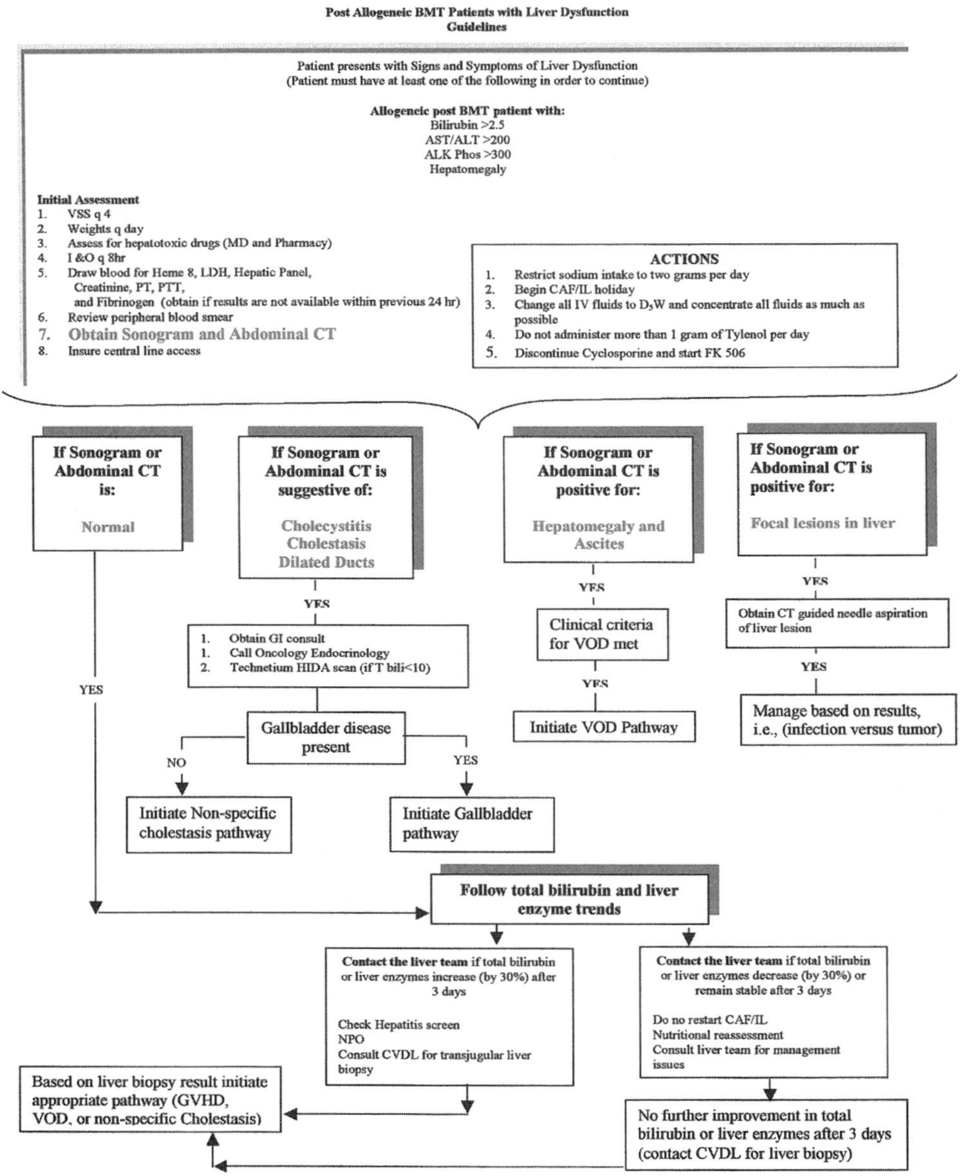
Post Allogeneic BMT Patients with Liver Dysfunction
Guidelines
Patient presents with Signs and Symptoms of Liver Dysfunction
(Patient must have at least one of the following in order to continue)
Allogeneic post BMT patient with:
Bilirubin >2.5
AST/ALT >200
ALK Phos >300
Hepatomegaly
Initial Assessment
1. VSS q 4
2. Weights q day
3. Assess for hepatotoxic drugs (MD and Pharmacy)
4. I &O q 8hr
5. Draw blood for Heme 8, LDH, Hepatic Panel, Creatinine, PT, PTT, and Fibrinogen (obtain if results are not available within previous 24 hr)
6. Review peripheral blood smear
7. Obtain Sonogram and Abdominal CT
8. Insure central line access
ACTIONS
1. Restrict sodium intake to two grams per day
2. Begin CAF/IL holiday
3. Change all IV fluids to D5W and concentrate all fluids as much as possible
4. Do not administer more than 1 gram of Tylenol per day
5. Discontinue Cyclosporine and start FK 506
If Sonogram or Abdominal CT is:
Normal
YES
If Sonogram or Abdominal CT is suggestive of:
Cholecystitis
Cholestasis
Dilated Ducts
YES
1. Obtain GI consult
1. Call Oncology Endocrinology
2. Technetium HIDA scan (if T bili<10)
Gallbladder disease present
NO
Initiate Non-specific cholestasis pathway
YES
Initiate Gallbladder pathway
If Sonogram or Abdominal CT is positive for:
Hepatomegaly and Ascites
YES
Clinical criteria for VOD met
YES
Initiate VOD Pathway
If Sonogram or Abdominal CT is positive for:
Focal lesions in liver
YES
Obtain CT guided needle aspiration of liver lesion
YES
Manage based on results, i.e., (infection versus tumor)
Follow total bilirubin and liver enzyme trends
Contact the liver team if total bilirubin or liver enzymes increase (by 30%) after 3 days
Check Hepatitis screen
NPO
Consult CVDL for transjugular liver biopsy
Contact the liver team if total bilirubin or liver enzymes decrease (by 30%) or remain stable after 3 days
Do no restart CAF/IL
Nutritional reassessment
Consult liver team for management issues
Based on liver biopsy result initiate appropriate pathway (GVHD, VOD, or non-specific Cholestasis)
No further improvement in total bilirubin or liver enzymes after 3 days (contact CVDL for liver biopsy)

sequencing, and timing the processes on a critical pathway, managers can target areas that are critical, measure variation, and try to make improvements. Once steps are taken to improve the process, performance measurements are repeated. Over time, variation will decrease, the time it took to complete the pathway will decrease, costs will decrease, and the quality of production will improve. Another approach to assessing variance is the development of performance measurements for the costs or time schedule for completion of the project. When these measurements exceed the pre-established thresholds, an analysis of the processes would be made to determine the cause of the variance (10).

In healthcare, a variance occurs when the patient's course of hospital stay, treatment plan, or expected outcomes do not conform to that of a critical pathway. Performance measurements may include financial, clinical, or quality measures. Financial measures include the projected length of stay, costs of the hospital stay, or utilization of resources for a specific diagnosis or procedure. Clinical measures relate to the processes or outcomes of care for a specific patient population. Quality measures such as complications or an unplanned return to the operating room or intensive care unit are also examples of variance from the pathway. Identification and analysis of the factors that contribute to variance and the interventions to improve those factors are the key features in process improvement and outcomes management.

Variances may be positive or negative, avoidable or unavoidable, and can be classified according to the sources of variance: patient/family, health/illness, caregiver/clinician, and hospital/community. A patient variance may be caused by an action or characteristic of the patient such as refusing a test, the complexity or severity of their medical condition, or their socioeconomic circumstances. Family actions/failure to act may also contribute to variances from the pathway. Examples of family variance may include their lack of availability for decision making or lack of resources to support the patient after discharge. Caregiver/clinician variances may include delays in discharge planning, failure to prescribe a recommended medication, excessive ordering of laboratory tests, or late discharge orders. Systems barriers, such as equipment failures, a lost laboratory result, a delayed consult, unavailable diagnostic testing on the weekends, or the

---

Figure 3 Clinical algorithm for post allogeneic bone marrow transplant patients with liver dysfunction. Definitions: BMT, bone marrow transplant; AST, aspartate aminotransferase; ALT, alanine aminotransferase; ALK, alkaline; VSS, vital signs; I&O, intake and output; LDH, lactate dehydrogenase; PT, prothrombin time; PTT, partial thromboplastin time; CT Scan, computed tomographic scan; CAF/IL holiday, complete alimentation formula/intralipids; IV, intravenous; D5W, dextrose 5% in water; HIDA, hepatoiminodiacetic acid; T bili, total bilirubin; VOD, veno-occlusive disease; GVHD, graft-versus-host disease; NPO, nothing per os (by mouth); CVDL, cardiovascular diagnostic laboratory.

lack of available general care beds to transfer a patient from the intensive care unit, can cause significant variances from the pathway. Other sources of variance can include the lack of adequate dialysis beds in the community, unavailable beds in a rehabilitation facility, or the shortage of registered nurses in home care agencies to deliver services needed by the patient after discharge from the hospital. All of these variances can have an impact on the efficiency, quality, and cost of care. Payers often deny payment to the hospital for what they perceive to be inefficiencies in care delivery and a waste of their financial resources.

When applied to healthcare, some physicians have raised concerns about the critical pathway technique. Every et al. (2) argue that unlike manufacturing, not all variation in patient care is negative. Individual patient factors may contribute to variation that cannot and should not be controlled by the system. Unlike manufacturing where products are standardized, patients are different and may not fit within the pathway.

Critical pathways are guidelines for patient care and should be flexible enough to be individualized to meet the patient's unique needs. Normal variation is expected among patients due to individual patient factors and should be anticipated in pathway development and implementation. There may also be variation that is not expected to occur normally during the care process, such as an exacerbation of congestive heart failure on the first postoperative day. In this situation, a patient may not be able to remain on a pathway and an individualized plan of care is developed for the patient. Data on individual patient variations that are not expected to occur should be aggregated and analyzed over time to determine if there are patterns or trends that identify opportunities to improve care or modify the pathway.

Goals of Critical Pathways

The specific goals of critical pathways when used to develop an interdisciplinary plan of care for a specific diagnosis or procedure usually include the following (1):

- Selecting the "best practice" based on available medical evidence when unnecessary variation in practice exists
- Defining the appropriate standards for the expected length of hospital stay and use of resources such as tests and treatments
- Examining the interrelations among the different steps in the care process to improve the coordination of care or decrease the time spent in the rate-limiting steps
- Identifying and resolving systems barriers
- Giving the interdisciplinary team caring for patients with a specific diagnosis or procedure a common game plan from which to view and understand their various roles in the overall care delivery process

- Enhancing communication and collaboration among the multidisciplinary care providers in the planning and delivery of care
- Decreasing documentation burdens
- Improving patient satisfaction with care by educating patients and their families about the plan of care and involving them more fully in its implementation
- Providing a framework for collecting data on the care process so that providers can learn how often and why patients do not follow an expected course during their hospitalization
- Operationalizing performance improvement at the direct patient care level
- Measuring and managing patient outcomes

CRITICAL CARE PATHWAY DEVELOPMENT AND IMPLEMENTATION PROCESS

Selecting a Diagnosis or Procedure

The selection of a diagnosis or procedure for which a pathway will be developed begins with a review of current practices. This review process may occur in a variety of ways. Typically, hospitals analyze the top 10 diagnosis related groups (DRGs) by department or service based on highest volume, cost, and length of stay. Other approaches include the identification of the diagnoses or procedures that are high risk, problem prone, or have complex medical management plans. There may be instances when the clinical team perceives there are significant variations in treatment regimens or inefficiencies in the care delivery processes. A thorough analysis of data for that specific diagnosis or procedure is conducted to validate these perceptions. The analysis may include a retrospective review of the medical records, discussions about current practice patterns with a team of key interdisciplinary clinicians involved in the care of that patient population, and a detailed descriptive analysis of the clinical and financial data available for the diagnosis group (DRG) or diagnosis/procedure classification (ICD-9). Financial data include length of stay, total charges or costs if available, types and volumes of diagnostic tests, treatments, therapies, pharmaceuticals, operating room and room charges, and denied payment days by the payer. Financial analysis may also include a comparison of the length of stay, case mix index, and charges with similar hospitals. Comparison of physician practices profiles for the same diagnosis or procedure may identify variations in practice and opportunities to standardize care. Quality indicators such as rates for complications, infection, mortality, and unplanned hospital readmissions are also reflective of current practices. Analyses of these data in the pathway development process provide a focus for the team to identify cost and practice patterns that need further investigation and help to identify opportunities for improving the processes and outcomes of care for this patient population.

A review of the literature for relevant research or clinical practice guidelines is an important step in analyzing current processes to determine if practice is evidence based. This step is also important to assure that the pathway developed by the team incorporates tests and treatments that are appropriate and cost effective. However, there may be situations in which there are no clinical protocols or clinical practice guidelines published in the literature to guide pathway development. The following is an example of how a multidisciplinary team addressed this dilemma for the post allogeneic bone marrow transplant patients with liver dysfunction at the Johns Hopkins Hospital Oncology Center, Baltimore, MD.

The hematological medical and nursing staff identified inconsistencies in the medical and nursing management of patients with liver dysfunction in the Oncology Center. These inconsistencies were evident by the variability in the types and number of diagnostic tests and laboratory tests ordered by the physicians. The high mortality rate for this patient population was also a concern of the clinicians. Based on these findings, a hematological multidisciplinary team consisting of three oncologists, a gastroenterologist, clinical nurses, nurse manager, and critical pathway facilitator developed a diagnostic algorithm that delineated the criteria for liver dysfunction and outlined a sequence of decisionmaking steps to guide the diagnosis, and management of patients with liver dysfunction. Four criteria for liver dysfunction were defined. If the patient met one of the criteria, specific monitoring, diagnostic and laboratory tests, radiological procedures, and pharmacological actions are initiated. One or more of six diagnostic conclusions could be made based on the results of the diagnostic tests: veno-occlusive disease (VOD), graft-versus-host disease (GVHD), gallbladder disease, nonspecific cholestasis, focal lesions in the liver, or no demonstrable pathology. Laboratory test results for total bilirubin and liver enzyme trends dictate subsequent patient management decisions that could potentially include a transjugular liver biopsy. Based on the results of these tests, the appropriate medical and nursing management of these patients was outlined on a critical pathway. This process of standardizing the clinical management of the patient with liver dysfunction resulted in the development of one diagnostic algorithm, four critical pathways, and three preprinted physician order sets. The diagnostic algorithm is presented in Figure 3.

Another approach hospitals have used to establish priorities for pathway development has been in response to the Centers for Medicare and Medicaid Services' (CMS, formerly Health Care Financing Administration) Health Care Quality Improvement Program for Medicare beneficiaries (12). Six clinical areas were identified by CMS as priorities for improvement due to their importance as causes of morbidity and mortality among the Medicare population and accounting for substantial numbers of hospitalizations and healthcare costs. These priorities include acute myocardial infarction, breast cancer, diabetes, heart failure, pneumonia, and stroke.

The Centers for Medicare and Medicaid Services conducted careful measurement of patterns of care for each diagnosis utilizing Medicare claims data. This analysis identified variation in practices across the country and opportunities to improve care. As a result, specific processes of care designed to improve patient outcomes were defined based on a review of the medical evidence by an expert panel of clinicians. Quality measures based on the evidence were developed for each diagnosis. For example, the process of care objectives defined to decrease the morbidity and mortality associated with community-acquired pneumonia in Medicare beneficiaries admitted to the hospital include

- To increase the number of inpatients who receive the initial antibiotic dose within 8 hr of hospital arrival
- To increase the use of initial antibiotic therapy consistent with current guidelines
- To increase the collection of blood cultures prior to the initial antibiotic dose
- To increase the number of hospitalized patients who are screened for or given pneumococcal and influenza vaccines

To achieve these objectives, it was expected that each hospital would develop a strategy to improve these processes of care in their setting. Critical pathways and physician order sets for these clinical priority areas have been the strategies implemented in many hospitals. Thus, these nationally defined clinical priorities have driven the establishment of the priorities for pathway development in many organizations.

Pathway Development Team

A successful pathway needs to be developed by a diverse team represented by all clinical disciplines involved in the care of patients with a specific diagnosis or procedure and who have an interest in continuously improving the quality of care for these patients. Each team member brings a unique clinical perspective to the multidisciplinary plan of care for that patient population. This multidisciplinary team lends credibility to the pathway and builds a foundation of support among all clinicians, particularly when the team is lead by a physician expert. Active physician participation and leadership are crucial to the successful development and implementation of the pathway. Depending on the diagnosis or procedure, other representatives may include a clinical nurse specialist or nurse practitioner, clinical nurse, nurse manager, social worker, pharmacist, pathologist, radiologist, dietician, respiratory therapist, physical and/or occupational therapist, home care nurse, and performance improvement/utilization management specialist. Financial analysts and medical record coders can also contribute significantly to the pathway development process.

The multidisciplinary team defines collaboratively what they hypothesize to be the best way to manage the care of patients with a specific diagnosis or procedure. They define the key clinical activities and sequence the activities to be most efficient and cost effective. Appropriate standards are defined for the length of stay, types and number of tests, treatments, medications, and other ancillary resources required to care for the patient. The team also defines boundaries of the pathway for the particular patient population. For example, the pathway may be limited to the episode of acute care hospitalization or it may extend from the inpatient to the outpatient settings, such as a clinic or home healthcare, in order to coordinate a smooth transition and appropriate follow-up care for the patient. The critical pathway team also identifies the outcomes to be measured, strategies for data collection, and the evaluation methods that will be used to determine the appropriateness and effectiveness of the care provided. Many times, additional management tools are developed in conjunction with the critical pathway. These tools may include preprinted physician order sets, clinical or diagnostic algorithms, patient/family teaching pathways, and preprinted discharge instructions.

The following is an example of how a multidisciplinary team responsible for the care of patients with community-acquired pneumonia determined how the clinical processes of care defined in the CMS Health Care Quality Improvement Program would be implemented in their hospital. Coordination of care among the hospital's emergency department, clinical laboratory, infectious disease service, and medical service where these patients were admitted was vital in order to achieve the process of care objectives. Clinicians representing all of these clinical areas were represented on the team. The team analyzed their current practices and the baseline data provided by the state peer review organization regarding their current performance in meeting the clinical objectives for community-acquired pneumonia. They then identified the following changes in the processes of care that needed to be made:

- Development of screening criteria to be used by the triage nurse in the emergency department to identify patients at risk for community-acquired pneumonia
- Implementation of procedures in the emergency department to expedite obtaining a chest x-ray, sputum specimens, and blood cultures on patients identified to be at risk
- Implementation of procedures in the clinical laboratory to expedite the analysis of sputum and blood cultures within a designated time frame

- Development of guidelines by the infectious disease and clinical laboratory physicians for antibiotic usage based on the organism
- Modification of patient flow in the emergency department to assure that patients with community-acquired pneumonia received their initial antibiotic dose within 8 hr of hospital arrival
- Development of criteria to guide decision making by the inpatient clinicians regarding the appropriate time for changing the antibiotic from intravenous to oral administration

The multidisciplinary team standardized the plan of care for these patients through the development of an algorithm for screening at triage and a critical pathway and preprinted physician order sets for the emergency department and the inpatient unit. An antibiotic reference was developed for physicians to guide the appropriate selection of antibiotics based on the organism. This reference was included on the pathway. The quality indicators defined by CMS for community-acquired pneumonia were included as the outcome measures for the pathway.

Pathway Approval Process

The final draft of the pathway and associated tools are reviewed and approved by various disciplines involved in the delivery of patient care for that diagnosis or procedure prior to implementation of the pathway. The extent of the approval process may vary by institution and could include representatives with a broader perspective within the organization. For example, the review board may include a clinical pharmacologist representing the pharmacy and therapeutics committee, the director of the clinical laboratory, and an attorney for the hospital.

The clinical pharmacologist reviews the medications that the pathway team has selected to be used in the care of these patients and either approves or makes recommendations based on the efficacy and cost effectiveness of alternative medications. Prevention of medication errors is a high priority in this review process. The clinical pharmacologist also focuses on the accuracy of the dosing, frequency of administration, route, and clarity of the preprinted physician orders that includes spelling and use of approved abbreviations.

The director of the clinical laboratory focuses on the appropriateness of selected laboratory tests, the frequency of testing, and the antibiotic selections. Questions are frequently raised regarding the rationale for the laboratory tests that were chosen. These questions may include the following: the necessity of the test, whether a panel of tests would be more appropriate than an individual test, the frequency of ordering the test, the necessity of ordering paired tests such as a prothrombin time/partial thromboplastin time (PT/PTT) and whether therapy will be changed based on one or both of the results, what evidence supports the use of the selected medication, and whether the medication needs therapeutic monitoring and the appropriate frequency of that monitoring. The appropriate use of antibiotics is a high priority in this review process because of the problems with antibiotic overuse, misuse, and drug-resistant organisms. The multidisciplinary team benefits from the clinical pathologist's clinical expertise and up-to-date knowledge of the evidence regarding the efficacy of antibiotics. Another benefit of obtaining approval for specific antibiotic usage during the pathway development step is that it eliminates a later step that the physician would have to take when an antibiotic requires approval by the Infectious Disease Service before it can be ordered.

The hospital attorney reviews the pathways and preprinted physician order sets for potential risk management issues. Each statement on the pathway and order set is critiqued for clarity. From a legal perspective, the pathway reflects the guideline of care for that diagnosis or procedure and must be able to be defended in a court of law.

The approval of pathways and order sets by the review board can prolong the process of pathway development because the reviewers frequently ask to review the medical research, protocols, or clinical practice guidelines used by the team to develop the pathway. The reviewers will consult with the physician leaders for the pathway when they need further clarification regarding the rationale for some aspect of the plan of care. However, the review process is an essential final step to ensure the plan of care is evidence based and safe for the patient.

The flowchart in Figure 4 outlines the pathway development process. It is important to recognize all the activities involved and the time it takes to complete each activity. Six months is the projected time frame to completely design and implement a new critical pathway at the Johns Hopkins Hospital. One of the major challenges in meeting this target is the limited availability of the multidisciplinary team members due to their competing clinical responsibilities.

Pathway Implementation

In order to optimize the adoption of critical pathways, an organization must first examine its capability for change, the availability of change agents, and its implementation strategies (13). Critical pathways should be thought of in terms of a conscious, deliberate, and collaborative plan to improve clinical, financial, patient-reported outcomes, and the efficiency of the system. As a result, a pathway often involves the implementation of changes in practice, clinical processes, technology, and clinician behavior. Acceptance and adherence to the changes defined on the pathway by all clinicians are essential for the pathway to be successful. To achieve this goal, the implementation plan should (1) take into consideration the factors and barriers that impede change, (2) anticipate potential reactions and

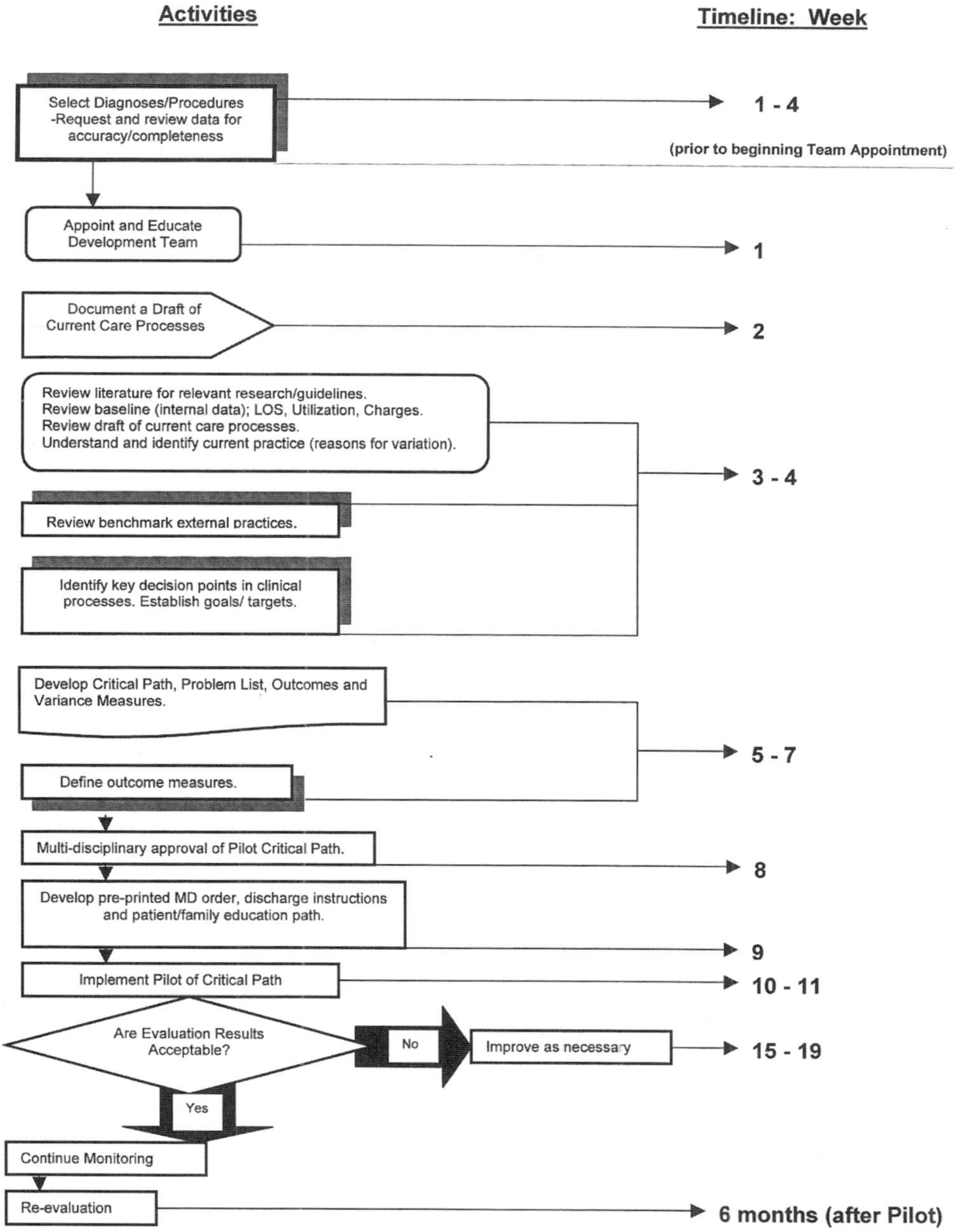

Figure 4 Critical path development process.

resistance of staff to change, (3) include interventions that target specific barriers to change and acceptance of pathways, and (4) include a committed team of clinical champions to promote and build support for the use of the pathway. Cabana et al. (14) developed a theoretical framework that identifies barriers to physician adherence to clinical practice guidelines in relation to behavior change. The authors of this chapter believe these barriers can also be applied to all clinicians' acceptance and adherence to critical pathways. Cabana et al.'s framework has been adapted and is presented in Figure 5. The barriers identified by Cabana et al. are discussed in more detail later in this chapter when the challenges to pathway development and implementation are presented.

Prior to implementation of a pathway, education of all hospital staff involved in the care of the patient population is vital. Nurses, physicians, and other care providers who have not been directly involved in the development of the pathway should understand and accept the goals of the pathway and the justification for the suggested length of hospital stay and care processes as a whole. The inclusion and exclusion criteria should be clearly defined as a guideline for the staff to ensure that the appropriate pathway is implemented for the right patient population. The inclusion criteria further defines subgroups of the patient population within a diagnostic or procedural category and may be further refined based on such things as the complexity level of the patient, results of a diagnostic test, or age groupings. Patients admitted with known complications or comorbidities are often excluded from the pathway since their anticipated clinical course may not be consistent with the pathway. It should be made clear to staff what constitutes removing the patient from a pathway, otherwise known as "falling off the pathway," and the actions to take when this occurs. "Falling off the pathway" means the plan of care outlined on the pathway is no longer appropriate for the patient due to the complexity or severity of the patient's clinical course. In these instances, an individualized plan of care must be developed to meet the unique needs of that patient.

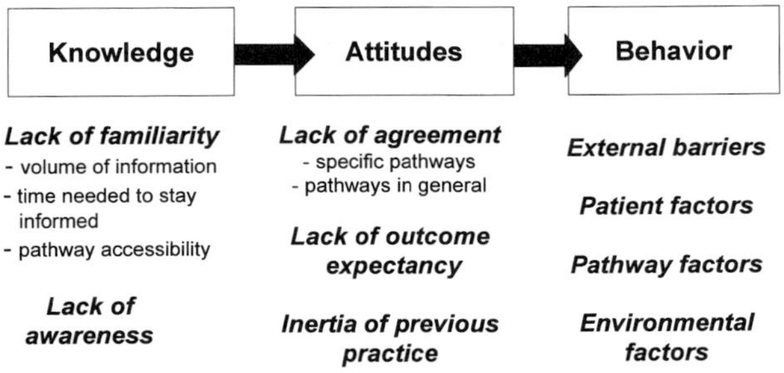

Figure 5 Barriers to clinician adherence to pathways. (Adapted from Ref. 14.)

Roles and responsibilities of the staff from each involved discipline must be clearly defined. Education should address who is responsible for initiating the pathway, how to document the pathway, and the mechanism for capturing data on variances or outcomes. The staff should be informed about how the outcomes of care will be measured and used to improve care. Educational sessions should continue on a regular basis even after pathways are implemented. This becomes extremely important as medical practices change and modifications to the pathway are required. Orientation of new employees and staff turnover will also necessitate more frequent educational sessions.

Clinical champions for each discipline involved in the pathway are key to successful implementation. The physician champion should be a clinical expert in the management of the diagnosis or procedure for which the pathway is developed and an opinion leader who is trusted by colleagues and able to build consensus for clinical change. Clinical champions in nursing and other involved disciplines are needed to promote the pathway, clarify questions, obtain feedback from clinicians regarding modifications that may be needed, and monitor the change process. Emphasis on how the pathway will benefit the patient as well as the staff is important. Benefits to the staff could include streamlined documentation, enhanced communication between clinicians, and an overall understanding of the plan of care and desired outcomes for the patient population.

Clinicians want to be assured that the critical pathways can be realistically implemented in the clinical setting and are dynamic enough to incorporate the latest medical evidence into clinical practice. The implementation plan should address these concerns by including a pilot evaluation of new pathways with a few patients to determine if the clinical processes defined by the team can be implemented effectively in the clinical setting. The pathway would be modified based on feedback from the clinicians utilizing the pathway during the pilot. After successful implementation, critical pathways should be reviewed and modified regularly based on changes in practice, new technology, and the availability of resources in other settings. A thorough analysis of pathway evaluation data and patient outcomes should drive any performance improvement initiatives and modifications to the pathway.

Critical pathways may focus on an episode of acute care or cover the continuum of care across many health care arenas such as a department, several hospital units, outpatient settings, or multiple hospitals. Once the pathway has been successfully implemented, one or several clinicians should be appointed to monitor the use of the pathway. At the Johns Hopkins Hospital, this responsibility is a shared responsibility between critical pathway facilitators, case managers, and senior staff nurses. Other hospitals have developed a case management program using case managers to follow the patient's progress on the pathway concurrently. Still other organizations many utilize a collaborative approach similar to that in place at the Vanderbilt University Medical Center, Nashville, TN, where case managers, social workers and utilization management nurses monitor specific patient populations. If pathways are shared by multiple hospitals or settings, a coordinator at each site is needed to develop and lead the implementation efforts and oversee the ongoing use of the pathway.

Finally, a critical pathway may be used as a part of a research study. The implementation plan in this instance would be developed as part of the research protocol. The research protocol would outline the expectations for the study, the roles of the key clinicians, and the activities that are expected during the training and implementation periods.

Challenges to Pathway Development and Implementation

One of the major challenges to pathway development and implementation is the complexity of medical diagnoses and their associated comorbidities and complications. Experience with pathways has demonstrated that surgical procedures lend themselves better to pathways than medical diagnoses because the anticipated course of care for a surgical procedure tends to be more clinically predictable. For most medical diagnoses, the greater heterogeneity among patients due to their comorbidities and disease progression makes it more difficult to translate patient care into pathways (1). Medical patients who have multiple diagnoses do not fit within any single standardized pathway. The severity of the patient's medical condition also determines whether the patient progresses according to the designated time frame of the pathway or requires additional ancillary resources beyond those defined on the pathway. The patient may also have other socioeconomic and psychological comorbidities that present additional challenges to adherence to the plan of care defined via the pathway.

Institutions deal with complex medical diagnoses in different ways. For example, some institutions decide not to develop highly complicated pathways, such as clinical trials for oncological diagnoses or post myocardial infarction with multiple organ insults. Other institutions establish specific exclusion criteria thereby targeting the medical pathway for a very select group of patients with few comorbidities and a minor level of disease severity. Other structured care methodologies, such as preprinted physician order sets, a treatment or diagnostic algorithm, or other clinical decision support systems that prompt compliance with medical therapies, may be more appropriate for medical patients than a critical pathway (3). An important step in addressing the challenges of developing a critical pathway for a medical diagnosis is to clearly define the clinical problem or the clinical practice that needs to be improved and then determine which structured care methodology is most appropriate for achieving the desired outcome.

The major challenges to pathway implementation are the barriers that limit or restrict the clinicians' acceptance and adherence to the multidisciplinary plan of care defined by the team. Cabana et al. (14) categorized these barriers into groups based on whether they affect physician knowledge, attitude, or behavior. In this chapter, the barriers are described in terms of how they apply to any clinicians' adherence to critical pathways.

First, the lack of awareness by the physicians or other clinicians that a pathway exists makes implementation difficult. Despite educational sessions that are provided when a pathway is initially implemented, turnover of staff can complicate sustained implementation. If clinicians are aware that a pathway exists but are not familiar with the content of the pathway, attempts at implementation and ongoing use will slowly erode. Implementation strategies that make the pathways and their goals highly visible and communicated throughout the organization are vitally important. Strategies include ongoing education, reminders, clinical champions, and integration of critical pathway outcomes and performance improvement initiatives into the organization's formalized performance improvement program.

Second, the lack of agreement among the clinicians with the multidisciplinary plan developed by the team can occur for a variety of reasons. There may be differences in the interpretation of the plan and/or disagreement as to its applicability to the patient population for which it was developed. Physicians may perceive that the pathway is oversimplified or represents "cookbook medicine" and reduces their professional autonomy in treating patients. A clinician may believe that the pathway lacks credibility and will not lead to improved outcomes. Disagreements about clinical practice need to be resolved before the pathway is implemented; otherwise, it will cause conflict between practitioners about patient care decisions. An explanation of the rationale for the development of the pathway and the goals to be achieved should be provided during the development and implementation phases.

Inertia of previous practice is another example of a barrier that can impede clinicians' adherence to pathways. As discussed earlier, pathways are deliberate plans to improve care that may involve change in practices, technology, or clinical processes. A change in practice requires a conscious effort and motivation to change on the part of the clinicians. This can be more difficult when there are time constraints and clinicians find that the familiar is the most expedient approach to the workload. A demonstration of how the changes in practice will improve patient outcomes is important in order to motivate the clinician to change behavior.

There are external barriers that may also impede the clinicians' adherence to a pathway. One such barrier may be the format of the pathway. Clinicians describe some pathway formats as cumbersome, inconvenient to use in the paper version, and too static to modify to fit individual patient needs. An automated medical record that incorporates pathways with prompts that increase the clinicians' awareness of the existence and content of the pathway, preprinted physician order sets, and links to clinical and financial outcomes could address this barrier. However, an organization's strategic plan for implementing automated systems is usually outside the control of the clinicians. The automation of critical pathways and preprinted order sets should be a future goal of healthcare organizations as they make decisions regarding electronic medical records and provider order entry systems.

Another proven challenge with critical pathways in the healthcare setting has been the approach and resources available to collect and analyze pathway variances. Although this step is important for identifying opportunities for improvement, it is challenging because the critical pathway is a series of time-associated actions and multiple data points can overwhelm data collection and analysis. The lack of integrated clinical and financial information systems compound the challenges of data collection and analysis. In order to address these challenges, key process and outcome measures for variance analysis must be selected carefully by the multidisciplinary team responsible for the development and implementation of the pathway, as these areas will become the focus for performance improvement. Priorities should be established to measure variances that are clinically critical to patient outcomes and/or result in substantial use of resources.

Requirements for Success

Physician leadership, particularly by the opinion leaders in the clinical specialty, is the primary driving force that leads to the acceptance and success of critical pathways. Physicians often express dissatisfaction with how patients are managed. An important strategy for garnering their leadership and commitment to the process is to address their goals to improve the quality, efficiency, and cost effectiveness of care. Additional goals can be achieved when physician champions utilize pathways to expand their knowledge about the financial implications of the care provided, to educate the payers about the treatment plan and management needs of atypical and complex procedures or diagnoses, to ensure timely involvement of key interdisciplinary staff, and to aid the novice and expert clinician to quickly assess where a patient should be in the treatment plan at any phase during the hospital encounter.

Another important requirement for the success of pathways is the commitment of the organization's administrative and clinical leadership to use critical pathways as a strategy to analyze clinical and financial practices and improve outcomes. Commitment to the performance improvement process via pathways should be evident in the strategic initiatives of the organization. The overall goals and objectives to be achieved by critical pathways should also be clearly defined. The development, implementation, and evaluation of patient care via the use of pathways require substantial institutional resources to be successful. The multidisciplinary team that develops the pathway must assume ownership and make an ongoing commitment to improving patient care based on the analyses of the clinical and financial outcomes.

A third requirement for success is the use of data. One strategy for gaining the clinicians' acceptance and use of the pathway is to demonstrate where there is a deficit in the performance of a clinical process or achievement of a desired patient outcome and how the pathway will improve the deficiency. This demonstration involves the use of baseline clinical data and comparative benchmarks that are accepted as credible by the clinicians. Interventions to address the performance problem should be determined by the data. Feedback should be provided to the clinicians as to whether the interventions made a difference in clinical practice and patient outcomes. Initiatives undertaken to improve performance should be achievable in a reasonable time frame and visible to the participants. This strategy builds support for successful implementation and use of pathways. It also demonstrates to the organizational leadership that resources devoted to critical pathways are worth the investment.

A final requirement for success is the alignment of incentives between the hospital and the physicians. This can be successfully accomplished in institutions that have implemented cost accounting systems that provide a mechanism for conducting detailed clinical and financial practice analyses. Analysis of clinical outcomes in conjunction with revenue and profit analysis of specific diagnostic or procedural categories helps to identify the areas that achieve the best clinical outcomes and are most profitable to the hospital. Understanding the financial and clinical impact of resource consumption, timing of tests, type of laboratory tests, and diagnostic procedures performed guides the clinicians in formulating plans to improve clinical and financial performance. An organizational strategy for clinical departments to share in the organization's profit margin provides incentives to the clinicians to be more fiscally responsible in clinical care. This can help to maintain a balance between quality and cost.

CRITICAL PATHWAY EVALUATION AND OUTCOMES

Outcomes refer to a measurable change in health status or behavior of patients as a result of an intervention. The evaluative part of the critical pathway process involves an analysis of key outcomes identified by the pathway development team. Desired and undesirable outcomes help to determine the effectiveness of the pathway as well as the next performance improvement strategy. The selection of a vital few outcomes that can be measured and understood well is more beneficial than the collection of data on so many outcomes that the analysis and interpretation become difficult and meaningless for the multidisciplinary team.

Analyses of patient outcomes provide the opportunity to demonstrate how specific practices contribute to patient care. The concept of outcomes management connects quality, cost, patient satisfaction, and the efficiency of the system (15). Therefore, indicators that measure cost, quality, and patient satisfaction should be the outcomes collected and analyzed for a pathway. Quality of life measures would be significant to measure if the pathway is developed for a patient population with a chronic condition or life-threatening diagnosis (16).

Outcomes can be classified into the five major groupings presented in Figure 6: clinical, financial, quality, variance analysis, and patient perception. Clinical outcomes are an assessment of how well the patient is able to function or responds physiologically or psychologically to medical and nursing interventions. Functional outcomes refer to the maintenance or improvement in the patient's physical functioning, such as their ability to perform day-to-day activities independently or with assistance. Financial outcomes reflect resource consumption, which can be measured by length of hospital stay, physician practice profiles, average charge per day, and denied payment days by the insurer. Laboratory testing is one of the more variable categories of charges because of practice variation among the physicians or service responsible for the patient. The financial implications of the types and frequency of laboratory tests should be taken into consideration when orders are written. Quality is influenced by the medical care delivered and is measured by events such as unplanned readmissions to the hospital, unscheduled returns to the emergency department or operating room, complications, and mortality rates. The patient's perceptions about their experiences during the hospital episode and their satisfaction with the care received and the providers of that care are important outcomes to measure. Examples of perceptual outcomes include satisfaction with: pain control, interpersonal interactions with clinicians and staff, access to care, or discharge readiness.

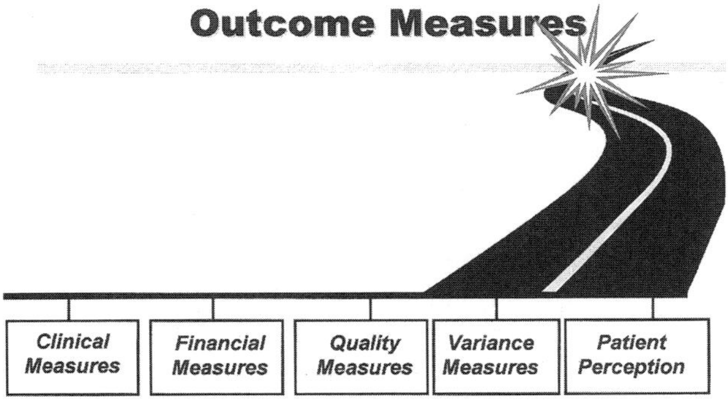

Figure 6 Classification of outcome measures.

The following is an example of the critical pathway outcomes that were identified by the multidisciplinary stroke team at the Johns Hopkins Hospital when a comprehensive stroke unit was established to provide state-of-the-art stroke therapy. Research studies have shown that comprehensive stroke programs decrease morbidity, mortality, and length of stay. An important strategy for standardizing the clinical practices in stroke care and incorporating the clinical processes recommended by the CMS's Health Care Quality Improvement Program for stroke was the development and implementation of two critical pathways. One pathway was for a stroke with deficit and the other was developed for transient ischemic attack. Clinical processes were defined on the pathways to guide the delivery of stroke care. Specific outcomes to measure the effectiveness of care were determined by the multidisciplinary stroke team. One clinical process was measured to assess the timeliness of obtaining diagnostic tests (for example, computed tomography [CT] and magnetic resonance imaging [MRI] scans, carotid duplex, transesophageal echocardiogram). It was important that these tests be completed within the time frame prescribed on the pathway because it would lead to an early determination of the location and etiology of stroke, the initiation of prompt treatment, and allow the patient to be discharged from the hospital within the designated length of stay on the pathways. The quality outcomes chosen for analysis were mortality rates, unplanned hospital readmissions, and complications. Mortality and unplanned hospital readmissions were selected based on findings in the literature that the rates for these outcome measures were high for stroke patients who were not clinically managed by a stroke team. Stroke complications were measured by rates of aspiration pneumonia, gastrointestinal bleeding, and deep venous thrombosis. The financial outcomes were measured by average length of stay, cost/charges per day, resource utilization, and profit/loss assessment for care of patients with a stroke. Clinical discharge outcomes included the proportion of eligible stroke patients without contraindications who were prescribed warfarin at discharge, the documentation of patient/caregiver education regarding warfarin, and planned follow-up of prothrombin time and international normalized ratio. These discharge outcomes were the CMS quality measures for stroke patients.

Many governing bodies, such as the Agency for Healthcare Research, the National Committee for Quality Assurance, the Joint Commission for Accreditation of Healthcare Organizations, and the Centers for Medicare and Medicaid Services, promote the measurement of outcomes to improve the quality of care. In the example of the community-acquired pneumonia, outcome measures were developed by the Centers for Medicare and Medicaid Services to monitor the performance of healthcare providers in improving the process of care objectives described earlier in this chapter. The following describes the completion of the performance improvement cycle for the community-acquired pneumonia example. Data were collected and reported on a quarterly basis to the multidisciplinary team to determine the effectiveness of the clinical processes that they implemented and to trend progress toward achieving the clinical objectives defined by CMS. Trend reports on performance are provided to each hospital on a regular basis by the state's peer review organization and include a comparison of their performance with that of other hospitals in the state. These data guide performance improvement initiatives.

ROLE OF CRITICAL PATHWAYS IN OUTCOMES MANAGEMENT

Critical pathways are tools that can operationalize outcomes management at the direct patient care level. Outcomes management is a comprehensive strategy designed to (1) provide clinicians with clinical practice guidelines and standards to assist in the process of delivering medical care, (2) provide skills and tools necessary to measure the clinical and functional status and well-being of a patient, (3) promote the development and use of large databases to conduct clinical and financial practice analysis, and (4) use outcomes information to guide clinical decision making (11). Outcomes management is achieved by applying the principles of quality improvement to improve the processes and outcomes of care. Systems breakdowns are best fixed through process improvement activities.

Quality improvement principles are based on three common process improvement steps: (1) understand the process, (2) design improvements into the process, and (3) measure performance to determine the effectiveness of the redesigned processes that have been implemented. Members of the interdisciplinary clinical team involved in patient management for a particular diagnosis or procedure are key participants in the process improvement steps. The relationship between the critical pathway and the cycle for performance improvement as defined by Deming's plan–do–check–act (PDCA) model is presented in Figure 7.

Outcomes management also requires behavior change on the part of the clinicians. Behavior modifications are best achieved by sharing credible clinical and individual performance data with clinicians. This may include the profiling of physician practices for compliance with recommended medical therapies and patterns of resource utilization. Comparison of an individual physician's performance with that of their peer physicians or with like institutions can also influence behavior change.

Each of these approaches to performance improvement requires different levels of analyses and strategies for communicating the information. The analyses are most effective when they are provided as information to help identify opportunities for managing and improving outcomes as opposed to a more negative connotation of punishment.

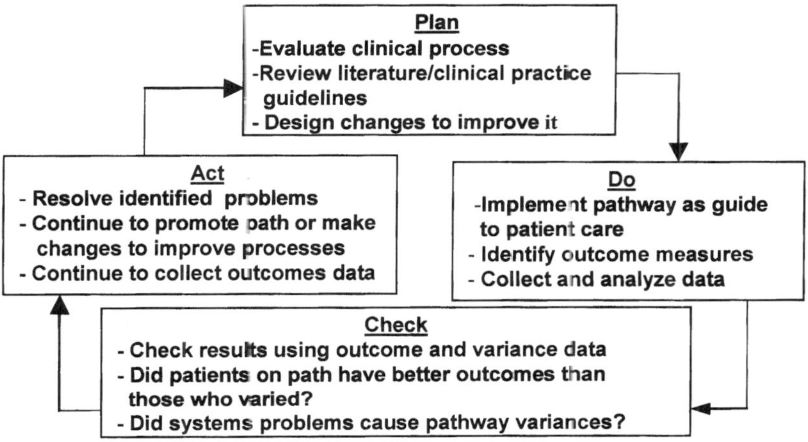

Figure 7 Critical pathways and performance improvement process.

EFFECTIVENESS OF PATHWAYS

The effectiveness of critical pathways to reduce costs and improve patient safety, quality, and outcomes is currently being debated in the medical literature. Early case reports from individual hospitals for the most part were positive (17). There have been an increasing number of empirical studies in the peer-reviewed literature suggesting that the implementation of critical pathways can result in shorter average lengths of stay and decreased costs while achieving similar patient outcomes (18–21). However, most of these observational studies are retrospective, uncontrolled before–after comparisons of a single pathway or a small group of pathways (22). The major criticism of the nonrandomized implementation of critical pathways is that it is difficult to differentiate the effects of the pathway from secular trends. Examples of secular trends that could be potential confounders affecting the results of the study include such things as changes in managed care policies or payment levels, changes in health system leadership or medical staff, or changes in core treatment processes within particular conditions.

Trowbridge and Weingarten (6) conducted a systematic review of pathways in the published literature and identified several randomized controlled trials that provided some evidence that pathways can be effective in influencing healthcare provider behavior. However, they concluded that the data were inconsistent in their effectiveness to reduce complications and improve other clinical outcomes. They found that there is very little information on the application of pathways to patient safety. Further research was recommended to determine the efficacy of pathways in reducing costs and improving patient safety, quality, and outcomes.

Further research is also needed to determine which elements of critical pathway development and implementation are the most important in determining their effectiveness (23). There are many benefits of bringing together a multidisciplinary team of clinicians to discuss patient care issues and focus on the development of a plan of care for a patient population that is efficient, cost effective, and evidence based. It is also important to understand the changes in the processes of care delivery that occur concurrently with pathway development. For example, in the case of the comprehensive stroke program, the Neurology Service restructured its approach to managing the patient population by establishing a dedicated stroke team of neurologists. A nursing unit dedicated to the care of stroke patients was created with a specially trained nursing staff. Additionally, in an attempt to improve the efficiency of care, the stroke team implemented daily multidisciplinary discharge planning rounds. This process educated the team members to the roles and contributions each discipline makes to the management of stroke patients. It also changed perceptions about care and involved disciplines that are not routinely viewed as instrumental in the care delivery process. Even though these benefits may not be captured by the outcomes typically measured for a pathway, they are a vital part in refining how care is delivered. As healthcare delivery becomes more complex and the need to maintain a balance between cost and quality becomes even greater, strategies for improving the communication and coordination of care among healthcare providers are vital. Tools and processes that effectively build bridges between research evidence and clinical practice are essential.

FUTURE OF PATHWAYS

The role of critical pathways and clinical practice guidelines in performance improvement is in an evolutionary process. Critical pathways were initially viewed as utilization guidelines focusing on the appropriate care setting or resource utilization, such as length of stay, diagnostic testing, medications, or use of therapies, and streamlining the processes of care to reduce delays and avoid redundancies. The integration of clinical practice guidelines and research findings with appropriate resource utilization is essential in order to implement evidence-based practices and to develop meaningful process and outcome measures. Guidelines help clinicians identify possible quality problems as a result of underuse, overuse, or inappropriate provision of care. Guidelines can also be used to determine priorities for improving or standardizing patterns of clinical care (7).

The principles of standardizing care that is most consistent with the available scientific evidence and expressing it in a way that is easy for the clinicians to use at the bedside are likely to remain important in the future. However, as clinical information systems become a reality, it is likely that critical pathways as we know them today will be replaced by point-of-care clinical decision support systems. Guidelines and other expressions of clinical content will become even more effective after information technology brings the right information to the right provider at the right time. Computerized decision algorithms that prompt the caregiver with real-time if/then choices specific to the patient's current needs will allow the development of treatment plans that are individualized to meet the patient's needs.

Finally, the development of healthcare information systems that can merge clinical and financial information will promote clinical and financial practice analyses to identify opportunities to improve care. A more comprehensive understanding of clinical practices and their cost implications will better facilitate a balance between cost and quality and improve patient outcomes.

REFERENCES

1. Pearson SD, Goulart-Fisher D, Lee TH. Critical pathways as a strategy for improving care: Problems and potential. Ann Intern Med 123:941–948, 1995.
2. Every NR, Hochman J, Becker R, Kopecky S, Cannon CP. Critical pathways: A review. Committee on Acute Cardiac Care, Council on Clinical Cardiology, American Heart Association. Circulation 101:461–465, 2000.
3. Weingarten S. Critical pathways: What do you do when they do not seem to work? Am J Med 110:224–225, 2001.
4. Coffey RJ, Richards JS, Remmert CS, LeRoy SS, Schoville RR, Baldwin PJ. An introduction to critical paths. Qual Manage Health Care 1:45–54, 1992.
5. Gaucher EJ, Coffey RJ. Total Quality in Healthcare: From Theory to Practice. Jossey-Bass, San Francisco, 1993, pp 469–478.
6. Trowbridge R, Weingarten S. Critical Pathways. In Evidence Report/Technology Assessment No. 3, Making Health Care Safer: A Critical Analysis of Patient Safety Practices. AHRQ Agency for Healthcare Research and Quality 01-E058, Rockville, MD, 2001.
7. Joint Commission on Accreditation of Healthcare Organizations. Selecting and Implementing Clinical Practice Guidelines in Hospitals, 2000, pp 1–6.
8. Field MJ, Lohr KN. Clinical Practice Guidelines: Directions for a New Program. National Academy Press, Washington, DC, 1990, pp 1–8.
9. Margolis CZ. In: Margolis CA, Cretin S, eds. Implementing Clinical Practice Guidelines. American Hospital Association, Chicago, 1999, pp 1–20.
10. Lambert LR. In: Dinsmore PC, eds. The AMA Handbook of Project Management. American Management Association, New York, 1993, pp 187–192.
11. Spath PL. In: Spath PL, eds. Clinical Paths: Tools for Outcomes Management. American Hospital Publishing, Chicago, 1994, pp 9–12.
12. U.S. Department of Health and Human Services. Health Care Quality Improvement Program. Health Care Financing Administration, Baltimore, MD, 2000.

13. Lichtman JH, Roumanis SA, Radford MJ, Riedinger MS, Weingarten S, Krumholz HM. Can practice guidelines be transported effectively to different settings? Results from a multicenter interventional study. Jt Comm J Qual Improv 27:42–53, 2001.
14. Cabana MD, Rand CS, Powe NR, Wu AW, Wilson MH, Abboud PC, Rubin HR. Why don't physicians follow clinical practice guidelines? A framework for improvement. JAMA 282:1458–1464, 1999.
15. Jones KR. Outcomes analysis: Methods and issues. Nurs Econ 11:145–152, 1993.
16. Erickson SM. The Vanderbilt model of outcomes management. Crit Care Nurs Clin North Am 10:13–20, 1998.
17. Spath PL, ed. Beyond Clinical Paths: Advanced Tools for Outcomes Management. American Hospital Publishing, Chicago, 1997.
18. Stanley AC, Barry M, Scott TE. Impact of a critical pathway on postoperative length of stay and outcomes after infrainguinal bypass. J Vasc Surg 27:1056–1064, 1998.
19. Levine PA. Otolaryngology. J Am Coll Surg 186:197–202, 1998.
20. Gerke ML. In: Spath PL, eds. Beyond Clinical Paths. Advanced Tools for Outcomes Management. American Hospital Publishing, Chicago, 1997, pp 53–69.
21. Zehr KJ, Dawson PB, Yang SC, Heitmiller RF. Standardized clinical care pathways for major thoracic cases reduce hospital costs. Ann Thorac Surg 66:914–919, 1998.
22. Conner D, Rifkin W, Silver A, Fansbaum B, Rose D. Critical pathways: How strong is the literature supporting their use? J Gen Intern Med 15(suppl 1):106, 2000.
23. Pearson SD, Kleefield SF, Soukop JR, Cook EF, Lee TH. Critical pathways intervention to reduce length of hospital stay. Am J Med 110:175–180, 2001.

7

Outcomes Management: The Cost–Quality Imperative

Patrice L. Spath
Brown-Spath and Associates, Forest Grove, Oregon, U.S.A.

OUTCOMES MANAGEMENT

The study of patient care outcomes and the effect of various healthcare interventions on outcomes has been actively pursued by the medical professions for more than 200 years. The goal of these studies has always been to improve patient outcomes. Today, more than ever before, healthcare professionals are collecting and analyzing information on the results of medical and surgical interventions. While the linkage of process to outcome is not a new science, it has assumed greater importance in today's healthcare economic climate. The need for detailed information on quality of care and outcomes is one result of the increased expectations of various stakeholders (patients, caregivers, payers, healthcare organizations) coupled with pressures to lessen costs. In this environment, "outcomes management" has flourished. In his classic article, Ellwood defined outcomes management as "a technology of patient experience designed to help patients, payers, and providers make rational medical care–related choices based on better insight into the effect of these choices on the patient's life" (1). Simply stated, outcomes management is the application of clinical, quality, and cost data in medical settings to change practice and/or demonstrate value. The technology of outcomes management relies on four strategies:

- Increased dependence on standards and guidelines
- Routine and systematic measurements of patient function and well-being, as well as disease-specific clinical outcomes
- Pooled process and outcome data

- Dissemination of study results to meet the needs of decision makers

What is the relevance of outcomes management to point-of-care (POC) testing? The answer is straightforward . . . the merits of POC testing can be evaluated when studying the effect of healthcare processes on patient outcomes. Caregivers can collectively assess such issues as

- Which POC tests work well and which do not?
- Is the technology beneficial and is it cost effective?
- Does POC testing improve quality of care?

All new technologies were once the subject of outcomes management efforts. For instance, the value of an early POC testing instrument, the thermometer, was widely debated by physicians. In the May 1867 issue of *The Medical and Surgical Reporter*, Dr. W. H. Draper wrote, "The recent introduction of the thermometer for the more accurate observation of the phenomena of fever, promises to be one of the most useful improvements that have ever been made in the study of disease. . . . Fever has usually been spoke of as one of the symptoms of disease; but until the introduction of the thermometer, we have never been able to study accurately the variations of this symptom in the natural progress and termination of different diseases" (2). Although the thermometer was invented by Gabriel Fahrenheit in 1724, it was not until the mid–nineteenth century that physicians were convinced of the clinical value of careful thermometrical observations. Physicians in the nineteenth century did not use the phrase "outcomes management," but they did spend considerable time evaluating the relationship between process and outcomes.

Outcomes management represents a growing area of research in medicine, with significant opportunities to improve efficiency, lessen waste, and provide a reasonable standard of care both to the patient's and the caregiver's satisfaction. This chapter explores the benefits of knowledge-based decisions and the steps of an outcomes management initiative. The techniques can be used to evaluate the effects of any healthcare process, including POC testing.

By gathering information about the value of POC testing, clinicians can discover better ways to practice medicine. Whether it is an anesthesiologist doing a blood gas in the operating room, a patient with diabetes measuring his own serum glucose, or an intensive care nurse conducting tests by the patient's bedside, outcomes management can help clinicians understand the impact of new technologies. Ultimately, a large number of POC tests may be just as commonplace as the thermometer.

DATA AND DECISION MAKING

In serving the needs of patients, clinicians practice an inexact science—one in which current knowledge often is not adequate to the task at hand and in which experience provides major guidance in selecting effective interventions. In many cases, the application of massive experience distilled through memory provides effective direction to the treatment of illness. When successful, the treatment decision is frequently recalled and the efficacy of clinical intuition hailed. When such decision making fails, it is rarely recalled.

Decision making that relies on recollections of personal experience and that of others is intuitive and subject to all of the fallible features of one's memory. We discount failures, recall successes, and apply various heuristic techniques that can bias the results. Heuristics, the cognitive framework people use as a guide in investigating or solving a problem, creates biases that affect what is remembered. For example, many people overestimate the risk inherent in taking a scheduled commercial airline flight, frequently overestimating the frequency of fatal accidents by factors of 10 or more (3). Why would such errors occur? One possible reason is what Tversky and Kahneman (4) called the availability heuristic. People are more likely to remember the salient events (e.g., those that were unusual, gained particular media coverage, or were particularly horrific) and therefore judge them to be more probable than is actually the case. Clearly people's heuristics and their associated biases can and do affect intuitive decision making. Quantification provides an effective antidote to such errors.

Why not just avoid the use of heuristics, thus avoiding the introduction of biases? This is not as easy as it appears. Simplification of our real world by various techniques (some biological and some learned) is necessitated by the severe limits of our cognitive systems. A particularly pertinent example is the limitation of our working (short-term) memory. In 1956 George Miller first reported that the size of this memory system was limited to about 7 ($\pm$2) "chunks" of information (5). Since 1956, it has become clear that the "chunks" may vary in size depending on the tasks involved and the training of the individual (6). However, it is evident that people's memory limitations restrict their ability to recognize all aspects of a complex situation. Because of this, humans must simplify situations in order to understand them. We create mental models because we quite simply have no other choice.

Decision making that is data based relies on experience that is recorded, quantified, and analyzed. Such decision making has the advantage of being less biased than intuitive decision making; however, accuracy comes at some expense. The first expense is that data-driven decisions may appear to lack the "human touch." This characteristic seems in direct opposition to the need that patients perceive healthcare providers as caring individuals.

The collection of data is also expensive in terms of monetary and human resources. The cost of planning, executing, analyzing, and documenting a study can be substantial. Finally, the most substantial cost associated with data-based decisions are the costs of poor planning. Inadequate planning can result in misdirected endeavors—causing wasted efforts or, worse yet, incorrect decisions.

It is not suggested that data-driven decision making supplant intuitive methods, but that the two approaches be combined. The best decisions combine the expertise of the specialist with the collection of critical data (7,8). Outcomes management is a technique that provides healthcare professionals with the critical data they need to make better patient care decisions.

THE OUTCOMES MANAGEMENT PROCESS

Outcomes management involves the collection, analysis, evaluation, and dissemination of information about the outcomes of medical or surgical interventions to improve the processes of healthcare. Outcomes management consists of four steps, illustrated in Figure 1. It starts with the selection of a study population of

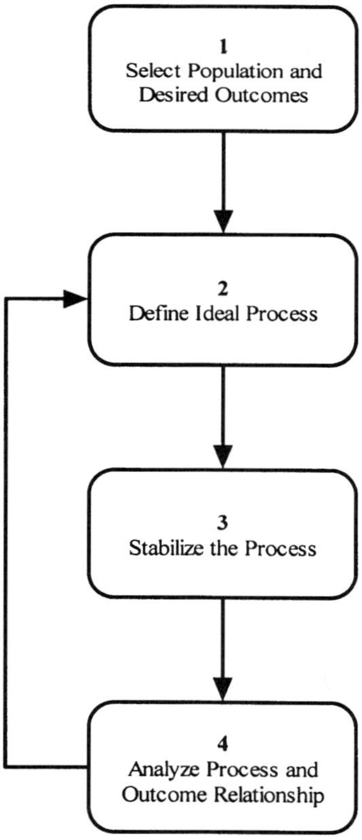

Figure 1 The steps of outcomes management.

patients and identification of desired outcomes. Next, the ideal process for achieving desired outcomes is defined. Information about the ideal process is disseminated to caregivers using a variety of tools and techniques. Once dissemination has occurred, data are gathered to determine whether or not the desired outcomes were actually achieved, and if not, why not. The information gathered during step four, the analysis phase, is used to improve upon the ideal process. Each step of an outcomes management project is presented in greater detail below.

Select Population and Desired Outcomes

The decision to conduct an outcomes management project is usually precipitated by the desire to improve quality of care and/or reduce costs for a particular patient population. Generally, the population represents a high-volume, high-risk, high-cost, or problem-prone group of patients. The reasons for choosing a patient population for an outcomes management study generally influences the outcomes of interest. For example, many hospitals have conducted outcomes management projects for patients that have severe congestive heart failure. These are "frequent flyer" patients with multiple high-cost hospital readmissions and emergency department visits. The outcome of interest in this patient population is primarily resource utilization (readmissions, length of hospital stay, emergency department charges, etc.).

An outcomes management initiative can also be initiated with the intent of improving patients' clinical and functional outcomes. For example, in 1993 five Kaiser Permanente Medical Centers in the San Francisco Bay area joined together to evaluate various strategies for modifying patients' coronary risk factors after myocardial infarction. The outcomes of interest were smoking cessation, plasma low-density lipoprotein (LDL) cholesterol levels, and patients' functional capacity 6 months after infarction (9).

Once the patient population and the outcomes of interest are identified, the goals of the outcomes management project must be clearly defined. Goals are specific, measurable, action statements that describe what the organization wants to achieve for the patient population. A goal is specific when everyone knows exactly what the outcomes management project is expected to accomplish. Being specific means spelling out the details of the goal. For example:

- "Improve patient outcomes" may be acceptable as a strategic objective, but it is too general for a population-specific outcomes management goal because it does not provide any definite information about what is to be accomplished.
- "Decrease the incidence of postoperative complications" is more specific because it narrows the scope of the desired outcome.
- "Reduce the number of patients admitted to the hospital for treatment of

community-acquired pneumonia by 20%" is the most specific because it clearly defines a measurable goal.

Goals for an outcomes management project involving congestive heart failure (CHF) might read as follows:

- Reduce hospital readmissions within 30 days for CHF-related diagnosis by 20%.
- Reduce patients' average length of hospital stay by 1.3 days.
- Reduce patients' visits to emergency department for CHF-related diagnosis by 20%.
- Increase patients' understanding of home care instructions by 20% (compared with baseline survey results).
- Increase patients' access to community resources by 30% (compared with baseline survey results).

Goals for an outcomes management project involving patients who have had a myocardial infarction might read as follows:

- Improve smoking cessation rate at 2 months post–myocardial infarction from the current 40% to 70%.
- Decrease patients' plasma LDL cholesterol levels at 6 months post–myocardial infarction from current average level of 3.56 mmol/L to an average level of 2.90 mmol/L.
- Improve patients' exercise tolerance at 6 months from current average level of 7.4 to an average level of 10 (metabolic equivalent—MET level; an index of the patient's functional capacity).

Define Ideal Process

Once everyone knows the goals of the outcomes management project, it's time to determine the best way to achieve those goals. In this project step, the ideal process for achieving desired outcomes in a specific patient population is defined. Selecting the ideal process involves an analysis of the current process to determine what improvements are needed. Aggregate data can be used to compare actual outcomes with expected outcomes. The clinicians must drill down into the process to identify practice variations that are influencing the outcomes of interest. Shown in Table 1 are data gathered during an outcomes management project involving patients admitted to the hospital for total hip replacement. Practice pattern variations are evident in the data. These could be unnecessary variations that affect patient length of stay. Further investigation will be needed to determine the ideal process.

Literature reviews are an important component of step two in an outcomes management project. Although record audits and aggregate data review can reveal

Table 1 Total Hip Replacement, January–June 2001

	Physician A (N = 27)	Physician B (N = 32)	Physician C (N = 29)	Physician D (N = 13)	Physician E (N = 46)	Physician F (N = 38)
Average length of stay	5.9	5.1	4.9	5.3	4.5	4.3
% admitted day of surgery	55.9%	60.3%	72.1%	66.9%	61.8%	78.3%
% preoperative antibiotics given	64.1%	93.4%	65.0%	82.5%	98.9%	100%
% patients with intraoperative complications	2.6%	0.5%	1.2%	0.8%	0%	1.3%
Average estimated blood loss during procedure (cc's)	574	480	560	420	490	522
% complications occurring in recovery room	5.0%	1.5%	3.2%	4.5%	1.2%	3.5%
Average length of time until postoperative pain medication is administered orally (hr/min)	14:01	11:30	9:47	12:22	9:05	9:57
Length of time after procedure patient is sitting at bedside (hr/min)	10:34	10:21	8:05	9:15	8:27	9:01
Length of time after procedure patient is ambulating any distance (with walker) (hr/min)	11:50	12:15	9:07	9:24	8:57	9:50
% patients began discharge planning before admission	68.1%	55.2%	89.1%	76.4%	82.6%	91.7%
% patients discharged to home with home care	72%	65%	71%	52%	61%	83%

Source: Patrice L. Spath, Brown-Spath and Associates, Forest Grove, OR.

current practices in one organization, these analyses do not provide sufficient information to establish an ideal process. Literature review involves gathering performance data from other organizations and reviewing clinical practice guidelines developed by national medical professional groups. This information is used to compare patient outcomes with what is being achieved by other practitioners and to identify evidence-based practice recommendations relevant to the population under study.

For example, in 1994, data gathered by clinicians at St. Luke's Episcopal Hospital in Houston, TX, showed that patients with a history of congestive heart failure who were older than 70 or who had previous heart surgery were spending a longer time on the ventilator following open heart surgery as compared with other patients. The healthcare team researched current literature to identify better interventions for these high-risk patients. The ideal patient care process included more timely respiratory interventions and more aggressive preoperative and postoperative teaching (10).

In the past 10–15 years, the availability of literature resources and evidence-based clinical practice guidelines has significantly increased. It is now easier for practitioners to find "best practice" recommendations. However, not all of these recommendations need to be incorporated into an organization's "ideal" patient care process. Each source, including clinical practice guidelines, must be carefully evaluated to determine if the recommendations are valid and whether they will be helpful in achieving desired outcomes. It is important to determine if researchers used an explicit and sensible process to identify, select, and combine literature and to assess the strength of the recommendations (11).

Once all available information relevant to the process of care is gathered and analyzed, the healthcare team is ready to define the ideal process for achieving desired outcomes for the patient population under study. This usually involves a consensus process whereby clinicians actively involved in the care of the target population reach an agreement. Preferably, those involved in defining the "ideal process" are recognized by their peers as being experienced and knowledgeable and are well respected. Barriers related to the examination of current practices and identification of "ideal practice" can also be reduced by the use of empirically based research methods, diligent attention to the reliability and validity of data collection and analysis, and effective communication (12).

An organization may choose to modify literature recommendations or published clinical practice guidelines for a variety of reasons, such as

- Published guidelines usually lack local clinical input. Physicians have confidence in guidelines that they or their peers take part in developing or that are developed by their professional organization. Guidelines adopted by a consensus of local physicians are more likely to be accepted.

- There may be controversy or lack of strong clinical evidence. All alternative treatments may not always be covered in research articles or guidelines. Caregivers may need to reach consensus at the local level.
- In some instances, clinical practice guidelines may allow choices among equally effective therapeutic options and caregivers may wish to narrow the choices. For example, a national guideline on the treatment of depression in primary care settings states: "No one antidepressant medication is clearly more effective than another. No single medication results in remission for all patients." The guideline lists several types of drugs that are considered equivalent in clinical effectiveness. In adapting this guideline, local caregivers may choose the least expensive class of drugs from the recommended list as its first-line treatment (13).

	ASSESSMENT PHASE	TREATMENT PHASE	DAY OF DISCHARGE
CONSULTS	• Old records • Evaluate legal status		
TESTS	• Thyroid Cascade • B12 • Folate • Fasting CBC, SMAC • U/A		
MEDS	Medication evaluation	Review of patient's medications and patient's response to medications (routine & as needed)	Discharge medications
TREATMENTS	Per multidisciplinary treatment plan	-------->	--------->
ACTIVITY	• Fall pre-cautions • Suicide precautions (if indicated)	---------->	---------->
NURSING TREATMENTS	• Zung Scale • Assess: suicide	---------->	• Zung Scale ---------->
REHAB SERVICE	• Occupational therapy evaluation • Social Service evaluation • Group assignment	• OT/SS summary • Group attendance	---------->
TEACHING	• Patient/caregiver/family orientation to program	Med/illness	----------> Discharge instructions
DISCHARGE PLANNING		• Determine discharge needs • Public Health Nurse assessment as needed	Complete referral forms. Confirm discharge plan w/team & family. Arrange transportation.

Figure 2 Clinical path for patients admitted to the hospital for treatment of depression disorder. (From Ref. 27.)

Initial Assessment: History, physical exam, PEF, SaO_2, & other tests as indicated.

Impending or Actual Respiratory Arrest
* HFN albuterol/Atrovent
* Start IV corticosteroid
* Intubation & ventilation with 100% O_2

Mild Exacerbation
(may be agitated, | RR, possible use of accessory muscles/suprasternal retractions, wheeze, | HR, PEF 80%, SaO_2 > 95%)
Standing Orders:
* PEF at assessment then after third HFN and at physician's discretion
* HFN albuterol/NS x 1
* Physician to evaluate response after 1" HFN
* Add Atrovent at physician discretion
* HFN albuterol q20 min. for a total of 3 treatments. Automatic reevaluation by respiratory therapist 20 min. after each HFN
* SaO_2 spot checks q20 min. & PRN
* Oxygen to keep SaO_2 > 90%
* Ongoing assessment

Moderate Exacerbation
(may be agitated, | RR, possible use of accessory muscles, prolonged expiratory phase, suprasternal retractions, wheeze, | HR, PEF 50-80%, SaO_2 > 91%)
Standing Orders:
* PEF at assessment then after third HFN and at physician's discretion
* HFN albuterol/NS x 1
* Physician to evaluate response after 1" HFN
* Add Atrovent at physician discretion
* HFN albuterol q20 min. for a total of 3 treatments. Automatic reevaluation by respiratory therapist 20 min. after each HFN
* SaO_2 spot checks q20 min. & PRN
* Oxygen to keep SaO_2 > 90%
* Ongoing assessment

After three treatments, start oral systemic corticosteriods if no improvement in PEF and/or symptoms. If conditions deteriorate, start IV corticosteriods.
* Ongoing assessment
* Repeat HFN q 1 hr for 1-3 hrs if there is controlled improvement

Severe Exacerbation
(agitated, dyspnea @ rest, high RR, use of accessory muscles, suprasternal retractions, inspiratory & expiratory wheeze, HR >120, pulsus paraoxus often present, PEF <50%, SaO_2 <91%)
Standing Orders:
* PEF at assessment then after third HFN and at physician's discretion
* HFN high dose albuterol/Atrovent x 1 then if poor response start continuous nebulization with albuterol
* Close supervision by physician
* Continuous supervision by respiratory therapist or nurse
* SaO_2 continuous
* Oxygen to keep SaO_2 > 90%
* Start IV corticosteroids
* Ongoing assessment

If **no improvement** after initial HFN, **admit** to ICU ASAP

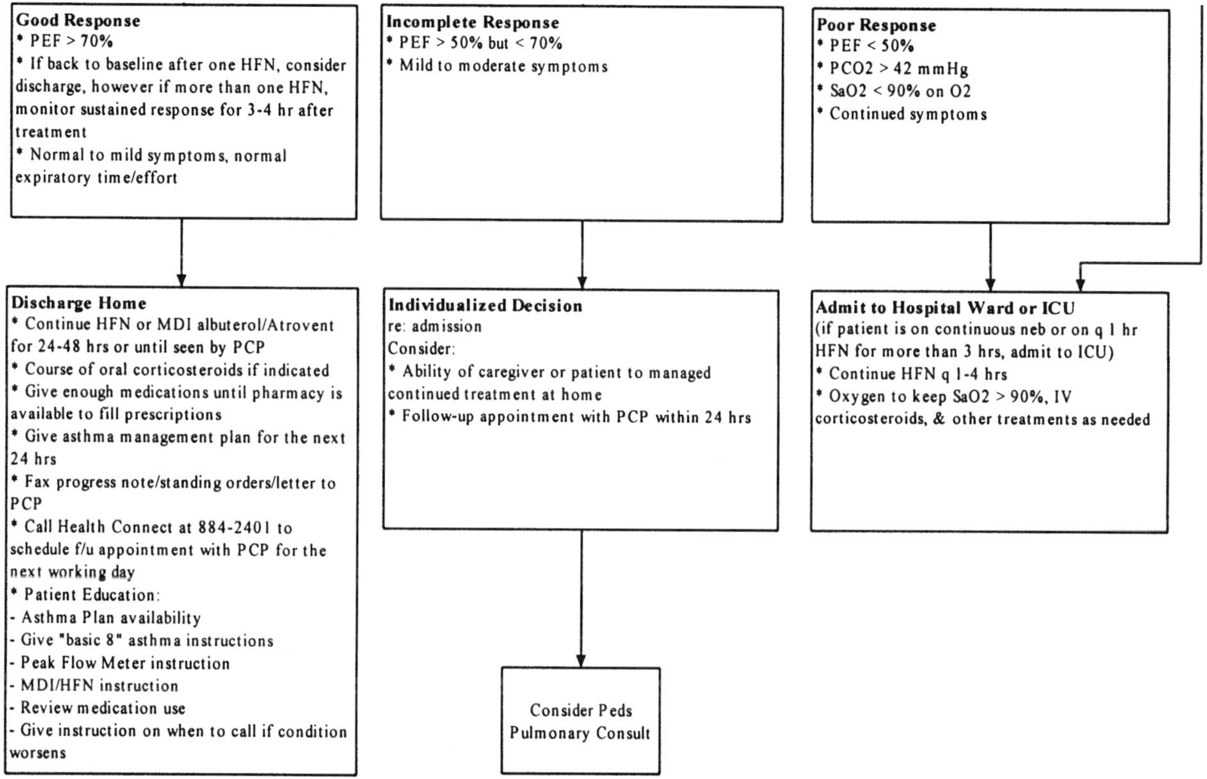

Figure 3 Managing pediatric patients with asthma in the emergency department. (From the University of Missouri Health Sciences Center, St. Louis, MO; © 1977 by the Curator of the University of Missouri, a public corporation.)

- Published recommendations may not adequately address the issue of cost effectiveness. In these instances, caregivers need to consider the local costs of alternative treatments in creating their "ideal process." Before incorporating POC testing into the "ideal process" the organization should perform a carefully detailed cost–benefit analysis comparing the current testing system with POC testing. This analysis should include a determination of the initial capital investment required and the ongoing costs for POC testing (14).
- Published recommendations may not apply to the demographical characteristics of the target population. Differences in patients' health need to be taken into account since socioeconomically different populations may have different incidence and prevalence rates of the disease. For example, research shows that Native American women require more frequent mammography screening due to their above-average incidence of breast cancer (15).
- Published recommendations may require modification based on the amount and type of health resources in the community. For example, several published studies have established that a pharmacist-managed anticoagulation service can prevent warfarin-related hospital admissions and improve the overall quality of patient care. (16–18) Communities with a sufficient number of trained pharmacists are more likely to establish such a clinic. However, those without enough trained pharmacists may decide to rely on other methods of patient education and ambulatory assessment of anticoagulation status.

Once everyone has agreed on the ideal process, it is documented. The process description may be illustrated as an algorithm (decision tree), a clinical path, a narrative treatment protocol, a computer-assisted guideline, a procedure, or in other formats. The organization selects the designs most applicable to the patient population and healthcare environment. For example, a hospital may choose to illustrate the ideal process using a clinical path wherein the care recommendations for every discipline can be listed for each day of the patient's stay. A clinical path that describes the care that should be provided to patients who are hospitalized for treatment of a depression disorder is shown in Figure 2. Some caregivers find it easier to follow "best practice" recommendations when they are presented in a clinical algorithm. This format illustrates the critical decisions and treatment options based on clinical findings. An algorithm describing the management of pediatric patients with asthma that present to the emergency department is shown in Figure 3. This algorithm is accompanied by the written drug dosage guidelines in Table 2. The algorithm and drug dosage guidelines were developed by clinicians at the University of Missouri Health Sciences Center and based on the Guidelines for the Diagnosis and Management of Asthma developed in 1997 by

Table 2 Dosages of Drugs for Asthma Exacerbations in Emergency Medical Care or Hospital

Medications	Children	Comments
Inhaled short-acting beta 2–agonists		
Albuterol —Nebulizer solution 0.15 mg/kg	0.15 mg/kg (minimum dose 2.5 mg) every 20 min. for 3 doses, then 0.15–.3 mg/kg up to 10 mg every 1–4 hours as needed, or by continuous nebulization at 5 mg/hr. 10 mg/hr OR 15 mg/hr.	Only selective beta 2–agonists are recommended. For optimal delivery, aerosols to minimum of 4 mL at gas flow of 6–8 L/min.
—MDI (90 mcg/puff)	4–8 puffs every 20 min. for 3 doses, then every 1–4 hours as needed.	As effective as nebulized therapy if is able to coordinate inhalation maneuver. Use spacer/holding chamber.
Systemic (injected) beta 2–agonists		
Epinephrine —1:1000 (1 mg/mL)	0.01 mg/kg up to 0.3–.0.5 mg every 20 min. for 3 doses sq.	No proven advantage of systemic therapy over aerosol.
Terbutaline —(1 mg/mL)	0.01 mg/kg every 20 min. for 3 doses, then every 2–6 hours as needed sq.	No proven advantage of systemic therapy over aerosol.
Anticholinergics		
Ipratropium bromide —Nebulizer solution (0.25 mg/mL)	0.25 mg every 20 min. for 3 doses, then every 2 to 4 hours.	May mix in same nebulizer with albuterol. Should not be used as first line therapy; should be added to beta 2–agonist therapy.
—MDI (18 mcg/puff)	4–8 puffs as needed.	Dose delivered from MDI is low and has not been studied in asthma exacerbation.
Corticosteroids		
Prednisone Methylprednisone Prednisolone	1 mg/kg every 6 hours for 48 hours then 1–2 mg/kg/day (maximum = 60 mg/day) in 2 divided doses until PEF 70% of predicted or personal best.	For outpatient "burst" use 40–60 mg in single or 2 divided doses for adults (children: 1–2 mg/kg/day, maximum 60 mg/day) for 3–10 days.

Note: No advantage has been found for higher dose corticosteroids in severe asthma exacerbations, nor is there any advantage for intravenous administration over oral therapy provided gastrointestinal transit time or absorption is not impaired. The usual regimen is to continue the frequent multiple daily dosing until the patient achieves an FEV, or PEF of 50 percent of predicted or personal best and then lower the dose to twice daily. This usually occurs within 48 hours. Therapy following a hospitalization or emergency department visit may last from 3 to 10 days. If patients are then started on inhaled corticosteroids, studies indicate there is no need to taper the systemic corticosteroid dose. If the follow-up systemic corticosteroid therapy is to be given once daily, one study indicates it may be more clinically effective to give the dose in the afternoon at around 3:00 p.m. (Beam et al. 1992).
Source: University of Missouri Health Sciences Center, St. Louis, MO.

an Expert Panel for the National Heart, Lung and Blood Institute of the National Institutes of Health (19).

Stabilize the Process

Once the ideal process has been defined it must be made available to caregivers. The goal is to reduce variation in the process by encouraging people to follow the ideal plan of care. While some variation is expected, ideally modifications are made only in response to unique patient factors and not atypical treatment choices by the caregiver. By stabilizing the process of care (minimizing unwarranted variation), improvements in quality and cost reductions can be realized. For example, LDS Hospital in Salt Lake City, UT, found that 80–100% compliance with their ventilator protocol for managing patients with adult respiratory distress syndrome yielded reduced costs and improved quality (20). Stabilized ventilator management cost about $120,000 per patient as compared with $160,000 per patient not managed according to the protocol. LDS Hospital physicians found that stabilizing the process resulted in a 44% survival rate for the patients managed according to the protocol, as compared with 38% survival for those not managed with the protocol.

Step three of the outcomes management project can be particularly challenging. Once the ideal process has been defined, the recommendations must be made available to clinicians. It is not enough to develop the ideal process—it must be visible to caregivers when they are making decisions. The reminder tools must also be "discipline friendly." The documentation tools and reminder systems that disciplines have traditionally used in their provision of patient care are each a little different. For example, hospital nurses are used to day-to-day patient care plans, Kardex forms, and flow sheets. Physicians have historically used standing orders, protocols, and preprinted forms (e.g., history/physical examination forms, test ordering forms) to remind them of important components of care and reduce repetitious writing. Other caregivers have designed documentation and reminder tools specific to their patient care roles. For example, pharmacists have their medication profiles and administration records. Physical therapists and other rehabilitative disciplines have their treatment records. Respiratory therapists seem to prefer flow sheets or predesigned charting records.

When designing discipline-friendly reminder tools, it is important to build on the commonplace. Caregivers are usually reluctant to relinquish their traditional forms in favor of ones they may find awkward or formats that appear to belong to another discipline. As computerization becomes more widely used in health services, including individual use of personal digital assistant devices, a broader range of reminder options is becoming available. If the ideal process addresses just one or two aspects of patient care, it may be best to display the recommendations as computer prompts or stickers placed in the patient's health record. An example of a reminder sticker placed in the records of patients in an intensive care unit is shown in Figure 4.

Documentation tools are a common technique for displaying patient care recommendations. Clinicians document the results of patient care on these forms and they also have ready access to treatment protocols. An example of such a tool is the TPA (blood clot dissolver) Infusion Record 90 Minute Protocol form shown in Figure 5. The TPA treatment protocol is incorporated into the form that nurses at the Regional Medical Center in Orangeburg, SC, use for documentation purposes. Physicians use the form to order appropriate preinfusion diagnostic studies and medications.

To minimize the need for duplicative documentation and improve physician access to "best practice" recommendations, many hospitals have developed preprinted physician orders. The ideal plan of care is incorporated into the list of orders. Physicians use the form to "check off" what they would like done for the patient. Sufficient space is provided on the form to add additional orders or remove those orders that may be inappropriate for a particular patient. In a hospital setting, preprinted physician orders may be used in conjunction with clinical paths, algorithms, and/or treatment protocols. A physician order sheet for pediatric patients admitted with diabetic ketoacidosis is shown in Figure 6. The physicians at William Beaumont Hospital in Royal Oak, MI, use this form, together with a clinical pathway, to promote ideal patient care practices. The order sets on the preprinted forms at William Beaumont Hospital will eventually be incorporated into a computerized physician order entry system.

> *Dear Doctor:*
>
> *Your patient is receiving parenteral H-2 receptor antagonist therapy (ranitidine- famotidine) apparently for stress ulcer prophylaxis. As your patient's condition improves, the need for parenteral agents for stress ulcer prophylaxis significantly decreases.*
>
> *It is suggested that reevaluation of parenteral H-2 receptor antagonist therapy take place when the patient is able to tolerate oral feedings, able to take oral therapy, or has been discharged from the ICU. Thank you for your cooperation.*
>
> *Your response is appreciated.*

Figure 4 Note placed in record of patient in the intensive care unit. (From Ref. 27.)

Date: ____ MD prescribing TPA: ____ @ ____ am/pm						
PRE-INFUSION	Pre-Infusion Diagnostic Studies:					
	[ ] Portable CXR	[ ] SMA-6			[ ] Fibrinogen	
	[ ] EKG	[ ] U/A			[ ] Troponin 1	
	[ ] CBC	[ ] CPK with Isoenzymes			[ ] Myoglobin	
	[ ] PT / PTT	[ ] LDH with Isoenzymes				
	Pre-Infusion Vital Signs: T: ____ P: ____ R: ____ B/P: ____ O2 Sat: ____					
IV INFUSION	**SITE**	**SOLUTION**	**JELCO SIZE**	**RATE**	**CONTROL DEVICE**	**NURSE**
	#1:					
	#2:					
	#3:					
	#4:					
	#5:					

MEDICATIONS	**TIME**	**MEDICATION**	**NURSE**	**IV #**
		Beta Blocker ____ mg IV / PO		
		Nitroglycerine Infusion (15mg/250cc/D5W) @ ____ micrograms/min		
		TPA Started 90 minute protocol via [ ] IVAC pump [ ] SIGMA pump 15 mg (V=15 cc) IV bolus over 1-3 minutes (R=450 cc/hr) 50 mg (V=50 cc) IV over 30 minutes (R=100 cc/hr) 35 mg (V=35cc) IV over 1 hour (R=35 cc/hr) 50 cc minibag of Normal Saline hung to flush tubing		
		TPA Ended		
		Heparin Bolus ____ units IV		
		Heparin Drip @ ____ cc/hr (____ units in ____ cc's D5W)		
		Additional prescribed medications: ____ ____	____ ____	____ ____
		[ ] ASA within 12 hours prior to admission [ ] ASA 1 po on admission [ ] Ascriptin 1 po on admission [ ] Baby ASA 1 po on admission		

POST	Post-Infusion Vital Signs: T: ____ P: ____ R: ____ B/P: ____ O2 Sat: ____ Post-Infusion labs ordered as prescribed per physician Bleeding Precautions: "No Venipunctures" Sign posted on door of room Patient teaching: ____ NURSE'S SIGNATURE: ____

Figure 5 TPA infusion record 90 minute protocol. (From the Regional Medical Center, Orangeburg, SC, 2001.)

ATTENTION PHYSICIAN: This preprinted form is available to facilitate patient care. This is not for pharmacy orders. Items preceded by ● will be implemented unless crossed out. Order other items by checking the box in front of the item and / or completing the blanks where necessary. If additional items are needed add them on the standard Doctors Order Sheet (Form 280)

INITIATION OF EC / PICU CLINICAL PATHWAY FOR PEDIATRIC DIABETIC KETOACIDOSIS

1. ● Admit to PICU Physician:
2. ● Institute Clinical Pathway for Diabetic Ketoacidosis
3. Allergies:
4. Labs in EC / PICU:
   - ● Serum Acetone
   - ● Venous pH
   - ● Lytes
   - ● Serum Glucose
   - ● CBC with diff.
   - ● Basic Metabolic Panel
   - ● UA
   - ☐ HCG
   - ☐ Phosphorous
   - ☐ Mg++
5. Routine Labs:
   - ● Glucose meter Q 1 hour while on IV insulin infusion
   - ● When off IV insulin infusion, change glucose monitoring to:
     - ● Glucose meter AC, HS, 2AM
     - ☐ Blood Glucose Q _____ hours
   - ● Lytes and Serum Glucose
     - ☐ Q 4 hours x 4, then Q 8 hours x 2
     - ☐ Q 2 hours x 4, then Q 8 hours x 2, then Q 8 hours x 2
   - ● Serum Acetone at _______ (time)
   - ☐ CBC with diff at _________ (time)
   - ☐ BUN & Creatinine at ________ (time)
   - ☐ Serum Osmolality
   - ☐ Hemoglobin A1C
   - ☐ ______________________________
   - ☐ ______________________________
6. Diet:
   - ☐ NPO
   - ☐ ___________ Clear Liquids
   - ☐ _________________________
7. Activity:
   - ☐ SBR
   - ☐ BRP
   - ☐ Up in chair as tolerated
8. Nursing Treatments:
   - ● Vital signs per routine
   - ● Neuro checks Q 2 hours x 8, then routine
   - ● Cardiorespiratory monitor
   - ● Continuous pulse oximetry
   - ● Strict I & O
   - ☐ O_2 at ____________________
   - ☐ Heparin lock for lab draws
   - ☐ Foley to dependent drainage
9.
10.
11.
12.
13.
14.
15.

Physician Assistant Signature	Date	Time	Physician Signature	Dr. Page No.	Date	Time
Noted by Unit Secretary	Date	Time	Noted by RN		Date	Time

Jan 01

Figure 6 Physician's order sheet for pediatric patients admitted for treatment of diabetic ketoacidosis. (From William Beaumont Hospital, Royal Oak, MI.)

After conducting several successful outcomes management initiatives, the Harvard Community Health Plan offered the following recommendations for designing effective reminder tools (21):

- Reminder systems should be considered as one of many potential solutions.
- Methods for implementing guidelines should be based on a thorough understanding of the causes of the problem and the potential effect of proposed remedies.
- Once implemented, reminder systems must be maintained to meet practitioners' and patients' needs.
- Continually monitor and improve the reminder systems.

Analyze Process and Outcome Relationship

At this point in the outcomes management project, the ideal process has been defined and it has been disseminated to the people involved in the process. The recommendations have been incorporated into various reminders that are well accepted and easily accessible by caregivers. Once this stage has been reached, the data collection and analysis process begins. Implementing the ideal process is part of an explicit, evidence-based process for evaluating and improving clinical practice. Information is gathered to determine:

- Is the ideal process actually being followed? If not, why not?
- Has the ideal process achieved desired results? Are the goals of the outcomes management project being met?
- What barriers may be still in place for achieving compliance with the ideal process and/or achieving desired goals?
- What changes need to be made in the ideal process to further improve patient outcomes?

The data that need to be gathered during this phase of the outcomes management project vary according to the project goals and scope of the processes involved. For example, emergency physicians practicing at Henry Ford Hospital, Detroit, MI, participated in an outcomes management project aimed at improving the diagnosis and treatment of patients with congestive heart failure. The ideal process being tested was the use of the bedside Triage BNP Test™, an immunoassay that measures the level of serum brain natriuretic peptide (BNP). The test results, available within 15 minutes, are used in conjunction with other tests and clinical findings to diagnose heart failure. Data were gathered to determine if the test results provided an accurate measurement of a patient's current cardiac function. Emergency physicians found that the Triage BNP Test allowed them to quickly and objectively determine whether a dyspneic patient's problem was attributable to congestive heart failure (22).

When there are many elements of care in the ideal process, a more extensive data collection and analysis process is required. For example, Abbott Northwestern Hospital and the Institute for Low Back Pain, in Minneapolis, MN, jointly sponsored an outcomes management project for patients undergoing spinal procedures (23). Project objectives were twofold:

- To improve the quality of patient care
- To improve the institution's competitive position in the marketplace

An extensive review of current inpatient practices was undertaken, along with literature reviews. Caregivers ultimately developed a "best practices" clinical path. Several process and outcome measurement data were gathered to evaluate the impact of the revised process of care. These data included

- Postoperative day when patients' parenteral fluids were discontinued
- Postoperative day when patients began oral pain medication
- Postoperative day when patients were allowed to sit on edge of bed and dangle legs
- Postoperative day when patients were allowed to walk
- Per patient operating room charges (broken down by type of charges)
- Per patient total hospital charges
- Per patient pharmacy charges
- Per patient ancillary test charges
- Average hospital length of stay
- Number of patients admitted the day of surgery
- Number of patients developing postoperative complications
- Number of patients with unplanned return to the operating room during same hospitalization
- Patients' functional status and quality of life following surgery
- Patient satisfaction with outpatient clinic wait times
- Patient satisfaction with clinic appointment wait times
- Patient satisfaction with amount of time spent with care provider
- Patient satisfaction with care provider's technical skills

Through an ongoing analysis of the inter-relationship of processes and outcomes, the care providers in Minneapolis are continually improving the care for patients who undergo spinal procedures.

Outcomes management is a continuous improvement cycle—with the feedback being used to update the ideal plan of care recommendations. An illustration of the outcomes management process was reported by EHS Hospitals in the Chicago area. After designing a clinical path for patients undergoing coronary artery bypass graft (CABG), surgery data were gathered to analyze the impact of patient extubation the morning after surgery versus extubation following recovery the same day as surgery. Study of these two practices revealed that same-day extubations were more cost effective, resulted in patient comfort improvements, and did not negatively impact outcomes. The revised CABG clinical path recommended patient extubation following the recovery period (24).

OUTCOMES MANAGEMENT: THE KEY TO IMPROVED QUALITY

The delivery of healthcare services will be subjected to innumerable reforms as the healthcare industry seeks to eliminate the serious shortcomings outlined in a recent Institute of Medicine report, *Crossing the Quality Chasm* (25). It is expected, however, that the emphasis on outcomes management will endure, as many see this approach to research as being key to improved cost efficiency and quality in the healthcare delivery system (26).

Once the patient population for the outcomes management project is selected, a multidisciplinary team of people involved in caring for these patients is formed. The team should be given objectively defined goals for the project. After studying the process as it currently exists, the outcomes management project team selects the actions necessary for achieving the goals. Any number of actions can be taken to achieve the goals of an outcomes management project. The team should focus on fundamental changes in systems that are most likely to produce positive long-term gains. They can do this by determining the barriers to goal attainment and then incrementally investing in strategies to achieve these goals. The project team must learn how to analyze practice pattern data to determine the best interventions and then monitor the success of various strategies. A successful outcomes management project requires more than good clinical skills. Each initiative requires timely feedback of process and outcome measures to the involved caregivers.

Much has been written about securing clinicians' compliance with practice guidelines and other "best practice" recommendations. However, it appears that defining ideal practices may be easier than getting clinicians to change their long-established habits. It appears that even when it is the right thing to do, caregivers resist change. There are two key factors that influence the caregiver's decision about adopting new practices. First, the practice changes that caregivers are asked to make must have been proven to be the right thing to do. Unless a valid research study has substantiated the benefits of the new way of doing things, it is hard to create much enthusiasm for change. Second, the caregivers being asked to change their practices must have personally agreed that it is the right thing to do. People should acknowledge that the practice change is a good thing for them and for their patients. If one or both of these criteria are not met, it is likely that there will be significant resistance to change. However, if both of these criteria have been met and caregivers still slip back into their old habits, then one is probably dealing with human errors. To reduce the chance of human errors, effective reminders must be developed.

Clinicians must be involved in all phases of outcomes management projects. Their advice, support, and expertise are crucial to the success of the project. Outcomes management represents a growing area of research in medicine, with significant opportunities to improve efficiency, lessen waste, and provide a reasonable standard of care both to the patient's and the caregiver's satisfaction. Regardless of how a healthcare organization implements outcomes-based practice, there's one certainty—valid, reliable and timely information about important clinical processes and patient outcomes will always be needed by caregivers.

REFERENCES

1. Ellwood P. Shattuck Lecture—Outcomes management: A technology of patient experience. N Engl J Med 318:1549–1556, 1988.
2. Draper WH. The thermometer in the diagnosis, prognosis, and treatment of disease. The Medical and Surgical Reporter 16:374–378, 1867.
3. Allman WF. Staying alive in the 20th century. Science 6:30–41, 1985.
4. Tversky A, Kahneman D. Judgment under uncertainty: Heuristics and biases. Science 85:1124–1131, 1974.
5. Miller GA. The magical number seven, plus or minus two: Some limits on our capacity for processing information. Psychol Rev 63:81–97, 1956.
6. Simon HA. The Sciences of the Artificial. 2d ed. MIT Press, Cambridge, MA, 1968.
7. Russo JE, Schoemaker PJH. Decision Traps: The Ten Barriers to Brilliant Decision-Making and How to Avoid Them. Doubleday, New York, 1989.
8. Schultz R. Unconventional Wisdom: Twelve Remarkable Innovators Tell How Intuition Can Revolutionize Decision Making. HarperCollins, New York, 1994.
9. DeBusk RF, Miller NH, Superko HR, Dennis CA, Thomas RJ, Lew HT, Berger WE III, Heller RS, Rompf J, Gee D, et al. A case-management system for coronary risk factor modification after acute myocardial infarction. Ann Intern Med 9:721–729, 1994.
10. Haefele M. Hospital finds success with CM approach on second try—Emphasis now on outcomes. Hosp Case Manage 2:21–26, 1994.
11. Guyatt GH, Haynes RB, Jaeschke RZ, Cook DJ, Green L, Naylor CD, Wilson MC, Richardson WS. Evidence-based medicine: Principles for applying the users' guides to patient care. JAMA 284:1290–1296, 2000.
12. Remus DR. Clinical practice improvement and plan of care approaches to outcomes management. In: Spath P, ed. Medical Effectiveness and Outcomes Management: Issues, Methods, and Case Studies. American Hospital Publishing, Chicago, 1996, pp 105–122.
13. Agency for Health Care Policy and Research. Depression in Primary Care: Vol 2.

Treatment of Major Depression. AHCPR 93-0551 U.S. Department of Health and Human Services, Agency for Health Care Policy and Research, Rockville, MD, 1993.
14. McConnell EA. Technology update: Hold the lab in the palm of your hand. Nurs Manage 30:57–59, 1999.
15. Nutting P. The danger of applying uniform clinical policies across populations: The case of breast cancer in American Indians. Am J Public Health 84:1631–1636, 1994.
16. Lee YP, Schommer JC. Effect of a pharmacist-managed anticoagulation clinic on Warfarin-related hospital admissions. Am J Health-Syst Pharm 53:1580–1583, 1996.
17. Pubentz MJ, Calcagno DE, Teeters JL. Improving warfarin anticoagulation in a community health setting. Pharm Pract Manage Q 18:1–16, 1998.
18. Kroner BA. Anticoagulation clinic in the VA Pittsburgh healthcare system. Pharm Pract Manage Q 18:17–33, 1998.
19. National Heart, Lung and Blood Institute. Guidelines for the Diagnosis and Management of Asthma. National Institutes of Health, Bethesda, MD, 1997.
20. James B. Implementing practice guidelines through clinical quality improvement. Frontiers Health Serv Manage 10:3–37, 1993.
21. Murrey KO, Gottlieb LK, Schoenbaum SC. Implementing clinical guidelines: A quality management approach to reminder systems. Qual Rev Bull 18:423–433, 1992.
22. Lang M. Bedside test could alter how patients are diagnosed and managed. COR Clin Excell 2001;2(2):6–8.
23. Dixon MD, Burton CV, Graham KJ, Roovers TJ. Outcome and effectiveness models in cardiovascular and spine services. In: Spath P, ed. Medical Effectiveness and Outcomes Management: Issues, Methods, and Case Studies. American Hospital Publishing, Chicago, 1996, pp 161–189.
24. Winter B. Collaboration—and trust—save four hospitals $896,000 on CABG patients. Hosp Case Manage 2:73–75, 1994.
25. Committee on Quality of Health Care in America, Institute of Medicine. Crossing the Quality Chasm: A New Health System for the 21st Century. National Academy Press, Washington, DC, 2001.
26. Alexander G, Clancy C. Practice-based research: Laboratories for health care reform. J Fam Pract 34:428–430, 1994.
27. Spath PL. Mastering Path-Based Patient Care. Forest Grove, OR, 1995.

8
Point-of-Care Decision Making, Adaptive Systems, and Outcomes Optimization (and the National Directives for Improved Healthcare)

Gerald J. Kost
University of California–Davis and University of California–Davis Health System, Davis, California, U.S.A.

GOAL AND OBJECTIVES

The goal of this chapter is to describe clinical approaches to optimizing point-of-care testing (POCT) for rapid decision making and improved medical and economic outcomes. The objectives of the chapter are

- To understand the national directives established by the Institute of Medicine (IOM) and the World Health Organization (WHO) for improving patient care
- To highlight the advantages and disadvantages of POCT, and to describe two essential performance attributes, therapeutic turnaround time (TTAT) and test clusters
- To illustrate the logic of adaptive POCT systems, including integrative strategies, performance maps, algorithms, and care paths, that blend rapid response testing effectively in critical care
- To arrive, based in part on the tenants of evidence-based medicine (EBM), at optimizing principles that will endure future advances in POCT and the demands of twenty-first century medicine

Chapter 4 discussed the recommendations in the first IOM monograph, *To Err Is Human: Building a Safer Health System* (1), for reducing medical errors and unnecessary deaths in the United States. Consistent with national concerns about safety, that chapter presented systems for preventing medical errors in POCT (2). This chapter takes a broader perspective, based primarily on directives for improving healthcare delivery in the recent IOM publication, *Crossing the Quality Chasm: A New Health System for the 21st Century* (3), and shows how to use adaptive POCT systems to improve patient outcomes.

NATIONAL DIRECTIVES AND THE ROLE OF POINT-OF-CARE TESTING

The Vision

The executive summary of the second IOM monograph from the Committee on Quality of Health Care in America addresses the future of U.S. healthcare (3) and states that despite revolutionary medical discoveries, the ". . . health system . . . frequently falls short in its ability to translate knowledge into practice, and to apply new technology safely and appropriately . . . [and] . . . does not, as a whole, make the best use of its resources." The executive summary also states that corrective actions are needed now. The IOM Committee envisions twenty-first century healthcare delivery that will provide evidence-based, patient-centered, and systems-oriented care equitably to those in need. The WHO shares this vision, clearly stated in a detailed report on improving health system performance worldwide (4) and in related POCT publications (5).

To foster continued growth of POCT in the United States and abroad, directors and coordinators of POCT programs, as well as POCT operators and consumers, have the challenge of appropriately applying POCT and carefully integrating rapid response services into clinical practice, while simultaneously conserving health system resources. According to the Department of Health and Human Services, national health spending in the United States approximates $1.3 trillion, or 13.2% of the nation's total output, with spiraling hospital and drug expenses recently generating the largest cost increases in nearly 10 years. Like the multidimensional objectives of improved performance and error reduction (see Chapter 4), optimizing the clinical benefits of POCT represents a difficult and necessary, but exciting task for readers and leaders, who together must assure that POCT does not become counterproductive to the directives of the IOM and WHO. In line with the IOM recommendations, POCT should be evidence-based, patient-centered, and systems-oriented.

The Institute of Medicine Agenda and Aims

Action items on the IOM agenda for change (3) pertinent to POCT include

- Customizing services based on patient needs and values
- Creating an infrastructure that supports evidence-based decision making

- Facilitating the use of information technology and free-flowing shared knowledge
- Preparing the workforce to better serve patients

The laboratory medicine workforce is shrinking rapidly and has entered virtually a state of national crisis. Therefore, POCT must blend with EBM (6) practiced by caregivers at the bedside and on site, and must fulfill the need for rapid diagnostic information in diagnosis, monitoring, and treatment, but still preserve the high standards of performance expected from accurate and precise testing, now customary in laboratory medicine. The performance improvement aims of the IOM encompass

- Safety
- Timeliness
- Patient-centering
- Effectiveness
- Efficiency
- Equity

These IOM action items and aims are worthy of any POCT program. They represent one of the most important rationales for the development and exposition of methods of optimizing POCT described in this chapter. However, each health system has unique attributes and requirements, and POCT, an emerging technology, has its advantages and disadvantages. Thus, the reader shares responsibility for creating or selecting POCT knowledge tools, and then adapting or customizing POC devices and knowledge tools to the local health system, clinical specialty, and sites of care, collectively covering an auspicious spectrum from critical care to the patient's home.

ADVANTAGES AND DISADVANTAGES OF POINT-OF-CARE TESTING

Table 1 outlines advantages and disadvantages of POCT. For each advantage, there tends to be an offsetting disadvantage, primarily attributable to the state-of-the-art of POC technologies. For example, POCT enjoys patient- and problem-focused test clusters, which work well, but on the other hand, test menus tend to be rather limited. They do not necessarily address the myriad of problems and difficulties that arise when the physician manages and treats patients in complex clinical crises. In critical care, clinical investigators have documented the fact that POCT decreases iatrogenic blood loss (7,8), but because for the most part, POCT uses whole blood analysis, problems occur with analytical performance.

Point-of-care testing provides fast TTAT, but because of the location of testing and other operational factors, there may be inadequate quality control

Table 1 The Advantages and Disadvantages of Point-of-Care Testing

Advantages	Disadvantages
Patient- and problem-focused test clusters	Limited test menus
Decreased iatrogenic blood loss	Poor analytic performance
Faster therapeutic turnaround time	Inadequate QC, PT, and documentation
Immediate information	Poor connectivity
Improved clinical decision making	Unauthorized testing
Improved medical outcomes	Increased costs of diagnostic testing

(QC), proficiency testing (PT), and documentation of test results in the medical record, resulting from insufficient connectivity (bidirectional communication between computerized information systems and remote devices). Point-of-care testing improves clinical decision making and medical outcomes, but the potential for risk from unauthorized testing and the costs of diagnostic tests, per se, increase. With these advantages and disadvantages in mind, let us review two fundamental principles of POCT practice that pave the way to performance monitoring, systems design, and outcomes optimization.

THERAPEUTIC TURNAROUND TIME

Several studies have shown that POCT improves turnaround time (9). More importantly, POCT improves TTAT, the time from test ordering to treatment of the patient (Figure 1). Either whole blood analysis or POCT can decrease TTAT, as shown by the shorter bars along the bottom left in Figure 1. Faster TTAT enhances convenience, conserves labor, increases clinician satisfaction, and improves patient care (10,11). Additionally, these efficiencies tend to decrease the duration of the third interval in Figure 1, the time from treatment to the desired outcome. Timeliness and early treatment generally help to improve outcomes, or at least diminish complications and unforeseen problems that delay favorable outcomes, prolong critical care, and waste medical and financial resources. Therefore, shortening TTAT, whether by means of in vitro POCT or alternate modalities, such as in vivo and ex vivo testing (12,13), has a high likelihood of improving medical and economic outcomes and represents an important principle of optimization of POCT.

TEST CLUSTERS

From the physician's perspective, POC test clusters, several of which have become readily available for use at the point of care, must cover vital functions

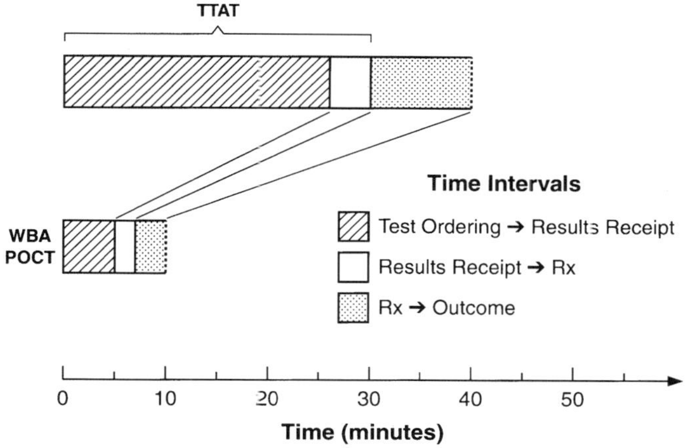

Figure 1 Therapeutic turnaround time. Therapeutic turnaround time (TTAT) is the time from test ordering to appropriate treatment (Rx). Point-of-care testing and whole blood analysis (WBA) shorten TTAT. The interval from treatment to outcome typically also decreases, thereby improving care. The TTAT is a valid medical surrogate for monitoring the performance of POCT and designing adaptive POCT systems.

and their diagnostic pivots (Table 2). For example, in acid–base management, analytes, such as pH, pCO_2, CO_2 content, end-tidal CO_2 tension, and bicarbonate, play an important role, while management of ventilation, oxygenation, and energy calls for timely knowledge of glucose, hemoglobin, pO_2, and O_2 saturation, as well as other physiological variables and parameters. Hence, test clusters represent valid criteria for the evaluation, selection, and implementation of POC instruments to assure that POCT will be clinically effective and efficacious. Therefore, the availability of appropriate test clusters at the point of care represents an important principle of optimization that helps blend POCT effectively into critical care and clinical practice.

ADAPTIVE POINT-OF-CARE TESTING SYSTEMS

Systems approaches to POCT (14) that build on the TTAT and test cluster concepts motivate careful clinical optimization using methods such as integrative strategies, performance maps, algorithms, and care paths. Please recognize that these methods and any guidelines that accompany them must make best use of new technologies, adapt to practice patterns, and evolve with the standard of care. Thus, in collaborative critical care, hospital, and clinic settings, optimal POCT contributes to the learning organization (15), a contextual role that calls for direc-

Table 2 Test Clusters

Vital function	Diagnostic pivots—physiological indicators
Energy	Glucose
	Hemoglobin
	pO_2
	O_2 saturation
Conduction	Potassium
	Sodium
	Ionized magnesium
	Ionized calcium
Contraction	Ionized calcium
	Ionized magnesium
Perfusion	Lactate
Acid–Base	pH
	pCO_2
	CO_2 content
	End-tidal CO_2 tension
	Bicarbonate
Osmolality	Measured osmolality
	Calculated osmolality
Hemostasis	Hematocrit
	Prothrombin time (PT), international normalized ratio (INR)
	Activated partial thromboplastin time (aPTT)
	Activated clotting time (ACT)
	Platelet count and function
	D-dimer
Homeostasis	Creatinine, urea nitrogen
	White blood cell count
	Chloride
	Inorganic phosphate
	B-type natriuretic peptide (BNP and pro-BNP)
	CO-oximetry variables
	Glycosylated hemoglobin, fructosamine, microalbumin
Biomarker	Cardiac injury and risk (myoglobin, CK-MB mass/isoforms, troponin I/T)
	Lipids (cholesterol, HDL, LDL, triglycerides)
	Cancer (prostate-specific antigen)
	Trauma (S 100 [brain injury marker])
	Bone formation and resorption
	Infection, sepsis, inflammation, and others (blood, CSF, body fluids, urine)
Birthing	Antenatal screening (genetic disorders)
	Prenatal testing (urine protein, plasma glucose)
	Delivery monitoring (fetal heart rate, newborn bilirubin)

tors, coordinators, and staff in the POCT program to develop requisite skills in team leadership, communication, management, and continuing education. Ultimately, the entire care team takes responsibility for the patient's outcome. *Outcomes integrate preceding effects.* Therefore, integrating POCT in adaptive systems will improve medical and economic outcomes. The next four sections illustrate the use of adaptive POCT system designs that have been shown effective in optimizing patient care.

Design I. Integrative Strategies

Steffes et al. (8) designed a prospective study to assess the merits of POCT integrated with an ordering protocol versus the use of conventional laboratory testing without whole blood analysis in a surgical intensive care unit (ICU) in a tertiary care university teaching hospital. The surgical ICU census averaged 14 patients, and the length of stay (LOS), 2.9 days. In response to mandated cost reduction, the surgical ICU, pediatric ICU (9 patients, 4.7 days average LOS), and medical ICU (9 patients, 3.9 days average LOS) were integrated by means of a protocol that delivered testing services to all three ICUs more promptly and efficiently.

Re-engineering included a new on-site surgical ICU laboratory positioned to serve all three ICUs and eliminate 10–20 min of transport time for most specimens; implementation of whole blood analysis; user-focused, service-specific order forms with very few ordering steps; mandatory daily renewal of test orders; temporal test sequences patterned for different problems (e.g., interval testing for glucose during insulin infusion in diabetic ketoacidosis); placement of whole blood analytes toward the top of the order form; a limited array of additional tests indicated by service; alternating testing schedules for workflow optimization; dynamic patient-focused test clusters (e.g., schedules for adult parenteral nutrition and modular enteral feeding); anticipation of test orders over 24-hr intervals and preparation of order entry, labels, and specimen containers in advance; preprinted minimum volume of blood required; transcription-free triplicate forms for the bedside care plan, laboratory, and medical record; and continuous interaction between nursing and laboratory staff.

The patient-focused, integrated approach decreased the number of procedural steps by 33%, allowed all routine tests to be performed at scheduled times, reduced the number of records or forms by 80% or more, and reduced the chance of mislabeling specimens (8). On the medical ICU, the number of tests per patient per 24 hr decreased. Figure 2 shows the impact of the integrated protocol on surgical ICU turnaround time (routine and emergency orders), sample volume, and blood removed, all of which improved significantly. The total amount of blood taken from the patient per 24 hr decreased by 63%, reflecting the use of 1-mL syringes and instructing nurses to match the minimum volumes preprinted on laboratory-generated labels when obtaining blood specimens. Preprinted labels

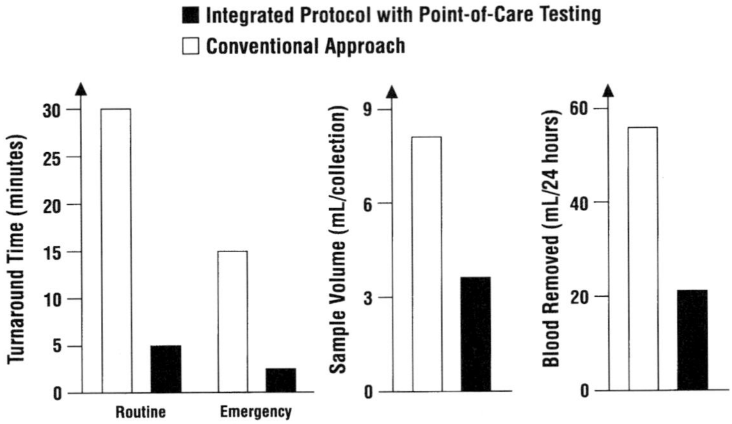

Figure 2 Integration saves time and conserves blood volume. An integrated protocol in conjunction with near-patient and on-site testing using whole blood analysis decreased response time for both routine and emergency test orders (left) and conserved blood volume per collection and per day (right) for patients in a surgical ICU. All changes were statistically significant. (Drawn from data from Ref 8.)

improved efficiency. Whole blood analysis facilitated small sample volume. The ICU personnel often combined separate blood collections into one.

Medical technologists who performed the testing could work more efficiently. They found added value and satisfaction. Physicians felt they saved time. Based on preanalytic, analytic, and postanalytic time saved, the investigators attributed substantial financial savings to the integrated strategy. These savings derived primarily from reduced stat and routine blood collections, streamlined order and specimen processing, decreased transport and transfusions, and enhanced personnel efficiency in both the clinical laboratory and the ICUs. First published in 1996, the integrated POCT approach has been expanded to serve a pediatric ICU. After several years of experience, supervisors feel that face-to-face interactions and communications save time not only at the point of care, but also in the conventional laboratory, and that these two elements represent pivotal attributes of hybrid staff and POCT integration in critical care. For other clinical models of effective integrative strategies using POCT, see Kost (16).

Design II. Performance Maps

Failure to notify physicians of critical test results in a timely fashion represents a serious problem in complex and busy healthcare systems. Emergency notification systems for critical test results are required in all hospitals. Critical limits define the boundaries of the low and high life-threatening values of laboratory test results (17–21). Critical results are those that fall outside these two levels. Hyponatremia is the single most common electrolyte disturbance in hospitalized patients (22). The objectives of treatment are to restore the sodium level at a safe rate and treat the underlying disease (23). Consider the stochastic flow of information during an episode of acute hyponatremia (Figure 3). Indecision as to what discrete low critical limit to select yields a potentially dysfunctional sequence of events that can produce high risk and poor outcomes. Hospitals select different critical limit thresholds (dashed lines) for emergency notification. Even within the same health system, thresholds may not be consistent.

The stepwise sequence to the right in Figure 3 may be complicated by misleading pseudohyponatremia (24–38) or by external defects, such as no action for undetected decreases in sodium levels, unsuccessful emergency notification of clinicians, or inability to rule out pseudohyponatremia. Rate-limiting steps in this awkward sequence increase the chances of encephalopathy, seizures, and respiratory failure, especially in vulnerable patients, such as women during or following surgery, when they may experience prolonged hospitalization and poor outcomes (39–49). Empiric treatment is dangerous and should not be undertaken

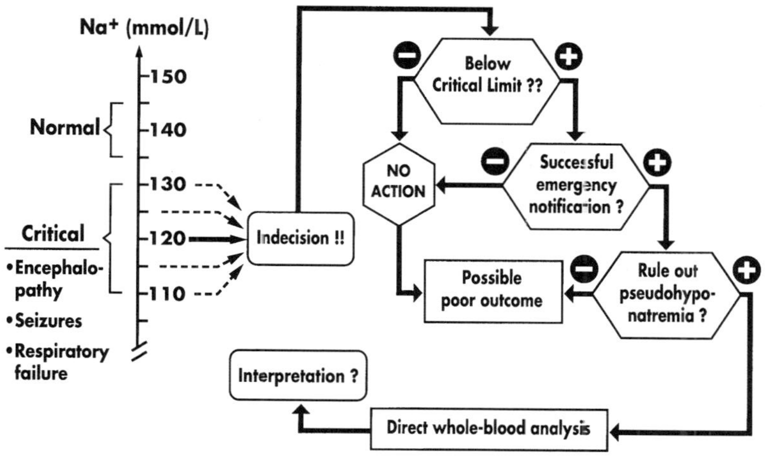

Figure 3 Emergency notification of critical test results for sodium. External defects in critical result notification occur frequently and are dangerous. This flowchart illustrates the potential mechanisms of errors. The vertical scale shows normal (135–145 mmol/L) and critical (mean 120 mmol/L) sodium levels (17,20). Please see Figure 4 and the text for explanation of how POCT can help improve performance.

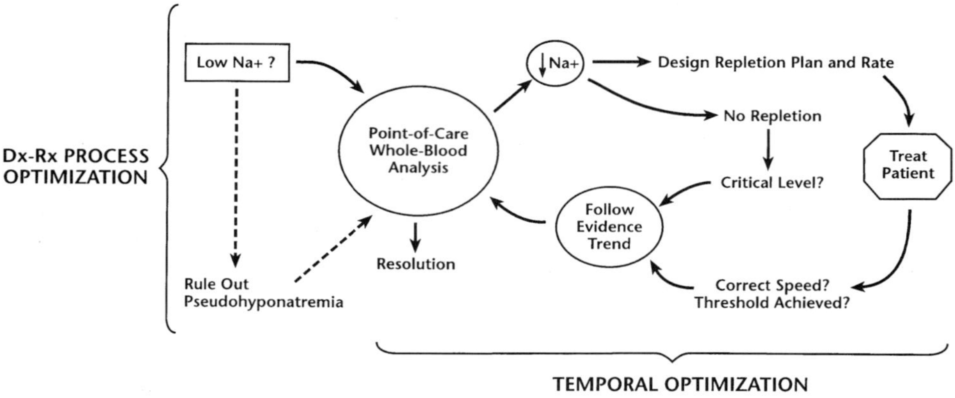

Figure 4 Performance map for acute hyponatremia. Point-of-care whole blood analysis obviates the problem of artifactual pseudohyponatremia and generates an evidence trail for prompt and efficacious treatment of hyponatremia in critically ill patients, often premenopausal women in surgery, who develop serious problems, such as encephalopathy, seizures, and respiratory failure.

(23). Unacceptable risks result from blind alleys in the logic of testing and from open loops in the knowledge feedback systems. These problems can be solved using POCT and a performance map approach.

Compare the performance map (Figure 4) designed for operating room and critical care settings where whole blood analysis is available on site. Point-of-care testing obviates the analytical problem of pseudohyponatremia and also provides the speed necessary to optimize the feedback loop of critical knowledge required for sodium repletion at a safe rate until a normal or near-normal sodium level is restored. See Engquist (22), Zaloga et al. (23), and Fraser and Arieff (46) for discussion of appropriate repletion rates. Diagnostic-therapeutic (Dx-Rx) process optimization (left bracket) and temporal optimization (bottom bracket) help prevent costly poor outcomes associated with acute hyponatremia.

Sodium represents a medical surrogate of sublethal and lethal events. Immediate knowledge of critical analyte levels through the use of POCT links temporal optimization and Dx-Rx process optimization. This linkage, easily visualized using the performance map approach, enhances medical synthesis and speeds decision making. Cost effectiveness derives from prevention of serious sequelae, or from their early detection and resolution through evidence-based treatment conducted in a timely manner. A similar performance map approach can be used for hypernatremia (50) and for the management of ionized hypocalcemia (51).

Design III. Algorithms

Despotis et al. (51–55) studied use of a transfusion algorithm for adult patients undergoing cardiac procedures with cardiopulmonary bypass (CPB). Subjects were selected from a large series of eligible patients ($n = 362$) if they had evidence of microvascular bleeding, and were divided into two groups. A standard therapy group ($n = 30$ patients) supported with conventional laboratory testing was compared with an algorithmic treatment group ($n = 36$ patients) supported with on-site hemostasis testing. An algorithm was used to guide therapy and to divert unwarranted transfusions. Platelet count, prothrombin time (PT), and activated partial thromboplastin time (aPTT) pivoted decision pathways in the algorithmic sequence leading to treatment. The algorithm can be found in Refs. 52 and 53, and, modified, in Refs. 56 and 57, which also describe specific POCT instruments and methods.

Despotis et al. (52,53) showed that on-site testing with algorithmic treatment yielded statistically significant improvements in intermediate outcomes. Figure 5 shows reduced use of fresh-frozen plasma (FFP), platelet, and red blood

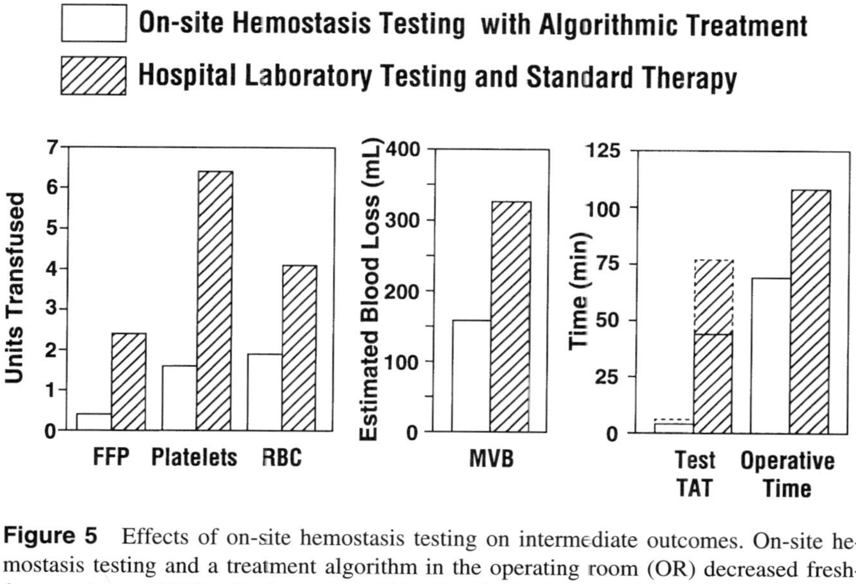

Figure 5 Effects of on-site hemostasis testing on intermediate outcomes. On-site hemostasis testing and a treatment algorithm in the operating room (OR) decreased fresh-frozen plasma (FFP), platelet, and red blood cell (RBC) transfusions. Estimated blood loss, turnaround time (TAT), and operative time also decreased. Changes were statistically significant ($p < 0.05$). The dashed lines show the 95th percentile for on-site turnaround time and the 90th percentile for laboratory turnaround time. (Drawn from research results from Ref. 52.)

cell (RBC) transfusions. Microvascular bleeding decreased from 326 to 158 mL, despite the more efficient use of blood products. Operative time decreased from 108 to 69 min. On-site testing provided a consistent TTAT of 4 min with a 95th percentile of only 6 min. In contrast, the response time for the standard laboratory approach averaged 44 min with a 90th percentile of 77 min. Although not statistically significant, there was a trend toward fewer re-explorations in the algorithmic treatment group (52). In this trial, use of POC diagnostics enabled physicians to differentiate microvascular bleeding from surgical bleeding and to change initial therapy in a substantial fraction of the patients.

A transfusion algorithm alone generally will streamline blood product utilization. Nonetheless, on-site testing plus algorithmic treatment significantly improved intermediate outcomes, decreased blood donor exposures (53), and generated a financial savings of $1504 per patient (54). According to Despotis et al. (57), identification of specific hemostasis defects optimizes transfusion- and pharmacological-based therapy in patients with nonsurgical coagulaopathic bleeding, while identification of patients with surgical sources of bleeding is expedited when coagulation test results are relatively normal in the presence of excessive bleeding. Nuttall et al. (58) recently demonstrated that the POCT-algorithmic systems approach is successful in reducing nonerythrocyte allogenic transfusion in the operating room and blood loss in the intensive care unit. For an example of the algorithmic approach applied to POC cardiac injury marker testing in acute myocardial infarction, see Ng et al. (59) and for further discussion of cardiac injury markers, see Logic Vignette A. below.

Design IV. Care Paths

Care paths (clinical management protocols with timeline tracking and quality monitoring) offer the prospect of enhancing performance while reducing healthcare costs. Closely related to algorithms, care paths, also known as care pathways, critical path/pathways (60), and practice guidelines, have become common for standardization of clinical practice, but do not appear frequently in the laboratory medicine literature (61). Indrikovs (62) recently reviewed useful POCT–care path synergies. While noting that the explicit use of POCT in care paths is not yet extensively developed or described, he concluded that "The true emphasis should not be on lowering the cost of laboratory testing or other diagnostic testing, but on using appropriate testing to lower the cost of an episode of care and the costs of managing disease." Evidence-based disease management and objective performance monitoring of episodes of care represent the forte of the care path approach, one that Indrikovs encourages laboratorians to support by actively participating in care path design and management for efficiency and timeliness in the hospital and other clinical settings.

In designing POCT for care paths, emphasis should be placed on intermediate outcomes, and conversely, where opportunities to improve intermediate outcomes exist, an EBM care path typically will improve outcomes through performance monitoring and iterative improvement in the pathway until it is effective, if not optimal. For example, rapid intraoperative parathyroid hormone (PTH) levels facilitate confirmation of removal of diseased gland in surgical parathyroidectomy following preoperative [^{99m}Tc]sestamibi scanning (63). Johnson et al. (64) screened patients first with [^{99m}Tc]sestamibi imaging, and then, parathyroidectomy was guided by two to five intraoperative PTH assays, available on site in 19 min (median). Savings from significantly fewer frozen sections ($p < 0.0001$), more frequent local anesthesia ($p < 0.001$), and shorter hospital stays ($p < 0.0001$) offset the costs of POCT. Median PTH decreased 88% (range 33–99%) from baseline. A $\geq$50% decrease in the PTH level within 10 min confirmed concise parathyroidectomy. Both length of stay and medical surrogates (i.e., frozen sections, local anesthesia, and unilateral exploration) were improved significantly compared with the control group, for whom POCT was not used. Temporal optimization through on-site PTH testing improved all these intermediate outcomes. Other care paths potentially improved using POCT can be found via the Internet and by consulting medical specialty groups, such as the Society of Critical Care Medicine (www.sccm.org) and Infectious Disease Society of America (www.idsociety.org) and their web sites.

FUTURE LOGIC FOR POINT-OF-CARE TESTING IN ADAPTIVE SYSTEMS

The systems approaches above show the validity and benefit of integrating POCT into clinical practice and of synthesizing test results directly with other patient data on site. Optimizing adaptive POCT systems means translating familiar laboratory science, such as evidence-based knowledge of the sensitivity, specificity, decision threshold, and predictive value for a single diagnostic test, often individually evaluated in isolation, into multidimensional outcomes logic by shrewdly selecting POCT test clusters (Figure 6) that provide simultaneous on-site measurements of several analytes in coherent medical systems. Statistical analysis of aggregate test cluster results and their trends is difficult and represents an excellent goal for future research exploration in POCT. Because of limited published evidence, the programming of POCT into complex adaptive systems often has been rooted primarily in intuition and experience, but in the future, should adhere to the tenants of EBM, that is, be based on documented evidence of efficacy to the extent feasible and practical in the actual clinical setting (9,65). Two brief vignettes, each illustrated with a logic Venn diagram, demonstrate the excit-

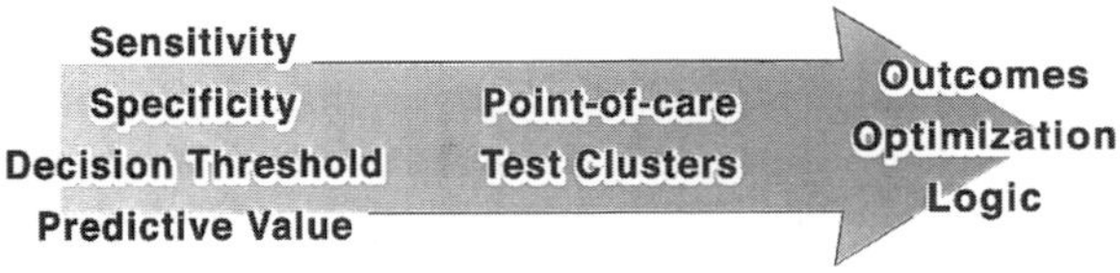

Figure 6 Transitions in logic levels for adaptive systems. The evidence-based evaluative metrics on the left represent the backbone of laboratory medicine practice. Point-of-care test clusters, which provide simultaneous measurements, transition these metrics toward complex adaptive systems and outcomes optimization (right), a challenging logic level that requires a high degree of collaborative problem solving at the bedside and on site.

ing challenges ahead when optimizing and managing POCT as a complex adaptive system (66).

Logic Vignette A: Consensus Guidelines versus Adaptive Systems

The first vignette involves cardiac injury markers and their implementation at the point of care (Figure 7). Current consensus guidelines recommend use of up to two cardiac injury markers with decision thresholds for acute myocardial infarction (AMI) at the 99th percentile of normal subjects and imprecision not greater than 10% (67). Well-established injury markers, such as myoglobin and

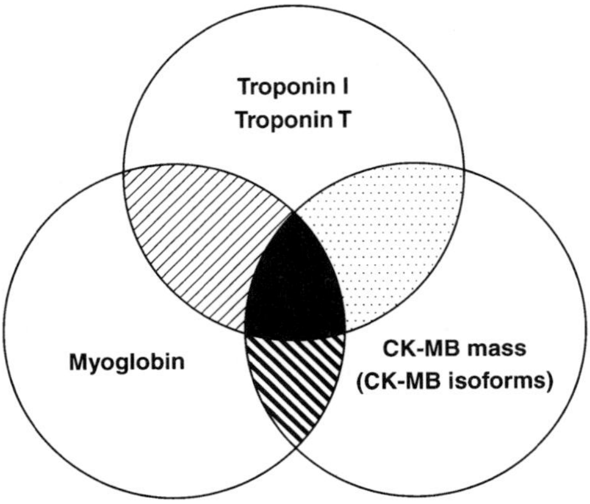

Figure 7 Logic template for cardiac injury marker testing.

creatine kinase-MB (CK-MB) (thick-striped overlapping area at the bottom of Figure 7) offer good sensitivity, but lack the specificity of cardiac troponin I or T testing needed to rule in AMI. Combining three cardiac injury markers (filled overlapping area in the middle of the Venn diagram) improves both negative and positive predictive value in patients with acute coronary syndrome (ACS) and provides the temporal span (temporal optimization) needed to rule in or rule out AMI, but may increase the costs of diagnostic testing, depending on the instrument format, whether POCT is used, and the extent of systems integration. Consensus guidelines for cardiac injury marker testing may omit algorithmic diagnosis and may not invoke the adaptive characteristics of systems thinking and the learning organization.

For POCT to be efficient, effective, economic, *and* efficacious, it must be integrative, algorithmic, performance map oriented, and/or care path based, that is, part of an adaptive system, with clinical experience at individual institutions considered in the selection of test clusters, instrument formats, and testing sites (68). That is, whether two or more markers are used, to optimize outcomes, POCT of cardiac injury markers should fit into practice patterns designed from evidence of proven benefit in the individual health system. Please consult the interesting recent contributions of Maisel et al. (59,69) for evidence of how POCT of cardiac injury markers with fast TTAT can be applied algorithmically and adaptively to generate improved outcomes and monetary savings in a systems approach to the diagnosis of patients with suspected AMI within 90 min. One can logically conclude that adaptive POCT systems need to become integral to consensus and practice guidelines.

Logic Vignette B: Static Evidence versus Dynamic Cascades

Consider the potential for development of adaptive POCT systems to improve the care of patients with sepsis (Figure 8). Optimal test clusters must integrate critical process steps in diagnosis, monitoring, and treatment to optimize outcomes. For the septic patient, time clearly is of the essence. Traditional microbiology laboratory methods of diagnosis, which require 24–48 hr or more, generally are too slow to prevent the high morbidity and mortality that can develop soon after admission of the patient because of poorly focused antimicrobial therapy initially. In this condition, critically optimized outcomes (filled overlapping area in Figure 8) result from rapidly diagnosing pathogens, immediately focusing antibiotics, and quickly interrupting cytokine and coagulation cascades (e.g., by administering activated protein C) to prevent the development of septic shock, multiple system organ failure, and possibly, death.

Sequential clinical events cascade in a distinctively dynamic and quickly evolving pattern in sepsis. Point-of-care testing potentially will fit into the ad-

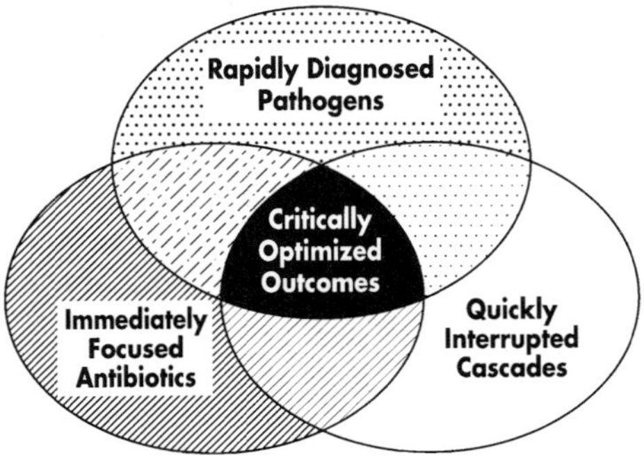

Figure 8 Critically optimized outcomes in sepsis.

vanced logic structure of sepsis diagnosis, monitoring, and therapy at various pathophysiological steps, but as yet, exactly how is not defined, understood, evaluated, or proven efficacious for patient care. Practice guidelines, such as those published by the Society of Critical Care Medicine and the International Sepsis Forum (70,71), are helpful and also dynamic, perpetually evolving to accommodate new knowledge. Sepsis calls for a *truly complex adaptive system* in which future POCT will be well suited, but not applied without extensive investigation and elucidation of the most effective and logical systems approaches that will benefit the patient optimally.

Adverse Surrogates and Outcomes Optimizers

Consideration of such difficult clinical problems as ACS and sepsis leads to identification of the necessary logic and role of POCT: rapid response diagnostic testing addresses the need for quickly attacking surrogates of adverse outcomes (Figure 9). Point-of-care testing helps target pathophysiological surrogates of adverse outcomes through early detection and correction, which facilitate prevention and optimization. Timely actions on medical surrogates decrease sublethal and lethal events. Reduced morbidity and mortality feed forward to improve integrated medical and economic outcomes. The challenge for POCT is to intercede at appropriate logic levels in quickly evolving sequences in critical care, and for POCT practitioners to design novel new optimization tools and adaptive POCT systems. In routine care, such systems are equally important and vital to maintaining the continuity of patient care. Hence, of necessity, the POCT coordinator of the future will design adaptive POCT systems and, along with the physician, will serve as an outcomes optimizer for those systems.

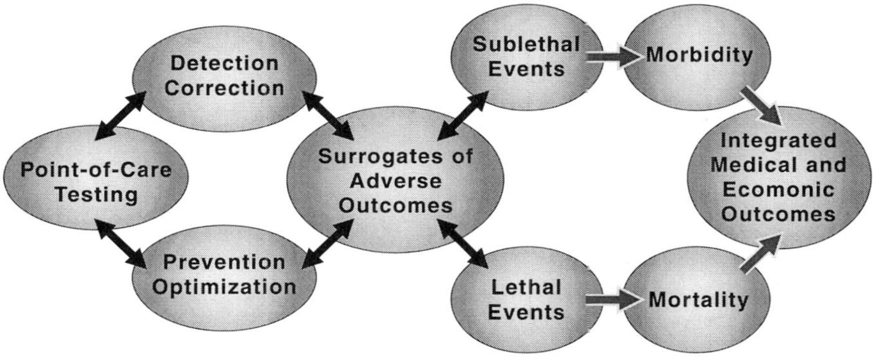

Figure 9 Surrogates of adverse outcomes. Point-of-care testing interrupts the feed forward of untoward episodes in care to poor medical and economic outcomes.

CONCLUSIONS AND RECOMMENDATIONS

As a new paradigm, POCT presents an apparent paradox of medical efficacy at higher cost per test versus offsetting collective benefits to the health system, such as timeliness, efficiency, patient centering, and overall cost effectiveness. These POCT benefits improve the performance of integrated decision making, while the mobility of POCT distributes services, thereby potentially improving equity of care, in line with the IOM and WHO directives. Collaborative teams (72) of clinicians and POCT practitioners have the challenge of focusing on priority medical conditions and providing leadership and stewardship, as recommended by the IOM (3), for optimization of outcomes through the following actions:

- Identification and delineation of goals and best practice guidelines
- Dissemination of those guidelines to professional communities and the general public
- Ongoing analysis and synthesis of medical evidence
- Development of decision support tools (e.g., integrative strategies, performance maps, algorithms, and care paths) to assist clinicians and patients in applying the evidence
- Development of quality measures and performance monitors for performance improvement in care processes and outcomes

The IOM Committee observed, "In the current health care system, scientific knowledge about best care is not applied systematically or expeditiously to clinical practice" and additionally, "More systematic approaches are needed to analyze and synthesize medical evidence for both clinicians and patients." The IOM also emphasized the importance of information technologies in solving communications problems. A recent report of the Agency for Healthcare Research and Quality states that one of the most distressing safety issues of the clinical encounter is the failure to follow up on diagnostic test results (73). Barriers to retrieving test results ranged from physician forgetfulness to a lack of cohesive communications. Immediate POC test results help alleviate these problems, and connectivity of POCT will advance diagnostic informatics and facilitate expansion of POCT as a complex adaptive knowledge system (74). With POC connectivity, substantial improvement in the immediacy, quality, safety, and continuity of bedside testing will be achieved in the next decade.

In summary, the strategies cited in this chapter illustrate that POCT provides optimal performance when adaptively systems-integrated into patient care processes. When optimally used, POCT will contribute, as envisioned by the WHO and the IOM, to a healthcare system ". . . that uses the best knowledge, that is focused intensely on patients, and that works across health care providers and settings" (3).

ACKNOWLEDGMENTS

I thank my wife, Angela, my son, Christopher, and my daughter, Laurie, for their help and inspiration. I am indebted also to the many generous students and colleagues who contributed to this work, portions of which were first published on-line via the World Wide Web (WWW) as an audiovisual educational presentation with accompanying text at www.poctctr.ucdavis.edu, the web site of the Point-of-Care Testing Center for Teaching and Research (POCT•CTR^{SM}). Table and figure concepts in this chapter and in the WWW media are used with the exclusive permission of Knowledge Optimization®, Davis, CA.

REFERENCES

1. Kohn LT, Corrigan JM, Donaldson MS, eds. Committee on Quality of Health Care in America, Institute of Medicine. To Err Is Human: Building a Safer Health System. National Academy Press, Washington, DC, 2000.
2. Kost GJ. Preventing medical errors in point-of-care testing: Security, validation, performance, safeguards, and connectivity. Arch Pathol Lab Med 125:1307–1315, 2001.
3. Richardson WL, Berwick DM, Bisgard JC, et al. Crossing the Quality Chasm: A New Health System for the 21st Century. National Academy Press, Washington, DC, 2001.
4. World Health Organization. Health Systems: Improving Performance. The World Health Report 2000. WHO, Geneva, Switzerland, 2000.

5. Tang Z, Louie RF, Kost GJ. Glucose meter measurements in point-of-care testing: Advantages and disadvantages in critical care. Global Health Care. World Medical Association, London, 2000, CD-ROM.
6. Sackett DL, Straus SE, Richardson WS, Rosenberg W, Haynes RB. Evidence-Based Medicine: How to Practice and Teach EBM. Churchill Livingstone, New York, 2000.
7. Salem M, Chernow B, Burke R, Stacey JA, Slogoff M, Sood S. Bedside diagnostic blood testing: Its accuracy, rapidity, and utility in blood conservation. JAMA 266: 382–389, 1991.
8. Steffes MW, Gillen JL, Fuhrman SA. Delivering clinical laboratory services to intensive care units. Clin Chem 42:387–391, 1996, and personal communication, 2001.
9. Kost GJ, Tran NK. Effects of POCT on time, process, decision making, treatment, and outcomes. In: Kost GJ, ed. Principles and Practice of Point-of-Care Testing. Lippincott/Williams & Wilkins, Philadelphia: 2002, Appendix I.
10. Mohammad AA, Summers H, Burchfield JE, Petersen JR, Bissell MG, Okorodudu AO. STAT turnaround time: Satellite and point-to-point testing. Lab Med 27:684–688, 1996.
11. Kilgore ML, Steindel SJ, Smith JA. Evaluating stat testing options in an academic health center: Therapeutic turnaround time and staff satisfaction. Clin Chem 44: 1597–1603, 1998.
12. Kost GJ, Hague C. The current and future status of critical care testing and patient monitoring. Pathology Patterns. Am J Clin Pathol 104(suppl 1):S2–S17, 1995.
13. Kost GJ, Hague C. In vitro, ex vivo, and in vivo biosensor systems. In: Kost GJ, ed. Handbook of Clinical Automation, Robotics, and Optimization. Wiley, New York, 1996, pp 648–753.
14. Kost GJ. The clinical systems manager: Optimizing point-of-care testing. Clin Lab Manage Rev 12:353–363, 1998.
15. Senge PM. The Fifth Discipline: The Art and Practice of the Learning Organization. Currency Doubleday, New York, 1990.
16. Kost GJ, ed. Principles and Practice of Point-of-Care Testing. Lippincott/Williams & Wilkins, Philadelphia, 2002.
17. Kost GJ. Critical limits for urgent clinician notification at US medical centers. JAMA 263:704–707, 1990.
18. Kost GJ. Critical limits for emergency clinician notification at United States children's hospitals. Pediatrics 88:597–603, 1991.
19. Kost GJ. The significance of ionized calcium in cardiac and critical care: Availability and critical limits at US medical centers and children's hospitals. Arch Pathol Lab Med 177:890–896, 1993.
20. Kost GJ. Using critical limits to improve patient outcome. Med Lab Observ 25:22–27, 1993.
21. Kost GJ. Designing critical limit systems for knowledge optimization. Arch Pathol Lab Med 120:616–618, 1996.
22. Engquist A. From plasma [Na^+] to diagnosis and treatment. Acta Anesthesiol Scand 39(suppl 107):273–279, 1995.
23. Zaloga GP, Kirby RR, Bernards WC, Layon AJ. Fluid and Electrolytes. In: Civetta

JM, Taylor RW, Kirby RR, eds. Critical Care. Lippincott-Raven, Philadelphia, 1997, pp 413–442.
24. Forrest ARW, Shenkin A. Dangerous pseudohyponatremia. Lancet 2:1256, 1980.
25. Frier BM, Steer CR, Baird JD, Bloomfield S. Misleading plasma electrolytes in diabetic children with severe hyperlipidemia. Arch Dis Child 55:771–775, 1980.
26. Nanji AA, Blank DW. Pseudohyponatremia and hyperviscosity. J Clin Pathol 36: 834–835, 1983.
27. Pain RW. Test and teach (41). Diagnosis: Hypertriglyceridemia with pseudohyponatremia in acute and chronic alcoholism. Pathology 15:331–334, 1983.
28. Aw TC, Keichle FL. Pseudohyponatremia. Am J Emerg Med 3:236–239, 1985.
29. Howard JM, Reed J. Pseudohyponatremia in acute hyperlipemic pancreatitis. A potential pitfall in therapy. Arch Surg 120:1053–1055, 1985.
30. Weisberg LS. Pseudohyponatremia: A reappraisal. Am J Med 86:315–318, 1989.
31. Kost GJ. Accurate and efficient diagnosis of hyperosmolar coma. Audio-Digest Intern Med Vol 38, no. 10, May 22, 1991.
32. Grateau G, Bachmeyer C, Taulera O, Sarfati G, Cremer G, Sereni D. Pseudohyponatremia and pseudohyperphosphatemia in a patient with human immunodeficiency virus infection. Nephron 46:640, 1993.
33. Vaswani SK, Sprague R. Pseudohyponatremia in multiple myeloma. South Med J 86:251–252, 1993.
34. Olivero JJ. Case in point. Pseudohyponatremia due to hyperproteinemia in multiple myeloma. Hosp Pract 29:61, 1994.
35. Sachs C, Levillain P. The real cause of discrepancy between plasma sodium results obtained by ISE and "dilution" techniques: An error in the dilution factor. AACC Electrolyte/Blood Gas Division Newsletter 9:2–4, 1994.
36. Lawn N, Wijdicks EF, Burritt MF. Intravenous immune globulin and pseudohyponatremia. NEJM 1998;339:632.
37. Ng SK. Intravenous immunoglobulin infusion causing pseudohyponatremia. Lupus 8:488–490, 1999.
38. Rosenthal R, Koelz A, Vogelbach P. Pseudohyponatremia. Schweizerische Medizinische Wochenschrift. J Suisse Med 130:161, 2000.
39. Ayus JC, Wheeler JM, Arieff AI. Postoperative hyponatremic encephalopathy in menstruant women. Ann Intern Med 117:891–897, 1992.
40. Singhi S, Dhawan A. Frequency and significance of electrolyte abnormalities in pneumonia. Indian Peds 29:734–740, 1992.
41. Singhi S, Prasad SVSS, Chugh KS. Hyponatremia in sick children: A marker of serious illness. Indian Peds 31:19–25, 1994.
42. Ayus JC, Arieff AI. Pulmonary complications of hyponatremic encephalopathy: Noncardiac pulmonary edema and hypercapnic respiratory failure. Chest 107:517–521, 1995.
43. Ayus CJ, Arieff AI. Brain damage and postoperative hyponatremia: The role of gender. Neurology 46:323–328, 1996.
44. Ayus JC, Arieff AI. Hyponatremia and myelinolysis. Ann Intern Med 127:163, 1997.
45. Ayus JC, Arieff AI. Postoperative hyponatremia. Ann Intern Med 126:1005–1006, 1997.

46. Fraser CL, Arieff AI. Epidemiology, pathophysiology, and management of hyponatremic encephalopathy. Am J Med 102:67–77, 1997.
47. Laureno R, Karp B. Myelinolysis after correction of hyponatremia. Ann Intern Med 126:57–62, 1997.
48. Arieff AI. Postoperative hyponatremic encephalopathy following elective surgery in children. Paediatr Anesth 81:1–4, 1998.
49. Arieff AI, Ayus JC. Hyponatremia. N Engl J Med 343:886, 2000.
50. Palevsky PM, Bhagrath R, Greenberg A. Hypernatremia in hospitalized patients. Ann Intern Med 124:197–203, 1996.
51. Kost GJ, Bullock J, Despotis GJ. On-site and near-patient testing in the operating room. In: Kost GJ, ed. Principles and Practice of Point-of-Care Testing. Lippincott/Williams & Wilkins, Philadelphia, 2002.
52. Despotis GJ, Santoro SA, Spitznagel E, et al. Prospective evaluation and clinical utility of on-site monitoring of coagulation in patients undergoing cardiac operation. J Thorac Cardiovasc Surg 107:271–279, 1994.
53. Despotis GJ, Grishaber JE, Goodnough LT. The effect of an intraoperative treatment algorithm on physicians' transfusion practice in cardiac surgery. Transfusion 34: 290–296, 1994.
54. Despotis GJ, Santoro SA, Spitznagel E, et al. On-site prothrombin time, activated partial thromboplastin time, and platelet count: A comparison between whole blood and laboratory assays with coagulation factor analysis in patients presenting for cardiac surgery. Anesthesiology 80:338–351, 1994.
55. Goodnough LT, Despotis GJ, Hogue CW, Ferguson TB. On the need for improved transfusion indicators in cardiac surgery. Ann Thorac Surg 60:473–480, 1995.
56. Despotis GJ, Joist JH, Goodnough LT. Monitoring of hemostasis in cardiac surgical patients: Impact of point-of-care testing on blood loss and transfusion outcomes. Clin Chem 43:1684–1696, 1997.
57. Despotis GJ, Skubas NJ, Goodnough LT. Optimal management of bleeding and transfusion in patients undergoing cardiac surgery. Sem Thorac Cardiovasc Surg 11: 84–104, 1999.
58. Nuttall GA, Oliver WC, Santrach PJ, et al. Efficacy of a simple intraoperative transfusion algorithm for nonerythrocyte component utilization after cardiopulmonary bypass. Anesthesiology 94:773–781, 2001.
59. Ng SM, Krishnaswamy P, Morrisey R, Clopton P, Fitzgerald R, Maisel AS. Ninety-minute critical pathway for chest pain evaluation. Am J Cardiol 88:611–617, 2001.
60. Kost GJ, Lathrop JP. Designing diagnostic testing for patient-focused care. Med Lab Observ 25(9S):16–26, 1993.
61. Kost GJ. National Guideline Clearinghouse. Web Site Review. Clin Chem 46:141–142, 2000.
62. Indrikovs AJ. The role of point-of-care testing in care paths. In: Kost GJ, ed. Principles and Practice of Point-of-Care Testing. Lippincott/Williams & Wilkins, Philadelphia, 2002.
63. Sokoll LJ, Donovan PI, Udelsman R. Point-of-care parathyroid hormone testing. In: Kost GJ, ed. Principles and Practice of Point-of-Care Testing. Lippincott/Williams & Wilkins, Philadelphia, 2002, case D.
64. Johnson LR, Doherty G, Lairmore T, et al. Evaluation of the performance and clini-

cal impact of a rapid intraoperative parathyroid hormone assay in conjunction with preioperative imaging and concise parathyroidectomy. Clin Chem 47:919–925, 2001.
65. Kost GJ, Tran NK. The economics of point-of-care testing. In: Kost GJ, ed. Principles and Practice of Point-of-Care Testing. Lippincott/Williams & Wilkins, Philadelphia, 2002, Appendix II.
66. Plsek P. Redesigning health care with insights from the science of complex adaptive systems. In: Richardson WL, Berwick DM, Bisgard JC, et al. Crossing the Quality Chasm: A New Health System for the 21st Century. National Academy Press, Washington, DC, 2001, pp 309–322.
67. Apple FS. On-site evaluation of chest pain using biomarkers of myocardial injury. In: Kost GJ, ed. Principles and Practice of Point-of-Care Testing. Lippincott/Williams & Wilkins, Philadelphia, 2002.
68. Kost GJ, Omand K, Kirk JD. A strategy for the use of cardiac injury markers (troponin I and T, creatine kinase-MB and mass, and myoglobin) in the diagnosis of acute myocardial infarction. Arch Pathol Lab Med 122:245–251, 1998.
69. Maisel A. Point-of-care diagnosis and management of myocardial infarction and congestive heart failure. In: Kost GJ, ed. Principles and Practice of Point-of-Care Testing. Lippincott/Williams & Wilkins, Philadelphia, 2002.
70. Lustbader DR. Severe sepsis and shock: Guidelines for management. 30th International Educational and Scientific Symposium of the Society of Critical Care Medicine. February 2001, www.sccm.org.
71. International Sepsis Forum. Guidelines for the management of severe sepsis and septic shock. Intens Care Med 27(suppl 1):S1–S134, 2001.
72. Kost GJ, Ehrmeyer SS, Chernow B, et al. The laboratory-clinical interface: Point-of-care testing. Chest 115:1140–1154, 1999.
73. Report on Patient Safety. Agency for Healthcare Research and Quality. AHRQ, Washington, DC, 2002, www.ahcpr.gov.
74. Kost GJ. Point-of-Care Testing ⇒ The Hybrid Laboratory ⇒ Knowledge Optimization. In: Kost GJ, ed. Handbook of Clinical Automation, Robotics, and Optimization. Wiley, New York, 1996, pp 757–838.

9

Point-of-Care Blood Gas and Electrolyte Testing: Its Effect on Patient Care and the Clinical Laboratory

Catherine J. Cox
Thermo BioStar, Inc., Boulder, Colorado, U.S.A.

INTRODUCTION

Performance of diagnostic tests at or near the bedside of patients has a long history in the practice of medicine. Works of art from the early ages depict medical practitioners observing various body fluids for properties that they noted to be associated with certain diseases. Over the years, research has elucidated the science behind these observations and then developed technology to measure these properties more precisely.

Measurement of blood gas values began about the same time the means to ventilate a patient with oxygen became available in the 1950s. As "ventilators" became more prevalent, a special subset of technicians came into being, respiratory therapists, who were trained in using the ventilators. It made sense that these technicians performed the blood gas analysis because results obtained were used by them to adjust the "settings" on the ventilators and to obtain the optimal oxygenation of the body. Of course, they placed these instruments in rooms near the intensive care units (ICUs), our first STAT laboratories. As cardiopulmonary resuscitation grew as a medical intervention, so did the need for other locations within the hospital to have blood gas determinations, especially operating rooms (ORs) and emergency rooms (ERs). Sometimes new laboratories were created, sometimes the existing STAT laboratories took on this additional work, and sometimes this testing was added to central laboratory sites (1).

The prevalence of blood gas laboratories grew even further as cardiac and transplantation surgery became more widespread in the 1960s through the 1980s. In addition to respiratory technicians, "perfusionists" (specialized technicians who operated vascular "bypass" instruments) and other medical technicians acquired these blood gas testing duties and skills. Instrumentation kept pace with medical need by the addition of whole blood electrolytes, portable instrumentation and in vivo sensors.

Over this same time, the proportion of critically ill patients in hospitals rose. This is reflected in test utilization statistics. Outside of fingerstick glucose measurement for the monitoring of diabetes, the most common panel of tests ordered in a hospital is probably an electrolyte panel consisting of some combination of sodium (Na), potassium (K), chloride (Cl), and bicarbonate (CO_2 or HCO_3). Depending on the instrumentation used to provide these results, and the clinical uses, the panel might also include glucose, creatinine, calcium (Ca), ionized calcium (iCa), lactate or even ionized magnesium (iMg). For a tertiary care hospital, the third or fourth most commonly ordered test combination is most likely "blood gases" (pO_2, pCO_2, HCO_3, pH) and their associated calculated parameters.

Blood Gas and Electrolytes in Critical Care

Many analytes are now available by a variety of methods at the point of care. Their direct costs are generally higher than tests performed in a centralized laboratory. Deciding which of these tests should be performed at the point of care is the goal of evidence-based medicine (EBM). Just because a test can be done at the bedside does not mean that this is the best place to do it. While a diabetic care unit may need rapid availability of glucose results, one does not see where they would need to have human chorionic gonadotropinin (HCG) levels for pregnancy testing at the bedside on a routine basis. In discussing the pros and cons of bedside blood gases and electrolytes and where they might best be placed, one must understand what these measurements tell a physician about the body, and the role routine measurement of them plays in monitoring and treating patients.

Electrolytes are essential for many body functions. They are a measure of cell membrane integrity, reflect renal function, and act as prime mediators of conduction and contractility of various muscles, such as the heart. Blood gases reflect oxygenation of tissues and the ability of the kidneys and lungs to regulate body pH through removal of CO_2 and bicarbonate.

Measurement of these analytes is therefore important in situations where any of these systems is compromised. Critically ill patients face several such situations, including shock, resuscitation, transfusion, acute myocardial infarction (AMI), trauma, cardiopulmonary bypass surgery, transplant, sepsis, acute respiratory distress syndrome (ARDS) and positive end-expiratory pressure (PEEP) (2,3).

It is not uncommon for major electrolyte imbalances to be present in these situations. Cardiac resuscitation is cation dependent (iCa, K, iMg). Decreased oxygen levels during cardiac arrest can lead to brain death. The infusion of large amounts of fluids that is common in both trauma and other surgeries can lead to a redistribution of plasma matrices and electrolyte levels. Anesthesia may change the kidney's ability to manage cation (potassium) balance. The high levels of potassium used in cardioplegia must be reversed at the end of surgery. Bypass pumps use cation-binding anticoagulants to prevent clotting. Insulin may be used to control glucose levels and affect potassium as a result. Use of a large number of citrated blood products may greatly reduce ionized calcium levels. Shock leads to inadequate perfusion of tissues. Depressed or impaired respiratory function is often a component of these critical situations and one must recognize respiratory acidosis and alkalosis as important factors in patient outcomes. Blood gas and electrolyte values in these situations can change quickly and must be responded to just as quickly in critical situations.

Changes in Perspective: Central Laboratories, Blood Gas Laboratories, and Point-of-Care Testing

In the late 1980s and the 1990s, two major events occurred to affect the practice of laboratory testing and medical care. First was implementation of the Clinical Laboratory Improvement Amendments of 1988 (CLIA'88), focused on improving the overall quality of laboratory testing. Second was acknowledgment of the spiraling cost of healthcare and major changes in how the federal government paid Medicare hospital bills.

The CLIA'88 revamped the regulatory environment of laboratory testing and essentially put laboratory testing under federal regulatory control. Its goal is to standardize quality, under the premise that all laboratory testing should be of equal quality no matter where it is performed or who is performing it. Faced with the need for written documentation and quality improvement measures, many small department laboratories within hospitals chose to close or limit their operations. Testing was either provided by the central laboratory or under central laboratory oversight.

Fiscal conservatism in the late 1980s and early 1990s by the federal government's Medicare program, followed by third party insurance groups in the private sector, reined in hospital spending and laboratory utilization. Diagnosis-related groups (DRGs), with a fixed reimbursement by diagnosis and not by the actual cost, turned hospital budgets upside down. All tests and procedures were now costs and not revenue. Performing more tests or consuming more products did not generate more revenue unless they resulted in a decrease in cost somewhere else. Hospital fiscal departments began to look at what it cost them to provide care and they also looked at who was spending in excess of the allotment. Up until this time, doing more testing was often equated with better medicine or a higher quality of medicine. Now medicine was being asked to justify that every component (cost) of care was critical to patient outcomes and quality.

Ordering patterns and other utilization measures were scrutinized to see where dollars were spent. Were these tests needed? Did they represent duplicate testing? What was their role in patient care? Individual physician ordering practices were also examined. Performance was being judged not just on patient outcomes, but also on the cost of that outcome. Third party payers were not going to sign contracts with hospitals or with doctors if the same or better outcome could be achieved at another institution, or from another doctor, at the same or even less cost.

When a physician requests that a new test be made available, its performance for a particular diagnosis or support role is now evaluated just as critically as the test itself is for accuracy and precision. Request for an added level of service, such as more frequent testing of batch assays or a faster turnaround time, are subject to the same analysis. In addition, current services and tests are reviewed to see if they meet the rigid standard of being cost effective.

On the clinical side, care units began to develop guidelines to decrease variability in delivery of care. This improved the overall quality, decreased errors, standardized treatment, and made caregiving more efficient and less costly. Included in these guidelines were basic laboratory tests and other procedures, in what situations they should be done and how frequently.

Outcomes of these endeavors were mixed. Changes were made with limited data on what their effects would be in reality. The laboratory and the clinical care unit often worked at cross-purposes to each other. Each section of hospital operations was making changes without consideration of their effects on the operations of the other sections. The laboratory focused on consolidation of services, reducing duplication of services (closing STAT laboratories), maximizing volume for lower costs of reagents, and increasing productivity of its workforce. Clinical units focused on standardizing care, developing care plans, streamlining processes, reassigning work, and improving outcomes. Other services decreased the frequency of transport routes or delivery to save on labor. So a plan to save money may not have saved money at all.

Evidence-Based Medicine and How It Applies to Critical Care Medicine

To meet the challenge of these issues, the principles of clinical decision analysis have been applied. Clinical decision analysis has been defined as "a systematic method of describing clinical problems in a quantitative fashion, identifying possible courses of action, assessing the probability and value of outcomes, and then making a calculation to select the optimal course of action" (4).

Well-designed studies employ these methods to demonstrate the costs and outcomes of medical practices. Using outcomes of such analysis to determine what practices to implement is known as evidence-based medicine. Evidence-based medicine is now widely used, not only to evaluate new technologies, but also to determine what healthcare plans will reimburse. Each test, procedure, or change in process is evaluated for its impact on patient care, patient outcome, efficiency, quality, and the cost of patient care, both individually and programwide. Inherent in this method is the understanding that cost in one department can contribute to overall savings in either another department or overall health care.

The reader is referred to previous chapters in this book for further information on evidence-based medicine and outcomes measurement.

So how has EBM been applied to critical care medicine and the issue of point-of-care blood gas and electrolyte availability? Evidence-based medicine requires that one quantitate the impact of a change. This might be in length of stay (LOS), cost of care or other outcome improvement. An early author of technology assessment in critical care medicine stated that "although technology accounts for only a small proportion of the direct costs of any critical care program, its indirect costs not only are substantial but usually define the greater issue" (5).

In the case of blood gas and electrolyte testing, such evaluations are especially difficult. Because blood gas technology is already widely available, its basic cost effectiveness in outcomes is not known. One can only access the effect of a methodology change and the usefulness of the test itself. A true EBM study would include a randomized clinical trial with and without such technologies. Patient care ethics have limited such studies.

Three approaches have been taken in such assessments: cost benefit analysis: i.e., benefits out-weigh cost; cost effectiveness: similar outcomes, one has less cost; and cost utility analysis: utility, or value of goods, to the individual outweighs price (5). Often a direct study of the technology cannot be done. As an alternative, modeling is used. Here researchers (5) attempt to judge the impact based on what would have happened if such a change were implemented. Sort of "hindsight applied to foresight." Crane (6) describes this process as "looking backward to look for trends and evidence of cause and effect relationships and then projecting forward in an effort to predict the future." By identifying the impact of each routine procedure on patient care, one can justify eliminating unnecessary use of resources.

OUTCOMES STUDIES

This section reviews various aspects of providing, or not providing, rapid blood gas and electrolyte testing and their impact on patient care, clinical practice, and clinical laboratory operations as reported in the literature and from my own experience. The studies are reviewed for their evidence of efficacy and outcomes documentation both for the laboratory and for the clinical unit using them.

Point-of-care literature over the past 10–12 yr has attempted to assess this technology. Most studies looked at cost effectiveness of point-of-care testing (POCT) versus the central laboratory. There was an underlying assumption that patient outcomes remained the same. In reviewing these studies, certain concepts of the role of blood gas and electrolytes test at the POC do take shape that will guide future assessments. Central is the issue of the benefits and the utility of POCT to clinicians.

Point-of-Care Testing: What It Is and How It Is Used

"Point-of-care" is a term that came into being in the 1990s. Prior to that, many laboratory tests were done at the bedside or near the patient. Fingerstick blood glucose determinations, urine dipstick testing, occult blood determinations, and fetal scalp pH were just a few of the tests performed by nonlaboratory staff on a clinical care unit. No one thought much about this testing. Many did not even know it was "lab" testing. Nursing ordered the supplies, nursing documented results in the chart, and the laboratory, for the most part, was puzzled when the floor complained that a laboratory result was different from a value the laboratory had no record of reporting. Laboratory instruments were bought without the knowledge of the laboratory, out of separate department budgets, under research grants, or by private foundation monies.

With the increased need for rapid blood gas and electrolyte results in critical care, new instruments were developed. These instruments were small, handheld, and portable—meant to be at the side of the OR table within easy reach of the anesthesiologist or the perfusionist. Justification for their acquisition was "need," the resources to purchase, personnel to operate it, and a place to put it. Results from this testing were recorded in the OR and other "procedure" reports. Billing may or may not have occurred. It might have been rolled up into the OR or room charges, billed individually, or billed as part of a procedure.

The CLIA'88 regulations and tightening of the Joint Commission on Accreditation of Healthcare Organizations (JACHO) laboratory quality standards made these practices unacceptable for "quality care." It was at this time that the central laboratory was given the management oversight of this testing. Once they got a handle on what testing was being done in the clinical units, they set up formal processes within their institutions to control and monitor the quality of such testing.

The Office of the Inspector General (OIG) also began looking for the connection between what was billed, what was reported, and what was ordered. Changes were made in how "charges" were to be reported. This POCT could no longer be "bundled" up into a room charge, nor could the cost of this testing continue to be borne by the hospital without accounting for it in an official manner. As hospitals, nursing, and laboratories struggled with how to "control" and "document" this testing, manufacturers began to develop instruments that could record data and "interface" or connect with other electronic record systems, such as medical records, billing, and laboratory. Technology also produced instruments, simple to use, easy to maintain, that would provide more tests at the bedside.

In assessing this type of testing, the laboratory looked at several aspects including reagent cost, labor, quality of results, errors, and turnaround time (TAT). The physicians who wanted this testing looked at TAT, convenience, satisfaction, length of stay, and patient care outcomes.

The Cost of Nonlaboratory Testing

There are several published studies evaluating the cost of POCT (7–16). Some of them limited their cost analysis to their own department budget, while others attempted to include the costs of other departments and previously unrecognized costs into the analysis. A traditional analysis would look at the cost of operating a large batch chemistry analyzer or a blood gas instrument in the central laboratory. This included moderate to high productivity by dedicated laboratory technicians, low reagent cost due to high-volume discounts, and minimal quality control (QC) requirements for a limited number of instruments. This "cost" was compared to the high cost of single-use reagents with low volume plus a QC program for multiple analyzers and multiple users. More sophisticated analysis included acquisition costs for POCT and inclusion of nonlaboratory labor, such as transportation and processing. Examples of some of these cost comparison studies for blood gas and electrolyte testing are listed in Table 1.

An undertone noted in many of these studies was a reflection of the rapid changes occurring in laboratory medicine and a natural resistance to change. Clinical laboratory literature often reflected the panic that many laboratories felt to this potential "loss of control" of testing that they had just "gotten back" from the medical and critical care departments. In the new budget consciousness, they saw the cost of the POCT instruments and their self-contained reagent units as being much larger than the costs of the central laboratory. Revenue dollars were also a concern. If the testing is no longer performed in the central laboratory, who incurs the expense of the reagents, the instruments, the operator labor, and the quality assurance (QA) labor (training, competency, regulatory)?

Blood gas and electrolytes are high-volume tests in a hospital, with most coming from a few critical care sites. If these high-volume tests are now done in other test locations, who performs testing for the low-volume sites? Is it the main laboratory? Without the high volume, fixed costs are now distributed over a small number of tests and the cost of an individual test rises. The central labora-

Table 1 Cost Comparison Studies

Test site type	POC		STAT lab		Central lab	
test panel	Lytes	ABG	Lytes	ABG	Lytes	ABG
Zolaga (7)		\$6.68[a]				\$11.07
Woo (8)	~\$10[b]				~\$3[b]	
Tsai (9)	\$14.37–\$16.67				\$11.14	
Winkleman (10)			\$8.98[c]			\$3.54
Nosanchuk (11)	\$45.23[d]				\$9.87[d]	
Fuhrman (12)			\$8.10[e]	\$5.74[e]	\$24.94	\$7.84
Demeritt (13)	\$6.49		\$39.96[f]		\$3.80	
Kiechle (14)			\$6.91–13.69[g]		\$8.76	
Bailey (15)[h]	\$7.41; \$6.95; \$7.25		\$8.97, \$14.48, \$122.38		\$14.42	
Kilgore (16)[i]		\$6.68 (\$8.60)		\$3.65 (\$6.12)		\$6.68 (\$9.72)

[a] Labor for POC not included.
[b] Direct labor and reagent costs.
[c] Reflects hand delivery of results and unfavorable reagent contract.
[d] Derived from total annual cost divided by annual volume (10 patients/shift/day = 10,950/year).
[e] Mobile lab on a cart. Sum of direct costs per test in equivalent panels.
[f] Low volume and low productivity.
[g] Range reflects specific sites: NICU lab using respiratory therapist and better utilization of labor versus OR lab with underutilized medical technologist.
[h] Laboratory components of cost per test ABG + Lyte panel; various prices for high-volume stat lab, perfusion lab, and low-volume PICU lab.
[i] Marginal costs only (average testing costs).

tory becomes less cost efficient. Faced with such apparent cost increase, it is not difficult to understand why the laboratory was resistant to implementing POCT.

None of these studies are directly comparable in what elements of cost were included, how costs were calculated, individual processes in each testing site, kinds of labor used, scope of processes included, or location and types of services provided to what clinical unit. These studies both support and disclaim the "cost effectiveness" of POCT. A meta-analysis of their outcomes fails to provide any insight into whether POCT is cost effective or not. One thing these studies did illustrate is that "cost" and "cost savings" differ from institution to institution and from site to site within an institution.

Based on these studies, EBM could not say that there is strong support for one type of testing or the other based on cost alone. The real question is not cost effectiveness, but cost benefit and utility. Is it strictly the cost of the reagents, or a wider view of cost to include the total cost of patient care that must be looked at?

Turnaround Time and Therapeutic Turnaround Time

The second major issue for POCT is turn around time and therapeutic turn around time (TTAT). Turnaround time is probably the number one reason given to justify the need for any POCT. Turnaround time is the time from action A to result in outcome B. For the laboratory, TAT is measured as the time from receipt of a sample in the laboratory to the time the result is available to the clinical user. This is something that the laboratory can measure and control.

Therapeutic turn around time is defined as the span between when the doctor decides to order a test and the time that the result of that test is acted upon by that doctor. It begins with the clinician recognizing the need for a laboratory measurement and ordering the test. Then there is the preanalytical process of obtaining the sample, completing any required paperwork, packaging the sample for transport, and transporting to the laboratory. Verification of receipt in the laboratory and other billing processes begin the laboratory TAT. The sample is queued for testing, analyzed, verified, and the results are transmitted back to the ordering location or doctor. While this is considered the end of laboratory-defined TAT, TTAT ends when the doctor acknowledges and acts on the results. At each step there is the possibility for a delay or error.

The issue of when does TAT or TTAT end is important and pertains to perception. The laboratory might very well consider that "STAT broadcast" via a computer or printer to the unit represents delivery of the result. This assumes that the printer is operational, that it has paper in it, that someone is there to see it print off and is available to deliver the result to the nurse or doctor taking care of the patient or to the ordering clinician. They may consider a phone call to the floor to be "delivery" of the test result. Again, this assumes that the physician is there to receive and act on the result. In fact, it has not reached the caregiver who will use it to alter patient care. The TTAT involves many departments and staff and is therefore much harder to measure.

Beginning in 1989, the College of American Pathologists (CAP) conducted periodic surveys of TAT via their quality assurance module "Q probe" (17). These surveys included monitoring by the laboratory of TAT and also polling different clinical groups on their expectations of TAT. While the reported laboratory TATs were very similar among like institutions, clinical requirements varied. What was adequate for one patient was not for another, and it depended on patient situations. If a patient is in cardiac arrest, then "immediate" is not soon enough; if it is routine monitoring for adjusting the ventilator, a longer time could be adequate. In general, laboratory TAT averaged 30–60 min for a STAT result and anywhere from 2–4 hr for a routine request. The clinicians, on the other hand, desired a TTAT anywhere from 5–15 min for STAT requests.

Laboratories intent on addressing this discrepancy looked at the steps involved in TAT to determine where it could be shortened and what was most economical. Some institutions moved testing closer to the patient with STAT laboratories. Others shortened the transport time between the patient and the laboratory with a pneumatic tube system. Another option is a rapid response section within the central laboratory to handle STAT samples only. Changes in the flow of samples to these rapid areas with shortened processing times and special identification of STAT samples, such as colored labels or transport containers, also improved TAT.

Some laboratories employed a mobile "laboratory on a cart" solution (12). The POCT instruments were placed on a cart and moved to different locations where needed. Staffing options varied with laboratory staff responding to a beeper and going to a particular location to perform testing, or laboratory staff performing the early morning routine high-volume work and letting the nursing staff perform the low-volume nonscheduled work that occurs during the day. The list of articles and letters commenting on how the central laboratory could decrease TAT with these changes, for less money than it would cost for POCT, is extensive and too numerous to list.

Still, physician satisfaction was lacking. The physicians kept asking for POCT and the laboratory kept saying it was too expensive. Feeding the cycle of dissatisfaction and frustration were reports from nonlaboratory journals and meetings on the benefits of POCT. The emergency, trauma, anesthesiology, obstetrics, neonatology, and critical care medicine literature were touting patient care improvements using these new technologies to manage their clinical practice. It is these reports from the clinical end users of laboratory testing that have kept up the demand for true POCT versus alternate site testing. Having a test available as near to the bedside as possible and a testing process that includes as few steps and as few manual (people) interventions as possible is inherently quicker and less prone to error.

Why is this difference in TAT and TTAT so important to critical care medicine and the issue behind blood gas and electrolyte point of care testing? Kost (18) discusses the concept of "physician capture." This is the amount of time that a clinician is able or willing to wait for a test result. If the TTAT is too great, physicians move on to another patient. The TTAT increases as the physician must be called back to the original patient when the results are available.

Popper (19) talks about the provider seeing many patients at once, switching back and forth between them as new data become available. This article notes the lack of recognizing the "cost" of this "switching time" and its implications on quality of care. Zaloga (7) notes that physicians often leave the work area before results are returned and that therapeutic decisions may be delayed while attempts are made to locate them. Schallom (20) weighs in on the view of nurses when physicians leave to attend other patients. In yet another article, Hines et al. (21) review what aspects of POCT enhance diagnosis and treatment of critically ill patients: less paperwork and streamlined patient management and the response time of physicians. From the clinicians' standpoint, they cannot afford to stand still for 15 min much less 60 min before proceeding with a course of action.

For anyone who has been a patient in a hospital, has functioned as a phlebotomist, or has worked in a laboratory, there is the daily routine called "morning draw" followed by "morning rounds." These two events are linked because one derives from the other. Doctors make rounds on their hospitalized patients early in the morning before going on to their offices to see other patients. This is when they write their orders and give instructions to nurses. In order to do this, they review the previous day's reports, including laboratory results, on how the patient responded to a course of therapy. Did the fever respond to antibiotics? Do they need to change the IV fluids or order other diagnostic tests? They want to look at recent results and not those from 24 hr ago. In order for them to have these results, phlebotomists go out early in the morning and draw patients' blood. The results are processed in a relatively quick fashion, usually in less than 2 hr, so that the reports can be on the charts for the doctors to review. The main reason for this early morning testing is to meet the therapeutic decision time of the physicians. The TAT and TTAT here are well defined and of a long enough time frame to be readily achievable. If it takes 2 hr to get a laboratory result from the central laboratory and the result is wanted at 8 AM, then the sample needs to be collected at 6 AM to meet this need. So TTAT is part need and part convenience of caregivers.

But can one measure the "cost" of a delayed TTAT to either the physician or patient care in general? Attempts to do this have been made by measuring the cost of defects in laboratory services, that is, failure to provide test results on time such that it leads to delays in other therapy. Fuhrman et al. (12) performed a frequency analysis to itemize key delays and defects in laboratory service delivery and the cost per defect. Included in these "defects" is the number of times a nurse, clerk, or physician calls the laboratory for results. They estimated the cost to be equal to one-fifth of an FTE (full time equivalent). Kiechle (22) presents information on the cost of internal failure (quality) compared with the cost of external failures (TAT) in laboratory testing. While POCT may have an increased number of internal failures requiring additional testing and increased costs 5× that of a central laboratory test, this is far surpassed by the 22× cost incurred by the clinical floor in delays of treatment based on laboratory results.

An example from my own experience involved a same day surgery center and the availability of electrolyte results. In this setting, physicians habitually fail to obtain certain laboratory tests (glucose, K, creatinine, BUN, etc.) prior to the day of surgery. Patients also tend not to arrive with an adequate lead time before surgery to obtain these results from the central laboratory (30-min TAT). Since the anesthesiologist is unable to evaluate them for type of anesthetic, surgical rooms and staff remained idle until the results are obtained. Each subsequent patient is delayed, leading to late surgeries and overtime costs, not to mention dissatisfaction of patients and surgeons alike. It was judged that the increased cost of POCT was marginal compared with the cost of other services.

Similarly, intensive care physicians are called to other care units to tend to patients with critical care needs (e.g., bone marrow transplant patients needing ventilator support). Having to leave their own unit to see a patient and then wait for laboratory results before they could treat that patient made them unavailable for treating other patients. To be as productive as possible, they insisted on POCT availability in these units. Without this technology, overall patient care would have suffered unless an additional physician were hired.

Point-of-care testing was implemented in an ER to impact the perceived TAT delay due to laboratory test results. Nurses are well aware of the need to get the patient diagnosed and on to the next care stop, whether admission or discharge. A common physician habit, before the advent of POCT, was to see the patient, give orders and then retreat to the lounge for dinner, knowing that they had at least 30–60 minutes before they would be able to decide the next step in caring for the patient. With POCT, laboratory results are available immediately and the nurses literally grab the doctor before they leave the area and press for new orders.

Unfortunately in this case, actual quantitation of these costs was not available to the laboratory for review for publication. Most literature is of a similar nature, personal experience of caregivers versus clinical studies. These anecdotes support the concepts of other authors that "physician capture" plays a major role in the efficiency of providing patient care. As this contributes to TTAT, it affects "cost," but measurement of that cost is difficult and only a few examples of such have been documented.

Length of Stay

Tying TAT and cost together, in another fashion, is the issue of length of stay. One claim of POCT is that the faster TAT will result in a decrease in LOS and therefore offer a cost savings. In addition, the cost saved in a decreased LOS will offset any increase in cost that POCT might incur. This argument is often brought up when talking about critical care units whose daily cost can be several thousands of dollars a day compared with the cost of a general medical bed.

How does TAT affect LOS in various situations? There are few comprehensive studies but numerous reports of isolated situations. Zaloga (23) reported on diabetic ketoacidosis and glucose levels from the central laboratory versus at the point of care. This study noted a significant decrease in ICU LOS from 2.5 to 1.5 days and in overall hospital stay from 8.0 days to 5.0 days when POCT glucose levels were available.

Demeritt (13) also noted a decrease in LOS when POCT was available on an orthopedic/neurology patient care unit. The LOS for "fracture" and "joint replacement" DRG codes decreased from 11.9 to 6.9 and 8.2 to 6.3, respectively. In this instance, the central laboratory was in a separate facility, at some distance from the care unit. Average TAT for nonurgent laboratory testing was close to 4 hr. Additional, undocumented reports state that POC blood gas and electrolyte results shorten the time to extubation of patients on respirators and therefore shortens LOS on ICUs.

Most literature in this area focuses on the ER LOS. Emergency rooms are busy places where the sickest patients are triaged to the front of the queue. As the number of beds occupied with patients awaiting test results increases, the LOS for other patients increases. The faster the disposition of the patient either to a hospital bed or to home, the quicker that bed becomes available for the next patient.

Review of the literature shows a general consensus of no significant decrease in overall ER LOS when using POCT. Parvin et al.'s (24) study notes that when the decision to admit or a particular treatment is dependent on the laboratory results, then laboratory TAT did delay treatment. Such instances were only noted in 3–4% of patients seen in the ER. Tsai et al. (9) report that test results affected the decision to admit in 28% of cases and that rapid test results would have resulted in an earlier intervention in 19% of cases. There was no effect on overall LOS. A more recent study by Asimos et al. (25) found that certain blood gas or electrolyte results "occasionally" reduce morbidity and conserve resources in "certain" situations.

From personal experience, POC blood gas and electrolyte testing was implemented in an ER to decrease LOS. It was hypothesized that the LOS is directly connected to laboratory test TAT. After implementation of POCT, the average LOS decreased by 16–20 min in the general ER. In follow-up analysis of why LOS did not decrease more, other delays were noted that were unaffected by rapid laboratory testing. Major areas included transportation to and from radiology and waiting for radiology reports to be delivered. If other laboratory tests were ordered, doing some by POCT did not impact LOS. Still, there was a need for rapid testing in a small subset of patients. The emergency department (ED) reevaluated the use of POCT, and POCT is now used only upon specific request by the caregiver. The ED physicians established guidelines based on analysis of which patients were most likely to benefit from such testing. This testing is predominantly glucose and potassium, in diabetic and dehydration patients. The effect on LOS and on cost is unknown.

Evidence-based medicine analysis would conclude that there is conflicting information on the utility of POCT blood gas and electrolytes on LOS. The POCT does seem to provide some benefit in time to decision for a small fraction of ER patients but there is no conclusive evidence of the cost effectiveness of POCT in these patients. A major hindrance is the lack of a direct link between such test results (TAT or TTAT) and patient outcome.

Quality: Errors and Their Effect on Outcomes

A third area of concern to POCT is the quality of the test results and the "error" rate of testing performed by nonlaboratory personnel. The most basic assessment of any test is its accuracy and precision in detecting disease. There are numerous reports in the literature on the various POCT devices and their performance compared with central laboratory methods and other POCT devices. The evaluation of these data is clear and unambiguous. A particular POCT device must first meet this expectation before it is considered for use and will not be discussed further. In general, they compare as well as other instruments do.

The second type of error is that incurred by the operator, in this case laboratory versus nonlaboratory. Laboratory technology is a profession that takes pride in their special training in handling patient specimens and performing testing according to regimented guidelines and procedures. Their job is not just to report the result but to report a correct result. And the rest of the medical profession depends on them to report laboratory results accurately, swiftly, and, when necessary, to note any abnormalities or disclaimers to the results. From the professional clinical laboratory perspective, delegating testing out to many nonlaboratory sites and many operators is inherently prone to errors and greater likelihood of harm to the patients than a longer TAT.

Several studies in the late 1980s reported on the performance of laboratory testing performed by laboratory-trained and non–laboratory-trained personnel, mostly physician's office laboratory (POL) testing (26,27). These studies involved general chemistry testing including electrolytes but not blood gases. By and large, the studies concluded that healthcare workers produced more variable results than trained technologists did. There was no mention if patient care was impacted from these variable results, only that they were different. It was also noted that the variability depended on the instrument.

Further support of the claim that nonlaboratory personnel cannot and should not be allowed to perform laboratory testing comes from, as yet unpublished, findings of a pilot study by the Centers for Medicare and Medicaid Services (CMS), formerly the Healthcare Finance Administration (HCFA), of laboratories operating under a "certificate of waiver." These laboratories, mainly POLs and not hospital based laboratories, were inspected for adherence to CLIA'88 regulations. A high rate of deficiencies was noted in failure to follow manufacturers instructions, quality assurance practices, quality control records, and proficiency testing.

Despite these findings, POCT is not decreasing in volume. Faced with the continued demand from clinical users, laboratories are developing processes to monitor and ensure the quality of such testing. Numerous books, articles, symposia, and professional workshops are now available on how to "manage" POCT (28–30). Manufacturers of POCT technology continue to developed better and more "foolproof" instruments with less variable results in the hands of different user types. Connectivity of POCT results to the central laboratory computer system has facilitated this undertaking. A central data storage system allows electronic comparisons of results, performed by both methods, on the same patients, in close time frame, as a QA monitor of nonlaboratory performance measure. Intermediary POCT data management systems now provide tools to monitor operator error in collecting the sample, loading the sample into the test devices, and interpreting error messages.

From a risk management perspective, a health system may not have the luxury of not implementing POCT in the hopes of avoiding "risk" (31). When and where POCT is considered state-of-the-art, lack of service may be a deviation from the standard of care! Rapid blood gas and electrolyte testing is fast becoming the norm and not the exception in many ICUs.

"Costs" and "Benefits"

Blood gases and electrolyte determinations form a core of laboratory measurements that can directly affect the course of therapy in very critical situations. Their availability at the bedside, and on demand, provides clinicians "value" in their care for such patients. There are numerous examples in the literature (32) where clinical units and the laboratory have worked together to meet the clinical needs of effective, efficient, and less expensive patient care using POCT blood gas and electrolytes.

For the central laboratory, high-volume STAT work has moved out to the care units. At Methodist Hospital (Indianapolis, IN), this alone decreased the ratio of STATs from over 50% to a more manageable 10–20%. This outcome supports the theory of "STAT abuse" (19) that tests are ordered STAT so that the result will arrive faster. In a centralized laboratory, a high volume of STATs end up being tested in the same fashion as routine tests, one after the other. The resulting effect is that as more STATs arrive in a given laboratory, the TAT increases, and as TAT increases, more STATs are ordered! This worsens patient outcomes through confusion over test priorities and degradation in analysis time (18).

Decreasing the number of "routine" STATs can result in a more efficient workflow, better ability to staff, and a reduction in the TAT for routine testing. At Methodist Hospital, moving the majority of STAT blood gas and electrolyte testing out of the laboratory did not result in a loss of jobs. Instead, the staff was deployed to areas of the laboratory performing more complex testing, and it allowed the laboratory to bring on new tests.

Implementing POCT as joint effort between laboratory and the clinical units has also increased the communication between these hospital departments. As laboratory testing became more complex and specialized, the tendency of the clinical units was to see it as a "black box," an entity they did not understand. Working together has connected laboratory technologists to the patient and their role in patient care.

For the clinicians, the availability of rapid, on request STAT results has increased their effectiveness and efficiency of patient care. While quality outcomes studies have not yet been performed to evaluate the effect of this on the cost of care or an improvement in patient care outcomes, physician and patient satisfaction has increased. Those who have benefited the most have been those who have changed their own practices of not only when they see patients, but what tests they order and how frequently.

CONCLUSION

Medicine is about information. Information that leads to a diagnosis; information that monitors the health status of a patient; information that improves quality of care, patient satisfaction, and better health outcomes. Information also has a propensity to degrade with time. Information that arrives late may be of no value at all (19). The rise of POCT is about information. Information received in a timely fashion that can be acted upon in just as timely a fashion. What is timely differs by diagnosis, treatment plan, and healthcare institution.

Blood gas and electrolyte testing in critical care areas is one such area where the balance between costs and benefits is tending toward POCT. While the evidence is not entirely clear-cut, it is gradually mounting that there are benefits to decreasing the TTAT of clinicians in such situations. More importantly, the indirect costs of not providing such rapid results will outweigh the direct costs of the instruments, reagents, and supporting infrastructure of POCT.

Evidence-based medicine will eventually help caregivers evaluate what is the balance between timeliness, cost, and quality in laboratory testing. The optimal situation will probably be a hybrid of interlinked centralized and decentralized instruments that reflect highly disparate needs regarding clinical information, decision making, and workflow (19). More and more studies are in progress that define the questions and arrive at answers. Meanwhile, in reviewing any of the literature, one must pay attention to the description of the institution and its layout, the patient population, the clinical laboratory and other outside forces that are acting on the practice of medicine including the need for cost containment, the need for more ICU beds, and the higher complexity of cases. One must also keep in mind the value of laboratory testing in terms of the "health loss cost of an untoward event." While testing may appear unnecessary when the results are normal and do not cause a change in treatment, the cost of not testing to someone with disease is significant (33).

REFERENCES

1. Hall J. Critical care medicine and acute-care laboratory. Clin Chem 36:1552–1556, 1990.
2. Shirrey T. Critical care profiling for informed treatment of the point of care. Am J Clin Pathol 104(suppl):S79–S87, 1995.
3. Castro H, Oropello J, Halpern N. Point-of-care testing in the intensive care unit: The intensive care physician's perspective. Am J Clin Pathol 104(suppl):S95–S99, 1995.
4. Sackett DL, Haynes RB, Tugwell P. Clinical Epidemiology: A Basic Science for Clinical Medicine. Little Brown, Boston, 1985, p 126.
5. Sibbald WJ, Escaf M, Clavin JE. How can new technology be introduced, evaluated, and financed in Critical Care? Clin Chem 36:1604–1611, 1990.
6. Crane VS. Economic Aspects of Clinical Decision Making: Applications of Clinical Decision Analysis. Am J Hosp Pharm 45:548–553, 1998.
7. Zaloga GP, Hill TR, Strickland RA, Kennedy D, Visser M, Ford K, Whitley J, Holt G, Booker C. Bedside gas and electrolyte monitoring in critically ill patients. Crit Care Med 17:920–925, 1989.
8. Woo J, McCabe JB, Chauncey D, Schug T, Henry JB. The evaluation of a portable chemical analyzer in the emergency department. Am J Clin Pathol 100:599–605, 1993.

9. Tsai WW, Nash DB, Seamonds B. Point of care versus central laboratory testing: An economic analysis in an academic medical center. Clin Ther 16:898–910, 1994.
10. Winkleman JW, Wybenga DR. Quantification of medical and operational factors determining central versus satellite laboratory testing of blood gases. Am J Clin Pathol 102:7–10, 1994.
11. Nosanchuk JS, Keefner R. Cost analysis of point-of-care laboratory testing in a community hospital. Am J Clin Pathol 103:240–243, 1995.
12. Fuhrman S, Travers EM, Handorf CR. The mobile laboratory in alternative site testing. Arch Pathol Lab Med 119:939–942, 1995.
13. Demeritt DM. Move from patient-focused care model to point-of-care testing: Transitioning of laboratory services. Clin Lab Manage Rev 10:568–581, 1996.
14. Kiechle FL, Aulakh V. Satellite Laboratories: A cost-benefit study. Med Lab Observ 28:44–50, 1998.
15. Bailey TM, Topham TM, Wantz S, Grant M, Cox CJ, Jones D, Zerbe T, Spears T. Laboratory process improvement through point-of-care testing. J Qual Improve 23: 362–380, 1997.
16. Kilgore ML, Steindel SJ, Smith JA. Cost analysis for decision support: The case of comparing centralized versus distributed methods for blood gas testing. J Health Care Manage 44:207–215, 1999.
17. Steindel S. Timeliness of clinical laboratory tests: A discussion based on five College of American Pathologists Q Probe studies. Arch Pathol Lab Med 119:918–923, 1995.
18. Kost G. The hybrid laboratory: Shifting the focus to the point of care. Med Lab Observ 24(suppl 9):S17–28, 1992.
19. Popper C. Using cost-effectiveness analysis to weigh testing decisions. Med Lab Observ 24(suppl 9):S29–35, 1992.
20. Schallom L, Point of care testing in critical care. Crit Care Nurs Clin North Am 11: 99–106, 1999.
21. Hines R, Mylott L, Barash PG. The evolving needs of critical care. Med Lab Observ 23(suppl):6–9, 1991.
22. Kiechle F. Comparing cost: point of care vs. central lab. Clin Lab Prod Jan:24, 2000.
23. Zolaga GP. Monitoring versus testing technologies: Present and future. Med Lab Observ 23(suppl):20–31, 1991.
24. Parvin C, Lo S, Deuser S, Weaver L, Lewis L, Scott M. Impact of point-of-care testing on patients' length of stay in a large emergency department. Clin Chem 42: 7111–717, 1996.
25. Asimos A, Gibbs M, Marx J, Jacobs G, Erwin R, Norton H, Tomason M. Value of point-of-care blood testing in emergent trauma management. J Trauma Inj Infect Crit Care 48:1101–1108, 2000.
26. Nanji AA, Poon R, Hinberg I. Quality of laboratory test results obtained by nontechnical personnel in a decentralized testing setting. Am J Clin Pathol 89:797–801, 1988.
27. Belsey R, Vandenbark M, Goitein RK, et al. Evaluation of a laboratory system intended for use in a physicians' offices: Reliability of results produced by health care workers without formal or professional laboratory training. JAMA 258:357–361, 1987.

28. Joint Commission on Accreditation of Healthcare Organizations. Quality Point of Care Testing. JCAHO, Chicago, 1999.
29. Price C, Hicks J. Point of Care Testing. AACC Press, Chicago, 1999.
30. Goldsmith B. Point of care testing: How laboratorians can ensure quality beyond the lab. Clinical Laboratory News 27:6–8, 2001.
31. Cooney MM. A collaborative approach to managing risk. Med Lab Observ 24(suppl):36–41, 1992.
32. Sandrick K. Moving blood gas testing to the point of care. CAP Today 14:37–42, 2000.
33. Hammond H. Applying the value-of-information paradigm to laboratory management. Clin Lab Manage Rev 10:98–102, 104–106, 1996.

10

Point-of-Care Testing in the Management of Diabetes Mellitus

William E. Winter
University of Florida, Gainesville, Florida, U.S.A.

DIABETES MELLITUS: DEFINITION AND ETIOLOGIES

This chapter deals with point-of-care testing (POCT) in the management of diabetes mellitus. Diabetes mellitus is a descriptive term for a large family of disorders involving carbohydrate dysmetabolism that are characterized by chronic hyperglycemia and the development of long-term microvascular, macrovascular, and neurological complications (1).

Most cases of diabetes result from a combination of insulin resistance and relative insulinopenia termed "type 2" diabetes (2). At least 80–90% of patients with type 2 diabetes are obese and increased free fatty acids are believed to contribute to the insulin-resistant state (3–5). Other factors that contribute to insulin resistance may include adipose tissue production of tumor necrosis factor-alpha (TNF-α) (6–7) and resistin (8).

Whereas type 2 diabetes was previously considered to be an exclusively adult disease, with the increasing severity and a rising prevalence of extreme obesity in children, type 2 diabetes has entered the world of the pediatrician (9–14). Like adults, type 2 diabetes in children is especially prevalent in minorities.

About 10% of cases of diabetes in the United States result from absolute insulinopenia: type 1 diabetes. Chronic, progressive autoimmune beta-cell destruction causes type 1 diabetes (15). Worldwide the incidences of type 1 and type 2 diabetes are rising.

DIABETES MELLITUS: CLINICAL IMPACT AND SCOPE OF THE PROBLEM

It is estimated that ~16 million Americans have diabetes or ~5.8% of our population. Yearly, ~800,000 people are diagnosed with diabetes: more than 2000 daily! In the United States, diabetes is the seventh leading cause of death and the sixth leading cause of death by disease. In 1996, based on death certificate data, diabetes contributed to more than 198,000 deaths. Compared with the general population, people affected with diabetes are 200–400% more likely to suffer from heart disease or stroke. In people ages 20–74, the leading cause of new cases of blindness is diabetes (~12,000–24,000 new cases of blindness yearly). The leading cause of end-stage renal disease is diabetes. Yearly, over 25,000 new cases of end-stage renal disease develop in people with diabetes. Approximately 2 in 3 people with diabetes are affected with mild to severe forms of diabetic neuropathy. Peripheral neuropathy can contribute to gangrene, necessitating lower limb amputations. In fact, the most frequent cause of nontraumatic lower limb amputations is diabetes. Among individuals affected with diabetes, >56,000 amputations are performed yearly.

In 1997, the total yearly cost of diabetes was estimated to be $98 billion ($44 billion in direct medical costs and $54 billion for indirect costs from disability and mortality). Also in 1997, healthcare costs for people with diabetes were almost 4 times as high as in unaffected Americans, respectively, $10,071 versus $2699.

DIABETES MELLITUS: OVERVIEW OF MANAGEMENT GOALS

In children, the initial goal in the management of diabetes is attaining normal growth and development. For both children and adults with diabetes, the next goal is the avoidance of the acute symptoms of diabetes (e.g., polyuria, polydipsia), diabetic ketoacidosis, hyperglycemic nonketotic coma, and hypoglycemia. Normalization of blood glucose, lipids, and blood pressure will assist in preventing the long-term complications of diabetes. Central laboratory and POCT play a major role in attaining these goals (16,17). Specialist care by endocrinologists or physicians with expertise in endocrine problems can also benefit outcomes (18). While diabetes can be managed effectively in the proper setting, many patients with diabetes do not achieve therapeutic targets (19).

A large industry has developed in response to the need to monitor blood glucose on a daily basis as part of routine diabetes management. Point-of-care testing of capillary glucose measurements is universally recommended for essentially all individuals with diabetes who can perform such testing. Based upon their blood glucose measurement, the informed patient can make real-time educated decisions about their diet, exercise needs, and insulin dose in an effort to normalize blood glucose.

There is a very strong impetus to improve diabetic glycemic control because microvascular and neuropathic complications are strongly correlated with the extent and duration of hyperglycemia. Furthermore, improved glycemic control lowers the risk of developing complications. The Diabetes Control and Complications Trial (DCCT) (20) demonstrated that "tight control" (e.g., an average hemoglobin A_{1c} of ~7% or less) in type 1 diabetes lowered the risk of developing microvascular and neuropathic complications. Hemoglobin A_{1c} is one form of glycohemoglobin.

Glycohemoglobin measurements represent an integrated assessment of glucose levels over the preceding 2–3 mo. Hemoglobin A_{1c} is the glycohemoglobin fraction that most closely correlates with average glucose levels. For every increase in the mean blood glucose of ~32 mg/dL, hemoglobin A_{1c} rises by ~1%.

In the DCCT (20), 1441 type 1 diabetes patients between the ages of 13 and 39 who had no diabetic complications or only background retinopathy were randomly prospectively assigned to receive standard care or intensive treatment. The DCCT lasted 9 yr. In the standard care group, the average hemoglobin A_{1c} was ~9% whereas the intensively treated group achieved a hemoglobin A_{1c} ~7%. This difference in mean hemoglobin A_{1c} of 2% was sufficient to lower the incidence of retinopathy, nephropathy, and neuropathy in the intensive treatment group by 50–65% compared with the standard treatment group.

The United Kingdom Prospective Diabetes Study (UKPDS) (21–24) showed that improved glycemic control in type 2 diabetes also decreased the risk of developing microvascular and neuropathic complications. The UKPDS was carried out over 20 yr with the results published in late 1998. Again, two treatment groups were identified: standard therapy and intensive therapy. Intensive therapy was sought using various combinations of oral agents and insulin. The mean hemoglobin A_{1c} in the standard therapy group in the UKPDS was 7.9% and the intensively treated group mean hemoglobin A_{1c} was 7.0%. Even though this difference in mean hemoglobin A_{1c} of 0.9% was smaller than the difference in hemoglobin A_{1c} achieved in the DCCT of 2.0%, the intensively treated patients in the UKPDS still suffered significantly lower rates of microvascular complications than individuals in the standard treatment group.

Neither the DCCT nor UKPDS conclusively demonstrated that improved control lowers the risk of developing macrovascular disease. There was a trend in the DCCT data suggesting lowered risk for coronary artery disease in intensively treated type 1 diabetes subjects. However, the DCCT was never designed to address prevention of macrovascular disease and the DCCT was a relatively short study in this regard as macrovascular disease usually does not develop in type 1 diabetes patients before 10–15 yr of disease duration. Since the DCCT concluded in 1993, the subjects involved in that study have been followed clinically. It is hoped that this follow-up will nonetheless prove that improved glycemic control lowers the frequency of macrovascular disease in type 1 diabetes.

In the UKPDS, myocardial infarction rates were reduced at $P = 0.052$ in the better controlled group. Again, longer follow-up may demonstrate a beneficial effect of improved control on preventing macrovascular disease. From the UKPDS, it was clearly shown that lowering blood pressure has a major effect in preventing macrovascular disease. Microvascular complications appear to be tightly linked to the mean blood glucose level multiplied by the duration of hyperglycemia. On the other hand, macrovascular disease in diabetes is more tightly linked to blood pressure, lipids, pro-coagulant status, and smoking than directly to glycemic levels. It is through the development of dyslipidemia from depressed insulin action and hypertension from diabetic nephropathy that diabetes, in part, appears to accelerate these classic atherosclerotic risk factors. Elevated plasminogen activator inhibitor (PAI-1) levels in insulin-resistant states and elevated fibrinogen levels in diabetes would be expected to predispose to accelerated atherosclerosis and arterial vascular thrombosis.

POINT-OF-CARE TESTING IN DIABETES MELLITUS: OVERVIEW

Having framed the discussion of glucose POCT in terms of disease management, POCT can provide vital information regarding glycemic monitoring, ketosis detection and monitoring, complications monitoring (e.g., microalbuminuria), and vascular risk factor assessment (e.g., lipids).

POINT-OF-CARE GLYCEMIC MONITORING

There are two aspects to glycemic monitoring: (1) the hour-to-hour or even minute-to-minute glucose monitoring that can be performed by a variety of handheld/bedside or body-worn devices and (2) intermediate- and long-term monitoring of integrated glycemic status. Intermediate-term monitoring of integrated glycemic status involves the measurement of glycosylated serum protein (also known as fructosamine). Long-term monitoring of integrated glycemic status is provided by measurement of glycohemoglobin.

The POCT devices commonly used for monitoring are not appropriate for diagnostic testing. If a clinic or physician's office laboratory wants to perform diagnostic testing, the analyzer must be U.S. Food and Drug Administration (FDA)-cleared for glucose measurement for the diagnosis of diabetes. One such analyzer that is small enough to take up little room in the clinic or physician's office laboratory is the Clinical Laboratory Improvement Amendments of 1988 (CLIA'88)-waived HemoCue B-Glucose Analyzer (HemoCue, Inc., Mission

Viejo, CA). HemoCue suggests multiplying the whole blood result by 1.11 for conversion to plasma if a plasma result is desired. This is based upon the International Federation of Clinical Chemistry and the American Association for Clinical Chemistry Critical Care and Point of Care Testing Division, 18th International Symposium, Helsingor, Denmark, June 1–4, 2000.

The HemoCue uses an absorbance (not reflectance) glucose dehydrogenase method that takes between 40 and 240 sec to report a result. Chemically, α-D-glucose is converted to β-D-glucose by mutarotase to speed the reaction because glucose dehydrogenase (GDH) is specific for β-D-glucose. Catalyzed by GDH, β-D-glucose becomes D-gluconolactone while oxidized nicotinamide adenine dinucleotide (NAD^+) is converted to reduced nicotinamide adenine dinucleotide (NADH). Catalyzed by diaphorase, NADH reacts with the chromogen MTT, a tetrazolium salt, to form NAD^+ and MTTH, a blue-colored formazan. The MTTH is then quantified photometrically at two wavelengths to yield a result. The manufacturer claims no interference from ascorbic acid, bilirubin, creatinine, or urea. The standard deviation is reported at $\leq$6 mg/dL.

POINT-OF-CARE GLYCEMIC MONITORING: GLUCOSE

Self-Monitoring of Blood Glucose

Self-monitoring of blood glucose (SMBG) is the single most important day-to-day metabolic parameter that must be assessed by the person affected with diabetes. This information allows the "committed" patient to make treatment decisions in concert with their healthcare team. All insulin-treated patients regardless of whether they are affected with type 1 or type 2 diabetes should optimally perform SMBG three or more times daily. For example, glucose should be monitored before meals and before bed, and more often if needed. The American Diabetes Association (ADA) recommends that SMBG be carried out at least three times per day (25). Non–insulin-treated type 2 diabetes patients should optimally monitor at least two times daily and over the course of a week monitor at different times of the day. The ADA states that the optimal frequency of monitoring in type 2 diabetes is unknown but should be frequent enough to facilitate reaching glucose goals. Self-monitoring of blood glucose is especially valuable when managing diabetes during pregnancy, in individuals with difficult-to-control diabetes or recurrent hypoglycemia, in patients prone to diabetic ketoacidosis (DKA), or in individuals undertaking a program of tight blood glucose control.

Bedside POCT for Glucose Measurement

Bedside POCT for glucose measurement is used in essentially every hospital in the United States and Canada. Such widely employed testing has created a huge market and has placed a substantial burden and demand for services on hospitals. An overview of currently available systems is presented in Table 1 (26).

Bedside glucose testing programs require substantial commitments from the hospital in terms of budget, laboratory personnel, nursing time, and compliance/regulatory overview. The greatest hospital glucose POCT challenges now revolve around the following issues: (1) ease of operator training, retraining, and competency testing; (2) lockout of inappropriate operators (operator identification); (3) appropriate quality control testing and device lockout when quality control is either not run or does not assay within appropriate ranges; (4) insurance of on-schedule proficiency testing; (5) patient and operator identification; (6) data recording: data uploading from the bedside to the hospital information system (HIS)/on-line medical record (OLMR); (7) options to upload other POCT data through the blood glucose meter; and (8) reimbursement and cost management.

To interface with the HIS, the glucose measuring devices are docked to an upload station or are attached by cable to an information-services port. The POCT blood glucose testing systems from several manufacturers including Abbott Diagnostics (Northridge, IL) and Roche Diagnostics (Indianapolis, IN) are interfacable and downloadable to the central hospital laboratory information system (LIS). Writing results into the bedside chart or patient's chart followed by hand entry of the data into the LIS must be considered an antiquated approach. Nevertheless, there are many centers where POCT glucose results never enter the medical record other than in the nursing notes or bedside chart. Other issues in hospital glucose POCT include infection control, bar code scanners for patient identification, the accuracy and precision of the testing, linearity, proficiency testing, size and weight of the devices, need for wireless communication and instantaneous result uploading to LIS/HIS, and wireless communication of laboratory results to physician handheld devices. Some POCT devices do have built-in bar code scanners for ease of operator and patient identification (e.g., Abbott Diagnostics Precision PCx). Cleverly, the Abbott Diagnostics docking device also serves as the battery recharger platform. Furthermore, data from other noninterfaced POCT devices can be hand-entered via the Precision PCx meter, furthering system connectivity. Abbott's Precision•Net software does interface with the LIS/HIS. The Abbott iStat can also perform POCT for glucose measurement. A discussion of the iStat is outside the realm of this chapter.

It is sometimes asked if diabetic patients can use their own meters when hospitalized. Most if not all institutions do not allow this practice as the patient's meter is not quality controlled similar to the institution's meters and the patient's meter may not be precise or accurate. Some institutions allow patients to use their own meters but the hospital does not use this data and repeats POCT for glucose with its own meters.

According to Merrill Lynch (27), the top four companies worldwide earn over \$3 billion yearly in the sales of glucose monitoring systems and strips for

Table 1 Hospital Bedside Glucose POCT Strip and Meter Systems

Manufacturer	System	Range (mg/dL)	Time	Neonatal use: well/sick	Known interferences/high altitude	Contraindications	Technology
Abbott Laboratories, MediSense Products	Precision PCx	20–600	20 sec	Yes/Yes	None/No	Hypovolemia/Shock	Glucose oxidase, electrode biosensor
Agilent Technologies	IRMA with Sure-Step Pro Module	0–500	<45 sec	Yes/Yes	NaF/No	—	Reflectance photometry, glucose oxidase
Bayer Corporation, Diagnostics Division	Glucometer Encore QA+	10–600	15–60 sec	Yes/Yes	NaF, NaI/No	Decreased peripheral perfusion	Hexokinase
GDS Technology	Stat-Site	50–500	2 min	No/No	Ascorbic acid/No	No	Reflectance photometry, glucose oxidase and peroxidase
HemoCue	HemoCue Glucose Analyzer	0–400	15–240 sec	Yes/Yes	None/No	No	Absorbance photometry, glucose dehydrogenase
Hypoguard	Assure	30–550	35 sec	No/No	L-dopa, dopamine/No	No	Glucose oxidase
	Supreme II	30–600	50 sec	No/No	Dopamine, ascorbate/No	No	Glucose oxidase
LifeScan	OT II Hospital	0–600	<45 sec	Yes/Yes	NaF/No	No	Reflectance photometry, glucose oxidase
	SureStep Pro	0–500	15–45 sec	Yes/Yes	NaF/No	Hypovolemia	Reflectance photometry, glucose oxidase
	SureStep FLEXX	0–500	≥15 sec	Yes/Yes	NaF/No	Hypovolemia	Reflectance photometry, glucose oxidase
Roche Diagnostics	Accu-Chek HQ	10–600	40 sec	Yes/Yes	Per labeling/Okay up to 10150 feet	Per labeling	Biosensor glucose dehydrogenase
	Accu-chek Inform (FDA-approval is pending)	10–600	40 sec	Yes/Yes	Per labeling/Okay up to 10150 feet	Per labeling	Biosensor glucose dehydrogenase
	AccuData GTS Plus	10–600	40 sec	Yes/Yes	Per labeling/Okay up to 10150 feet	Per labeling	Biosensor glucose dehydrogenase

POCT and SMBG. The market shares are distributed as follows: Roche 31% ($1.065 million), LifeScan 27% ($975 million), Bayer 18% ($675 million), Abbott/MediSense 12% ($495 million), and other companies 12%.

Chemistry and Technology: Methods of Glucose Measurement

Introduction

Classic analytical approaches to the determination of glucose include the hexokinase, glucose oxidase, and glucose dehydrogenase enzymatic methods, and the *o*-toluidine colorimetric method. The hexokinase method is considered by some to be the reference method for glucose measurement. Neither the hexokinase method nor *o*-toluidine colorimetric method are used in POCT strip devices.

Differences in reference ranges exist among whole blood, serum/plasma, and capillary glucose values. Whole blood glucose values are lower than serum or plasma values because whole blood has less water by percent than serum or plasma. Serum or plasma glucose concentrations are ~10–15% higher than those of whole blood. Capillary blood is comparable to arterial blood in glucose concentration. Arterial blood glucose is 2–3 mg/dL greater than venous blood glucose in the fasting state. After a glucose load, glucose concentrations may be ~15% higher in capillary blood than in venous blood, presumably because tissues clear glucose after a meal. While all POCT devices for patient use measure whole blood glucose, many newer instruments report the glucose result interpolated to a plasma result.

The SMBG systems for patient use or hospital bedside use usually employ a plastic strip and pad or capillary port to which capillary blood is applied. By necessity, patients must use a microlancet or device with a spring-loaded microlancet to draw a drop of blood from the side of the finger or other site. Avoiding the most sensitive portion of the fingertip minimizes discomfort and averts the development of a callus directly over the fingertip. Although meters were uncommon 15 yr ago, essentially all diabetic patients performing SMBG now have a meter to read their blood glucose concentration. All currently used testing systems do not require that the strip be washed with water or wiped before measurement. With the present generation of meters, the strip is usually inserted into the meter, and after blood is applied to the strip being drawn by capillary action, no patient manipulation is required because the meter self-times and displays the glucose value. Some meters can alert the patient if inadequate sample volume has been applied to the strip (a very desirable instrument characteristic).

In place of the meter measuring the glucose concentration, some strips can be read visually. Examples of visually interpreted strips include Chemstrip bG by Roche Diagnostics, Glucostix Reagent Strips by Bayer Corporation, Diagnostics

Division, and Select GT Strips and Supreme Strips by Hypoguard. Other systems, in addition to glucose, may measure analytes other than glucose (e.g., blood ketones). An overview of POCT devices for glucose measurement is presented in Table 2 (28).

Chemistry and Technologies

The glucose oxidase (GO) method is a popular technique for measuring POCT blood glucose concentrations. This was the first method used for POCT. Because glucose oxidase is specific for β-D-glucose, mutarotase can be included in reagent mixtures to accelerate the interconversion of α-D-glucose and β-D-glucose. Without mutarotase, reaction time must be extended to allow for spontaneous interconversion; otherwise, glucose concentrations will be underestimated.

Several analytic variations are employed in POCT devices. In the most senior colorimetric version, GO oxidizes glucose to gluconic acid and produces hydrogen peroxide (H_2O_2). Catalyzed by peroxidase, H_2O_2 reacts with a chromogen to form a colored product. Bilirubin, ascorbic acid, uric acid, and glutathione inhibit the peroxidase reaction, leading to a negative bias in the glucose measurement in such circumstances. The SureStep system glucose oxidase reaction, as depicted below, is an example of a colorimetric (a.k.a., spectrophotometric or photometric) glucose oxidase method:

$$\text{Glucose} + \text{FAD} \xrightarrow{\text{glucose oxidase}} \text{gluconic acid} + \text{FADH}_2$$

$$\text{FADH}_2 + \text{O}_2 \xrightarrow{\text{glucose oxidase}} \text{FAD} + \text{H}_2\text{O}_2$$

$$\text{H}_2\text{O}_2 + \text{MBTH-R} \xrightarrow{\text{HRP}} \text{MBTH-R}^+$$

$$\text{MBTH-R}^+ + \text{ANS} + \tfrac{1}{2}\text{O}_2 \rightarrow \text{blue-green dye}$$

Abbreviations: ANS = 8-anilino-1-napthalenesulfonic acid; FAD = flavin adenine dinucleotide; $FADH_2$ = reduced form of FAD; HRP = horse radish peroxidase; MBTH-R = meta[3-methyl 2-benzothiazolinone hydrazone] N-sulfonyl benzenesulfonic acid; $MBTH\text{-}R^+$ = oxidized form of MBTH.

The most modern SMBG strips can be used with any whole blood specimen, whether arterial, venous, or capillary, and are suitable for use in neonates. In general, anticoagulated specimens should not be used for blood glucose testing in POCT devices. Oxygen is required for glucose oxidation in most older glucose oxidase SMBG strip systems (as depicted above), and in most circumstances, capillary blood is rich in oxygen. Although older systems were not intended for use with venous blood, there was usually a good correlation between venous serum or plasma glucose and capillary glucose unless hypoxemia was present.

Table 2 Summary of Pertinent Information Concerning Currently Available POCT Glucose Strip and Meter Systems

Manufacturer	System	Strip	Range	Time	Calibration	Control(s) supplied	Technology	Other features
Abbott Laboratories, MediSense Products	ExacTech	ExacTech	40–450	30 sec	Calibrator w/strips	Yes	Biosensor (electrochemical glucose oxidase) system	Credit-card size
	ExacTech RSG	ExacTech RSG	40–450	30 sec	Automatic calibration	Yes	Biosensor (electrochemical glucose oxidase) system	Requires no calibration
	MediSense 2 Card	MediSense 2, Precision QID	20–600	20 sec	Calibrator w/strips	Yes	Biosensor: amperometric ferricinium glucose oxidase	Large display window
	MediSense 2 Pen	MediSense 2, Precision QID	20–600	20 sec	Calibrator w/strips	Yes	Biosensor: amperometric ferricinium glucose oxidase	Pen-size
	Precision Xtra	Precision Xtra	20–500	20 sec (ketones; 30 sec)	Calibrator w/strips	3 Levels	TrueMeasure: proprietary chemistry	Measures blood glucose and ketones; data downloaded to PC or MD office; lighting features; spotlight, backlit display screen, glow-in-the dark case
	Sof-Tact Diabetes Management System	Sof-Tact	30–450	20 sec	Calibrator w/strips	3 Levels	Biosensor system	Forearm/upper arm testing; lancet and strip in 1 device w/1 motion
Amira Medical	AtLast Blood Glucose System	AtLast Test Strip	40–400	≤15 sec	Calibrator chip w/strips	Yes	Colorimetric reaction	Meter + lancet; nonfinger draw site

Bayer Corporation, Diagnostics Division	GlucometerDEX	GlucometerDEX test Sensors (10/cartridge)	20–600	30 sec	Automatic calibration	3 Levels	Electrochemical using glucose oxidase	10 tests/cartridge; includes lancet as part of glucometer
	Glucometer Elite	Glucometer Elite	20–600	30 sec	Strip calibration	Yes	Electrochemical using glucose oxidase	No buttons; Bayer's easiest self-test system
	Glucometer Elite XL	Glucometer Elite	20–600	30 sec	Strip calibration	Yes	Electrochemical using glucose oxidase	No buttons, larger memory than Elite
	Glucometer Encore Diabetes Care System	Glucometer Encore	10–600	15 sec	Single button cal. by lot of strips	Yes	Hexokinase, colorimetric	Permanent battery
Home Diagnostics, Inc.	Prestige IQ	Prestige Smart System	25–600	10–50 sec	Standard strip	Yes	Glucose oxidase, colorimetric	Large display, Internet data uploading
	Prestige LX	Prestige Smart System	25–600	10–50 sec	Standard strip	Yes	Glucose oxidase, colorimetric	Large display, no Internet data upload
Hypoguard	Assure	Assure	30–550	35 sec	Calibrator w/strips	Yes	Biosensor, glucose oxidase	Large touch screen display
	Assure II	Assure II	30–550	30 sec	Calibrator w/strips	Yes	Biosensor	Simple 2-step procedure
	Supreme II	Supreme	30–600	50 sec	Built-in single button	Yes	Glucose oxidase	Large display
LifeScan	One Touch Basic	One Touch	0–600	45 sec	Built-in single button	Yes	Photometric glucose oxidase	No software (see "FastTake")
	One Touch FastTake	FastTake	20–600	15 sec	Built-in single button	Yes	Electrochemical glucose oxidase	Alternate-site testing; Touch Software provided
	One Touch Profile	One Touch	0–600	45 sec	Built-in single button	Yes	Photometric glucose oxidase	Large display
	One Touch SureStep	SureStep	0–500	15–30 sec	Built-in single button	Yes	Photometric glucose oxidase	Large display, data download to PC
	One Touch Ultra	One Touch Ultra	20–600	5 sec	Built-in single button	Yes	Electrochemical glucose oxidase	Alternate-site testing; Touch Software provided
LXN Corporation	Duet Diabetes Control	Duet	20–600	8–30 sec	Use code button set strip lot	Yes	Photometric glucose oxidase	For use in physician's office laboratory; measures fructosamine with separate strip
	In Charge Diabetes System	In Charge	20–600	5–20 sec	Use code button set strip lot	Not stated	Photometric glucose oxidase	For patient use; measures fructosamine with separate strip

Table 2 Continued

Manufacturer	System	Strip	Range	Time	Calibration	Control(s) supplied	Technology	Other features
Polymer Technology Systems	BioScanner 2000	BioScanner Glucose strip	20–600	30–60 sec	Automatic calibration via MEMo chip	Optional	Photometric glucose oxidase	Can also measure; cholesterol, ketones, triglyceride and HDL-C
Roche Diagnostics	Accu-Chek Active	Accu-Chek Active	10–600	5 sec	Snap-in code key	Yes	Photometry glucose oxidase	Data are downloadable
	Accu-Chek Advantage	Accu-Chek Advantage or Comfort Curve	10–600	26 sec	Snap-in code key	Yes	Electrochemical using glucose dehydrogenase	Data are downloadable; Comfort Curve uses palladium electrodes
	Accu-Chek Complete	Accu-Chek Advantage or Comfort Curve	10–600	26 sec	Automatic	Yes	Electrochemical using glucose dehydrogenase	Software available to upload data to PC or healthcare team
	Accu-Chek Voicemate	Accu-Chek Comfort Curve	10–600	20 sec	Snap-in code key	Yes	Electrochemical using glucose dehydrogenase	The meter is the Advantage; voice guided for blind or visually impaired
QuestStar Medical	CheckMate Plus	CheckMate Plus	25–500	15–70 sec	Automatic	Yes	Glucose oxidase/peroxidase	Built-in lancing device, data port for PC downloading
TheraSense	FreeStyle	FreeStyle	20–500	15 sec	Built-in button	Yes	Coulometric method	Alternate-site testing
Wal-Mart Pharmacies	ReliOn	ReliOn	20–600	20 sec	Calibrator w/strips	No	Biosensor	External appearance is very similar to ExaTech

If venous blood from a hypoxic subject or a patient in shock was applied to older SMBG strips (such as in an intensive care unit), there could be insufficient oxygen present in the sample, leading to an underestimation of blood glucose. Likewise, in patients with severe dehydration, hypotension, shock, or peripheral vascular disease, low flow could lead to depressed capillary glucose concentrations compared with venous samples. In shock, there is poor peripheral perfusion. Because hypoxia in such systems can produce negative biases, glucose oxidase devices should not be used to measure glucose when patients are hypoxic. In addition, capillary blood should not be used for glucose testing in any POCT device when patients demonstrate poor peripheral perfusion.

Other glucose oxidase methods offer amperometric analyses where the chemical reactions produce a flow of electrons with current being measured by the analyzer. Ferrocyanide (e.g., Glucometer Elite) or ferrocene (e.g., Precision PCx, Precision QID) become electron sources. The Glucometer Elite reactions are depicted below:

$$\text{Glucose} + \text{FAD} \xrightarrow{\text{glucose oxidase}} \text{gluconic acid} + \text{FADH}_2$$

$$\text{FADH}_2 + \text{ferricyanide} \xrightarrow{\text{glucose oxidase}} \text{ferrocyanide} + \text{FAD}$$

$$\text{Ferrocyanide} \rightarrow \text{ferricyanide} + e^-$$

$$\text{FADH}_2 + \text{O}_2 \xrightarrow{\qquad\qquad} \text{FAD} + \text{H}_2\text{O}_2$$

In the Precision PCx and Precision QID, ferricinium replaces ferricyanide:

$$\text{Glucose} + \text{FAD} \xrightarrow{\text{glucose oxidase}} \text{gluconic acid} + \text{FADH}_2$$

$$\text{FADH}_2 + \text{ferricinium} \xrightarrow{\text{glucose oxidase}} \text{ferrocene} + \text{FAD}$$

$$\text{Ferrocene} \rightarrow \text{ferricinium} + e^-$$

$$\text{FADH}_2 + \text{O}_2 \xrightarrow{\qquad\qquad} \text{FAD} + \text{H}_2\text{O}_2$$

In these SMBG strip glucose oxidase reactions that use ferricyanide or ferricinium instead of oxygen, hypoxemia will produce a false positive bias in glucose concentrations. Also, at altitudes $\gtrsim$1524 m where atmospheric oxygen is reduced, glucose oxidase ferricyanide/ferricinium systems display a false positive bias in the measurement of glucose.

The newest blood glucose detection systems use an electrochemical biosensor based on a glucose dehydrogenase reaction that is not affected by oxygen availability. Glucose dehydrogenase catalyzes the formation of glucono-*d*-lactone from glucose while NAD^+ is reduced to NADH. Like the glucose oxidase method, mutarotase can be used to speed the conversion of α-D-glucose to β-D-glucose. The glucose dehydrogenase assays are highly specific for glucose and show good agreement with the hexokinase assay. The glucose dehydrogenase reaction is depicted below:

$$\text{Glucose} + \text{NAD}^+ \xrightarrow{\text{GDH}} \text{D-glucono-}d\text{-lactone} + \text{NADH} + \text{H}^+$$

For example, the reactions used in the Advantage H and Comfort curve strips utilizing the GHD employ electrochemical detection (amperometry) (PQQ = pyrroloquinoline; $PQQH_2$ = reduced form of pyrroloquinoline):

$$\text{Glucose} + \text{PQQ} \xrightarrow{\text{GDH}} \text{gluconic acid} + \text{PQQH}_2$$

$$\text{PQQH}_2 + \text{ferricyanide} \xrightarrow{\text{GDH}} \text{ferrocyanide} + \text{PQQ}$$

$$\text{Ferrocyanide} \rightarrow \text{ferricyanide} + e^-$$

Technological Innovations and Limitations

Newer GO and GDH strips draw into the strip the proper volume of sample from the blood drop formed from lancing the skin, and determine that the sample volume is adequate before reporting a result. Some analyzers simultaneously lance the skin and apply blood to the strip for analysis (e.g., MediSense Sof-Tact system, Abbott Laboratories; GlucometerDex system, Bayer Corporation, Diagnostics Division; CheckMate, QuestStar Medical) while other systems include both the lancet and the strip but the operator must apply the blood to the strip (e.g., AtLast®, Amira Medical, Scotts Valley, CA; FreeStyle™, TheraSense, Inc., Alameda, CA).

Several newer systems allow blood to be drawn from sites other than the fingers (e.g., forearm) (AtLast system; TheraSense FreeStyle; OneTouch® Ultra, Lifescan, Johnson & Johnson, Milpitas, CA; Sof-Tact, Medisense, Abbott Diagnostics). The skin of the dorsal and lateral forearm or thumb base is less sensitive to pain than the fingertips. Another novel system approach to patient POCT includes a blood glucose monitor combined with an insulin doser (Induo™, Lifescan, Johnson & Johnson; and Novo Nordisk, Princeton, NJ). Despite the tenderness induced by repetitive puncture of fingertips, there is no evidence of injury to local microcirculation (29).

Concerning alternate-site testing, there can be a 5- to 20-min lag between changes in fingerstick glucose and the alternate-site glucose result (30). A significant delay in the detection of hypoglycemia using arm monitoring was reported by Jungheim and Koschinsky (31). Among various puncture sites, other investigators, in contrast, have not documented a significant gradient among capillary, venous, or interstitial fluid glucose (32).

Alternative site testing is contraindicated when patients are hypovolemic, hypotensive or are in shock. In a study from Tang et al. (33), hypoxia or hyperoxia did not significantly influence glucose determined with the GDH-based amperometric test strips and had minimal influences on GO-based photometric test strips. Increased oxygen tension decreased glucose measured with GO-based amperometric test strips. The authors recommended using oxygen-independent test strips for POC glucose testing in critically ill and other patients with high or unpredictable blood pO_2 levels. Kurahashi et al. (34) have proposed to correct measured blood glucose concentrations depending upon the sample oxygen tension [$glucose_{corrected} = glucose_{glucometer} + (0.1 \times pO_2) + 16$]. Oxygen therapy and hyperbaric chambers can produce hyperoxia.

Depending on the system, if the hematocrit is <20–25% or >60–65%, the estimate of plasma glucose from capillary/whole blood glucose will not be accurate (35,36). With anemia, the fraction of the whole blood that is plasma increases, and this increase leads to a false elevation in the capillary blood glucose determination of $\geq$10%. With polycythemia, the fraction of the whole blood that is plasma decreases, and this decrease leads to a false depression in the capillary blood glucose determination of $\leq$15%. Temperature can also affect testing and, in extremes of temperature, the design limits of the meter must not be exceeded.

When employed by properly instructed individuals, SMBG meters exhibit coefficients of variation of 2–5%. Nevertheless, in practice, up to half of all results may vary more than 20% from simultaneous values reported by a central laboratory. This emphasizes the need for proper training, instrument maintenance, and yearly validation of the monitor's performance compared with the central laboratory. Thus at least yearly, SMBG-measured glucose and a simultaneous plasma or serum glucose should be compared to confirm that the glucose meter is functioning properly. Controls are supplied by nearly all meter manufacturers; however, from the author's clinical experience, patients are essentially never instructed to measure controls to determine if their meters are performing properly.

Continuous Glucose Monitoring

The Continuous Glucose Monitoring System (CGMS™) (MiniMed, Northridge, CA) and the GlucoWatch® (Cygnus, Redwood City, CA) are the only ambulatory devices available that can continuously monitor glucose over 12 or more hours. There are indwelling vascular devices to measure blood glucose continually (37). However because of their complexity, it is not appropriate to include such invasive devices in discussions of POCT in this chapter.

It must be recognized that these ingenious new continuous glucose monitoring devices are problem-solving tools that, at the present time, are not usually intended for 24/7/365 use by patients. Both devices provide profiles of interstitial fluid glucose levels that the patient and physician can later use for assessment of glycemic control to lower mean plasma glucose, avoid hypoglycemia, manage glucose in pregnancy, and lower hemoglobin A_{1c}. Both systems offer potential advances in recognizing otherwise unrecorded hyperglycemia, unrecognized hypoglycemia, Somogyi rebound hyperglycemia, and the dawn phenomenon.

Continuous Glucose Monitoring System

Produced by MiniMed, Inc., a company with a comparatively long tradition of manufacturing continuous subcutaneous insulin infusion (CSII) pumps, the CGMS involves placing under the skin a small needle that is attached by a wire to a control module (38). Typically, the needle is inserted under the skin overlying the abdomen. The needle contains the electrochemical microelectrode sensor that is thinly coated with glucose oxidase beneath a biocompatible membrane. The measurement of the interstitial fluid glucose is changed into an electronic signal and stored in the pager-sized control module, which can be worn on the patient's belt. The patient does not have access to the CGMS glucose results while they are wearing the device.

A glucose reading is taken every 10 sec and the measurements are averaged and recorded for 5-min intervals (288 measurements per day). In studies of anesthetized dogs, there was a 5- to 12-min delay between changes in blood glucose and interstitial fluid glucose levels (39). These researchers concluded that "differences between plasma and interstitial fluid glucose will not be a significant obstacle in advancing the use of interstitial fluid as an alternative to blood glucose measurements."

The glucose range reported by CGMS spans 40–400 mg/dL. The device is calibrated with fingerstick blood glucose measurements 2–4 times daily. The patient can key in event codes such as meals, exercise, and insulin dosages. The control module is docked to the Com-Station in order to transmit data to a personal computer for analysis. Software then generates graphs and statistics in a report format.

Clarke error grid analysis has shown that 96% of CGMS-SMBG pairs fall within clinically acceptable regions (40). An uncontrolled study from Bode et al. (41) demonstrated that CGMS could assist in lowering hemoglobin A_{1c} concentrations. Similarly Kaufman et al. (42) showed that use of CGMS contributed to a decline in hemoglobin A_{1c} in children. In a very small sample of study subjects, Chase et al. (43) described a trend for lower hemoglobin A_{1c} levels in children using CGMS versus children who did not use CGMS. Using the CGMS in children even in "good" glycemic control, Boland et al. (44) detected episodic nocturnal hypoglycemia and postprandial hyperglycemia that was not otherwise evident with routine monitoring. Otherwise unexpected hypoglycemia and hyperglycemia were also reported by Phillips et al. (45) through the use of CMGS.

The CGMS device is owned by the clinic or treating physician and is "dispensed" to patients as needed. The monitor list price is near $2000 and the Com-Station costs ~$400. Additional startup supplies cost ~$600. Each glucose sensor is ~$30. MiniMed suggests a charge to the patient of $400 for monitoring.

GlucoWatch

Manufactured by Cygnus, Inc., the GlucoWatch is a noninvasive reverse-iontophoresis/electrochemical interstitial fluid glucose–measuring system that is configured similarly to a wristwatch that consists of the Biographer and the detection device, the AutoSensor (46). The gel collection disks are part of the single-use, disposable AutoSensor unit. The AutoSensor snaps into the Biographer. AutoSensors should be stored refrigerated. At room temperature, AutoSensors are stable for up to 1 mo.

Two electrodes that are part of the gel collection disks are positioned against the skin. Excess hair should be shaved off and the pads should not be applied over skin that is in any way damaged. The device uses reverse iontophoresis to collect interstitial fluid glucose samples through this intact skin. Glucose is drawn to the cathode along with cations. Glucose is aggregated in the disks that contain glucose oxidase, generating H_2O_2. A biosensor in contact with the gel collection disks ascertains the H_2O_2 ($H_2O_2 \rightarrow H_2O + 2H^+ + 2e^-$) and develops an electronic signal recorded by the nonreplaceable Biographer unit.

Analytically, there can be considerable biases reported by the GlucoWatch. Tolazamide and dopamine can affect Biographer readings. However, acetaminophen does not interfere (47).

Initially, there is a 3-hr period when the GlucoWatch is calibrated against the subject's capillary glucose level obtained by fingerstick. Thereafter, the GlucoWatch measures blood glucose every 20 min for up to 12 continuous hours. The matter of reporting plasma versus whole blood glucose is a function of the fingerstick meter used for calibration. If the meter used for calibration reports glucose as a whole blood result, so will the GlucoWatch after calibration. On the other hand, if the calibration meter reports glucose as a plasma result, after calibration the GlucoWatch will report plasma levels.

The "data density" provided by the GlucoWatch is only one-quarter of that of the CGMS where glucose would be measured 144 times in 12 hours instead of 36 times with the GlucoWatch. However, the GlucoWatch can be programmed to alert the wearer by sound if the glucose level exceeds preset limits or exceeds a preset rate of decline in blood glucose. The GlucoWatch detects more episodes of hypoglycemia than traditional SMBG (48).

Up to 4000 glucose results can be stored in the Biographer's memory. Results are examined by touching a button. Patient events can be entered reflecting meals, exercise, and injections. At the present time, the data from the GlucoWatch does not appear to be downloadable to a personal computer or Web site for data analysis.

While the GlucoWatch provides important information regarding trends, acute glycemic problems should be managed by performing fingerstick SMBG. Such situations include times when the Biographer must be calibrated, when clinical symptoms do not match GlucoWatch results, or when patients consider making prompt alterations in insulin dosing or other therapies.

Sweating and device movement along the skin can interfere with the sensing apparatus. Cygnus, Inc. reports that ~25% of Biographer uses terminate prematurely and that ~20% of readings are skipped. Cygnus, Inc. also reports that most individuals using the GlucoWatch experience erythema and edema at the testing site. However, severe irritation is seen at no more than 2% of placement sites. Because of the skin and analytical limitations, the author anticipates that initial GlucoWatch use will be limited to episodic problem solving. The manufacturer stresses that the GlucoWatch is not to be used without concurrent fingerstick SMBG.

Error grid analysis found that ~96% of GlucoWatch results were acceptable (49). Mean error between measurements was ~16%. GlucoWatch results lagged behind blood glucose levels by ~18 min. Correlation of GlucoWatch glucose and HemoCue analyzer glucose results in the clinic setting was acceptable ($r = 0.90$) (50). Overall analytical performance is satisfactory for monitoring trends (51).

The GlucoWatch is expected to sell for ~$250 with AutoSensors costing ~$4 each. Presently, the GlucoWatch is approved for individuals age 18 and older. Cygnus, Inc. has submitted data to the FDA seeking approval of the device for use in children ages 7–17.

Minimally Invasive Technologies for Measuring Glucose

Many new technologies are under development that noninvasively or nearly noninvasively measure glucose similar, in spirit, to the relatively noninvasive GlucoWatch. Other than the GlucoWatch, none of these noninvasive technologies are FDA-approved.

In development or under hypothetical consideration are three general approaches to noninvasive (NI) or nearly noninvasive (NNI) measurement of glucose in the body: NI analysis of body fluids, NNI analysis of body fluids, and NI spectrophotometric techniques involving skin, mucosa, or the eye. New technologies for drawing capillary blood are also under development such as the use of erbium:YAG lasers (52).

The first technique involves analyzing fluids that can be completely noninvasively obtained, such as tears. Chen et al. (53) describe the measurement of tear glucose in nanoliter sample volumes using capillary electrophoresis with laser-induced fluorescence detection (CE/LIF). Clearly, this instrumentation is not adaptable for POCT. Secondly, the correlation between tear glucose and blood glucose was poor. This technology would appear to have little or no hope of being used in the near term for POCT.

Whereas saliva can be noninvasively obtained, the correlation between parotid fluid glucose and blood glucose is no more than $r = 0.52$, indicating that such fluid analysis is unsuitable for estimating blood glucose (54). One paper suggests that glucose does not appear in salivary fluid until the blood glucose exceeds 180–270 mg/dL (55). Sweat is another fluid that can be obtained noninvasively (56). However there is no recent literature on this topic.

The NNI analysis of body fluids for glucose concentration involves the analysis of interstitial fluid obtained by microlaser puncture of skin, creating micropores. Theoretically, the skin puncture is not so deep as to contact pain nerve endings, making the sample acquisition painless. The interstitial fluid is then obtained by reverse iontophoresis, exudation, or suction into a microassay device for glucose measurement. This is the approach being sought by SpectRx, Inc. (Norcross, GA) (http://www.spectrx.com). Abbott Laboratories/MediSense is a partner with SpectRx, Inc. in this development process. Integ Inc. (http://www.integonline.com/) is also working on analysis of interstitial fluid glucose.

Spectrophotometric techniques are being investigated for their ability to measure glucose in skin (57), within mucosa surfaces, or in the eye. Various regions of the electromagnetic spectrum have been studied for their applicability to measuring glucose, including mid-infrared radiation (Mid-IR) spectroscopy, near-infrared radiation (Near-IR) spectroscopy, radio wave impedance, and optical rotation of polarized light. For example, regarding the eye, a light beam can be emitted into the anterior chamber (58) or aqueous humor to measure the absorption of light by glucose (59–61). Whether the technique involves skin, mucosa of the mouth or tongue, anterior chamber fluid (62), or aqueous humor, the concept is that sophisticated analysis of spectra of reflected radiation or spontaneously emitted radiation (e.g., heat) can be correlated with glucose concentrations in the body to create a totally noninvasive glucose meter. One NI project in development from the Futrex company (http://www.futrex.com/glucose.html) is fancifully named "The DREAM BEAM Analyzer."

There is one NI technology besides the GlucoWatch that claims to be governmentally approved. The Diasensor literature states that it is approved for use in the 15-nation European Union. However, current discussions available on the Internet suggest that the device does not work (http://www.childrenwithdiabetes.com/d 06 e10.htm).

The Diasensor is approximately the size of a toaster oven and reportedly costs several thousands of dollars. From its size, the Diasensor is not portable. The Diasensor shines infrared light into the subject's skin and measures the light that is scattered back out of the skin. The Diasensor must be individually calibrated to each patient although the Diasensor Web site [http://www.diasensor.com/] does not describe how this calibration is achieved.

According to the manufacturer, the individual who wishes to measure their blood glucose with the Diasensor lays their forearm upon the arm tray. In 3 min, blood glucose is measured. The device is described by the manufacturer as a ". . . trending device. It provides the user with averages of glucose test results obtained at up to nine clinically relevant times of the day (e.g., fasting, pre-meal, post-meal and bedtime) over at least 15 to 30-day periods." As marketed, the Diasensor is not intended as a replacement for fingerstick SMBG. The question then arises: If the Diasensor does not replace SMBG, what value does the Diasensor provide? The Diasensor was first submitted for FDA approval in 1996. As of January 2001, there had not been a new submission to the FDA for review of the product.

At this time, spectroscopy of oral mucosa (63) or the tongue (64) is not a promising technology but might be improved with sophisticated data transformation (65). In conjunction with Roche Diagnostics, SpectRx is working on the Accu-Chek D-Tector for diabetes screening. This desktop device shines blue light into the lens of the eye and analyzes the returned light to differentiate diabetic and nondiabetic individuals. InLight Solutions (Albuquerque, NM) (www.rgmt.com) in collaboration with LifeScan is another company that is studying the application of spectroscopy to glucose measurement.

All of these NI or NNI approaches are highly theoretical (66–68) except for the GlucoWatch, which is FDA approved. There are several excellent reviews concerning NI and NNI testing to which the reader is referred (69–71).

Reference Ranges

Normal fasting plasma glucose is less than 110 mg/dL. Fasting plasma glucose between 110 and 125 mg/dL is termed impaired fasting glucose (IFG). Fasting plasma glucose equal to or greater than 126 mg/dL represents hyperglycemia. In adults after a 75-g oral glucose load and in children after a 1.75-g/kg load (to a maximum of 75 g), the 2-hr plasma glucose is normally less than 140 mg/dL. Impaired glucose tolerance is present when the 2-hr plasma glucose is 140–199 mg/dL. Two-hour plasma glucose levels of 200 mg/dL or greater represent hyperglycemia. Random plasma glucose levels are normally less than 200 mg/dL. Random plasma glucose levels 200 mg/dL or greater, associated with symptoms of diabetes, represent hyperglycemia. Diabetes is diagnosed when hyperglycemia is identified on two more occasions (e.g., two or more separate days). However, diabetic ketoacidosis or hyperglycemic nonketotic coma are sufficient to diagnose diabetes.

Table 3 Glycemic Goals in the Management of Diabetes

	Plasma glucose (mg/dL)		Whole blood glucose (mg/dL)	
	Average preprandial	Average bedtime	Average preprandial	Average bedtime
Normal	<110	<120	<100	<110
Goal	90–130	110–150	80–120	100–140
Action	<90; >150	<110; >180	<80; >140	<100; >160

The goal of SMBG is to achieve normal or nearly normal glucose levels, thereby lowering hemoglobin A_{1c} (as a reflection of improved control) and subsequent risk for diabetic complications. Glycemic control goals are outlined in Table 3.

Further Comments Regarding POCT for Glucose

To reap the benefits of SMBG, the healthcare team should authorize and instruct patients to make alterations in their exercise habits, diets, and medications to optimize diabetes control. Many clinics furnish algorithms that permit patients to alter their insulin doses, meals, and exercise plans based on trends in blood glucose concentrations (72).

When choosing a SMBG metering system, the following questions should be reviewed to match the correct system to the correct patient:

- How sophisticated a system is appropriate?
- Should the monitor be buttonless and only turned on when a strip is inserted?
- What memory capacity should the meter have?
- Can the meter record patient events?
- Are the data downloadable to a personal computer or via the Internet?
- Should the meter be able to signal the user if the small volume applied is insufficient?
- Do glucose measurements only begin after the strip is full of blood?
- What blood volume is acceptable for testing?
- Should a meter be chosen that can use sites other than the fingertips?
- Should strips be individually packaged?
- Can the meter system use both alternative sites and fingertips for blood lanceting?
- Does the meter provide both lanceting and glucose testing capacities?
- Does the meter simultaneously lance the skin and apply the glucose to the strip?

- Can blood be applied to the strip when the strip is outside the meter?
- Can strips other than those produced by the device manufacturer be used (e.g., Excel strips in the Glucometer Elite meter)?
- What range of blood glucose values needs to be detectable?
- How accurate and precise should the meter be?
- Will controls be run by the patient?
- How is the instrument calibrated?
- Can the meter be used by visually impaired individuals?
- Does the meter instruct the individual in its use via a display?
- How large should the display be?
- Should the meter have lighting features that allow it to be used in the dark?
- What type of battery is desired? Should the battery be "lifelong," replaceable, or rechargeable?
- How large is the meter and its carrying case?
- Does the meter measure any analytes other than glucose?
- Is instruction available in languages other than English?
- Are the device and strips covered by the patient's insurance company (since 1998, Medicare has covered the cost of meters and strips for all diabetic recipients)?

Simple errors in SMBG might be avoided by proper patient instruction. For example, Stewart and Khardori (73) report on an elderly man who "experienced" repeated episodes of severe hyperglycemia that were not confirmed upon retesting some time later. Upon review by the patient's daughter, the meter was being occasionally read upside down by the patient and his wife. Likewise, coexisting or pre-existing conditions can remarkably effect glucose results. Pseudohypoglycemia has been reported in a woman with Raynaud's phenomenon (74). Physicians should develop a skills checklist that can be used during the training of their patients in performing SMBG.

Within hospitals, POCT for glucose was reported for ~10% of all admissions at Massachusetts General Hospital (75). Bedside glucose testing was, on average, 9% costlier than central laboratory glucose testing. The major cost of bedside testing was labor at ~80% of total expenses. Despite higher costs, POCT for electrolytes in one study demonstrated a turnaround time ~14% of that of the central laboratory (8 versus 59 min) (76). Because POCT can be up to fourfold more expensive than central laboratory testing, cost must be a concern when considering POC service (77). Also, increased utilization of POCT may drive costs up and not down as central laboratory utilization may not fall as the frequency of POCT rises. For inpatients, what is often not considered is the fact that somebody does need to perform the POCT when ordered: this means increased burden on the nursing staff or respiratory care staff. In light of the nationwide nursing shortage, adding more responsibilities to an already overworked nursing staff may not be prudent.

While implantation of monitors into body cavities is certainly a novel idea, this concept does not fall under the umbrella of POCT. A final word on urine glucose testing: other than in patients who for some reason cannot perform SMBG, urine glucose testing has no role in the diagnosis or monitoring of diabetes. It is appropriate that glucose testing be continued as part of routine urinalyses; however, urine glucose testing is not part of routine diabetes management.

Most POCT devices designed to measure glucose do perform satisfactorily if acceptable bias is defined as ±20 mg/dL for glucose levels less than 100 mg/dL and ±20% for glucose levels 100 mg/dL and greater (78). However if acceptable bias is defined as ±5%, most devices are not accurate. Studies of hospital-based bedside POCT for glucose illustrate the need to improve quality control compliance (79). Decisions concerning acceptable precision goals should involve discussions with clinicians (80). Whether considering the hospital or home, producing acceptable glucose results at the POC is still very challenging (81–83). Boyd and Bruns (84) point out that meters that meet today's somewhat lax analytical performance guidelines can lead to insulin dosing errors. Furthermore, if bias and imprecision were both 5% or less, more than 75% of patients in clinical situations would be satisfied with such performance (85). Manufacturers should strive to produce POCT meter and strip systems with biases and imprecision ≤5% (86). For perspective, based particularly on the recent study by Harris (87), there are few data that prove that SMBG in type 2 diabetes actually improves outcomes (88).

POINT-OF-CARE GLYCEMIC MONITORING: FRUCTOSAMINE

Chemistry

The nonenzymatic addition of glucose to proteins is known as glycation or glycosylation. Via glycosylation of hemoglobin, glycohemoglobin is formed. Glycohemoglobin measurements represent an index of long-term glycemic status extending over the previous 2–3 mo. For intermediate-term glycemic monitoring, measurement of glycosylated serum protein can be accomplished. The addition of glucose to protein produces a chemical structure similar to fructose and, therefore, glycosylated serum protein is commonly referred to as "fructosamine." In a colorimetric technique, fructosamine concentrations are determined by reacting serum with nitroblue tetrazolium under basic conditions. The ketoamine linkages of fructosamine reduce nitroblue tetrazolium to formazan dye, which absorbs near 550 nm.

Fructosamine is the sum of all serum glycosylated proteins. Because albumin is the most abundant serum protein, glycosylated albumin is the major contributor to fructosamine. Because albumin's half-life is ~17 days (range 15–20 days), fructosamine reflects glucose control over a 2–3 wk time span (89). In nondiabetic individuals, up to 8% of serum albumin is glycosylated. However, in persons with diabetes, up to 25% of serum albumin may be glycosylated. Fructosamine is stable at room temperature for 2–4 hr. Refrigerated fructosamine is stable for 4–7 days and frozen fructosamine is stable for 4–5 wk.

POCT Technology

Until recently, fructosamine measurements have been available only from reference laboratories and some hospital laboratories. Fructosamine measurements were first introduced clinically in the early 1980s. In our experience at the University of Florida, there has been little clinical demand for fructosamine measurements even from the obstetrics service.

In 1997, a point-of-care device for fructosamine measurement in the physician's office became available from LXN Corporation (San Diego, CA). The system for at-home use was introduced in late 1999. The FDA has approved these devices for use in adults but not in children or in pregnancy. GlucoProtein® is the term that LXN Corporation uses for fructosamine. LXN Corporation has combined fructosamine and capillary blood glucose measurements into a single device. These combined systems are marketed as the IN CHARGE™ 2-Test Diabetes Control System for patient self-testing and as the Duet™ Diabetes Control System for in-office testing. These tests use capillary blood.

Initially, the instrument is turned on and a GlucoProtein test strip is inserted into the instrument. Capillary blood is obtained using a finger lancet and is taken up into a sampling straw via capillary action. Via the straw, the blood is then applied to the strip. The GlucoProtein strip consists of the following layers: sample cup, screen, blood separation layer that provides plasma, a buffer layer, a dye layer, and finally a Mylar™ window. The GlucoProtein assay takes approximately 4 min.

GlucoProtein results are comparable to laboratory reference methods of fructosamine measurement (90). From data provided by LXN Corporation in their advertising, professionals performing the GlucoProtein test compared with the venipuncture Roche®ROTAG fructosamine assay displayed a correlation coefficient of 0.771 with the following regression equation: y (GlucoProtein) = 0.821 x (ROTAG fructosamine) + 63.88. Nonprofessional GlucoProtein users performed similarly in comparison to the ROTAG fructosamine method: $r = 0.75$, $y = 0.798\,x + 69.58$. Concerning GlucoProtein results, nonprofessionals and professionals correlated satisfactorily ($r = 0.867$, $y = 0.846\,x + 45.329$). Correlation coefficients of 0.80 (91) and 0.72 (92) have been reported comparing central laboratory fructosamine measurements with those of the fingerstick GlucoProtein method.

The GlucoProtein test is CLIA waived for in-office testing. Normal and high controls for the GlucoProtein in-office Duet Diabetes Control System are employed. The meter stores GlucoProtein (and glucose) control results in memory with time and date. No data are published in the literature concerning the reproducibility of GlucoProtein measurements. Automated fructosamine measurements on venous blood can display within-run precision less than 3% (0.9–3%) and between-run precision of 2.5–5.6% (93). An older fructosamine method using commercially available reagents run on an IL Multistat III centrifugal analyzer exhibited within- and between-batch precision of <4% (94).

Training and customer support provided by LXN Corporation include an instructional videotape, a user's manual, and materials for in-service and certification programs. Regarding professional education and support, LXN Corporation furnishes CEU programs for Certified Diabetes Educators and Pharmacists. There is a 24-hr technical service phone number. LXN Corporation claims that monitors and supplies are replaced in a timely manner. Use of the sampling straw provides a measure of infection control as patient's fingers are not directly applied to the meter. The IN CHARGE Monitor stores the last 50 GlucoProtein test results in memory. LXN Corporation reports that software will soon be available that will allow users to automatically upload and chart their test results using LXN's Web site.

The IN CHARGE Diabetes Control System has a suggested list price of $79.95. Six GlucoProtein test strips have a suggested list price of $24.95 and the value pack of 50 glucose test strips and four GlucoProtein test strips has a suggested list price of $36.95. Concerning the in-office Duet Diabetes Control System, the Medicare reimbursement in most states is $20.83.

Reference Ranges and Interferences

It is controversial whether fructosamine reference ranges should be corrected for total protein or albumin concentrations. In comparison, glycohemoglobin is always reported as a percent of total hemoglobin and never as an absolute concentration. GlucoProtein is reported as an absolute concentration (μmol/L).

LXN Corporation states in their literature that GlucoProtein results above 380 μmol/L indicate poor control whereas results below 310 μmol/L indicate good control (95). Unfortunately no peer-reviewed reference is provided to support the use of these guidelines. In LXN Corporation literature a fructosamine level of 380 μmol/L is equated with an average glucose of ~230 mg/dL and a hemoglobin A_{1c} of ~9.6%. A fructosamine level of 310 μmol/L is equated with an average glucose of ~170 mg/dL and a hemoglobin A_{1c} of ~7.6%. LXN Corporation does reference two sources to document these relationships among average glucose, hemoglobin A_{1c}, and fructosamine. However one of these sources (96) was not found in an on-line search of the medical literature (PubMed) and the other reference (97) did not provide data on the stated relationships. Therefore, there are few or no data available to this author validating the GlucoProtein interpretations or relationship of fructosamine concentration to hemoglobin A_{1c} or average glucose. For comparison, Quest Diagnostics provides a fructosamine reference range of 174–286 μmol/L (98).

Using a first-generation fructosamine assay, a 30 mg/dL rise in glucose increased fructosamine by 180 μmol/L (99). However it is important to note that first-generation assays provided fructosamine measurements that are ~10 times higher than the present second-generation assays. Also using a first generation assay, another author determined that for every rise in hemoglobin A_{1c} of 1%, fructosamine rose by 250 μmol/L (100).

Another point of contention is the choice of 380 and 310 μmol/L as levels above which glycemic control is defined as poor and below which glycemic control is defined as good, respectively. The corresponding hemoglobin A_{1c} values (according to LXN Corporation) of ~9.6% and ~7.6% are considerably above the ADA recommended cutpoints when therapy should be altered [(e.g., a hemoglobin A_{1c} >8%) or the desirable hemoglobin A_{1c} (e.g., target hemoglobin A_{1c} <7%)].

Concerning reference ranges, fructosamine in nondiabetic children is ~5% lower than in adults, whereas fructosamine is lower in alcoholics, pregnant women, and obese individuals. Peritoneal dialysis raises fructosamine in nondiabetic individuals. Because serum albumin is the major contributor to fructosamine, changes in albumin concentration or half-life may affect the fructosamine concentration. Conditions with shortened albumin half-life may provide a falsely decreased fructosamine level. Such conditions include nephrosis, protein-losing enteropathy, and burns. Reduced albumin half-life may also occur with malnutrition when albumin is being consumed by the body as a ready source of amino acids. If serum albumin is <3 g/dL, experts advise against measuring fructosamine. Other conditions that may invalidate fructosamine measurements include hepatic cirrhosis, rapid changes in acute phase reactants, and dysproteinemias. Technically, in the first-generation fructosamine assays, elevated immunoglobulin A concentrations caused a false elevation in fructosamine.

The current second generation of fructosamine assays have been improved over the first-generation assays by including uricase to eliminate uric acid interference, increasing detergent concentrations (e.g., TX-100) to minimize lipid interferences, calibrating with glycated lysine, and developing and adopting an industry standard. These changes have reduced fructosamine levels to ~10% of the first generation levels.

Indications for Testing

Fructosamine measurements may be helpful when patients are undergoing intensive short-term therapy to correct hyperglycemia (for example, during pregnancy) (101). Fructosamine measurements are also useful in the assessment of glycemic control in patients with SS, CC, or SC hemoglobinopathies in whom hemoglobin A_{1c} cannot be measured or in cases of altered red blood cell (RBC) half-life. Examples of conditions in which RBC half-life is altered include splenectomy with prolonged RBC half-life and hemolysis with shortened RBC half-life.

Other than the above indications, "there is a lack of consensus on its [fructosamine's] clinical utility" (102). Even in cases in which fructosamine is used as an index of short-term glycemic control, the ADA states that further studies are needed to determine if fructosamine provides "useful information" (103). The American Association of Clinical Endocrinologists (AACE) recommends regular glycohemoglobin and fructosamine measurements (104). However, AACE provides no references to substantiate their recommendation concerning fructosamine testing. The manufacturer of GlucoProtein contends that weekly measurements of fructosamine provide valuable information in the management of the patient's diabetes. This remains an unsettled and controversial issue (105).

Similar to hemoglobin A_{1c}, a fructosamine level within the reference range cannot exclude diabetes. Fructosamine measurements should not be used to screen for diabetes.

Relationship of Fructosamine to Diabetic Complications and Glycemic Control

Whereas there are excellent data from the DCCT and UKPDS that lowering hemoglobin A_{1c} lowers the risk of microvascular and neurological complications, data are lacking that demonstrate that lowering fructosamine levels reduces the risk of developing long-term complications (106). At the LXN Corporation Web site (http://www.lxncorp.com), an educational program regarding type 2 diabetes states "And like HbA_{1c}, elevated fructosamine levels signify an increased risk of developing complications, including heart disease." The reference for this statement is given as http://heartinfo.org/reutersnews/t0304-2f.htm. However, that URL is currently inactive. Thus, there is no available scientific, peer-reviewed data demonstrating that fructosamine levels are related to the development of heart disease.

There are preliminary data that measuring fructosamine may assist in improving metabolic control. A 1999 paper (107) reported that 20 type 2 diabetes patients who performed weekly fingerstick fructosamine measurements over 6 wk displayed significant declines in fasting glucose (~205 to ~145 mg/dL,

P = <0.001) and fingerstick fructosamine levels (~365 to ~315 μmol/L, P = <0.001). However, no control group was reported. Thus, it is not possible to determine which specific intervention was responsible for the improvement in metabolic control witnessed by these investigators. Another uncontrolled study published in 2001 (108) showed reductions in mean glucose by 27% and fructosamine by 17% when a combined glucose/fructosamine metering system was employed.

In 2000, Edelman et al. (109) reported on their studies randomizing 25 diabetic patients with initial hemoglobin A_{1c} levels over 8% to one of two groups: ≤4 times per day self-monitoring of blood glucose with one follow-up visit at 3 mo, versus ≤4 times per day SMBG with weekly fructosamine measurements and phone contact if the fructosamine level exceeded 350 μmol/L. The patient group that performed weekly fructosamine measurements and had access to professional phone contact to guide interventions did exhibit significant declines in hemoglobin A_{1c} (mean values: 9.2 to 8.0%, P = <0.0001) whereas the routinely managed patients did not display a significant decline in hemoglobin A_{1c} (mean values: 9.4 to 9.1%, P = NS). However it is impossible to judge from the study design whether it was frequent contact with the healthcare team or the fructosamine measurements (or both) that actually lead to improved control.

In contrast to these suggestive but not definitive studies concerning the value of GlucoProtein testing, Petitti et al. (110) found that the addition of GlucoProtein testing to routine glucose monitoring did not improve glycemic control. Petitti et al. studied 140 type 2 diabetes patients with initial hemoglobin A_{1c} levels of 8% or greater. What makes this study superior to the studies of Cefalu et al. (107) and Edelman et al. (109) is that in Petitti et al.'s study the only apparent difference between study groups was the addition of fingerstick fructosamine measurements. Otherwise, SMBG and clinical contact were reported to be identical. After 3 mo of follow-up, hemoglobin A_{1c} had declined in the control group by 0.8% and had declined in the fructosamine-monitored group by 0.5% (P = >0.2). At 6 mo, the control group had an even greater decline in hemoglobin A_{1c} (1.2%) than the fructosamine-monitored group (0.7%, P = 0.04).

Summarizing a very limited body of literature, there are no data that measuring fructosamine leads to a decline in complication rates. While it is hoped that the use of GlucoProtein measurements will independently improve glycemic control, the definitive data to support this hypothesis are lacking. It has been also proposed that serial fructosamine measurements may be most useful in assessing short-term diabetic control. Data to demonstrate this benefit are anxiously awaited.

Further Comments Regarding POCT for Fructosamine

There are many limitations to both capillary blood glucose monitoring (e.g., SMBG) and hemoglobin A_{1c} measurements. Self-monitoring of blood glucose requires 2–4 or more measurements per day that all involve drawing a drop of blood with a lancet. As was discussed above, POCT for glucose can display considerable biases compared with central laboratory glucose measurements. Nevertheless, for daily diabetes management, SMBG is critical when combined with an algorithm to treat hyperglycemia or hypoglycemia.

Glycosylated hemoglobin measurements including hemoglobin A_{1c} are expensive, not standardized nationally, and are generally unavailable at the POC unless the DCA2000 POCT analyzer or A_{1c}Now devices are employed. Compared with hemoglobin A_{1c}, fructosamine is a simpler assay, provides a short turnaround time when measured using the POC GlucoProtein test, is relatively inexpensive compared with central laboratory testing, is not subject to the same interferences as glycosylated hemoglobin, and changes more rapidly than hemoglobin A_{1c} in response to changes in glycemic status (111). The fact that fructosamine changes more rapidly than hemoglobin A_{1c} means that fructosamine provides more rapid feedback concerning short-term changes in glycemic control. By its nature, fructosamine is not affected by changes in hemoglobin turnover rates or hemoglobinopathies.

Many of the criticisms discussed regarding GlucoProtein are not unique to fingerstick fructosamine measurements and reflect a general ambivalence in the literature concerning the usefulness of any fructosamine measurement. In the world of evidence-based medicine, the need for fructosamine measurements outside of limited clinical circumstances (e.g., lack of hemoglobin A and pregnancy) is unproven.

POINT-OF-CARE GLYCEMIC MONITORING: GLYCOHEMOGLOBIN

Chemistry

As noted above, the nonenzymatic addition of glucose to blood proteins provides a measure of blood glucose. The level of glycohemoglobin in the circulation is proportional to the extent to which blood glucose is elevated and the duration of time over which the glucose is elevated (112). Elevated glycohemoglobin concentrations predict an increased risk for microvascular and neuropathic complications, whereas reductions in glycohemoglobin concentrations predict reduced risks for such complications (113).

Hemoglobin glycation occurs in the erythrocytes of both nondiabetic and diabetic subjects. Because of chronic hyperglycemia, glycohemoglobin levels are elevated above the reference range in diabetic people. There was no objective method to determine patients' long-term glycemic control until the development of assays for glycohemoglobin.

Prior to the development of SMBG systems, subjects with diabetes semiquantitatively ascertained how much glucose was lost in their urine and chronicled this information in a booklet. Conceptually, the urine glucose reflected the serum glucose. Nevertheless, the correlation between the two assessments was crude at best, and the necessity for urine glucose measurement was eliminated with the acceptance and implementation of SMBG. Even with the availability of SMBG, patients can fail to perform SMBG, can perform SMBG incorrectly, or can falsify their written records. These critiques of SMBG require the availability of independent measures of glycemia, such as glycohemoglobin.

A brief review of hemoglobin and glycohemoglobin terminology is useful. Hemoglobin A (e.g., "adult" hemoglobin) is the major form of hemoglobin after ~2 mo of age. By ~8 mo of age hemoglobin F (e.g., "fetal" hemoglobin) is <5% and by 12 years of age hemoglobin F is near adult levels, i.e., <2%. Non-glycosylated hemoglobin A can be referred to as hemoglobin A_0. In adults, ~97% of hemoglobin is hemoglobin A (or A_0; α_2, β_2), 2.5% is hemoglobin A_2 (α_2, δ_2), and 0.5% is hemoglobin F (α_2, γ_2).

Glycohemoglobin (sometimes abbreviated GHb) is a general term for hemoglobin with nonenzymatically bound glucose exhibiting a ketoamine structure. Glycohemoglobin includes glycosylated hemoglobin A and non-A hemoglobins. Total GHb describes all forms of glycosylated hemoglobin measured by affinity chromatography methods. Glycosylated hemoglobin A is termed hemoglobin A_1.

Hemoglobins A_{1a}, A_{1b}, and A_{1c} make up hemoglobin A_1. Hemoglobin A_{1a} contains two subfractions: A_{1a1} and A_{1a2}. Fructose-1,6-diphosphate is bound to the β-chain in hemoglobin A_{1a1} whereas in hemoglobin A_{1a2}, glucose 6-phosphate is bound to the β-chain. The structure of hemoglobin A_{1b} is controversial. A 1991 paper reported that hemoglobin A_{1b} was a ketoamine-linked pyruvic acid at the amino end of the hemoglobin β-chain (114). Glucose is attached to the NH_2-terminal valine of the hemoglobin β-chain in hemoglobin A_{1c}. Whereas sugars are less often added to the α-chain or ε-NH_2-lysine groups, sugars are preferentially added to hemoglobin at the NH_2-terminus making hemoglobin A_{1c}, the major contributer to hemoglobin A_1. Hemoglobin A_{1c} fraction usually represents 75–80% of hemoglobin A_1.

At the biochemical level, when glucose first reacts with the amine group of hemoglobin, a reversible (labile) product is formed termed an aldimine or Schiff base. The aldimine is sometimes designated pre–hemoglobin A_{1c} (the labile fraction). A ketoamine is then formed via a further nonreversible Amadori rearrangement. Glycohemoglobin assays must exclude measurement of the labile fraction, otherwise wide daily intraindividual fluctuations appear because variations in ambient glucose levels influence the labile fraction. The labile fraction can represent 5–8% of hemoglobin A_1 in nondiabetic control subjects. In individuals with diabetes, the labile fraction can even approach 30%. Without exclusion of the labile fraction, false conclusions can be reached regarding glycemic control.

Many methods have been developed to measure glycohemoglobin and its derivatives. A review of all such methods is beyond the scope of this chapter but they are well reviewed in other sources (97,115). It is important to note that the reference method is measurement of hemoglobin A_{1c} by high-performance liquid chromatography (HPLC) using an ion-exchange column. This was the hemoglobin A_{1c} method employed in the Diabetes Control and Complications Trial. The major POCT methods are immunoassay (DCA2000, Bayer Laboratories, Tarrytown, NY), column chromatography (Micromat®II and DiaSTAT®, Bio-Rad, Hercules, CA) and immunoassay plus chemistry technology (A_{1c}Now, Metrika, Sunnyvale, CA). In addition to the DCA2000, Bayer Laboratories offers the DCA2000+®, which can measure, in addition to hemoglobin A_{1c}, urinary albumin and creatinine to determine microalbumin excretion using a specially designed cartridge for urine testing. Of these methods, only the A_{1c}Now test is applicable to home use by diabetes patients (see below).

Regardless of the technique used to measure glycated hemoglobins (minicolumn or HPLC, boron-affinity, ion-exchange, immunoassay, or electrophoresis), the standard of excellence is traceability to the HPLC method. Colorimetric glycohemoglobin assays report "total GHb." Affinity chromatography minicolumn measurements also report "total GHb." Electrophoresis methods determine hemoglobin A_1. Ion-exchange chromatography minicolumns measure either hemoglobin A_1 or hemoglobin A_{1c}. Ion-exchange HPLC and immunoassays determine hemoglobin A_{1c}. Assays that demonstrate traceability to the HPLC method that acceptably minimize bias and exhibit satisfactory precision can be accredited by the National Glycohemoglobin Standardization Program (NGSP) (http://www.missouri.edu/~diabetes/ngsp/index.html). A certificate of traceability to the DCCT reference method is issued to manufacturers or laboratories that successfully complete the certification process.

Standardization of hemoglobin A_{1c} results is especially important when therapeutic guidelines are based upon hemoglobin A_{1c} measurements. In addition to the efforts of the NGSP, standardization may be afforded by cross-methods calibration (116,117). To aid in these efforts, lyophilized calibrators are stable for as long as 5 yr (118). Without industry-wide standardization practices for glycohemoglobin measurements, changing glycohemoglobin methods can produce significant variations in the reported results (119).

Whereas there are many field methods and one reference method (HPLC) for glycohemoglobin, there is no accepted definitive method for the measurement of hemoglobin A_{1c}. Researchers are working on a mass spectroscopy method as a definitive method for the measurement of hemoglobin A_{1c}.

POCT Technology

There are three devices to consider that can be used to determine hemoglobin A_{1c} at the POC. The DCA2000 employs an immunoassay technique to measure hemoglobin A_{1c} as does the A_{1c}Now, whereas the Micromat II and DiaSTAT use column chromatography. Only the A_{1c}Now test is applicable to home use by diabetic patients.

Immunoassay POC Devices

A_{1c} At-Home Test™. The Beckin-Dickenson (B-D) A_{1c} At-Home Test allows patients to obtain a blood specimen at home and mail this specimen to a central laboratory for analysis. Although the testing is not performed at the POC, the sample is obtained at the POC. The kit includes a lancet, test paper, instructions and a prepaid mailer. Two drops of blood are placed on the test paper, are allowed to dry overnight, and are then mailed to the central laboratory. Patients can be enrolled in a postal program to receive new test kits every 3–6 mo. The arrival of the kit prompts the patient to obtain a specimen and submit the specimen for testing. Patients who fail to submit a blood sample for At-Home Test hemoglobin A_{1c} can be contacted by phone or by mail.

The At-Home Test laboratory uses an immunoassay system from Roche Diagnostics (Roche Unimate immunoassay). This immunoassay for hemoglobin A_{1c} is measured using the Roche Cobas Mira analyzer. At-Home Test adjusts the immunoassay hemoglobin A_{1c} measurement to an HPLC hemoglobin A_{1c} using the following regression equation: HPLC = 0.899 Roche Unimate + 1.34 (B-D data: 98A1CDMO43E1). The At-Home Test hemoglobin A_{1c} measurement compares favorably with the venipuncture Roche Unimate immunoassay hemoglobin A_{1c} (Roche Unimate = 0.869 At-Home Test + 0.948).

A PubMed National Library of Medicine search reveals one peer-reviewed article that deals with the analytical performance of the B-D A_{1c} At-Home results (120). Correlation with the Cobas Integra hemoglobin A_{1c} assay was satisfactory ($r^2 = 94.7\%$). The coefficient of variation for 3-day sample results with 10-day sample results was acceptable (2.7%). The authors report that there were no clinically significant differences in samples aged 3–10 days, between venous or capillary blood samples, or from freezing and thawing or prolonged exposure of dried blood samples to elevated temperatures prior to assay. Conceptually, this combination of convenient, minimally invasive sample acquisition at home combined with central laboratory accuracy and precision should be very attractive to the patient and the healthcare provider.

Single At-Home A_{1c} tests cost ~\$25 with a \$3.00 shipping and handling fee. Other "at-home" mail-in kits are advertised on the Web (e.g., Accu-Base Hemoglobin A_{1c} Sample Collection Kit, Diabetes Technologies, Inc., Thomasville, GA; Appraise Hemoglobin A_{1c} Diabetes Monitoring System, ChoicePoint Health Systems Inc., Olathe, KS; BioSafe Home HbA_{1c} Kit, BIOSAFE, Lake Forest, IL). However, few specifics concerning these latter options are available. Their costs vary between \$20 and \$40 per hemoglobin A_{1c} measurement.

DCA2000. Monoclonal antibody technology is utilized by the DCA2000. In the reaction cell, anti–hemoglobin A_{1c} monoclonal antibody binds to a particle coated with hemoglobin A_{1c}. Because antibodies are bivalent (e.g., have two antigen-binding sites), cross-linking of the particles occurs and subsequently causes light scattering. When the patient sample is added, the patient's own hemoglobin A_{1c} competes with the bound hemoglobin A_{1c} for antibody binding and less particle cross-linking and less light scatter occur. This technique correlates satisfactorily with HPLC measurement of hemoglobin A_{1c}.

The DCA2000 test uses fingerstick whole blood. After the capillary tube is filled with fingerstick blood, the sample-filled capillary holder is placed into the reagent cartridge. The reagent cartridge is self-contained and requires no reagent handling, mixing, or preparation. The sample-loaded cartridge is passed through the instrument's integral bar-code reader to automatically calibrate the instrument. The cartridge is next placed into the instrument, the buffer is released by removal of the pull tab on the cartridge, and the instrument door is closed. After this point, no further operator intervention is required other than the eventual disposal of the cartridge. Analysis time is approximately 6 min. The internal memory will hold 16 results. The instrument screen displays all instructions, calibration status, and results.

For hemoglobin A (i.e., AA), the regression was DCA2000 hemoglobin $A_{1c} = 0.96 * \text{Diamat hemoglobin } A_{1c} + 0.54$ ($r = 0.98$) (121). For hemoglobin AS (i.e., sickle cell trait), the regression was DCA2000 hemoglobin $A_{1c} = 1.14 * \text{Diamat hemoglobin } A_{1c} - 0.82$ ($r = 0.97$). However, for hemoglobin AC (i.e., hemoglobin C trait), there were biases of 8.4 and 10.4% at hemoglobin A_{1c} levels of 7 and 9% (DCA2000 hemoglobin $A_{1c} = 1.17 * \text{Diamat hemoglobin } A_{1c} - 0.61$; $r = 0.96$). This does not meet NGSP criteria for comparability to the DCCT method. In one report, structural hemoglobin variants did not interfere with hemoglobin A_{1c} levels measured with the DCA2000 (122). However in another report, hemoglobin C trait displayed positive biases as much as 10.4% (123). The precision of the DCA2000 approaches that of some central laboratory hemoglobin A_{1c} methods. At hemoglobin A_{1c} levels of 5.4 and 13.0%, intra-assay coefficients of variation are 1.6 and 3.0%, whereas interassay coefficients of variation are reported at 4.2 and 3.8% (124). Analytical performance in physician office laboratories (125) and community settings (126) has been acceptable.

A_{1c}Now. The A_{1c}Now device is a new FDA-approved, CLIA-waived single-use disposal system that is used to measure hemoglobin A_{1c} in physician offices or at home. For home use, patients must obtain a prescription from their physician for the device. Because of the infrequent need to measure hemoglobin A_{1c} (e.g., every 2–3 mo), the manufacturer judged that there was no need to maintain an independent meter, and it was advantageous to produce a completely self-contained disposal device. Current CPT codes useful for billing include

83036 QW—Glycated hemoglobin and 36415—Venipuncture for fingerstick. The cost per device is <$20. The A_{1c}Now 03003 A_{1c}Now Monitoring Kit includes 10 single-use HbA_{1c} monitors and 10 sample dilution kits.

Mechanistically, the device must be at room temperature for 30 min. At room temperature, the device is stable for up to 30 days assuming that the overall expiration date for the device is not exceeded. The device should be stored at 2–8°C. Once the sealed plastic bag containing the device is opened, testing must begin within 15 min. A lancet is used to draw a drop of fingerstick blood and 10 μL is taken up into a horizontal pipette by capillary action. Venous blood can also be used. For hemoglobin A_{1c} testing, venous blood is stable for 8 hr at room temperature or 2 wk refrigerated.

Either from the capillary pipette or, for venous blood using a standard laboratory pipette, 10 μL of blood is added to the dilution buffer. Presumably the dilution buffer lyses the subject's red blood cells. The recapped tube containing dilution buffer is shaken vigorously 6–8 times. The specially designed transfer pipette is used to place a specific volume of diluted sample into the meter sample well. To do this, the top bulb of the transfer pipette is squeezed and placed into the tube with dilution buffer containing the patient's lysed sample. As the bulb is released, diluted sample is drawn into the transfer pipette. Next, the transfer pipette is positioned above the sample well and the bulb is squeezed all at once to deliver sample to the sample well. The diluted sample should be used within 2 hr of preparation. The transfer pipette is designed in a fashion not to deliver excessive diluted sample to the meter. The manufacturer states that the device senses inadequate sample volume. When sample delivery occurs, the device self-activates. This procedure is illustrated in detail in order to stress the relative complexity of the sample delivery process. Nevertheless, the device is CLIA-waived.

Once the sample is loaded, the device is not further disturbed until a result is reported on the LCD screen. As the device turns itself on with sample delivery, there are no buttons to push. No result is reported if there is a QC failure. In such a case, an error code is displayed. Assay time is ~8 min. The device will display the result for 1 wk.

The A_{1c}Now device utilizes MODM™ (micro-optical detection method) technology. Within the device, there are two strips so that hemoglobin A_{1c} can be measured in duplicate and the results are averaged. Initially, hemoglobin A_{1c} in the patient's sample is bound by sheep polyclonal anti–hemoglobin A_{1c} antibodies to which blue-microparticles have been attached. This complex migrates along each of the two strips and is captured in "Test Zone 1." Specific further information about the hemoglobin A_{1c} assay is not provided by the manufacturer. It is possible that the A_{1c}Now device uses anti–hemoglobin A_{1c} antibodies bound to the strip to capture the blue-microparticle–labeled hemoglobin A_{1c} and that the blue color is measured spectrophotometrically. Other similar devices (e.g., for measurement of troponin T) have a capture antibody adhered to the strip. No interferences are reported for bilirubin levels up to 20 mg/dL, triglycerides to 3000 mg/dL, hemoglobin to 500 mg/dL or ascorbic acid to 5 mg/dL.

Total hemoglobin is determined by oxidizing hemoglobin to methemoglobin. Presumably using another spectrophotometer at the "second test zone," the red-brown color of methemoglobin is measured as an index of total hemoglobin. A_{1c}Now uses calibrators with values assigned by a NGSP-certified laboratory that uses a Tosoh A_{1c} 2.2 Plus instrument. Therefore, the A_{1c}Now hemoglobin A_{1c} results are traceable to the DCCT. However, the device itself is not certified by the NGSP. In part, this is because the reproducibility of the A_{1c}Now hemoglobin A_{1c} results is >5% (see below). The range of reported hemoglobin A_{1c} results is 3–15% and the assay is stated to be valid for hematocrits between 20 and 60%.

The device does carry out internal QC checks before reporting a result and has built-in controls. Manufacturer's data demonstrate a device failure rate of 3% (A_{1c}Now HbA_{1c} accuracy and precision studies. Metrika 90086 Rev. A). Concerning precision, reported coefficients of variation (CV) were 9.7% at a mean hemoglobin A_{1c} of 5.8%, and 9.5% at a mean hemoglobin A_{1c} of 10.7%. From other manufacturer data, precision is recorded as follows: at a mean hemoglobin A_{1c} of 4.7%, the CV was 10.2%; at a mean hemoglobin A_{1c} of 6.2%, the CV was 7.7%; and at a mean hemoglobin A_{1c} of 8.6%, the CV was 8.9%. Stivers et al. report coefficients of variation between 5 and 9% (127).

The manufacturer does recommend that external controls be run in physician's offices upon receipt of a new shipment and at regular intervals "determined by the laboratory," when room temperature storage conditions have been exceeded, to train or retrain operators when the regular operator of the kit changes, and when A_{1c}Now test results do not match the clinical status of the patient. The manufacturer does not supply controls and recommends that such materials should be purchased from other vendors.

Regarding analytical accuracy, from manufacturer data for nonprofessionals using the A_{1c}Now device, percent-biases at hemoglobin A_{1c} levels of 6, 7, and 9% were reported at, respectively, −0.2, −1.0, and −2.1%. Bias was similar for professional users (i.e., 1.8, 0.1, and −2.1%). From company data, compared with the Tosoh HPLC measurement (x-axis) for 258 samples, the regression equation was y (A_{1c}Now) $= 0.9431\,x + 0.3487$. The correlation coefficient was 0.92. For 50 samples compared with the Bio-Rad DiaSTAT method by Stivers et al. (127), the correlation coefficient was 0.935 with the following regression equation: $y = 0.994\,x + 0.003$.

In contrast to HPLC methods, A_{1c}Now does not identify hemoglobins F, S, or C. Incorrect hemoglobin A_{1c} results (falsely low) may occur in individuals with hemoglobin AS, AC, or high levels of hemoglobin F. Recognizing that 8% of African-Americans have sickle trait (hemoglobin AS), this limitation must be considered when the patient's clinical glycemic status and A_{1c}Now result are discordant.

Column Chromatography POC Devices

Bio-Rad offers two analyzers that can be operated at the POC. The Micromat II is designed for low-volume testing environments, whereas the DiaSTAT is a modest-volume, small-laboratory device. The Primus CLC330 analyzer has been used at the POC successfully in one pilot study in Australia (128). However this borate-affinity HPLC device is really a very sophisticated central laboratory analyzer that would not be readily adaptable to low-volume testing environments such as a clinic or physician's office laboratory. The Primus CLC330 analyzer is certified by the NGSP.

Micromat II Assay. The 5-min, 10-μL blood sample Micromat II assay employs affinity chromatography. In Europe, this test is offered by Provalis Diagnostics Ltd. as Glycosal™. Operationally, the Micromat II utilizes a disposable, single-use test cartridge and a small nondisposable photometric instrument named the HaemaQuant™ from Chelsea Instruments (London, UK). After the HaemaQuant is turned on, the test cartridge is placed into the HaemaQuant. Ten microliters of blood is diluted into sample buffer where red blood cell hemolysis is accomplished and hemoglobin is mixed with the affinity matrix. After a 1-min incubation, the entire contents are added to the test cartridge. This is advantageous compared with the A_{1c} At-Home test where another aliquoting step is required for sample introduction into the meter.

With addition of the diluted patient sample, the cartridge is rotated and a wash buffer tube appears during this rotation step. This buffer is then poured into the cartridge. After 30 sec, the cartridge is rotated again and the elution buffer tube appears. This buffer is then poured into the cartridge. One minute later, the cartridge is rotated a final time and removed. Upon removal, the LCD screen displays the hemoglobin A_{1c} result.

Comparing the Micromat II assay with the DCA2000, the A_{1c} At-Home test, or the A_{1c}Now test, the Micromat II is clearly much more complicated to run, reflecting its use only in physician office laboratories. To accomplish rapid, simple testing, it is unclear why the Micromat II would be chosen over either the DCA2000 analyzer or the A_{1c}Now test. The Micromat II procedure appears to be relatively complicated for a POCT device. During the incubation periods, the operator will need to attend essentially exclusively to the testing procedure. Assuming that the operator earns $12/hr, the assay time costs $1 of operator time. This does not include the time to initially obtain the specimen. A printer is available for creating hardcopies of test results.

The linear limits of hemoglobin A_{1c} measurements span 3–18% (129). This reference is the only peer-reviewed article available on the Micromat II/Glycosal analyzer. Mean coefficients of variation were less than 5%. Comparisons with the Bio-Rad Variant HPLC analyzer and Pharmacia Mono-S HPLC analyzer were favorable, with correlation coefficients, respectively, of 0.98 and >0.98. However, the Micromat II exhibited a negative bias compared with both HPLC systems. In a group of 54 subjects with diabetes, the Micromat II hemoglobin A_{1c} results were ≥0.52% lower than the HPLC results near hemoglobin A_{1c} results of ~7%. Although the Bio-Rad Web site (http://www.bio-rad.com) states that the Micromat II is certified by the NGSP, the device is not listed at the NGSP web site as being certified in 2001. The NGSP requires that manufacturers recertify their devices yearly. It is interesting that in an editorial that accompanies the above referenced article (130), the need for hemoglobin A_{1c} testing by patients was stressed.

DiaSTAT Analyzer. The DiaSTAT liquid chromatography analyzer is really a compact version of Bio-Rad's HPLC systems that are used in larger central hospital laboratories and reference laboratories (e.g., the Variant™, Variant II™, MDMS™, and DIAMAT™ analyzers). One hundred and 500 test reagent test kits are available. In fact, the DiaSTAT analyzer can be used in a hospital laboratory in addition to a clinic or physician office laboratory. The DiaSTAT analyzer has been certified by the NGSP to be traceable to the DCCT reference method and values.

The operator is directed to run the analyzer from a touch screen. Blood sample preparation is one step. Assay time is 10 min and samples are batched. The DiaSTAT reports hemoglobin A_{1c} results even in the presence of hemoglobins S and C. The analyzer prints the chromatographic tracing.

This is a very sophisticated monitor and it may be inappropriate to include such a device in discussions of POCT devices. Because of the expense of the analyzer and the anticipated maintenance requirements, the DiaSTAT analyzer might only be appropriate for very large diabetes clinics or smaller hospital laboratories that wish to employ a method that measures hemiglobin A_{1c} chromatographically. The A_{1c}Now test or DCA2000 appear to be much more adaptable to the physician's office laboratory. In PubMed, no articles are identified that report on the performance of the DiaSTAT analyzer.

Reference Ranges and Relationship of Glycohemoglobin to Diabetic Complications

The usual upper limit of normal for most assays for hemoglobin A_{1c} is near 6.0%. Total glycohemoglobin assays display reference ranges near 8.5% as more forms of glycated hemoglobin are measured in such assays. The ADA has recommended that the hemoglobin A_{1c} goal for the care of diabetic individuals represent a value of <7%. This cutpoint defining desirable glycemic control was primarily chosen because the DCCT "tight"-control group achieved an average hemoglobin A_{1c} of ~7%. The DCCT concluded that, even without achieving a normal hemoglobin A_{1c}, better glycemic control (e.g., blood glucose levels closer to normal) reduced the danger of developing microvascular and neuropathic complications. Because a hemoglobin A_{1c} of ~9% did represent a significant risk for microvascular and neuropathic complications, the ADA recommends currently that action be taken to improve glycemic control when the hemoglobin A_{1c} exceeds 8%.

Another important point that the DCCT demonstrated is that tight control can be achieved and tight control can be maintained for long periods of time (e.g., years). The price of tight control, however, is an increased frequency and severity of hypoglycemic reactions. There was a two- to threefold higher risk of hypoglycemia in tightly controlled individuals than traditionally controlled individuals as well as a 4.5-kg average weight gain in the tightly controlled DCCT patients. The other price of tight control involves increased expense and personal time spent on diabetes care. The DCCT support network for achieving good control was very extensive and involved a multitalented team including doctors, nurses, dieticians, etc. Such teams of professionals are often not available to individuals with diabetes at an affordable price. The UKPDS substantiated the findings of the DCCT in individuals with type 2 diabetes.

In the summer of 2001, the American Association of Clinical Endocrinologists and the American College of Endocrinology recommended a more stringent hemoglobin A_{1c} cutpoint of <6.5% to define the goal of diabetic therapy. This may not be an unreasonable goal as the UKPDS showed that microvascular and macrovascular complications first appeared at hemoglobin A_{1c} levels of 6.5%.

Indications for Testing

As discussed in the previous section, glycemic control clearly makes a difference in the long run as to whether microvascular and neuropathic complications occur in both type 1 and type 2 diabetes. The DCCT and UKPDS are both very clear on this point: control does make a difference! As an assessment of glycemic control over the previous 2–3 mo, the standard of care as recommended by the ADA is that hemoglobin A_{1c} be measured every 2–3 mo. If control is "satisfactory," hemoglobin A_{1c} can be measured every 6 mo.

A novel use of hemoglobin A_{1c} and fructosamine measurements has been proposed by Cohen et al. (131): the glycosylation gap. The glycosylation gap was defined as the difference between the hemoglobin A_{1c} predicted from the fructosamine measurement using population data and the measured hemoglobin A_{1c}. The glycosylation gap correlated better with nephropathy than either hemoglobin A_{1c} or fructosamine measurements alone. The value of the "glycosylation" gap requires independent validation.

Limitations of Hemoglobin A_{1c} Measurements in Diagnosis of Diabetes

Hemoglobin A_{1c} should not be used for diabetes screening or diagnosis. As illustrated in Table 4 (132), a hemoglobin A_{1c} cutoff just above the upper limit of

Table 4 Hemoglobin A_{1c} Sensitivity and Specificity for the Diagnosis of Diabetes

SD >mean	Positive cutoff HbA_{1c}	Diagnosis of diabetes[a] Sensitivity (%)	Specificity (%)
1	5.6	83.4	84.4
2	6.1	63.2	97.4
3	6.5	42.8	99.6
4	7.0	28.3	99.9

[a] Fasting plasma glucose ≥ 126 mg/dL.

normal (6.1%) does not provide sufficient sensitivity to diagnose diabetes, although specificity for the diagnosis of diabetes was satisfactory. Nevertheless, it is clear that not all individuals with an elevated hemoglobin A_{1c} display fasting hyperglycemia (Table 5) (133). Of 1565 adults tested for diabetes, whereas 54 (3.4%) displayed fasting hyperglycemia, another 18 (1.1%) individuals exhibited fasting glucose levels below 126 mg/dL and had an elevated hemoglobin A_{1c}.

Whereas hemoglobin A_{1c} can be measured at the POC as an extremely important part of diabetes management, hemoglobin A_{1c} measurements should not be used to screen for diabetes. Excluding cases of prolonged red blood cell half-life (e.g., splenectomy) that falsely elevate hemoglobin A_{1c}, elevated hemoglobin A_{1c} levels are usually most consistent with diabetes. However because hemoglobin A_{1c} is not universally elevated at the time of diagnosis of diabetes, a normal hemoglobin A_{1c} cannot be used to exclude the diagnosis of diabetes.

Table 5 Fasting Plasma Glucose and Hemoglobin A_{1c} in the Diagnosis of Diabetes

	No. studied	No. diagnosed with diabetes via FPG[a]	HbA_{1c}[b]	Both
Men	766	17	11	12
(%)		2.2%	1.4%	1.6%
(% of DM)		42.5%	27.5%	30%
Women	799	13	7	12
(%)		1.6%	0.9%	1.5%
(% of DM)		40.6%	21.9%	37.5%

[a] Fasting plasma glucose ≥ 126 mg/dL.
[b] Hemoglobin A_{1c} ≥ 6.1%.

Biological variation does affect hemoglobin A_{1c} measurements. For example, increased red blood cell half-life (RBC-$T_{1/2}$) increases hemoglobin A_{1c} and decreased RBC-$T_{1/2}$ decreases hemoglobin A_{1c}. Examples of conditions that shorten RBC-$T_{1/2}$ include autoimmune hemolytic anemias, mechanical hemolysis from a prosthetic heart valve, and genetic hemolytic states such as ovalocytosis, elliptocytosis, and glucose-6-phosphate dehydrogenase deficiency. Also among different individuals in the population, there are variable rates of hemoglobin glycosylation that can affect hemoglobin A_{1c} levels (134–136). Hemoglobin A_{1c} values among nondiabetic individuals vary widely; however, intraindividual variation is small.

Using a hemoglobin A_{1c} cutoff for diabetes of 6.1%, compared with fasting plasma glucose levels of $\geq$126 mg/dL, hemoglobin A_{1c} measurements displayed a sensitivity of only 63% (132). This means that ~4 in 10 in people with fasting hyperglycemia would be missed by hemoglobin A_{1c} testing. If the definition of diabetes is expanded to include individuals with nondiagnostic fasting plasma glucose levels (e.g., <126 mg/dL) and a hemoglobin $A_{1c} \geq 6.1\%$, measuring hemoglobin A_{1c} will increase the yield of subjects diagnosed with diabetes by about 30% (133).

Besides the poor sensitivity of hemoglobin A_{1c} measurements for the diagnosis of diabetes, there is a lack of glycohemoglobin method standardization worldwide. Most laboratories in the United States measure hemoglobin A_{1c} using immunoassay procedures. The ADA recommends that all measurements of glycohemoglobin be traceable to a hemoglobin A_{1c} standard that is measured by high-performance liquid chromatography as directed by the National Glycohemoglobin Standardization Program (http://web.missouri.edu/~diabetes/ngsp.html). The NGSP awards manufacturers a "certificate of traceability to the DCCT reference method" if rigorous accuracy and precision criteria are achieved in measuring hemoglobin A_{1c}. Unfortunately not all hemoglobin A_{1c} assays are certified by the NGSP. Also, NGSP certification must be maintained yearly.

Another issue in considering hemoglobin A_{1c} as a diagnostic test for diabetes is the precision of hemoglobin A_{1c} assays. In general, other than hemoglobin A_{1c} measured by HPLC, all other hemoglobin A_{1c} assays are less precise than plasma glucose measurements. This makes a strong case for plasma glucose as the best diagnostic tool as it is the most precise measure of the glycemic state of the patient.

It can be argued that glucose measurements are superior diagnostically to hemoglobin A_{1c} assays because glucose measurements are relatively inexpensive. Measurement of hemoglobin A_{1c} is very expensive compared with glucose measurements. If measurement of hemoglobin A_{1c} became the standard of practice for the diagnosis of diabetes, most of the world would not be able to afford to pay for such diagnostic testing. Because type 2 diabetes is rising in frequency worldwide at an explosive rate, the use of the least expensive (and accurate) method of diagnosis must be fostered worldwide. Epidemiological studies also demand that the diagnosis of diabetes be made on the same biochemical bases whether the patient lives in the United States or in Bangladesh.

While "hemoglobin A_{1c}" protagonists may state that diabetes is only present when hemoglobin A_{1c} levels are elevated, diabetes is really a disease of chronic hyperglycemia and not "hyper-hemoglobin A_{1c}-emia." Elevated hemoglobin A_{1c} is a consequence of diabetes but is not "diabetes" itself. Complications of diabetes are caused by hyperglycemia; elevated hemoglobin A_{1c} is the consequence of diabetes and not the cause of diabetes. It is possible that in the future the ADA will expand the definition of diabetes to include individuals solely with elevated hemoglobin A_{1c} measurements; however, in the short term, it is unlikely that hemoglobin A_{1c} measurements will replace glucose measurements as the primary tools in diagnosing diabetes.

Further Comments Regarding POCT for Glycohemoglobin

There is strong evidence that patient outcomes are improved when glycohemoglobin test results are available when a patient is seen by their physician. Cagliero et al. (137) conducted a trial in which type 1 and insulin-treated type 2 diabetes patients were randomized to a control group or to the experimental group where hemoglobin A_{1c} testing was performed at the POC. The hemoglobin A_{1c} results were then immediately available for the patient–physician encounter. Whereas the control group (without the benefit of immediate hemoglobin A_{1c} results) experienced no significant decline in hemoglobin A_{1c} results, at 6 and 12 mo hemoglobin A_{1c} in the experimental group declined by 0.57 and 0.40%, respectively. In a retrospective chart review (138), for type 2 diabetes patients over age 65, the availability of hemoglobin A_{1c} results at the time of the clinic visit contributed to a 12-mo decline in hemoglobin A_{1c} of 1.03%. In contrast, when hemoglobin A_{1c} results were not available for 2–3 days following the visit, patients achieved only a 0.33% decline in hemoglobin A_{1c} over 12 mo. Regrettably, these differences did not reach statistical significance due, in part, to the small sample size of the study. Nevertheless, an accompanying editorial spoke out in favor of rapid availability of hemoglobin A_{1c} results (139). Pope et al. (140) reported that the availability of hemoglobin A_{1c} results at the POC allowed therapeutic adjustments in 50% of their subjects at the time of their visit.

These data support the concept that POCT for hemoglobin A_{1c} (or glycohemoglobin) should lead to better diabetes management and convenience for physicians and their patients. With the hemoglobin A_{1c} results in-hand, physicians can immediately counsel their patients at the time of their visit instead of waiting several days for the central laboratory hemoglobin A_{1c} results. When data are delayed, there is the added problem of actually reaching the patient to discuss the appropriate follow-up. This can consume substantial amounts of physician or staff time. It is possible to contact the patient by phone to discuss laboratory results after their visit. Alternative, less personal, interactions involve use of fax communication or e-mail. However, these convenient, yet impersonal, communications lack the warmth, humanity, and conviction that can be imparted in person at the time of the patient's visit. The most effective means of communication is face-to-face encounters in the office or clinic. Thus, the laboratory studies must be performed prior to the visit or all of the pertinent laboratory work must be performed on the same day as the patient's visit.

While the testing institution's cost per test expense for hemoglobin A_{1c} at the POC will likely be greater than the central laboratory costs, the actual patient charge for hemoglobin A_{1c} POCT may be equal to that of the central laboratory or even less than the central laboratory if devices such as the DCA2000 or A_{1c}Now tests are used. A major issue regarding costs-versus-charges is the degree to which POC hemoglobin A_{1c} testing will be reimbursed by government and third party payers. There are many studies showing that hemoglobin A_{1c} testing is underutilized. Point-of-care testing might improve utilization of this important test.

Between the DCA2000 analyzer and the A_{1c}Now device, the A_{1c}Now test is clearly the simplest test platform available and is expected to capture a sizable portion of the market. Certainly there is no capital investment for the A_{1c}Now device other than purchasing the device. The DCA2000 (or DCA2000+) is a substantial investment, although less expensive than the Micromat II or DiaSTAT devices. However, if patients (and their physicians) can be convinced to mail-in blood samples before their clinic visits, the A_{1c}At-Home test (or similar tests) provides the technical advantages of central laboratory analysis with low cost per test. With mail-in formats, reproducibility of testing can be maintained even if a patient changes practitioners as the central testing laboratory for mail-in-programs should stay constant. At the University of Florida when our central laboratory attempted to introduce a mail-in hemoglobin A_{1c} program, we were, unfortunately, unable to convince our institutional diabetes practitioners to use the program and thus the program never went into operation.

Regardless of how hemoglobin A_{1c} is measured, its measurement does not instruct patients on how to improve their glycemic control (141). Improved glycemic control requires the development of an intervention plan created by the healthcare team and the patient and implemented by the patient. Knowledge of hemoglobin A_{1c} is only helpful when it leads to a change in diabetes management if the hemoglobin A_{1c} is above the desirable range. In addition to decreasing the rates of microvascular and neuropathic complications, lowering of hemoglobin A_{1c} levels is associated with considerable health care savings (142). Using a method traceable to the DCCT methodology, when the hemoglobin A_{1c} is $>8\%$, the ADA advises that "action" be taken to improve the patient's glycemic control. The current ADA goal of therapy is to achieve a hemoglobin A_{1c} of <7%.

POINT-OF-CARE KETOSIS DETECTION AND MONITORING

Chemistry

Ketone bodies are formed physiologically in cases of fasting and starvation, or pathologically in states of severe insulinopenia or alcoholic ketoacidosis. Ketone bodies are formed by the partial oxidation of free fatty acids. During fasting when insulin levels are suppressed, hormone-sensitive lipase in adipose tissue is not suppressed. Thus, adipose tissue triglycerides are broken down into glycerol, free fatty acids, and monoglycerides. The free fatty acids are released into the circulation where they are transported, in part, by albumin to the liver. In insulinopenic conditions, the liver utilizes free fatty acids for ketone production.

When the rate of production of ketone bodies exceeds the rate of clearance of ketone bodies, ketonuria immediately occurs because there is no renal threshold for ketones as opposed to glucose. The renal threshold for glucose is between 150 and 180 mg/dL in most people. With low levels of ketosis, ketonuria is detectable but ketonemia (elevated ketones in the blood) does not develop. However, as ketosis worsens (e.g., in poorly treated or untreated type 1 diabetes), ketonemia can complicate the medical condition of the patient, leading to nausea and acidosis (e.g., ketoacidosis). The two main ketone bodies are beta-hydroxybutyric acid (βHB) and acetoacetic acid. Spontaneous decarboxylation of acetoacetate produces acetone. Acetone excretion through the lungs produces a fruity smell detectable in exhaled breath. The predominant ketone body is βHB.

Ketones can be detected using Acetest tablets. The tablet contains nitroprusside, lactose, disodium phosphate, and glycine. In the presence of glycine, acetoacetate and to a lesser extent acetone, react with nitroprusside forming a lavender-purple complex. Nitroprusside does not react with βHB. Lactose increases the color and optimum pH is afforded by disodium phosphate. Urine dipsticks and Ketostix use nitroprusside embedded in a pad. Gerhardt's test, in which acetoacetate reacts with ferric chloride, is not specific for ketones and cannot be recommended.

In the case of urine testing, a drop of urine is placed directly on the tablet. For serum testing, the tablet is crushed and a drop of serum is added. The color is read at 30 sec, 2 min, and 10 min. By comparing the color intensity to a standard chart, the relative positivity of the sample can be graded. In cases of ketoacidosis, the predominant ketoacid is βHB and thus Acetest testing can underestimate the severity of ketosis. At our institution in a recent case of severe diabetic ketoacidosis, we observed the situation where urine ketones became transiently negative while serum levels of βHB were greatly elevated. Thus it is possible to theoretically miss ketosis when nitroprusside is used to test for ketones, emphasizing the potential value of serum βHB measurement.

The best method to assess ketonemia is the measurement of serum βHB. The KetoSite automated assay is summarized below:

$$\beta\text{HB} + \text{NAD}^+ \xrightarrow{\beta\text{HB dehydrogenase}} \text{acetoacetate} + \text{NADH} + \text{H}^+$$

$$\text{NADH} + \text{NBT} \xrightarrow{\text{Diaphorase}} \text{NAD}^+ + \text{reduced NBT (purple color)}$$

POCT Technology

Urine or serum testing with Acetest tablets or urine testing via dipstick or Ketostix are straightforward techniques. There are three more sophisticated POCT options for ketone measurement in blood: the BioScanner 2000 (Polymer Technology Systems, Inc., Indianapolis, IN), the KetoSite instrument (Stanbio Laboratory, San Antonio, TX) and the Precision Xtra POCT device (Abbott/MediSense).

Using reflectance photometer analysis of capillary blood, the BioScanner 2000 can measure glucose and lipids in addition to ketones. The meter is available for use by professionals or patients. A meter-inserted "MEMo chip" is employed to calibrate the meter for the desired assay. The manufacturer's Web site (http://www.bioscanner2000.com) does not describe the chemistry used in measuring ketones and a search of PubMed failed to identify any articles using the key word "bioscanner." Therefore, many specifics concerning this device are unknown, including analytical performance, linearity, correlation with other ketone assays, reportable range, etc. Nevertheless, the device and its strip system are FDA-approved. Polymer Technology Systems, Inc. advertises the BioScanner 2000 meter at ~$150.

The KetoSite strip uses the enzyme βHB dehydrogenase to measure serum, plasma, or whole blood βHB. The chemistry for the reactions is as described above in the previous section. The KetoSite strip is placed in the StatSite analyzer and 25 μL of blood is applied. After ~2 min, a result is reported. The correlation between the GDS enzymatic βHB method and the KetoSite measurement is satisfactory (slope = 0.986 and intercept = 0.04; $r = 0.975$). Coefficients of variation are ~6–7%. The StatSite device can also measure glucose with the GlucoSite strip.

The Abbott/MediSense Precision Xtra meter measures βHB. The precise chemistry is not described in their advertisements. This strip employs "TrueMeasure technology." These strips are novel in that they allow not only sample volume detection but also allow the addition of a second drop of blood to minimize strip wastage. Once sufficient blood is present, the chemical reactions then begin.

Reference Ranges and Interferences

Normal urine and serum from a nonfasting individual should be negative for ketones by Acetest and dipstick. The BioScanner 2000 literature does not provide a reference range for blood ketones. The KetoSite system describes a reference range of 0.02–0.27 mM for βHB. Above 0.27 mM, ketosis is present; above 5 mM, ketoacidosis is possible. The upper linear limit of this assay is 2 mM. Above 2 mM, the sample must be diluted with diluent supplied by the manufacturer. For the Precision Xtra, normal βHB is less than 0.6 mmol/L. Moderate βHB elevations are between 0.6 and 1.5 mmol/L. Between βHB levels of 1.6 and 3.0 mmol/L (e.g., "high" blood βHB levels) patients are at risk for diabetic ketoacidosis (DKA). Beta-hydroxybutyric acid concentrations >3.0 mmol/L are consistent with metabolic acidosis.

When using the nitroprusside-glycine reaction to measure ketones, false positive reactions can occur with drugs that contain free sulfhydryl groups (e.g., penicillamine, cysteine, acetylcysteine, dimercaprol, captopril) (143,144), very large quantities of phenylketones, or, for urine specimens, samples where 8-hydroxyquinoline was added as a preservative.

Concerning interferences in the measurement of βHB, acetoacetate decreases the measured level of βHB. No notable interference is described for the following substances: ascorbic acid at 3 mg/dL, bilirubin at 10 mg/dL, creatinine at 5 mg/dL, glucose at 2000 mg/dL, or uric acid at 16 mg/dL.

Indications for Testing

Patients are generally advised to check for ketosis if they are pregnant, acutely ill, stressed, feel nauseated, vomit, experience abdominal pain, or their blood glucose consistently exceeds 300 mg/dL. The presence of ketosis in a patient with type 1 diabetes signals the need to administer additional insulin to shut off ketogenesis. Aggressive insulin administration and monitoring can prevent the development of full-blown DKA. One in 200 children with DKA die, whereas 10–15% of adults succumb when acutely ill with DKA. It is advised that βHB be monitored during the treatment of DKA (145). In epileptic individuals treated with a ketogenic diet, βHB levels have been followed (146). While POCT measurements of blood βHB are quite novel, there are no data that blood βHB testing is superior to urine ketone testing at the POC other than when drug interferences are potentially present (147). Nevertheless, POCT βHB testing is very convenient (148).

Because the reagents can deteriorate with exposure to air, individually packaged strips should be used or patients should be meticulous in tightly closing test strip containers every time they are opened. This can also be said for blood glucose testing strips.

CONCLUDING REMARKS CONCERNING POINT-OF-CARE TESTING FOR DIABETES

Limitations of POCT Glucose Measurements in Diagnosis of Diabetes

In contrast to disease management, POCT measurements of blood glucose do not have a routine role in the diagnosis of diabetes or in screening for diabetes. Outside of the settings of DKA and hyperglycemic nonketotic coma (HNKC), for the diagnosis of diabetes the American Diabetes Association requires that glucose be measured by central laboratory methods or comparable methods that display high levels of accuracy and precision. As discussed above, the diagnosis of diabetes depends on the recognition of hyperglycemia on at least two separate occasions, e.g., on two separate days. The preferred specimen is plasma obtained from blood drawn into a gray top tube. Gray top tubes contain sodium fluoride or iodoacetate that poisons oxidative metabolism and either potassium or sodium oxalate that serves as an anticoagulant. After 1 hr, further glucose metabolism is blocked by sodium fluoride or iodoacetate, and plasma glucose levels are then stable for up to 24 hr even at room temperature.

Hyperglycemia is defined as a morning plasma glucose level of 126 mg/dL or greater obtained in the fasting state, during an oral glucose tolerance test (OGTT) a 2-hr plasma glucose level of 200 mg/dL or greater, or a random glucose level of 200 mg/dL or greater when the subject has symptoms of diabetes such as polyuria, polydipsia, polyphagia, and/or weight loss. Since many laboratories measure serum glucose in place of, or in addition to, plasma glucose, serum measurements can be used for diagnostic purposes if the blood is assayed within 1 hr of being drawn or if serum separator tubes are used and the blood is spun within 1 hr of being drawn.

Regarding the diagnosis of diabetes, POCT devices should not be used because, in general, glucose point-of-care testing using fingerstick analyzers is neither sufficiently accurate nor sufficiently precise to be employed in the diagnosis of diabetes. Many POCT devices used to measure fingerstick glucose levels display biases of up to 20 mg/dL at glucose values less than 100 mg/dL and biases of up to 20% at glucose values of 100 mg/dL or greater. On the other hand, typical coefficients of variation for central laboratory analyzers measuring glucose are 4–5% or less. Proficiency testing provided by the College of American Pathologists requires that bias from the group mean not exceed 6% for central laboratories. One POCT device that can be used for the diagnosis of diabetes is the HemoCue B-Glucose analyzer.

A recurrent point of confusion in assessing glucose levels reported by handheld devices is whether the result reported by the meter is a capillary (whole blood) result or the plasma equivalent. While all such handheld devices use capillary whole blood, some analyzers report glucose values as capillary whole blood whereas other devices report plasma glucose extrapolated from the capillary whole blood glucose measurement. Whole blood or capillary glucose levels are 10–15% lower than plasma or serum glucose values because the aqueous portion of whole blood is lower than the aqueous portion of plasma or serum. Capillary measurements of glucose are subject to tissue fluid artifact, are subject to hemoconcentration from low flow, are affected by hemocrit, and following carbohydrate loads, capillary glucose can be ~20 mg/dL greater than venous whole blood measurements. Venous whole blood is also not recommended for diagnostic purposes because whole blood glucose measurements are affected by hematocrit similar to capillary measurements.

Limitations of POCT Glucose Measurements in Diabetes Screening

For the same reasons that handheld glucose monitors should not be used to diagnose hyperglycemia, handheld glucose monitors should not be used to screen for type 2 diabetes. Near the critical cutpoint of 126 mg/dL, if the handheld glucose monitor displays a bias of ±20%, a substantial number of individuals will be misclassified as either hyperglycemic or not hyperglycemic. The ADA recommends that all adults age 45 and above should be screened for elevations in venous fasting plasma glucose every 3 yr. When individuals are at increased risk for diabetes, the ADA recommends that screening be initiated prior to age 45. The American Association of Clinical Endocrinologists states that high-risk individuals should be screened for diabetes beginning at age 30.

High risk for type 2 diabetes is defined as a positive family history of diabetes in a first-degree relative, belonging to a high-risk minority group (e.g., African American, Hispanic American, Native American, Asian American, or Pacific Islander), obesity (>20% above ideal body weight or a body mass index [BMI] ≥27), dyslipidemia (e.g., triglycerides ≥250 mg/dL; hypoalphalipoproteinemia (HDL-C ≤35 mg/dL), hypertension (≥140/90), giving birth to an infant >9 lb or being diagnosed with gestational diabetes, polycystic ovary syndrome, or previously identified impaired fasting glucose (IFG) or impaired glucose tolerance (IGT). IFG is a fasting plasma glucose level of 110–125 mg/dL. IGT is a 2-hr plasma glucose level during an OGTT of 140–199 mg/dL.

Because of their ease of use and low cost per test compared with venipuncture and central laboratory analysis, handheld glucose POCT devices are often employed in community health fairs that include diabetes screening. In addition to concerns about the accuracy and precision of such devices for screening, community screening is not recommended by the ADA. This may appear surprising recognizing the ADA's interest in diabetes screening using fasting plasma glucose measurements. The ADA does not recommend community screening because random glucose measurements, whether performed on a handheld device or in a central laboratory, are difficult to interpret even if accurate. If the plasma glucose level is <110 mg/dL, the glucose is normal and in the absence of diabetic symptoms, no further testing is indicated for another 3 yr. Community screening is not encouraged because it is unproven that community screening is cost effective. Most "community" screening programs are, in fact, sought out by people who already know their health status and community screening usually misses the people who need most to be tested.

POINT-OF-CARE TESTING FOR DIABETES MANAGEMENT

The benefit of lowering hemoglobin A_{1c} in the prevention of microvascular and neuropathic complications is undeniable. Lowering mean plasma glucose is reflected in lower hemoglobin A_{1c} levels. There is a fair correlation between mean plasma glucose and hemoglobin A_{1c} (Table 6). The goal of diabetes care is to lower hemoglobin A_{1c} to less than 7%. Achieving lower hemoglobin A_{1c} values is a major challenge.

For hospital POCT for blood glucose or other diabetes tests, there are many potential sources of error, including failure to document results, errors in patient and operator identification, and failure to follow procedures, such as not performing appropriate quality control or releasing results even when quality control is out of range. Although manufacturers might lead consumers and nonpathologist

Table 6 Relationship Between Hemoglobin A_{1c} and Mean Blood Glucose (MBG)

HbA_{1c} (%)	MBG[a] (mg/dL)	Interpretation
4	61	Nondiabetic range
5	92	
6	124	
7	156	ADA target
8	188	Action suggested
9	219	
10	251	
11	283	
12	314	
13	346	
14	378	

[a] Capillary whole blood glucose (plasma glucose values would be approximately 10–15% higher).

physicians to believe the contrary, there is nothing simple about the basic technology required to measure blood glucose accurately and precisely much less hemoglobin A_{1c}, fructosamine, or βHB. Traditional approaches to error reduction, such as education, feedback, financial penalties or incentives, and administrative rules, have not always been successful. Alternate approaches to error prevention may best focus on further simplifying medical devices, providing computer oversight of all procedures, continuous process monitoring technology, and more immediate operator alerts when errors are detected. Besides their primary healthcare providers, Web-interfaced services (e.g., lifechart.com; note: no endorsement of this Web site is made or implied) are available to help patients manage their diabetes. Errors in SMBG must also be addressed by the practitioner and patient.

Regardless of the monitoring systems employed, there is no substitute for frequent contact between the patient and the healthcare team. Kaufman et al. (149) demonstrated that pediatric patients who visited clinic 3–4 times per year had, on average, hemoglobin A_{1c} levels 0.7% lower than children that visited clinic only 1–2 times per year. Clearly in the DCCT, the multidisciplinary "tight control" approach achieved hemoglobin A_{1c} levels proportionately ~27% lower than the routinely managed group.

At the time of the patient's clinic visit, laboratory results should be available to the physician. While POCT is usually more expensive than central laboratory testing, patient convenience is a significant issue in achieving high rates of patient and clinician satisfaction with laboratory services. There are no universal credos that exist for the site of testing: certainly POCT will continue to expand, become more accurate and precise, will be easier to use, and will challenge the dominance of the central laboratory. The SMBG remains a keystone in the everyday management of diabetes. Despite this optimism, the general role of POCT in reducing length of stay, at least in the emergency room, still remains to be proven (150). Developing proper outcome indicators for future studies is important (151). Process enhancement can improve bedside POCT for glucose (152). Harmonization of results among POCT analyzers as well as harmonization with the central laboratory is important for bedside POCT programs in hospitals.

REFERENCES

1. American Diabetes Association. Clinical Practice Recommendations 2001. Expert Committee: Report of the expert committee on the diagnosis and classification of diabetes mellitus. Diabetes Care 24(suppl 1):S5–S20, 2001.
2. DeFronzo, RA. The triumvirate: β-cell, muscle, liver. Diabetes 37:667–687, 1988.
3. Roden M, Price TB, Perseghin G, et al. Mechanism of free fatty acid–induced insulin resistance in humans. J Clin Invest 97:2859–2865, 1996.

4. Rebrin K, Steil GM, Getty L, et al. Free fatty acid as a link in the regulation of hepatic glucose output by peripheral insulin. Diabetes 44:1038–1045, 1995.
5. Sindelar DK, Chu CA, Rohlie M, et al. The role of fatty acids in mediating the effects of peripheral insulin on hepatic glucose production in the conscious dog. Diabetes 46:187–196, 1997.
6. Hotamisligil GS, Shargill NS, Spiegelman BM. Adipose expression of tumor necrosis factor-alpha: Direct role in obesity-linked insulin resistance. Science 259: 87–91, 1993.
7. Hotamisligil GS, Spiegelman BM. Tumor necrosis factor alpha: A key component of the obesity-diabetes link. Diabetes 43:1271–1278, 1994.
8. Steppan CM, Bailey ST, Bhat S, Brown EJ, Banerjee RR, Wright CM, Patel HR, Ahima RS, Lazar MA. The hormone resistin links obesity to diabetes. Nature 409: 307–312, 2001.
9. Glaser N, Jones KL. Non–insulin dependent diabetes mellitus in children and adolescents. Adv Pediatr 43:359–396, 1996.
10. Pinhas-Hamiel O, Dolan LM, Daniels SR. Increased incidence of non–insulin dependent diabetes mellitus among adolescents. J Pediatr 128:608–615, 1996.
11. Glaser NS. Non–insulin dependent diabetes mellitus in childhood and adolescence. Pediatr Clin North Am 44(2):307–337, 1997.
12. Jones KL. Non–insulin dependent diabetes in children and adolescents: The therapeutic challenge. Clin Pediatr 2:103–110, 1998.
13. Rosenbloom AL, House DV, Winter WE. Non–insulin dependent diabetes mellitus (NIDDM) in minority youth: Research priorities and needs. Clin Pediatr 37:143–152, 1998.
14. Rosenbloom AL, Joe JR, Young RS, Winter WE. Emerging epidemic of type 2 diabetes in youth. Diabetes Care 22:345–354, 1999.
15. Marker J, Maclaren N. Immunopathology of immune-mediated (type 1) diabetes. Clin Lab Med 21:15–30, 2001.
16. Emancipator K. Laboratory diagnosis and monitoring of diabetes mellitus. Am J Clin Pathol 112:665–674, 1999.
17. Charles MA. Diabetes and the laboratorian: Opportunities for a new role. Med Lab Observ May:16–24, 2001.
18. Levetan CS. The value of the clinical endocrinologist in the new millennium. Endocrinologist 11:137–145, 2001.
19. Peters AL. Diabetes disease management: Past, present, and future. Endocrinologist 11:86–93, 2001.
20. Diabetes Control and Complications Trial Research Group. The effect of intensive treatment of diabetes on the development and progression of long-term complications in insulin-dependent diabetes mellitus. N Engl J Med 329:977–986, 1993.
21. United Kingdom Prospective Diabetes Study Group. Intensive blood-glucose control with sulphonylureas or insulin compared with conventional treatment and risk of complications in patients with type 2 diabetes. UKPDS 33. Lancet 352:837–853, 1998.
22. United Kingdom Prospective Diabetes Study Group. Effect of intensive blood-glucose control with metformin on complications in overweight patients with type 2 diabetes. UKPDS 34. Lancet 352:854–865, 1998.

23. United Kingdom Prospective Diabetes Study Group. Tight blood pressure control and risk of macrovascular and microvascular complications in type 2 diabetes. UKPDS 38. Br Med J 317:703–713, 1998.
24. American Diabetes Association. Implications of the United Kingdom Prospective Diabetes Study. Diabetes Care 21(12):2180–2184, 1998.
25. American Diabetes Association. Tests of glycemia in diabetes. Diabetes Care 24(suppl 1):S80–S82, 2001.
26. Table. CAP Today 15(12):26–34, 2001.
27. Borgert N. Diabetes epidemic pushes glucose point-of-care testing. Clin Lab Prod Sept:34, 2001.
28. American Diabetes Association. Resource Guide 2002. Diabetes Forecast (suppl): 44–47, 2002.
29. De Graaff JC, Hemmes GJ, Bruin T, Ubbink DT, Michels RP, Jacobs MJ, Sanders GT. Influence of repetitive finger puncturing on skin perfusion and capillary blood analysis in patients with diabetes mellitus. Clin Chem 45:2200–2206, 1999.
30. McGarraugh G, Price D, Schwartz S, Weinstein R. Physiologic influences on off-finger glucose testing. Diabetes Technol Ther 3:367–376, 2001.
31. Jungheim K, Koschinsky T. Risky delay of hypoglycemia detection by glucose monitoring at the arm. Diabetes Care 24:1303–1306, 2001.
32. Thennadil SN, Rennert JL, Wenzel BJ, Hazen KH, Ruchti TL, Block MB. Comparison of glucose concentrations in interstitial fluid, and capillary and venous blood during rapid changes in blood glucose levels. Diabetes Technol Ther 3:357–365, 2001.
33. Tang Z, Louie RF, Lee JH, Lee DM, Miller EE, Kost GJ. Oxygen effects on glucose meter measurements with glucose dehydrogenase- and oxidase-based test strips for point-of-care testing. Crit Care Med 29:1062–1070, 2001.
34. Kurahashi K, Maruta H, Usuda Y, Ohtsuka M. Influence of blood sample oxygen tension on blood glucose concentration measured using an enzyme-electrode method. Crit Care Med 25:231–235, 1997.
35. Louie RF, Tang Z, Sutton DV, Lee JH, Kost GJ. Point-of-care glucose testing: Effects of critical care variables, influence of reference instruments, and a modular glucose meter design. Arch Pathol Lab Med 124:257–266, 2000.
36. Tang Z, Lee JH, Louie RF, Kost GJ. Effects of different hematocrit levels on glucose measurements with handheld meters for point-of-care testing. Arch Pathol Lab Med 124:1135–1140, 2000.
37. Coss-Bu JA, Jefferson LS, Stone-McCord S, Ou CN, Watrin C, Sachdeva R, Copeland KC. Evaluation of a real-time blood glucose monitor in children with diabetic ketoacidosis. Diabetes Res Clin Pract 44:175–181, 1999.
38. Mastrototaro J. The MiniMed continuous glucose monitoring system (CGMS). J Pediatr Endocrinol Metab 12(suppl 3):751–758, 1999.
39. Rebrin K, Steil GM. Can interstitial glucose assessment replace blood glucose measurements? Diabetes Technol Ther 2:461–472, 2000.
40. Gross TM, Bode BW, Einhorn D, Kayne DM, Reed JH, White NH, Mastrototaro JJ. Performance evaluation of the MiniMed continuous glucose monitoring system during patient home use. Diabetes Technol Ther 2:49–56, 2000.
41. Bode BW, Gross TM, Thornton KR, Mastrototaro JJ. Continuous glucose monitor-

ing used to adjust diabetes therapy improves glycosylated hemoglobin: A pilot study. Diabetes Res Clin Pract 46:183–190, 1999.
42. Kaufman FR, Gibson LC, Halvorson M, Carpenter S, Fisher LK, Pitukcheewanont P. A pilot study of the continuous glucose monitoring system: Clinical decisions and glycemic control after its use in pediatric type 1 diabetic subjects. Diabetes Care 24:2030–2034, 2001.
43. Chase HP, Kim LM, Owen SL, MacKenzie TA, Klingensmith GJ, Murtfeldt R, Garg SK. Continuous subcutaneous glucose monitoring in children with type 1 diabetes. Pediatrics 107:222–226, 2001.
44. Boland E, Monsod T, Delucia M, Brandt CA, Fernando S, Tamborlane WV. Limitations of conventional methods of self-monitoring of blood glucose: Lessons learned from 3 days of continuous glucose sensing in pediatric patients with type 1 diabetes. Diabetes Care 24:1858–1862, 2001.
45. Phillips M, Benzaquen H, Shalitin S, Galatzer A, Fayman G. Use of continuous glucose sensor for monitoring intensive diabetic control of children and adolescents with type 1 diabetes. Pediatr Res 49:96A, 2001.
46. Tierney MJ, Tamada JA, Potts RO, Eastman RC, Pitzer K, Ackerman NR, Fermi SJ. The GlucoWatch biographer: A frequent automatic and noninvasive glucose monitor. Ann Med 32:632–641, 2000.
47. Tierney MJ, Garg S, Ackerman NR, Fermi SJ, Kennedy J, Lopatin M, Potts RO, Tamada JA. Effect of acetaminophen on the accuracy of glucose measurements obtained with the GlucoWatch biographer. Diabetes Technol Ther 2:199–207, 2000.
48. Pitzer KR, Desai S, Dunn T, Edelman S, Jayalakshmi Y, Kennedy J, Tamada JA, Potts RO. Detection of hypoglycemia with the GlucoWatch biographer. Diabetes Care 24:881–885, 2001.
49. Tamada JA, Garg S, Jovanovic L, Pitzer KR, Fermi S, Potts RO. Noninvasive glucose monitoring: Comprehensive clinical results. Cygnus Research Team. JAMA 17;282:1839–1844, 1999.
50. Garg SK, Potts RO, Ackerman NR, Fermi SJ, Tamada JA, Chase HP. Correlation of fingerstick blood glucose measurements with GlucoWatch biographer glucose results in young subjects with type 1 diabetes. Diabetes Care 22:1708–1714, 1999.
51. Tierney MJ, Tamada JA, Potts RO, Jovanovic L, Garg S. Clinical evaluation of the GlucoWatch biographer: A continual, non-invasive glucose monitor for patients with diabetes. Biosens Bioelectron 16:621–629, 2001.
52. Fonseca V, Hinson J, Pappas A, Waner M, Flock S. An erbium: YAG laser to obtain capillary blood samples without a needle for point-of-care laboratory testing. Arch Pathol Lab Med 121:685–688, 1997.
53. Chen R, Jin Z, Colon LA. Analysis of tear fluid by CE/LIF: A noninvasive approach for glucose monitoring. J Capillary Electrophor 3:243–248, 1996.
54. Borg Andersson A, Birkhed D, Berntorp K, Lindgarde F, Matsson L. Glucose concentration in parotid saliva after glucose/food intake in individuals with glucose intolerance and diabetes mellitus. J Oral Sci 106:931–937, 1998.
55. Reuterving CO, Reuterving G, Hagg E, Ericson T. Salivary flow rate and salivary glucose concentration in patients with diabetes mellitus influence of severity of diabetes. Diabetes Metab 13:457–462, 1987.

56. Ginsberg BH. An overview of minimally invasive technologies. Clin Chem 38: 1596–1600, 1992.
57. Heinemann L, Kramer U, Klotzer HM, Hein M, Volz D, Hermann M, Heise T, Rave K. Noninvasive glucose measurement by monitoring of scattering coefficient during oral glucose tolerance tests. Non-Invasive Task Force. Diabetes Technol Ther 2:211–220, 2000.
58. Cote GL, Fox MD, Northrop RB. Noninvasive optical polarimetric glucose sensing using a true phase measurement technique. IEEE Trans Biomed Eng 39:752–766, 1992.
59. Borchert MS, Storrie-Lombardi MC, Lambert JL. A noninvasive glucose monitor: Preliminary results in rabbits. Diabetes Technol Ther 1:145–5, 1999.
60. March WF. A noninvasive ocular glucose sensor. Diabetes Technol Ther 3:209–210, 2001.
61. Cameron BD, Baba JS, Cote GL. Measurement of the glucose transport time delay between the blood and aqueous humor of the eye for the eventual development of a noninvasive glucose sensor. Diabetes Technol Ther 3:201–207, 2001.
62. Cameron BD, Gorde HW, Satheesan B, Cote GL. The use of polarized laser light through the eye for noninvasive glucose monitoring. Diabetes Technol Ther 1:135–143, 1999.
63. Heise HM, Marbach R. Human oral mucosa studies with varying blood glucose concentration by non-invasive ATR-FT-IR-spectroscopy. Cell Mol Biol (Noisy-le-grand) 44:899–912, 1998.
64. Burmeister JJ, Arnold MA, Small GW. Noninvasive blood glucose measurements by near-infrared transmission spectroscopy across human tongues. Diabetes Technol Ther 2:5–16, 2000.
65. Kajiwara K, Uemura T, Kishikawa H, Nishida K, Hashiguchi Y, Uehara M, Sakakida M, Ichinose K, Shichiri M. Noninvasive measurement of blood glucose concentrations by analysing Fourier transform infra-red absorbance spectra through oral mucosa. Med Biol Eng Comput 31(suppl):S17–S22, 1993.
66. MacKenzie HA, Ashton HS, Spiers S, Shen Y, Freeborn SS, Hannigan J, Lindberg J, Rae P. Advances in photoacoustic noninvasive glucose testing. Clin Chem 45: 1587–1595, 1999.
67. Burmeister JJ, Arnold MA. Evaluation of measurement sites for noninvasive blood glucose sensing with near-infrared transmission spectroscopy. Clin Chem 45: 1621–1627, 1999.
68. Malin SF, Ruchti TL, Blank TB, Thennadil SN, Monfre SL. Noninvasive prediction of glucose by near-infrared diffuse reflectance spectroscopy. Clin Chem 45:1651–1658, 1999.
69. Klonoff DC. Noninvasive blood glucose monitoring. Diabetes Care 20:433–437, 1997.
70. Marwick C. Development of noninvasive methods to monitor blood glucose levels in people with diabetes. JAMA 280:312–313, 1998.
71. Khalil OS. Spectroscopic and clinical aspects of noninvasive glucose measurements. Clin Chem 45:165–177, 1999.
72. Albisser AM, En Chao SC, Parson ID, Sperlich M. Information technology and home glucose clamping. Diabetes Technol Ther 3:377–386, 2001.

73. Steward DE, Khardori R. An avoidable cause of false home glucose measurements. Diabetes Care 24:794, 2001.
74. Rushakoff RJ, Lewis SB. Case of pseudohypoglycemia. Diabetes Care 24:2157–2158, 2001.
75. Lee-Lewandrowski E, Laposata M, Eschenbach K, Camooso C, Nathan DM, Godine JE, Hurxthal K, Goff J, Lewandrowski K. Utilization and cost analysis of bedside capillary glucose testing in a large teaching hospital: Implications for managing point of care testing. Am J Med 97:222–230, 1994.
76. Tsai WW, Nash DB, Seamonds B, Weir GJ. Point-of-care versus central laboratory testing: An economic analysis in an academic medical center. Clin Ther 16:898–910, 1994.
77. Nosanchuk JS, Keefner R. Cost analysis of point-of-care laboratory testing in a community hospital. Am J Clin Pathol 103:240–243, 1995.
78a. Ross D, Heinemann L, Chantelau EA. Short-term evaluation of an electro-chemical system (ExacTech) for blood glucose monitoring. Diabetes Res Clin Pract 10:281–285, 1990.
78b. Rheney CC, Kirk JK. Performance of three blood glucose meters. Ann Pharmacother 34:317–321, 2000.
78c. Li K-L, Huang H-S, Lin J-D, Huang B-Y, Huang M-J, Wang P-W. Comparing self-monitoring blood glucose devices. Lab Med 25:585–593, 1994.
79. Jones BA, Howanitz PJ. Bedside glucose monitoring quality control practices. A College of American Pathologists Q-Probes study of program quality control documentation, program characteristics, and accuracy performance in 544 institutions. Arch Pathol Lab Med 120:339–345, 1996.
80. Watts NB. Reproducibility (precision) in alternate site testing: A clinician's perspective. Arch Pathol Lab Med 119:914–917, 1995.
81. Bennett BD. Blood glucose determination: Point of care testing. South Med J 90: 678–680, 1997.
82. Brunner GA, Ellmerer M, Sendlhofer G, Wutte A, Trajanoski Z, Schaupp L, Quehenberger F, Wach P, Krejs GJ, Pieber TR. Validation of home blood glucose meters with respect to clinical and analytical approaches. Diabetes Care 21:585–590, 1998.
83. Du Plessis M, Ubbink JB, Vermaak WJ. Analytical quality of near-patient blood cholesterol and glucose determinations. Clin Chem 46:1085–1090, 2000.
84. Boyd JC, Bruns DE. Quality specifications for glucose meters: Assessment by simulation modeling of errors in insulin dose. Clin Chem 47:209–214, 2001.
85. Skeie S, Thue G, Sandberg S. Patient-derived quality specifications for instruments used in self-monitoring of blood glucose. Clin Chem 47:67–73, 2001.
86. Geffken G, Winter WE. Hardware and software in diabetes mellitus: Performance characteristics of hand-held glucose testing devices and the application of glycemic testing to patients' daily diabetes management. Clin Chem 47:11–12, 2001.
87. Harris MI. Frequency of blood glucose monitoring in relation to glycemic control in patients with type 2 diabetes. Diabetes Care 24:979–982, 2001.
88. Kennedy L. Self-monitoring of blood glucose in type 2 diabetes: Time for evidence of efficacy. Diabetes Care 24:977–978, 2001.

89. Armbruster DA. Fructosamine: Structure, analysis, and clinical usefulness. Clin Chem 33:2153–2163, 1987.
90. U.S. Food and Drug Administration. The LXN Fructosamine Test System. 510(k) file K962597. USFDA, Washington, DC, 1997.
91. Cefalu WT, Wang ZQ, Redmon E, Bell-Farrow AD, McBride D, King T. Clinical validity of a self-test fructosamine in outpatient diabetic management. Diabetes Technol Ther 1:435–441, 1999.
92. Edelman SV, Callahan P, Deeb LC. Multisite evaluation of a new diabetes self-test for glucose and glycated protein (fructosamine). Diabetes Technol Ther 2:233–238, 2000.
93. Ng WY, Lui KF, Thai AC. An improved colorimetric assay for fructosamine. Ann Acad Med Singapore 19:480–483, 1990.
94. Glikmanas G, Sarmini H, Bigorie B, Haioun B, Gouget B, Truchaud A. Evaluation of Roche fructosamine test: Use for diabetic patient monitoring. Clin Biochem 21: 319–321, 1988.
95. Guidance document for healthcare professionals, using the GlucoProtein test in diabetes management. LXN Corporation, San Diego, CA, 1998.
96. Glauber H, Welch S. Fructosamine, a new test for assessing diabetes control. NWP J Clin Pract 1:11–12, 1994.
97. Goldstein DE, Little RR, Lorenz RA, Malone JI, Nathan D, Peterson CM. Tests of glycemia in diabetes. Diabetes Care 18:896–909, 1995.
98. The 1998/1999 Quest Diagnostics Nichols Institute Reference Manual. Quest Diagnostics, San Juan Capistrano, CA, 1998, p 132.
99. Gebhart SS, Wheaton RN, Mullins RE, Austin GE. A comparison of home glucose monitoring with determinations of hemoglobin A_{1c}, total glycated hemoglobin, fructosamine, and random serum glucose in diabetic patients. Arch Intern Med 151: 1133–1337, 1991.
100. Daubresse JC, Laurent E, Ligny C, Bailly A, Lemy C, Duchateau A, Meunier JC. The usefulness of fructosamine determination in diabetic patients and relation to metabolic control. Diabetes Metab 13:217–221, 1987.
101. Cefalu WT, Prather KL, Chester DL, Wheeler CJ, Biswas M, Pernoll ML. Total serum glycosylated proteins in detection and monitoring of gestational diabetes. Diabetes Care 13:872–875, 1990.
102. Sacks DB. Carbohydrates. In: Burtis CA, Ashwood ER (eds.). Tietz Textbook of Clinical Chemistry. 3rd ed, Saunders, Philadelphia, 1999, p 796.
103. American Diabetes Association. Tests of glycemia in diabetes. Diabetes Care 24(suppl 1):S80–S82, 2001.
104. American Association of Clinical Endocrinologists. Medical guidelines for the management of diabetes mellitus: The AACE system of intensive diabetes self-management—2000 update. Endocr Pract 6:42–84, 2000.
105. Goldstein DE, Little RR. Monitoring glycemia in diabetes. Endocrinol Metab Clin North Am 26:475–486, 1997.
106. American Diabetes Association. Tests of glycemia in diabetes. Diabetes Care 24(suppl 1):S80–S82, 2001.
107. Cefalu WT, Wang ZQ, Redmon E, Bell-Farrow AD, McBride D, King T. Clinical

validity of a self-test fructosamine in outpatient diabetic management. Diabetes Technol Ther 1:435–441, 1999.
108. Carter AW, Borchardt N, Cooney M, Greene D. Dual-test monitoring of hyperglycemia using daily glucose and weekly fructosamine values. Diabetes Technol Ther 3:399–408, 2001.
109. Edelman SV, Callahan P, Deeb LC. Multisite evaluation of a new diabetes self-test for glucose and glycated protein (fructosamine). Diabetes Technol Ther 2:233–238, 2000.
110. Petitti DB, Contreras R, Dudl J. Randomized trial of fructosamine home monitoring in patients with diabetes. Eff Clin Pract 4:18–23, 2001.
111. Koch DD. Fructosamine. Clin Chem News April:8–9, 1990.
112. Schwartz JG. The role of glycohemoglobin and other proteins in diabetes management. Diabetes Rev 3:269–287, 1995.
113. Krishnamurti U, Steffes MW. Glycohemoglobin: A primary predictor of the development or reversal of complications of diabetes mellitus. Clin Chem 47:1157–1165, 2001.
114. Prome D, Blouquit Y, Ponthus C, Prome JC, Rosa J. Structure of the human adult hemoglobin minor fraction A_{1b} by electrospray and secondary ion mass spectrometry. Pyruvic acid as amino-terminal blocking group. J Biol Chem 266:13050–13054, 1991.
115. Schwartz JG. The role of glycohemoglobin and other proteins in diabetes management. Diabetes Rev 3:269–287, 1995.
116. Weykamp CW, Penders TJ, Miedema K, Muskiet FA, van der Slik W. Standardization of glycohemoglobin results and reference values in whole blood studied in 103 laboratories using 20 methods. Clin Chem 41:82–86, 1995.
117. Steffes MW. Glycemic control: Perhaps we can define it, but can we measure it? Clin Chem 41:180–181, 1995.
118. Weykamp CW, Penders TJ, Muskiet FA, van der Slik W. Evaluation of a reference material for glycated haemoglobin. Eur J Clin Chem Clin Biochem 34:67–72, 1996.
119. Turpeinen U, Karjalainen U, Stenman UH. Three assays for glycohemoglobin compared. Clin Chem 41:191–195, 1995.
120. Parkes J, Ray R, Kerestan S, Davis H, Ginsberg B. Prospective evaluation of accuracy, precision, and reproducibility of an at-home hemoglobin A_{1c} sampling kit. Diabetes Technol Ther 1:411–419, 1999.
121. Roberts WL, McCraw M, Cook CB. Effects of sickle cell trait and hemoglobin C trait on determinations of HbA_{1c} by an immunoassay method. Diabetes Care 21: 983–986, 1998.
122. Blakney GB, Higgins TN, Holmes DJ. Comparison of hemoglobin A_{1c} results by two different methods on patients with structural hemoglobin variants. Clin Biochem 31:619–626, 1998.
123. Roberts WL, Craw M, Cook CB. Effects of sickle cell trait and hemoglobin C trait on determinations of HbA_{1c} by an immunoassay method. Diabetes Care 21:983–986, 1998.
124. Rumley AG, Kilpatrick ES, Dominiczak MH, Small M. Evaluation of glycaemic

control limits using the Ames DCA2000 HbA_{1c} analyser. Diabetic Med 10:976–979, 1993.

125. Guthrie R, Hellman R, Kilo C, Hiar CE, Crowley LE, Childs B, Fisher R, Pinson MB, Suttner A, Vittori C. A multisite physician's office laboratory evaluation of an immunological method for the measurement of HbA_{1c}. Diabetes Care 15:1494–1498, 1992.
126. Carter JS, Houston CA, Gilliland SS, Perez GE, Owen CL, Pathak DR, Little RR. Rapid HbA_{1c} testing in a community setting. Diabetes Care 19:764–767, 1996.
127. Stivers CR, Baddam SR, Clark AL, Ammirati EB, Irvin BR, Blatt JM. A miniaturized self-contained single-use disposable quantitative test for hemoglobin A_{1c} in blood at the point of care. Diabetes Technol Ther 2:517–526, 2000.
128. Phillipov G, Charles P, Beng C, Phillips PJ. Alternate site testing for HbA_{1c} using the Primus CLC330 GHb analyzer. Diabetes Care 20:607–609, 1997.
129. Stevenson T. Glycosal: The first rapid, point-of-care test for the determination of hemoglobin A_{1c} in patients with diabetes. Diabetes Technol Ther 1:425–431, 1999.
130. Peterson CM. Glycosal. Commentary. Diabetes Technol Ther 1:433–434, 1999.
131. Cohen RM, Holmes YR, Chenier TC, Joiner CH. Discordance between hemoglobin A_{1c} and fructosamine: The glycosylation gap and its role in complications in type 1 diabetes. Diabetes 50(suppl 2):A62, 2001.
132. Rohlfing CL, Little RR, Wiedmeyer HM, England JD, Madsen R, Harris MI, Flegal KM, Eberhardt MS, Goldstein DE. Use of GHb (HbA_{1c}) in screening for undiagnosed diabetes in the U.S. population. Diabetes Care 23:187–191, 2000.
133. Takahashi Y, Noda M, Tsugane S, Kuzuya T, Ito C, Kadowaki T. Prevalence of diabetes estimated by plasma glucose criteria combined with standardized measurement of HbA_{1c} among health checkup participants on Miyako Island, Japan. Diabetes Care 23:1092–1096, 2000.
134. Modan M, Meytes D, Rozeman P, Yosef SB, Sehayek E, Yosef NB, Lusky A, Halkin H. Significance of high HbA_1 levels in normal glucose tolerance. Diabetes Care 11:422–428, 1988.
135. Kilpatrick ES, Maylor PW, Keevil BG. Biological variation of glycated hemoglobin. Implications for diabetes screening and monitoring. Diabetes Care 21:261–264, 1988.
136. Wiener K, Roberts NB. The relative merits of haemoglobin A_{1c} and fasting plasma glucose as first-line diagnostic tests for diabetes mellitus in non-pregnant subjects. Diabetic Med 15:558–563, 1998.
137. Cagliero E, Levina EV, Nathan DM. Immediate feedback of HbA_{1c} levels improves glycemic control in type 1 and insulin-treated type 2 diabetic patients. Diabetes Care 22:1785–1789, 1999.
138. Ferenczi A, Reddy K, Lorber DL. Effect of immediate hemoglobin A_{1c} results on treatment decisions in office practice. Endocr Pract 7:85–88, 2001.
139. Lichtenstein LS. Rapid availability of hemoglobin A_{1c} value in the care of patients with diabetes. Endocr Pract 7:143–144, 2001.
140. Pope RM, Apps JM, Page MD, Allen K, Bodansky HJ. A novel device for the rapid in-clinic measurement of haemoglobin A_{1c}. Diabetic Med 10:260–263, 1993.
141. Porter KH, Myers GL. Implications of point-of-care testing for hemoglobin A_{1c}. Diabetes Technol Ther 2:527–528, 2000.

142. Menzin J, Langley-Hawthorne C, Friedman M, Boulanger L, Cavanaugh R. Potential short-term economic benefits of improved glycemic control: A managed care perspective. Diabetes Care 24:51–55, 2001.
143. Csako G, Elin RJ. Unrecognized false-positive ketones from drugs containing free-sulfhydryl group(s). JAMA 269:1634, 1993.
144. Csako G, Elin RJ. Spurious ketonuria due to captopril and other free sulfhydryl drugs. Diabetes Care 19:673–674, 1996.
145. Rosenbloom AL, Hanas R. Diabetic ketoacidosis (DKA): Treatment guidelines. Clin Pediatr (Phila) 35:261–266, 1996.
146. Gilbert DL, Swink TD, Casey J, Pyzik P, Freeman JM. Blood β-OH butyrate levels and management of the ketogenic diet. Ann Neurol 42:502, 1997.
147. Laffel L. Sick-day management in type 1 diabetes. Endocrinol Metab Clin North Am 29:707–723, 2000.
148. Wallace TM, Meston NM, Gardner SG, Matthews DR. The hospital and home use of a 30-second hand-held blood ketone meter: Guidelines for clinical practice. Diabetic Med 18:640–645, 2001.
149. Kaufman FR, Halvorson M, Carpenter S. Association between diabetes control and visits to a multidisciplinary pediatric diabetes clinic. Pediatrics 103:948–951, 1999.
150. Parvin CA, Lo SF, Deuser SM, Weaver LG, Lewis LM, Scott MG. Impact of point-of-care testing on patients' length of stay in a large emergency department. Clin Chem 42:711–717, 1996.
151. Collier CP, Houlden RL, Gleeson KA, Patrzykat A, Rhymer SL. A survey to identify potential outcome indicators for a hospital blood glucose monitoring program. Clin Biochem 31:263–268, 1998.
152. Lewandrowski E, Mac Millan D, Misiano D, Tochka L, Lewandrowski K. Process improvement for bedside capillary glucose testing in a large academic medical center: The impact of new technology on point-of-care testing. Clin Chim Acta 307:175–179, 2001.

11

Outcomes-Based Evaluation of Dipstick Urinalysis

William Clarke and Darryl Erik Palmer-Toy*
Johns Hopkins Medical Institutions, Baltimore, Maryland, U.S.A.

Dipstick urinalysis (DUA) is one of the cornerstones of point-of-care testing—relatively inexpensive, robust, easy to perform, painless to the patient, and available worldwide. Almost since the inception of the Clinistix (Ames Co., Elkhardt, IN) in 1956, DUA has been a staple for community health and preoperative screening, and in the workup of urinary tract and systemic diseases. Yet, the real clinical utility of DUA is more often assumed than proven. In this chapter, we progress through each component of DUA, to review the physiological and analytical considerations and then to discuss the literature on the efficacy of each component in the screening of various populations and in the workup of specific disorders.

Evidence from the literature was evaluated both with regard to the design of the study that supports the evidence and the recommendations gleaned from the evidence in the study. The recommendations are characterized as either supporting or discrediting the practice in question in standard patient care according to the following scale:

A: Good evidence to support the inclusion of the practice
B: Fair evidence to support the inclusion of the practice
C: Insufficient evidence to support the inclusion or exclusion of the practice
D: Fair evidence to support the exclusion of the practice
E: Good evidence to support the exclusion of the practice

* *Current affiliation*: Massachusetts General Hospital, Boston, Massachusetts, U.S.A.

In addition, the level of evidence in the papers is described as being level I, II, or III. Level I evidence is characterized as coming from at least one properly randomized controlled trial. Evidence from trials that are not randomized, such as well-designed cohort or case-control studies, is classified as level II. Opinions of respected authorities, anecdotal evidence from clinical experience, or reports from a panel of experts are considered to be level III evidence. A table summarizing the relevant references and the level of evidence for each study, as well as our recommendations, is presented in each section.

To ensure a systematic review of the literature, the National Library of Medicine/MEDLINE database was searched using the keywords indicated in Table 1. The search was limited to human studies, and articles were chosen for more careful reading based upon their titles and abstracts. Additional searches were performed cross-referencing specific disorders and DUA components. Some foreign language entries were cited based upon their English abstracts, but these were not read completely.

Table 1 Keywords Used in Systematic MEDLINE Search for Dipstick Urinalysis Literature

Urinalysis AND	(Outcome OR outcomes)
Urine specific gravity AND	(Specificity OR diagnostic accuracy OR evidence based medicine)
Urine pH AND	(Specificity OR diagnostic accuracy OR evidence based medicine)
Proteinuria AND	(Specificity OR diagnostic accuracy OR evidence based medicine)
(Urine blood OR hematuria) AND	(Specificity OR diagnostic accuracy OR evidence based medicine)
Hemoglobinuria AND	(Specificity OR diagnostic accuracy OR evidence based medicine)
Urobilinogen AND	(Specificity OR diagnostic accuracy OR evidence based medicine)
(Urine bilirubin OR bilirubinuria) AND	(Specificity OR diagnostic accuracy OR evidence based medicine)
(Glucosuria OR glycosuria OR urine glucose) AND	(Specificity OR diagnostic accuracy OR evidence based medicine)
(Ketonuria OR urine ketones) AND	(Specificity OR diagnostic accuracy OR evidence based medicine)
(Pyuria OR leukocyte esterase OR urine nitrite) AND	(Specificity OR diagnostic accuracy OR evidence based medicine)

PATIENT SCREENING WITH DUA

Dipstick urinalysis has been widely used as a screening tool in two major contexts: screening the general population and screening inpatients. Where the reports of DUA screening focus on specific components of DUA, they are discussed in the corresponding sections below. However, many of the patient screening studies by DUA or full urinalysis have provided no more information than the frequency of abnormal results, without specifying the type of abnormality (Table 2).

Preoperative testing was long used as both an element of comprehensive care as well as insurance against operative misadventure. Dipstick urinalysis was viewed as something of a catchall. In a study of 3375 oral and maxillofacial surgical outpatients, preoperative screens by DUA revealed 91 patients with unexpected abnormalities (2.7%) (1). The yields of abnormal urinalysis (DUA and/or microscopic) results in review of 11 preoperative screening studies range from 2.4–39.2%, while 0.1–16.6% resulted in a change in management (2). Several of the studies separately examined "routine" DUA (i.e., testing was not indicated by information obtained from a careful history, review of systems, and physical examination). For routine DUA with abnormal results, the yields drop to 1–18.0% abnormal with only 1.0–2.8% resulting in a change of management.

Other studies confirm the limited impact of DUA on outpatient and inpa-

Table 2 Evidence of Clinical Utility of Dipstick Urinalysis for Patient Screening

Reference	Total DUA abnormal	Routine DUA abnormal	Change in patient management	Evidence level	Recommendation grade
Outpatient screening					D
Fraser et al. (3)	7%	—	0.5%	II	
Boland et al. (4)	—	13.8%	1.1%	II	
Preoperative screening					D
Gold and Wolfersberger (1)	—	2.7%	—	II	
Velanovich (10)	—	—	—	II	
Munro et al. (2)	2.4–39.2%	1.0–18.1%	1–1.3%	II	
Other admission screening					D
Del Mar and Badger (5)	9.2%	—	0.7%	II	
Berber and McFeeley (6)	7.8%	—	0.8%	II	
Mitchell and Stapleton (7)	—	20%	0.8%	II	
Swingler (8)	32.6%	—	0%	II	

tient care. An Australian study of 2600 outpatients screened by DUA identified 316 abnormal results for 182 patients (7%), but only 13 abnormalities had a significant bearing on diagnosis or management (0.5%) (3). Among 100 adult ambulatory patients at the Mayo Clinic, 12 of 87 (13.8%) urinalyses were abnormal, resulting in two additional evaluations and one new diagnosis. Urinalysis was deemed by the authors as inferior to all other case finding modalities evaluated except for the electrocardiogram in terms of diagnostic yield (4). Of 2294 admission DUA at a large private Australian hospital, 9% yielded predictable abnormalities and 4% yielded unexpected abnormalities, but 24% of the unexpected abnormalities were later attributed to sample contamination (5). Urinalyses performed on 515 patients admitted to a Canadian psychiatric hospital had a 7.8% yield for abnormal results, but only 0.8% changed management (6). Among pediatric admissions, routine DUA performed on 732 American children found a 20% prevalence of abnormal results, but management was only altered in 0.8% of patients (7). At a South African children's hospital, 76 of 233 (32.6%) admission urinalyses were abnormal, but only two (0.9%) patients' care was changed (8).

The limited impact of routine DUA on patient management is generally viewed as a strong argument against routine patient testing. However, a few important assumptions are made in this focus on routine screening: namely, that physicians are adept at recognizing appropriate indications for ordering urinalyses, and that patients are capable of providing histories and reviews of systems upon admission. Many of the "indicated" urinalyses that discovered abnormalities may have been "routine" to the clinicians who ordered them. There is also an implicit cost–benefit ratio in each study's interpretation. It is easy to denounce a practice that produces no change in management, but much harder to do so in the face of small but definite management changes. One analysis of routine pediatric admission DUA estimated that $3911 was spent per urinary tract infection (UTI) diagnosed (7). Another study estimated that $1.5M would be spent on preoperative DUA per UTI-related complication avoided (9). However, the ultimate argument against routine testing may be that abnormal preoperative urinalyses are not associated with any kind of postoperative complication or mortality, based upon multivariate analysis of 520 patients undergoing elective surgery at a San Francisco hospital (10).

Another important problem uncovered by these studies is that most abnormal DUA results from patient screening are not noted or adequately addressed in the chart (5–8,11,12). Several explanations have been advanced for this negligence. This may reflect that the patients' physicians anticipate some abnormalities identified by urinalysis. However, the basis for anticipating these abnormalities was not apparent upon systemic review of the charts by the various study authors. Another possibility is that physicians distrust DUA results when the clinical picture is inconsistent. They may view the costs of delaying a scheduled procedure and working up an unanticipated DUA result as prohibitive. However, this deliberate disregard of an abnormal result certainly should be explained in the chart. More likely, the caregivers never checked the results. Therefore, much of the implied shortcomings of DUA in patient management may represent a flaw in test utilization, rather than a limitation of DUA itself.

pH

Urine pH is dependent on the ability of the kidneys to maintain hydrogen ion concentration in plasma and extracellular fluid; perturbations of acid–base balance in the body are reflected in urine pH. The measurable range of pH in urine using a reagent dipstick is 4.5–8.0, whereas urine pH typically ranges somewhere from 5–6. However, there are no "normal" values for urinary pH; other factors must be considered alongside the pH such as acid–base content of blood, renal function, infection status, dietary intake, and age.

Determination of urinary pH can sometimes indicate the presence of a renal disorder; if the urinary pH does not reflect systemic conditions, then kidney dysfunction is suspected. Proximal tubule acidosis is characterized by reabsorptive dysfunction, so bicarbonate ions are wasted (e.g., Fanconi's syndrome) and urinary pH is decreased. Renal insufficiency is characterized by a decreased ability to excrete acid, leading to systemic acidosis. Because acid cannot be excreted, the blood becomes more acidic but the urinary pH cannot be lowered beyond 6–6.5, so both the titratable acidity along with ammonium ion (NH_4^+) concentration are decreased. In cases of urinary tract infection, bacterial metabolism of urea leads to increased urine pH.

In order to measure urinary pH on a reagent dipstick, multiple colorimetric indicators are used. The measurement is made in 1-unit increments by colorimetric comparison to a pH chart, with the colors progressing from orange to yellow to green to deep blue. The main interference with dipstick measurement of urine pH is reagent runover from an adjacent test pad on the strip. A protein analysis pad is directly next to the pH pad and is buffered at pH 3. If the strip is excessively wet and some pH 3 buffer runs into the pH area, the pH will be falsely lowered. Any pH-altering foods or drugs that are ingested prior to analysis can mask an underlying condition by temporarily shifting the acidity of the specimen. Bacterial contamination will cause a pH increase upon standing, in fact, a sample with pH of greater than 8.5 is considered improperly preserved and not fit for analysis. On the other hand, large amounts of glucose in urine (as in diabetes mellitus) can be metabolized by bacteria in the urine to acids and alcohols, which will artifactually lower the pH of the specimen. A urine sample left standing uncovered can lose carbon dioxide to the atmosphere and become more alkaline.

Few studies examine the effect that measurement of urine pH has on patient

Table 3 Evidence of Clinical Utility of Dipstick Urinalysis for Urine pH

Reference	Sensitivity	Specificity	PPV	NPV	Evidence level	Recommendation grade
Screening						D
Fraser et al. (3)	—	—	—	—	II	
Assessing renal tubular function						D
Skinner et al. (15)	—	—	—	—	II	
Recurrence of stones						B
Hussain et al. (16)	?	?	?	?	II	

outcomes (Table 3). Measurement and control of urinary pH are primarily important in treatment of renal stone formation and urinary tract infection. Outcomes research involving urinalysis generally is focused on protein, blood, glucose, ketones, and leukocytes; when pH is noted, it sometimes is not even recorded (13). One issue is that urine pH values for most patients are not really different from those found in healthy individuals (3). Population variance in urine pH may be attributable to differences in dietary protein, sodium, and potassium (14).

One group has studied the specificity of pH measurements in assessing distal renal tubular function in children (15). Early morning samples were collected and tested to evaluate urinary acidification in renal and metabolic disorders; however, their conclusion was that pH testing in children was not a useful screening technique in this capacity. Urine pH measurements may have a role in the management of kidney stones. The urine pH of 239 patients with renal and ureteric calculi associated with renal failure was evaluated before definitive surgery, serially after 24 hr and then every week for 6 wk. Urine pH $\leq$6 was found to be a favorable prognostic factor (16). This result may depend on the type of stone afflicting the patient, as treatment to prevent uric acid stone recurrence involves alkalinizing the urine.

SPECIFIC GRAVITY

Urine specific gravity (USG) provides an estimate of the proportion of dissolved solids in urine, giving an indication of the ability of the kidney to concentrate or dilute urine. Renal disease and dysregulation of antidiuretic hormone (ADH) are two major causes of inability to concentrate or dilute urine. Normally, USG ranges from 1.010–1.025. Low USG (hyposthenuria), defined as ranging from 1.001–1.003 is usually present in patients with diabetes insipidus or other renal dysfunction in which the kidney has lost the ability to concentrate urine. High

USG usually occurs due to excessive loss of water due to the loss of diluting ability in the kidney. Isosthenuria is urine of fixed specific gravity regardless of fluid loss or intake, usually at a value of 1.007, and occurs in cases of severe renal damage.

Urine specific gravity is most commonly measured by a chemical approximation using the urine dipstick, but can be more accurately measured using a hydrometer or refractometer. The specific gravity estimate of dipstick urinalysis is based on a pKa change of pretreated electrolytes in relation to the ionic concentration of the sample. High specific gravity results from an increased electrolyte concentration, which lowers the pKa of the electrolyte. This in turn causes the pH to decrease. The indicator changes color in relation to the ionic translation, which corresponds to specific gravity values. The reagent is sensitive to the number of ions in the urine specimen, so the results must be corrected for the pH of the urine (17). High levels of proteins in the urine will interfere with reagent strip measurements because they carry multiply charged groups per molecule.

As with pH measurement, USG is not a urine test that is often evaluated in the context of patient outcomes (Table 4). One study found no utility of urine osmolality in the evaluation of renal tubular function (15). Urine specific gravity has been given mixed reviews as a measure of hydration status. In studies of fit individuals, USG was very sensitive to changes of hydration status in one study (18), but was shown to lag behind plasma osmolality with acute dehydration and rehydration according to another study (19). Plasma osmolality has consistently been shown to be the best marker of hydration status. In the more clinically relevant population of acutely dehydrated children, 40 children who required intravenous fluid resuscitation were examined by several laboratory measures. Urine specific gravity was poorly predictive of fluid deficits (20).

Table 4 Evidence of Clinical Utility of Dipstick Urinalysis for Urine Specific Gravity

Reference	Sensitivity	Specificity	PPV	NPV	Evidence level	Recommendation grade
Assessing renal tubular function						D
Skinner et al. (15)	—	—	—	—	II	
Assessing hydration						C
Armstrong et al. (18)	—	—	—	—	II	
Popovsky et al. (19)	—	—	—	—	II	
Teach et al. (20)	?	?	?	?	II	
Assessing sample integrity						B
Cook et al. (21)	—	—	—	—	III	
Clarke et al. (22)	—	—	—	—	III	

Another important semi-clinical role for USG is in the identification of adulterated specimens (21,22). However, no studies have shown a significant correlation between USG measurements and patient outcomes.

PROTEIN

Of the tests available on the urine dipstick, protein analysis is the most indicative of intrinsic renal disease or dysfunction. Small amounts of protein from plasma and the urinary tract are commonly present in urine. The amount of each protein filtered diminishes with increasing size and more negative charge. About one-third of excreted protein is albumin and another third is the Tamm-Horsfall protein secreted by the distal tubule and the ascending loop of Henle. Proteins have a low maximal tubular reabsorption rate, so the mechanism is quickly saturated and changes in protein status, either filtration or production, are reflected early in urine samples. With normal urine flow, the typical protein concentration is less than 8–10 mg/dL. Dehydration or strenuous exercise can cause trace elevated protein in healthy individuals. More positive dipstick protein results are generally considered significant and should be confirmed by a second method. Precipitating factors include hemorrhage, salt depletion, febrile illness, or renal ischemia. Normalization of protein measurements using specific gravity resulted in improved reproducibility and reduction of false negatives (23).

Benign postural proteinuria is usually diagnosed if the first morning urine specimen is negative, but a second sample obtained after the subject has been standing tests positive for protein. Benign proteinuria also occurs in pregnancy due to increased filtered protein levels. With renal infection or inflammation, there is characteristically proteinuria along with pyuria. Diabetic nephropathy results in small but consistent amounts of albumin excreted in urine. This "microalbuminuria" can be more sensitively detected using specialized dipsticks. Toxins may cause proteinuria by inhibition of renal tubular reabsorption.

The reagent strip method for detecting proteins in urine takes advantage of the protein error of pH indicators: certain pH indicators change color in the presence or absence of protein, even when the pH remains constant. The protein strip test area is buffered with citrate to a constant low pH; therefore, any color change is dependent only on the presence and concentration of protein in the specimen. The color change is from yellow to varying shades of green, detecting a range from 5–70 mg/dL protein. The reagent strip method is more sensitive to albumin than to globulins, Bence-Jones protein, or mucoproteins, which can be grossly underestimated.

Extended immersion in the specimen can lead to leaching of the buffer from the reagent pad, which will increase pH, and a color change will occur giving a false positive. In highly alkaline urine, the buffer will be overwhelmed and the pH will rise, causing a color change not related to protein. High salt concentrations decrease the sensitivity of the reagent strip. Substances that alter urine color can also interfere with DUA interpretation.

Dipstick measurement of proteinuria as a screening tool for the general population, as opposed to symptom-specific patient populations, is of uncertain value (Table 5). The U.S. Preventive Health Service does not recommend screening in their 1989 review of the literature, despite the prevalence and positive predictive value (PPV) of proteinuria for possible significant disease ranging from 0.4–1.85% and 9–62%, respectively, for adults and 0.5–6.0% and 1–11%, respectively, for children (24). They determined that <1.5% of those with DUA positive for proteinuria have serious and treatable urinary tract disorders. Screening of approximately 21,000 healthy Israelis with DUA identified proteinuria in 4.9% of men and 3.9% of women (25). This was the most common abnormality

Table 5 Evidence for Clinical Utility of Dipstick Urinalysis for Urine Protein

Reference	Sensitivity (%)	Specificity (%)	PPV (%)	NPV (%)	Evidence level	Recommendation grade
Population screening						C
Woolhandler et al. (24)	—	—	1–62	—	II	
Carel et al. (25)	—	—	—	—	II	
Pugia et al. (26)	—	—	—	—	II	
Murakimi (27)	—	—	—	—	II	
Iwata et al. (29)	—	—	—	—	II	
Kawamura et al. (28)	20–94	—	—	—	II	
Patient screening						C
Kroenke et al. (31)	—	—	—	—	II	
Mitchell and Stapleton (7)	—	—	—	—	II	
Akin et al. (32)	—	—	—	—	II	
Fraser et al. (3)	—	—	—	—	II	
Del Mar and Badger (5)	—	—	—	—	II	
Berber and McFeeley (6)	—	—	—	—	II	
Gold and Wolfersberger (1)	—	—	—	—	II	
Hypertension in pregnancy						D
Barton et al. (33)	—	—	—	—	II	
Brown and Buddle (34)	—	—	60	87	II	
Meyer et al. (35)	—	—	—	—	II	
Saudan et al. (36)	—	—	—	—	—	
Microalbuminuria in diabetics						B
Bouhanick et al. (37)	76	81	69	—	II	
Poulsen et al. (38)	91	85	—	95	II	
Pugia et al. (39)	—	—	87	—	II	
Sacks et al. (40)						
Lung cancer versus benign pulmonary disease						B
Pedersen and Milman (41)	30	91	88	38	II	

found in men and the second most common abnormality identified in women. No outcome information was provided. Screening of over 6000 Japanese schoolchildren identified a 2.1% prevalence of albuminuria and a 4.3% prevalence of proteinuria (26). This prevalence is high relative to another mass screening of Japanese elementary and junior high schoolchildren, which yielded a prevalence of proteinuria of approximately 0.11 and 0.48%, respectively (27). In one of the largest series, 26,082 healthy Japanese adults were screened by DUA (28). Of these subjects, 3.7% of men and 3.0% of women had proteinuria. In men, the prevalence increased with age, up to 9.9% for men over age 70, but this trend was less clear in women because of a relatively high incidence in the 20- to 29-year-olds. In addition, the authors surveyed 158,426 subjects who participated in this screen between 1971 and 1990 at 2 yr after their DUA. From this group, they identified 230 patients with renal disease out of 93,917 respondents. Proteinuria of trace or greater was present on prior screen in 17 of 18 (94%) who developed renal failure, 37 of 53 (70%) who developed glomerulonephritis, 19 of 64 (30%) who developed renal or bladder tumors, and 27 of 138 (20%) who developed renal stones. In another Japanese public health study, proteinuria was associated with significantly higher mortality in women (29). There is a definite, but more modest, association of trace proteinuria and cardiovascular disease mortality for women, and all cause mortality in both men and women, among the Framingham Study cohort (30).

Screening patients is also of unclear value. One study of 746 routine admission urinalyses in an American community hospital utility revealed only two (0.27%) where patient management was altered due to proteinuria (31). Screening routine DUA performed upon admission to an American children's hospital found a 4% incidence of proteinuria (7). Among preoperative testing results at a California hospital, 16 of 123 (13%) routine and 29 of 120 (24%) indicated DUA were positive for proteinuria (32). Six of the 16 patients with positive routine DUA were negative for protein on repeat testing. An Australian study of 2600 outpatients screened by DUA revealed 129 (5%) instances of proteinuria (3). Twenty-seven of 2294 (1.2%) admission DUA at a large private Australian hospital were unexpectedly positive for proteinuria (5). Urinalyses performed on 515 patients admitted to a Canadian psychiatric hospital resulted in one case of proteinuria, which was negative on repeat testing (6). In a study of 3375 oral and maxillofacial surgical outpatients, preoperative screens by DUA revealed 40 patients (1.2%) with unexpected proteinuria of 3+ or greater (1).

Detection of proteinuria in hypertensive pregnant women is significant because it signals an increased risk for both maternal and fetal complications. Development of 1+ proteinuria in pregnant women with mild gestational hypertension remote from term is associated with an earlier gestational age at delivery, lower birth weight, and an increased incidence of small-for-gestational-age newborns (33). A study found a PPV of 60% for dipstick protein measurements and a negative predictive value (NPV) of 87% in predicting proteinuria by quantitative urine protein analysis on a 24-hr collection, leading to the conclusion that dipstick testing is not reliable enough to replace 24-hr urine collection and testing (34). Another group compared quantitative urine protein analysis on 300 24-hr collections from hypertensive pregnant women to DUA proteinuria measurements on spot urines during the 24-hr collection. They found the spot urine DUA with trace or 1+ had a 92% PPV for ≥300 mg/day proteinuria, but that the spot urine DUA with <1+ proteinuria had only a 34% NPV (35). In contrast, DUA of 103 hypertensive pregnant Australian women had a 48% PPV and 98–100% NPV for proteinuria by visual inspection and a 74% PPV and 98–100% NPV by optical reader as compared with quantitative urine protein analysis (36).

The main utility of DUA for protein may be the detection of albuminuria in diabetic patients, which can signal the development of diabetic nephropathy. A urinary albumin excretion rate of 30–300 mg/day or 30–300 μg/mg creatinine defines microalbuminuria. About 80% of type 1 diabetics and 20–40% of type 2 diabetics who manifest microalbuminuria will progress to overt nephropathy, which may be preventable if treatment is initiated in time. Testing for microalbuminuria using the standard protein error of indicators method yielded a specificity of 81% and a sensitivity of 76% as well as a PPV of 69% (37). Other methods of albumin detection, including immunochromatographic and dye binding, have been incorporated into alternative dipstick tests with varying success. The immunochemical dipstick in the hands of laboratory technicians shows promise for detection of microalbuminuria in random urine samples with a sensitivity of 91% and specificity of 85% and a NPV of 95% when compared with 24-hr urinary albumin concentration (38). The semiquantitative dipstick based on dye binding correctly identified urines as having <20 mg/L or ≥20 mg/L with an accuracy of 87% (39). Clearly the modified dipstick methods have greater potential for microalbuminuria screening than dipsticks based on the protein error of pH indicators. The National Academy of Clinical Biochemistry (NACB) recommends periodic DUA to test for albuminuria in diabetic adults, but they suggest that negative results should be followed by quantitative assays for microalbuminuria, as current DUA are insufficiently sensitive for reliable screening (40).

In an entirely different vein, detection of proteinuria has shown to be significant in oncology patients. One study has revealed that the prevalence of proteinuria is higher in lung cancer patients than those with benign pulmonary disease (41). Furthermore, proteinuria predicted poorer survival time, higher stage, and worse histological type.

BLOOD/HEMOGLOBIN

An increased number of erythrocytes (RBC) in urine is referred to as hematuria, which is different from the presence of hemoglobin in urine (hemoglobinuria). Hematuria is fairly common in patients, while hemoglobinuria is uncommon and the presence of myoglobin in urine (myoglobinuria) is even more rare. Both hemoglobin and myoglobin produce clear urine of a dark red color while hematuria gives a red, cloudy urine. Normally, there may be up to 5 RBC per high-powered field (hpf) (dipsticks are calibrated in microscopic terms), but there is no free hemoglobin in urine because any that is liberated from systemic hemolysis binds to serum haptoglobin. Abnormal amounts of red cells in the urine are a common finding. Isolated hemoglobinuria is an indicator significant intravascular hemolysis, which then exceeds the binding capacity of haptoglobin (hemoglobinemia) as well as the tubular resorption capacity and ends up in urine. Red blood cell lysis in urine will produce a mixture of hematuria and hemoglobinuria.

Hematuria is often indicative of damage from trauma to the kidneys or glomerular dysfunction. Major causes of hematuria include formation of renal calculi, glomerulonephritis, tumors, trauma, pyelonephritis, and exposure to toxins. Glomerular causes of hematuria can be diagnosed microscopically by the presence of distorted erythrocytes. Hematuria of renal origin is generally accompanied by proteinuria and erythrocyte casts; if it is from urinary tract bleeding or inflammation, then proteinuria is usually not present.

The reagent strip method for detection of hemoglobin in urine is based on a peroxidase reaction. Heme-containing substances (e.g., hemoglobin, myoglobin, and red blood cells) act as an oxidant to change the color of the indicator when peroxide is present. The oxidation caused by hemoglobin or myoglobin is reflected in a color change from yellow to green to dark blue. Intact red blood cells lyse when they contact the pad giving a speckled pattern. Low levels of hematuria can be missed if only the reagent strip is used without microscopic evaluation. The sensitivity of the reagent strip is reduced in specimens with high specific gravity or in the presence of ascorbic acid. A large amount of nitrate in urine slows the kinetics of the peroxidase reaction and delays the test result or causes a false negative if the test is read at the recommended time interval. False positives can occur with oxidizing contaminants such as bleach, as well as the presence of vegetable or microbial peroxidases. In women, a clean-catch specimen is necessary to prevent possible menstrual contamination of the sample.

Studies of the clinical utility for dipstick hematuria tests fall under two general categories, comparison of the DUA with urine microscopy for detection of blood and relation of hemoglobin dipstick results to patient diagnosis (Table 6). Although the causes of hematuria include malignancies of the prostate, bladder, and kidney, as well as nephrotic syndrome and urinary tract infection, the majority of studies concerning outcomes of hemoglobin dipsticks are performed in the context of UTI detection. One study demonstrated a sensitivity of 86% and a specificity of 85% for hematuria using DUA versus microscopy, and concluded that if hematuria is suspected then cytoscopy should be performed regardless of the DUA result (42). Another study determined similar specificity and sensitivity, but concluded that when considered in conjunction with improved

Table 6 Evidence for Clinical Utility of Dipstick Urinalysis for Hematuria

Reference	Sensitivity (%)	Specificity (%)	PPV (%)	NPV (%)	Evidence level	Recommendation grade
Prediction of microscopic hematuria						B
Gleeson et al. (42)	86	85	—	—	I	
Craver et al. (43)	88	75	29	98	II	
Bonnardeaux et al. (44)	75	89	28	98	I	
Jou and Powers (50)	—	—	—	—	I	
Goldner et al. (45)	80	69	67	81	II	
Daum et al. (46)	100	59	61	100	II	
Chadhoke and McAninch (47)	97.5	97.5	—	—	II	
Kennedy et al. (48)	68	95	77	92	II	
Moore and Robinson (49)	100	99.3	—	—	III	
Population screening						C
Woolhandler et al. (24)	—	—	6–58	—	II	
Carel et al. (25)	—	—	—	—	II	
Murakimi (27)	—	—	—	—	II	
Kawamura et al. (28)	11–42	—	—	—	II	
Anosike et al. (51)	41	82	—	—		
Mafe (52)	69	—	—	—		
Patient screening						D
Gold and Wolfersberger (1)	—	—	—	—	II	
Lawrence and Kroenke (12)	—	—	—	—	II	
Mitchell and Stapleton (7)	—	—	—	—	II	
Swinger (8)	—	—	—	—	II	
Akin et al. (32)	—	—	—	—	II	
Fraser et al. (3)	—	—	—	—	II	
Del Mar and Badger (5)	—	—	—	—	II	
Berber and McFeeley (6)	—	—	—	—	II	
Kaplan et al. (53)	—	—	16	—	I	
Khadra et al. (54)	—	—	18.7	—	II	
Screening trauma patients for intra-abdominal injury						B
Isaacman et al. (55)	97.8–100	64	13	100	II	
Ford et al. (57)	60	79.2	—	—	II	

turnaround time (TAT) DUA screening was a reasonable approach (43). Yet, a different study demonstrated that there was a 27% discordance between dipstick and microscopic urinalysis of abnormal urines, with most of the discrepancies due to false positives from the dipstick testing (44). In a review of 169 blunt trauma workups, one group found that DUA had a sensitivity of 80% and a specificity of only 69% relative to microscopic urinalysis (45). Yet another review of 178 blunt abdominal trauma workups revealed that DUA was 100% sensitive, but only 58.6% specific relative to microscopic results (46). As in the previous study, they found little correlation between level of positivity and microscopic results. A study of 339 abdominal trauma patients with radiographic correlation found that DUA has a sensitivity and a specificity of 97.5% relative to microscopic urinalysis (47). The largest abdominal trauma series of 1485 patients found a sensitivity of 80% and a specificity of only 69% relative to microscopic urinalysis, but used an unusually low criteria of 1 RBC/hpf to define a positive microscopic result (48). They noted that there were no cases of missed injury among the 100 false negatives. In a laboratory concordance study, another group found that DUA was 100% sensitive and 99.3% specific relative to microscopic results (49). They found that N-Multistix™ were less reliable after 4 mo of air exposure. A randomized controlled study reported that in 94% of patients examined using DUA no significant change in management occurred with subsequent microscopic urinalysis (50). The authors argued that DUA for hematuria is an efficient method that saves both cost and time.

As a screening tool, the utility of hematuria detection is equally contentious. The U.S. Preventive Health Service does not recommend screening for hematuria in their 1989 review of the literature, despite the prevalences and positive predictive values for possible significant disease ranging from 0.2–33.8% and 6–58%, respectively, for adults and 0.3–1.0% and 10–15%, respectively, for children (24). Here they determined that fewer than 2% of those with DUA positive for hematuria have serious and treatable urinary tract disease. Screening of approximately 21,000 healthy Israelis with DUA identified hematuria in 2.6% of men and 8.1% of women (25). This was the second most common abnormality found in men and the most common abnormality identified in women. No outcome information was provided. Screening of Japanese elementary and junior high schoolchildren yielded a prevalence of hematuria of approximately 0.53 and 0.98%, respectively (27). In one of the largest series, 26,082 healthy Japanese, results were screened by DUA (28). Of these subjects, 3.4% of men and 12.9% of women had hematuria. In men, the prevalence increased with age, up to 4.6% for men over age 70. In addition, the authors surveyed 158,426 subjects who participated in this screen between 1971 and 1990 at 2 yr after their DUA. From this group, they identified 230 patients with renal disease out of 93,917 respondents. Hematuria of trace or greater was present in only 2 of 18 (11%) who developed renal failure, 22 of 53 (42%) who developed glomerulonephritis, 16 of 64 (25%) who developed renal or bladder tumors, and 29 of 138 (21%) who developed renal stones. The authors recommend using proteinuria rather than hematuria as a prognostic indicator of urinary tract disease. Particularly high yields for hematuria are obtained by DUA screening of African children, due to the presence of *Schistosoma haematobium* infection (51,52).

Screening patients using DUA is also of unclear value. Preoperative screening of 3375 outpatients identified one (<0.1%) with hematuria (1). Another series of 180 routine preoperative urinalyses identified two with hematuria (1.1%), neither of which was appropriately documented (12). Routine DUA performed upon admission to an American children's hospital found a 9% incidence of hematuria (7). At a South African children's hospital, 8 of 233 (3.4%) admission DUA were positive for hematuria, but all were ignored (8). Among admission testing results at a California hospital, 7 of 123 (6%) routine and 14 of 120 (12%) indicated DUA were positive for hematuria (32). Four of the seven patients with positive routine DUA were negative for hematuria on repeat testing. An Australian study of 2600 outpatients screened by DUA revealed 49 (1.9%) instances of hematuria (3). Seventy-four of 2294 (3.2%) admission DUA at a large private Australian hospital were unexpectedly positive for hematuria (5). Urinalyses performed on 515 patients admitted to a Canadian psychiatric hospital resulted in five cases of proteinuria, three of which were negative on repeat testing (6). A 1997 study examining the utility of asymptomatic DUA screening suggests a false positive/transient hematuria rate of almost 88%, leading to unnecessary evaluation and patient anxiety as well as increased cost (53). In contrast, a 2000 study involving 1930 patients demonstrated that significant disease was found in 18.7% of the patients with microscopic hematuria (54).

Dipstick urinalysis for hematuria may be most useful in the assessment of trauma patients. In a combined retrospective and prospective study of pediatric trauma patients, the combination of physical examination and urinalysis proved 97.8–100% sensitive to intra-abdominal injury (IAI) (55). Another study that compared physical examination and urinalysis for hematuria found a sensitivity of 93% with a NPV of 93%, comparable to computed tomography (56). In a retrospective study of 100 pediatric trauma patients, DUA alone proved 60% sensitive and 79.2% specific for IAI and retroperitoneal injury (57). Absent significant hematuria (≥100 RBC/hpf), there is little likelihood (4%) of a positive finding in intravenous pyelography in patients with suspected blunt renal injuries (58).

BILIRUBIN AND UROBILINOGEN

Dipstick urinalysis generally includes both urine bilirubin and urobilinogen. Urine bilirubin is conjugated bilirubin, derived from hepatic metabolism of the breakdown products of hemoglobin and the hemoproteins. Most conjugated bilirubin is secreted in the bile, but with hepatic disease, some diffuses out of the hepatocytes and into the blood, ultimately to be filtered by the kidneys. No bilirubin is present in normal urine. Most of the conjugated bilirubin excreted in the bile is metabolized by bacteria to a family of compounds known as urobilinogen. Some of the urobilinogen seeps into the bloodstream via the enterohepatic circulation, also to be filtered by the kidneys. Normal urine urobilinogen levels may reach 1 mg/dL.

The pathophysiology of these analytes suggests a potential diagnostic dyad: urine bilirubin should be elevated in any form of conjugated hyperbilirubinemia, especially if biliary obstruction is present, but usually not in intravascular hemolysis. Urobilinogen should be increased in both conjugated hyperbilirubinemia and in intravascular hemolysis, but diminished in obstructive jaundice. In practice, the DUA are calibrated so that the urobilinogen levels of normal individuals will often be undetectable, so the absence of urobilinogen cannot be conclusively demonstrated.

Bilirubin is measured in urine through colorimetric assays. Urine bilirubin dipstick tests use the "diazo" reaction. Bilirubin is coupled with a diazonium compound in acidified medium to produce a color change, which can be quite subtle. Oxidation, photoisomerization, or deconjugation of bilirubin in the specimen can cause false negatives, as can elevated nitrite or vitamin C levels. Stool contamination, mefenamic acid, thorazine, and chlorpromazine can cause false positives. Urobilinogen is measured through a colorimetric assay that couples the molecules either to the Ehrlich's reagent in acidified medium or a diazonium compound. In patients receiving antibiotics, the intestinal flora may be reduced, and lower urobilinogen levels may occur. Porphyrins or phenazopyridine can also cross-react with Ehrlich's reagent, causing false positives, while nitrite, vitamin C, or formalin preservative can cause false negative results.

One important clinical scenario in which urine bilirubin and urobilinogen may have utility is in the identification of subclinical liver disease (Table 7). As a surrogate for liver disease, Binder et al. (60) correlated DUA with serum "liver function" tests (LFTs) for a prospective series of 324 patients presenting to an Emergency Department with any indication for LFTs and DUA. Initially, they included serum aspartate aminotransferase (AST), alkaline phosphatase (ALP), and bilirubin levels, and prothrombin and partial thromboplastin times (59), but in their largest series, the coagulation parameters were omitted (60). They used

Table 7 Evidence for Clinical Utility of Dipstick Urinalysis of Urine Bilirubin (B) and Urobilinogen (U)

Reference	Sensitivity (%)	Specificity (%)	PPV (%)	NPV (%)	Evidence level	Recommendation grade
Abnormalities in serum "liver function" tests						E
Binder et al. (61)	B 47; U 48	B 89; U 90	B 88; U 88	B 49; U 52	II	
Hypertensive disorders of pregnancy						D
Schrocksnadel et al. (65)	—	—	—	—	II	

a higher than normal urine urobilinogen threshold of 3 mg/dL or greater to define an abnormal result in order to optimize diagnostic accuracy and predictive value. While either urine bilirubin or urobilinogen was relatively sensitive (76–78%) for hyperbilirubinemia, both were less sensitive for AST or ALP abnormalities (47–48% for any LFT abnormality). The two tests were 89–90% specific for any LFT abnormality, with correspondingly high positive predictive values of 88%, yet the negative predictive values were only 49–52% (61). Hence, the authors deemed these tests unsuitable for screening purposes, but warned that any abnormal DUA bilirubin or urobilinogen results warrant follow-up. The diagnostic utility of the urine tests in disjunctive combination (either/or/both) was not assessed, but they are likely to be highly redundant. Urobilinogen has little utility in screening the general outpatient population, even among patients with liver disease, according to the Japanese literature (62–64).

In the context of hemolysis detection, Austrian investigators compared DUA and other laboratory parameters in distinguishing 166 women with hypertensive disorders of pregnancy versus 179 healthy pregnant controls. Neither urine bilirubin nor urobilinogen predicted hypertensive disorders and were only significantly elevated in patients with clinically severe hemolysis (65).

GLUCOSE AND KETONES

Dipstick urinalyses for glucose and ketones have long been used for detection and monitoring of diabetes mellitus. Normally, almost all of the glucose filtered by the glomeruli is reabsorbed by the proximal tubule. However, when the plasma glucose exceeds about 180 mg/dL, glucosuria occurs. Urine glucose can vary depending on glomerular blood flow, tubular reabsorption, and urine flow. Ketones, or ketone bodies, are intermediates of fat metabolism and do not normally appear in urine. In carbohydrate-deficient metabolism, such as starvation or uncontrolled diabetes mellitus, fat becomes the major source of energy. With the increase in fatty acid metabolism, acetyl coenzyme A (acetyl CoA) is produced in excess of the metabolic capacity, and ketone intermediates accumulate. In ketonuria, three forms appear in urine: acetoacetic acid (20%), acetone (2%), and 3-hydroxybutyrate (about 78%). Acetoacetic acid reversibly forms 3-hydroxybutyrate, a portion of which then goes on to irreversibly form acetone.

The most common cause of glucosuria is diabetes mellitus. In diabetes, glucosuria is often accompanied by polyuria and increased thirst, along with metabolic acidosis. Other conditions in which systemic hyperglycemia and glycosuria are encountered include pituitary and adrenal disorders, pancreatic disease or tumors, brain injury or tumor, hypothalmic disease, and asphyxia. Metabolic disturbances in burns, infection, fractures, uremia, and acute myocardial infarction (AMI) can also increase glucose levels. Liver disease, glycogen storage disease, obesity, and certain drugs (e.g., thiazides, corticosteroids, adrenocorticotropic hormone, and birth control pills) can also cause glucosuria.

Glucosuria without accompanying hyperglycemia is sometimes referred to as benign glucosuria, but actually it can be indicative of renal dysfunction. Specifically, glucosuria determined to be renal in origin is characteristic of conditions that affect tubular reabsorption (e.g., Fanconi's syndrome). Inherited renal glucosuria is uncommon and is generally specific for glucose as opposed to other sugars excreted in urine. Pregnancy increases glomerular filtration rate, which can introduce more glucose into the filtrate than can be reabsorbed. This is particularly pronounced in the third trimester of pregnancy, but can be identified by a low plasma glucose concentration. Persistent glucosuria in pregnant women, however, warrants monitoring for gestational diabetes. Urine glucose testing was popular for home testing of diabetic patients, but this has largely been replaced by home blood glucometry, which was thought to more quickly and accurately reflect poor diabetic control.

Ketonuria is manifested in any state or disorder that results in increased fat metabolism: diabetes, carbohydrate restriction, starvation (anorexia/bulimia), acute febrile illness, hypothermia, diarrhea, vomiting, or excessive strenuous exercise. Excretion of ketones in neonates could indicate an inherited metabolic disease. Ketone testing is the most valuable in management of diabetic patients. A positive result can be interpreted to indicate insufficient insulin dosage. Ketonuria can precede ketoacidosis, which can serve as a warning of an impending diabetic coma. An increased level of ketones leads to electrolyte imbalance, dehydration, and acidosis that can develop into a coma. Generally, a large amount of ketones is seen in urine before a buildup of ketones in the blood (ketosis) occurs. Urine ketone reagent strips do not correlate well with blood ketone analyses.

On the urinalysis dipstick, glucose is detected using a glucose oxidase reaction. The peroxide produced is cleaved by peroxidase in the presence of a chromagen to produce a color change. This test is sensitive down to a glucose concentration of 0.1 g/dL. There are multiple manufacturers of urinalysis dipsticks with each one using their chromagen of choice for the glucose test, the most common being *o*-toluidine (pink to purple), potassium iodide (blue to brown) and aminopropyl-carbazol (yellow to orange-brown). Urine glucose levels are reported qualitatively in terms of trace, 1+, 2+, 3+, or 4+, and interpreted by comparison to a color chart and ranging from 0.1–2 g/dL. Specialized glucose dipsticks have been developed with pads of varying sensitivity that can give semiquantitative results ranging from 0.06–5.0 g/dL.

Despite the highly specific nature of the glucose oxidase test, there are a few interferences that cause false positives. Contamination of the container with strongly oxidizing cleaning agents could give a false positive if a residue were left behind. The presence of ketones (ketonuria) in the specimen suppresses the glucose reaction. High specific gravity in urine or exposure of the reagent strips to humidity can diminish the reactivity of the strips as well (66). The use of sodium fluoride as a preservative can give false negative results. Many false negatives occur from unpreserved samples that are left at room temperature for an hour or more, allowing bacterial proliferation that metabolizes glucose from the sample. Endogenous compounds that prevent oxidation of the chromagen and give falsely negative results include ascorbic acid, 5-hydroxyindoleacetic acid, and homogentistic acid. Medications that can produce false negative results include aspirin and levodopa.

On most glucose dipstick tests, ketone coanalysis is performed. The reagent strip method of ketone detection is based on the nitroprusside (sodium nitroferricyanide) reaction for ketones. In the presence of glycine, sodium nitroferricyanide reacts with acetoacetic acid and acetone to form a violet dye. The test is able to detect 10 mg/dL of acetoacetic acid and 70 mg/dL acetone in solution. Results are reported as negative, 1+, 2+, and 3+. The 3-hydroxybutyrate is not detected, but this is generally considered unimportant because when one compound is present, all are usually present. Ketonuria by DUA is often confirmed by a more sensitive method, but this is probably unnecessary for any result greater than trace positive (67).

In samples that are not analyzed immediately or are improperly stored, false negatives can occur if ketones have evaporated. Bacterial breakdown of acetoacetic acid in solution can also cause false negative results. The reagent strips are highly sensitive to moisture and so can lose reactivity and become less sensitive. Phenylketone can cause false positive values, as well as 8-hydroxyquinilone or L-dopa. Colorimetric interference can come from pthalein dyes or acetylcysteine that cause a red color and interfere with the colorimetric results of the reagent strip. The antihypertensive drugs methyldopa and captopril also give false positive results. In lactic acidosis, 3-hydroxybutyrate is the major component of ketones in the sample and so may be missed by the nitroprusside test.

Given the high prevalence of type 2 diabetes millitus, and the demonstrated benefits of early recognition and treatment, there is substantial motivation to screen the population at large. However, it is understood that glucosuria and ketonuria will not be sensitive to the earliest manifestations of the disease: impaired glucose tolerance and elevated fasting glucose. Furthermore, correlation between blood glucose levels and urine glucose levels is not good (68). Screening of approximately 21,000 healthy Israelis with DUA identified glucosuria in 0.6% of men and women and ketonuria in 0.4% of men and 0.5% of women (25). Three different approaches of DUA glucosuria screening were employed in populations from 10 countries: fasting, postprandial, and postglucose load (1 g glucose/kg body weight) (69) (Table 8). Using a diagnostic standard for diabetes of blood glucose $\geq$150 mg/dL at 2 hr postglucose load, sensitivities, specificities, and positive predictive values were 35.3%, 99.7%, and 92.3% for fasting glucosuria; 38.9%, 97.6%, and 45.7% for postprandial glucosuria; and 67.0%, 94.0%,

Table 8 Evidence for Clinical Utility of Dipstick Urinalysis for Urine Glucose (UG) and Ketones (UK)

Reference	Sensitivity (%)	Specificity (%)	PPV (%)	NPV (%)	Evidence level	Recommendation grade
UG for screening for type 2 diabetes mellitus						C
West and Kalbfleisch (69)	35–67	94–100	40–92	—	II	
Andersson et al. 1993	18	99	53	—	II	
Hanson et al. (75)	64	99	80	—	II	
Forrest et al. (71)	7	98	—	—	II	
Davies et al. (73)	43	98	58	—	II	
UG for self-monitoring in type 2 diabetes mellitus						C
Miles et al. (80)	—	—	—	—	I	
Starostina et al. (81)	—	—	—	—	I	
Fontbonne et al. (83)	—	—	—	—	I	
Sacks et al. (40)	—	—	—	—	III	
Coster et al. (84)	—	—	—	—	II	
Patrick et al. (85)	—	—	—	—	II	
UG for screening for gestational diabetes mellitus						E
Watson (92)	27	83	7	96	II	
Hooper (93)	36	98	27	99	II	
UK for screening for type 1 diabetes mellitus						D
Savova et al. (94)	86.5	—	—	—	II	
Levy-Marchal et al. (95)	83.8	—	—	—	II	
UK to exclude diabetic ketoacidosis						C
Sacks et al. (40)	—	—	—	—	III	
Schwab et al. (103)	95	80	63	98	II	
Papadakis and Grunfeld (104)	—	—	—	—	II	

and 40.4% for postglucose load glucosuria. These performance characteristics were broken down on a nation-by-nation basis and the tests were found to perform better as the severity of the typical diabetic increased. In a study of random venous blood and urine from 1092 Scandinavian outpatients, multiple brands of dipsticks were evaluated and found to be 30–59% sensitive and 97–99% specific relative to oral glucose tolerance test (OGTT) results, while random blood screening was 95% sensitive with comparable specificity (70). Another study of fasting and postglucose load glucosuria found a 16.7% sensitivity and a 98.0% specificity fasting versus 72.7% sensitivity and 77.4% specificity postglucose load (71). The Japanese literature on occupational screening of 671 adults confirms these trends, albeit with somewhat better sensitivity (72). Using glucosuria of 40 mg/dL as a

cutoff with fasting or 2 hr after a 75-g glucose load, they achieved sensitivities of 84% (males) and 100% (females) and specificities of 71% (males) and 92% (females) relative to the OGTT. But fasting, the sensitivities fell to 11% (males) and 0% (females). In another Japanese public health study, glucosuria was associated with significantly higher mortality in men (29). A more convenient approach to glucosuria was taken by a British group who used 1 hr postprandial self-screening for glycosuria by DUA to achieve 43% sensitivity, 98% specificity, and 53% positive predictive value (73). Yet, a Danish group employing a similar approach found 21% sensitivity, 99% specificity, and 47% positive predictive value and 97% negative predictive value among 3041 respondents (74). Using random glucosuria, an American group found 64% sensitivity and 98% specificity with DUA (75). However, in a review of six studies of glucosuria-based screening, the American result was by far the most sensitive (76). The reviewers concluded that glucosuria screening by any approach was too insensitive to compete with fasting blood glucose measurements.

Screening patients for glycosuria is also of unclear value. Routine DUA performed upon admission to an American children's hospital found a 4.5% incidence of glucosuria (7). Among admission testing results at a California hospital, 6 of 123 (6%) routine and 25 of 120 (12%) indicated DUA were positive for glucosuria, while 3 of 123 (6%) routine and 4 of 120 (12%) indicated DUA were positive for ketonuria (32). Four of the six patients with positive routine DUA were negative for glucosuria on repeat testing. An Australian study of 2600 outpatients screened by DUA revealed 28 (1.0%) instances of glucosuria (3). Twenty of 2294 (0.9%) admission DUA at a large private Australian hospital were unexpectedly positive for glucosuria (5). Urinalyses performed on 515 patients admitted to a Canadian psychiatric hospital resulted in two cases of glucosuria, neither of which prompted further testing (6).

In testing "high-risk" patients, the performance of DUA is substantially better than among the general population. An Italian study of 110 high-risk patients found 1 hr postprandial glucosuria to be 100% sensitive, 44% specific, and to have 23% positive and 100% negative predictive values, respectively, in patients over age 50 (77). In patients under age 50, fasting glucosuria was 100% sensitive, 96% specific, and had 33% positive and 100% negative predictive values, respectively.

Dipstick urinalysis for glycosuria was formerly a mainstay of self-monitoring by diabetics, but this has been largely supplanted by POCT for blood glucose. Some of the drawbacks of using glucosuria are obvious, such as relatively high level of blood glucose that would be reached before glucosuria occurs. Other problems are more subtle, such as the difficulties that people with diabetic retinopathy may have in reading dipstick color changes (78). The most critical limitation is that DUA is unable to identify hypoglycemia, a major concern among insulin users. Among diabetics in third world countries, DUA has demonstrated comparable performance to fingerstick blood glucose monitoring in identifying "clinically significant" hyperglycemia (defined as >180 mg/dL) at a fraction of the cost (79). On a randomized crossover trial of 150 consecutive newly diagnosed, non–insulin-dependent, British diabetics, no significant difference was seen in glycemic control (measured by glycated hemoglobin), change in body mass index, or quality of life score between those monitoring by urine or blood glucose (80). Slightly more patients chose blood glucose monitoring in the end (48% blood, 42% urine, 10% both). Other randomized controlled clinical trials from Russia (81), America (82), and France (83) all failed to show any benefit of blood testing over urine testing. Despite the evidence showing lack of additional benefit, the NACB recommends blood glucose over urine glucose for self-monitoring by type 2 diabetics (40). It is worth noting that there is controversy whether any benefit is accrued from self-monitoring by type 2 diabetics, either by blood or urine glucose (81,83–85).

There is substantial evidence that gestational diabetes mellitus (GDM) is associated with adverse maternal and fetal outcomes (86–89). Several guidelines recommend screening for glucosuria at each prenatal visit to detect GDM (90,91). However, one study of 3217 pregnancies found that only first- and second-trimester glucosuria is predictive of GDM. Moreover, there is evidence that glycosuria is an insensitive and nonspecific finding. Dipstick urinalysis was used to screen for glycosuria at each prenatal visit for 500 consecutive pregnancies at a U.S. Army hospital (92). Gestational diabetes mellitus was diagnosed in 22 women by a 50-g oral glucose tolerance test at 28 wk of gestation. Of these, only six (27%) had DUA positive for glucose, and only four (18%) had severe glycosuria. Moreover, 79 other pregnant women had positive results, and 15 had severe glycosuria. Another study that reviewed 610 antepartum records in an Atlanta, GA hospital found that glucosuria was present in 4 of 15 patients with GDM and in 11 of 595 patients without GDM (93).

Glycosuria and ketonuria in a dehydrated, panting child represents a classical presentation of type 1 diabetes mellitus. In series of new onset type 1 diabetic children, ketonuria was present in 86.5% of 1248 Bulgarian children (94), and 83.8% of 340 French children (95). Ketonuria at presentation was not found to be helpful in predicting the need for insulin treatment over the next several months (96–98), but it was associated with lower IQ at 1 yr after diagnosis (99). The prevalence of type 2 diabetes is increasing in children, particularly among obese adolescents. Ketonuria is relatively uncommon (38%) among 55 Mexican children and African-American (42%) children with new onset type 2 diabetes (100,101).

After diagnosis, the impact of DUA for ketonuria is unclear. In a 24-hr study of 10 otherwise healthy, but poorly controlled diabetics, only 43% of episodes of elevated plasma beta-hydroxybutyrate were accompanied by ketonuria (102). However, a prospective study of 697 patients with known diabetes and hyperglycemia found that a positive DUA for ketonuria was highly sensitive for diabetic ketoacidosis (DKA), and had a high negative predictive value (103). In a review of ketonuria testing among 135 hospitalized type 2 diabetics, 26% had ketonuria during their hospitalization, but 23% of these results were not acknowledged in the charts, and in no case did progress notes link ketonuria to a change in care (104). The NACB does not recommend using DUA for ketonuria in the diagnosis or monitoring of DKA (40).

Ketonuria is often assessed in pregnant women as a marker of starvation and dehydration, although it may occur sporadically in normal pregnancies (105). In post-term pregnancy, ketonuria is associated with more than twice the risk of oligohydramnios and nonreactive nonstress tests, although the benefits of treating ketonuria have not yet been evaluated (106).

Ketogenic diets are sometimes prescribed for seizure control. Ketonuria of 3+ to 4+ by DUA was found to necessary, but not sufficient for seizure control in epileptic children (107). In their study of 42 children initiating ketogenic diet therapy, 4+ ketonuria corresponded to 2 mmol/L of blood beta-hydroxybutyrate, but blood beta-hydroxybutyrate levels of 4 mmol/L were necessary for adequate seizure control.

LEUKOCYTE ESTERASE AND NITRITE

Leukocyte esterases are found in the primary granules of neutrophils. Urinary leukocyte esterase activity signifies the presence of intact or lysed neutrophils. Urinary nitrite usually comes from nitrate reduction by enteric gram-negative rods (especially *E. coli*). Together these tests are used to screen for urinary tract infections.

Esterase activity is measured through the conversion of indoxyl carbonic acid ester on the dipstick into indigo, a process accelerated by diazonium salts in the reagent pad. Elevated urine specific gravity, albumin, glucose, ascorbic acid, or oxalic acid can suppress the reaction, as can the antibiotics cephalothin, cephalexin, or tetracycline. Nitrite couples with *p*-arsanilic acid in a separate reagent pad to form a diazonium compound, which couples in turn with a benzoquinoline to produce a red chromagen. If the dipstick is exposed to prolonged humidity during storage, false negatives can occur. Elevated urine specific gravity or ascorbic acid can suppress the reaction.

There are also physiological interferences. Vaginal contamination can be rich in neutrophils, and can mimic pyuria. Some urinary pathogens do not reduce nitrate, including *Candida albicans*, *Chlamydia urethritis*, and many gram-positive cocci. If the urine does not spend sufficient time in the bladder, false negatives can occur.

Table 9 Evidence for Clinical Utility of Urine Leukocyte Esterase and/or Nitrite

Reference	Sensitivity (%)	Specificity (%)	PPV (%)	NPV (%)	Evidence level	Recommendation grade
Urinary tract infections						D
Pels et al. (109)	70–100	60–98	40.8–44.4	94.3–99.9	III	
Hurlbut et al. (108)	—	—	—	—	III	
Gorelick and Shaw (111)	88	93	—	—	III	
Roberts (112)	—	—	—	—	III	
Jou and Powers (50)	—	—	—	—	I	

The merits of leukocyte esterase and nitrite for UTI screening have been extensively debated (Table 9). Generally, most studies have examined the disjunctive (either/or/both) combination of leukocyte esterase and nitrite to determine a positive screen, and have compared the results with urine microscopy using urine culture as a gold standard. In a meta-analysis of 51 studies, literature ranges for UTI diagnostic sensitivity spanned from 50 to >99%, and from 20 to >95% for specificity (108). From their analysis, the authors concluded that the negative predictive value of DUA was too low to exclude UTI in a patient with high a priori likelihood of infection (e.g., symptomatic women). The U.S. Preventive Health Services review of DUA in adult UTI found sensitivities ranging from 70–100% and specificities ranging from 60–98 for the disjunctive combination (109). Based on prevalences for different populations, positive predictive value ranged from 0.8% in nondiabetic men under age 60 to 44.4% for the institutional elderly, with negative predictive values of 99.9% and 94.3%, respectively, for these same groups. For comparison, another study has found that simple inspection of urine clarity has a 97.3% negative predictive value (110). The U.S. Preventive Health Services recommended that pregnant women be screened for UTI by urine culture instead of DUA or microscopic urinalysis, and that asymptomatic nondiabetic, nonpregnant adults under age 60 should not be screened at all. A review of the literature on screening tests for UTI in children found that DUA and urine Gram's stain performed similarly, and both were superior to standard microscopic urinalysis (111). The American Academy of Pediatrics recommends that febrile infants and young children have their urine cultured, and if urinalysis is to be done, it should consist of a Gram's stain of unspun urine rather than DUA or standard microscopic urinalysis (112). The sensitivity and specificity of DUA were estimated at 88% and 93% for the disjunctive combination. The literature is also divided as to whether DUA or microscopic urinalysis is superior in symptomatic adults, but a randomized clinical trial concluded that microscopy results altered management in only 6% of patients screened by DUA (50).

REFERENCES

1. Gold BD, Wolfersberger WH. Findings from routine urinalysis and hematocrit on ambulatory oral and maxillofacial surgery patients. J Oral Surg 38:677–678, 1980.
2. Munro J, Booth A, Nicholl J. Routine preoperative testing: A systematic review of the evidence. Health Technol Assess 1:i–iv,1–62, 1997.
3. Fraser CG, Smith BC, and Peake MJ. Effectiveness of an outpatient urine screening program. Clin Chem 23:2216–2218, 1977.
4. Boland BJ, Wollan PC, Silverstein MD. Review of systems, physical examination, and routine tests for case-finding in ambulatory patients. Am J Med Sci 309:194–200, 1995.
5. Del Mar C, Badger P. The place of routine urine testing on admission to hospital. Med J Aust 151:151–153, 1989.
6. Berber MJ, McFeely N. Efficacy of routine admission urinalyses in psychiatric hospitals. Can J Psychiatry 36:190–193, 1991.
7. Mitchell N, Stapleton FB. Routine admission urinalysis examination in pediatric patients: A poor value. Pediatrics 86:345–349, 1990.
8. Swingler GH. The impact of routine admission tests on the care of Third-World children. S Afr Med J 75:578–580, 1989.
9. Lawrence VA, Gafni A, Gross M. The unproven utility of the preoperative urinalysis: Economic evaluation. J Clin Epidemiol 42:1185–1192, 1989.
10. Velanovich V. The value of routine preoperative laboratory testing in predicting postoperative complications: A multivariate analysis. Surgery 109:236–243, 1991.
11. Heimann GA, Frohlich J, Bernstein M. Physicians' response to abnormal results of routine urinalysis. Can Med Assoc J 115:1094–1095, 1976.
12. Lawrence VA, Kroenke K. The unproven utility of preoperative urinalysis: Clinical use. Arch Intern Med 148:1370–1373, 1988.
13. Rumley A. Urine dipstick testing: Comparison of results obtained by visual reading and with the Bayer CLINITEK 50. Ann Clin Biochem 37:220–221, 2000.
14. Hongo T, Ohtsuka R, Inaoka T, Kawabe T, Akimichi T, Kuchikura Y, Suda K, Tohyama C, Suzuki T. Health status comparison by urinalysis (dipstick test) among four populations in Papua New Guinea. Asia Pac J Public Health 7:165–172, 1994.
15. Skinner R, Cole M, Pearson AD, Coulthard MG, Craft AW. Specificity of pH and osmolality of early morning urine sample in assessing distal renal tubular function in children: Results in healthy children. Br Med J 312:1337–1338, 1996.
16. Hussain M, Ali B, Ahmed S, Zafar N, Naqvi SA, Rizvi SA. Prediction of renal function recovery in obstructive renal failure due to stones. J Pak Med Assoc 47: 159–161, 1997.
17. Hennequin C, Daudon M, Phung T, Lacour B, Jungers P. Evaluation of the lithogenic risk in renal lithiasis: Value of urine density measurement. Presse Med 24: 1559–1562, 1995.
18. Armstrong LE, Soto JA, Hacker FT Jr, Casa DJ, Kavouras SA, Maresh CM. Urinary indices during dehydration, exercise, and rehydration. Int J Sport Nutr 8:345–355, 1998.

19. Popowski LA, Oppliger RA, Patrick Lambert G, Johnson RF, Kim Johnson A, Gisolf CV. Blood and urinary measures of hydration status during progressive acute dehydration. Med Sci Sports Exerc 33:747–753, 2001.
20. Teach SJ, Yates EW, Feld LG. Laboratory predictors of fluid deficit in acutely dehydrated children. Clin Pediatr (Phila) 36:395–400, 1997.
21. Cook JD, Caplan YH, LoDico CP, Bush DM. The characterization of human urine for specimen validity determination in workplace drug testing: A review. J Anal Toxicol 24:579–588, 2000.
22. Clarke W, Klein W, Palmer-Toy DE. Athletic drug testing. Ther Drug Monit Toxicol 21:221–234, 2000.
23. Newman DJ, Pugia MJ, Lott JA, Wallace JF, Hiar AM. Urinary protein and albumin excretion corrected by creatinine and specific gravity. Clin Chim Acta 294:139–155, 2000.
24. Woolhandler S, Pels RJ, Bor DH, Himmelstein DU, Lawrence RS. Dipstick urinalysis screening of asymptomatic adults for urinary tract disorders. I. Hematuria and proteinuria. JAMA 262:1214–1219, 1989.
25. Carel RS, Silverberg DS, Kaminsky R, Aviram A. Routine urinalysis (dipstick) findings in mass screening of healthy adults. Clin Chem 33:2106–2108, 1987.
26. Pugia MJ, Lott JA, Kajima J, Saambe T, Sasaki M, Kuromoto K, Nakamura R, Fusegawa H, Ohta Y. Screening school children for albuminuria, proteinuria and occult blood with dipsticks. Clin Chem Lab Med 37:149–157, 1999.
27. Murakami M. Screening for proteinuria and hematuria in school children—methods and results. Acta Paediatr Jpn 32:682–689, 1990.
28. Kawamura T, Ohta T, Ohno Y, Wakai K, Aoki R, Tamakoshi A, Maeda K, Mizuno Y. Significance of urinalysis for subsequent kidney and urinary tract disorders in mass screening of adults. Intern Med 34:475–480, 1995.
29. Iwata K, Yamasaki T, Saito H, Ito S, Fukahori M, Nakazato T, Nagao S. [Results of annual health examination for the aged provided by the law that are predictive of increased mortality risk]. Nippon Koshu Eisei Zasshi 41:1065–1072, 1994.
30. Culleton BF, Larson MG, Parfrey PS, Kannel WB, Levy D. Proteinuria as a risk factor for cardiovascular disease and mortality in older people: A prospective study. Am J Med 109:1–8, 2000.
31. Kroenke K, Hanley JF, Copley JB, Matthews JI, Davis CE, Foulks CJ, Carpenter JL. The admission urinalysis: Impact on patient care. J Gen Intern Med 1:238–242, 1986.
32. Akin BV, Hubbell FA, Frye EB, Rucker L, Friis R. Efficacy of the routine admission urinalysis. Am J Med 82:719–722, 1987.
33. Barton JR, O'Brien JM, Bergauer NK, Jacques DL, Sibai BM. Mild gestational hypertension remote from term: Progression and outcome. Am J Obstet Gynecol 184:979–983, 2001.
34. Brown MA, Buddle ML. Inadequacy of dipstick proteinuria in hypertensive pregnancy. Aust NZ J Obstet Gynaecol 35:366–369, 1995.
35. Meyer NL, Mercer BM, Friedman SA, Sibai BM. Urinary dipstick protein: A poor predictor of absent or severe proteinuria. Am J Obstet Gynecol 170:137–141, 1994.

36. Saudan PJ, Brown MA, Farrell T, Shaw L. Improved methods of assessing proteinuria in hypertensive pregnancy. Br J Obstet Gynaecol 104:1159–1164, 1997.
37. Bouhanick B, Berrut G, Chameau AM, et al. Predictive value of testing random urine sample to detect microalbuminuria in diabetic subjects during outpatient visit. Diabetes Metab 18:54–58, 1992.
38. Poulsen PL, Hansen B, Amby T, et al. Evaluation of a dipstick test for microalbuminuria in three different clinical settings, including the correlation with urinary albumin excretion rate. Diabetes Metab 18:395–400, 1992.
39. Pugia MJ, Lott JA, Clark LW, et al. Comparison of urine dipsticks with quantitative methods for microalbuminuria. Eur J Clin Chem Clin Biochem 35:693–700, 1997.
40. Sacks DB, Bruns DE, Goldstein DE, Maclaren NK, McDonald JM, Parrott M. Guidelines and recommendations for laboratory analysis in the diagnosis and management of diabetes mellitus. Clin Chem 48:436–472, 2002.
41. Pedersen LM, Milman N. Prevalence and prognostic significance of proteinuria in patients with lung cancer. Acta Oncol 35:691–695, 1996.
42. Gleeson MJ, Connolly J, Grainger R, et al. Comparison of reagent strip (dipstick) and microscopic haematuria in urological outpatients. Br J Urol 72:594–946, 1993.
43. Craver RD, Abermanis JG. Dipstick only urinalysis screen for the pediatric emergency room. Pediatr Nephrol 11:331–333, 1997.
44. Bonnardeaux A, Somerville P, Kaye M. A study on the reliability of dipstick urinalysis. Clin Nephrol 41:167–172, 1994.
45. Goldner AP, Mayron R, Ruiz E. Are urine dipsticks reliable indicators of hematuria in blunt trauma patients? Ann Emerg Med 14:580–582, 1985.
46. Daum GS, Krolikowski FJ, Reuter KL, Colby JM, Silva WM. Dipstick evaluation of hematuria in abdominal trauma. Am J Clin Pathol 89:538–542, 1988.
47. Chandhoke PS, McAninch JW. Detection and significance of microscopic hematuria in patients with blunt renal trauma. J Urol 140:16–18, 1988.
48. Kennedy TJ, McConnell JD, Thal ER. Urine dipstick vs. microscopic urinalysis in the evaluation of abdominal trauma. J Trauma 28:615–617, 1988.
49. Moore GP, Robinson M. Do urine dipsticks reliably predict microhematuria? The bloody truth! Ann Emerg Med 17:257–260, 1988.
50. Jou WW, Powers RD. Utility of dipstick urinalysis as a guide to management of adults with suspected infection or hematuria. South Med J 91:266–269, 1998.
51. Anosike JC, Nwoke BE, Njoku AJ. The validity of haematuria in the community diagnosis of urinary schistosomiasis infections. J Helminthol 75:223–225, 2001.
52. Mafe MA. The diagnostic potential of three indirect tests for urinary schistosomiasis in Nigeria. Acta Trop 68:277–284, 1997.
53. Kaplan RE, Springate JE, Feld LG. Screening dipstick urinalysis: A time to change. Pediatrics 100:919–921, 1997.
54. Khadra MH, Pickard RS, Charlton M, et al. A prospective analysis of 1930 patients with hematuria to evaluate current diagnostic practice. J Urol 163:524–527, 2000.
55. Isaacman DJ, Scarfone RJ, Kost SI, Gochman RF, Davis HW, Bernardo LM, Nakayama DK. Utility of routine laboratory testing for detecting intra-abdominal injury in the pediatric trauma patient. Pediatrics 92:691–694, 1993.
56. Richards JR, Derlet RW. Computed tomography and blunt abdominal injury:

Patient selection based on examination, haematocrit and haematuria. Injury 28: 181–185, 1997.
57. Ford EG, Karamanoukian HL, McGrath N, Mahour GH. Emergency center laboratory evaluation of pediatric trauma victims. Am Surg 56:752–757, 1990.
58. Hashmi A, Klassen T. Correlation between urinalysis and intravenous pyelography in pediatric abdominal trauma. J Emerg Med 13:255–258, 1995.
59. Kupka T, Binder LS, Smith DA, Nelson BK, Wainscott MP, Glass BA. Accuracy of urine urobilinogen and bilirubin assays in predicting liver function test abnormalities. Ann Emerg Med 16:1231–1235, 1987.
60. Binder L, Smith D, Kupka T, Nelson B, Glass B, Wainscott M, Haynes J. Failure of prediction of liver function test abnormalities with the urine urobilinogen and urine bilirubin assays. Arch Pathol Lab Med 113:73–76, 1989.
61. Binder L, Smith D, Kupka T, Nelson B, Glass B, Wainscott M, Haynes J. Abnormalities of urine urobilinogen and urine bilirubin assays and their relation to abnormal results of serum liver function tests. South Med J 81:1229–1232, 1988.
62. Kuwajima M. [Clinical usefulness of essential laboratory tests]. Rinsho Byori 40: 489–493, 1992.
63. Takemura Y, Kobayashi H, Kugai N, Sekiguchi S. [The results of the "essential laboratory tests" applied to new outpatients—Re-evaluation of diagnostic efficiencies of the test items]. Rinsho Byori 44:555–563, 1996.
64. Takemura Y. [Assessment of the guidelines for efficacious utilization of laboratory tests in primary care medicine]. Rinsho Byori 45:342–346, 1997.
65. Schrocksnadel H, Sitte B, Steckel-Berger G, Dapunt O. Hemolysis in hypertensive disorders of pregnancy. Gynecol Obstet Invest 34:211–216, 1992.
66. Cohen HT, Spiegel DM. Air-exposed urine dipsticks give false-positive results for glucose and false-negative results for blood. Am J Clin Pathol 96:398–400, 1991.
67. Abdelaziz HM, Billett HH. Follow-up testing for ketonuria. Is it necessary? Am J Clin Pathol 101:346–348, 1994.
68. Morris LR, McGee JA, Kitabchi AE. Correlation between plasma and urine glucose in diabetes. Ann Intern Med 94:469–471, 1981.
69. West KM, Kalbfleisch JM. Sensitivity and specificity of five screening tests for diabetes in ten countries. Diabetes 20:289–296, 1971.
70. Bitzen PO, Schersten B. Assessment of laboratory methods for detection of unsuspected diabetes in primary health care. Scand J Prim Health Care 4:85–95, 1986.
71. Forrest RD, Jackson CA, Yudkin JS. The glycohaemoglobin assay as a screening test for diabetes mellitus: The Islington Diabetes Survey. Diabetic Med 4:254–259, 1987.
72. Shinozaki T, Yamaoka K, Yano E. Validity of urinary glucose test for diabetes screening in workplace regular medical checkups. Nippon Koshu Eisei Zasshi 46: 790–798, 1999.
73. Davies MJ, Williams DR, Metcalfe J, Day JL. Community screening for non–insulin-dependent diabetes mellitus: Self-testing for post-prandial glycosuria. Q J Med 86:677–684, 1993.
74. Friderichsen B, Maunsbach M. Glycosuric tests should not be employed in population screenings for NIDDM. J Public Health Med 19:55–60, 1997.
75. Hanson RL, Nelson RG, McCance DR, Beart JA, Charles MA, Pettitt DJ, Knowler

WC. Comparison of screening tests for non–insulin-dependent diabetes mellitus. Arch Intern Med 153:2133–2140, 1993.
76. Engelgau MM, Narayan KM, Herman WH. Screening for type 2 diabetes. Diabetes Care 23:1563–1580, 2000 (erratum in: Diabetes Care 23:1868–1869, 2000).
77. Tosetti C, Brunetti R, Evangelisti A, Napoli A. Relevance of postprandial glycosuria in survey for diabetes mellitus. Minerva Med 87:505–508, 1996.
78. Bresnick GH, Groo A, Palta M, Korth K. Urinary glucose testing inaccuracies among diabetic patients. Effect of acquired color vision deficiency caused by diabetic retinopathy. Arch Ophthalmol 102:1489–1496, 1984.
79. Feleke Y, Abdulkadir J. Urine glucose testing: Another look at its relevance when blood glucose monitoring is unaffordable. Ethiop Med J 36:93–99, 1998.
80. Miles P, Everett J, Murphy J, Kerr D. Comparison of blood or urine testing by patients with newly diagnosed non–insulin dependent diabetes: Patient survey after randomized crossover trial. Br Med J 315:348–349, 1997 (erratum in: Br Med J 316:195, 1998).
81. Starostina EG, Antsiferov M, Galstyan GR, Trautner C, Jorgens V, Bott U, Muhlhauser I, Berger M, Dedov II. Effectiveness and cost-benefit analysis of intensive treatment and teaching programmes for type 1 (insulin-dependent) diabetes mellitus in Moscow—Blood glucose versus urine glucose self-monitoring. Diabetologia 37: 170–176, 1994.
82. Allen BT, DeLong ER, Feussner JR. Impact of glucose self-monitoring on non–insulin-treated patients with type II diabetes mellitus. Randomized controlled trial comparing blood and urine testing. Diabetes Care 13:1044–1050, 1990.
83. Fontbonne A, Billault B, Acosta M, Percheron C, Varenne P, Besse A, Eschwege E, Monnier L, Slama G, Passa P. Is glucose self-monitoring beneficial in non–insulin-treated diabetic patients? Results of a randomized comparative trial. Diabetes Metab 15:255–260, 1989.
84. Coster S, Gulliford MC, Seed PT, Powrie JK, Swaminathan R. Self-monitoring in type 2 diabetes mellitus: A meta-analysis. Diabetic Med 17:755–761, 2000.
85. Patrick AW, Gill GV, MacFarlane IA, Cullen A, Power E, Wallymahmed M. Home glucose monitoring in type 2 diabetes: Is it a waste of time? Diabetic Med 11:62–65, 1994.
86. Vambergue M, Nuttens C, Verier-Mine O, Dognin C, Cappoen JP, Fontaine P. Is mild gestational hyperglycaemia associated with maternal and neonatal complications? The Diagest Study. Diabetic Med 17:203–208, 2000.
87. Pettitt DJ, Bennett PH, Saad MF, Charles MA, Nelson RG, Knowler WC. Abnormal glucose tolerance during pregnancy in Pima Indian women. Long-term effects on offspring. Diabetes 40:126–130, 1991.
88. O'Sullivan JB, Charles D, Mahan CM, Dandrow RV. Gestational diabetes and perinatal mortality rate. Am J Obstet Gynecol 116:901–904, 1973.
89. Jensen DM, Sørensen B, Feilberg-Jørgensen N, Westergaard JG, Beck-Nielsen H. Maternal and perinatal outcomes in 143 Danish women with gestational diabetes mellitus and 143 controls with a similar risk profile. Diabetic Med 17:281–286, 2000.
90. Jardine-Brown C, Dawson A, Dodds R, Gamsu H, Giumer M, Hall M. Report of the Pregnancy and Neonatal Care Group. Diabetic Med 13(suppl):S43–S53, 1996.

91. Scottish Intercollegiate Guidelines Network. Management of Diabetes in Pregnancy. Scottish Intercollegiate Guidelines Network, Edinburgh, 1996, pp 24–26.
92. Watson WJ. Screening for glycosuria during pregnancy. South Med J 83:156–158, 1990.
93. Hooper DE. Detecting GD and preeclampsia. Effectiveness of routine urine screening for glucose and protein. J Reprod Med 41:885–888, 1996.
94. Savova R, Popova G, Koprivarova K, Konstantinova M, Angelova B, Atanasova M, Goranova S, Christov V, Kalinov K. Clinical and laboratory characteristics of type I (insulin dependent) diabetes mellitus at presentation among Bulgarian children. Diabetes Res Clin Pract 34(suppl):S159–S163, 1996.
95. Levy-Marchal C, Papoz L, de Beaufort C, Doutreix J, Froment V, Voirin J, Czernichow P. Clinical and laboratory features of type 1 diabetic children at the time of diagnosis. Diabetic Med 9:279–284, 1992.
96. Hother-Nielsen O, Faber O, Sorensen NS, Beck-Nielsen H. Classification of newly diagnosed diabetic patients as insulin-requiring or non–insulin-requiring based on clinical and biochemical variables. Diabetes Care 11:531–537, 1988.
97. MacIver DH, McNally PG, Shaw DE, Hearnshaw JR. Predicting future treatment of diabetes mellitus from characteristics available at presentation. Diabetic Med 5: 766–770, 1988.
98. Guerrero F, Ortego J, Cordoba JA, Giron JA, Freire JM, Aguilar M. Clinical parameters (body mass index and age) are the best predictors for the need of insulin therapy during the first 18 months of diabetes mellitus in young adult patients. Horm Metab Res 32:185–189, 2000.
99. Rovet JF, Ehrlich RM, Czuchta D. Intellectual characteristics of diabetic children at diagnosis and one year later. J Pediatr Psychol 15:775–788, 1990.
100. Neufeld ND, Raffel LJ, Landon C, Chen YD, Vadheim CM. Early presentation of type 2 diabetes in Mexican-American youth. Diabetes Care 21:80–86, 1998.
101. Pinhas-Hamiel O, Dolan LM, Zeitler PS. Diabetic ketoacidosis among obese African-American adolescents with NIDDM. Diabetes Care 20:484–486, 1997.
102. MacGillivray MH, Li PK, Lee JT, Mills BJ, Voorhess ML, Putnam TI, Schaefer PA. Elevated plasma beta-hydroxybutyrate concentrations without ketonuria in healthy insulin-dependent diabetic patients. J Clin Endocrinol Metab 54:665–668, 1982.
103. Schwab TM, Hendey GW, Soliz TC. Screening for ketonemia in patients with diabetes. Ann Emerg Med 34:342–346, 1999.
104. Papadakis M, Grunfeld C. Ketonuria in hospitalized patients with non–insulin-dependent diabetes mellitus. Diabetes Care 9:596–600, 1986.
105. Chez RA, Curcio FD III. Ketonuria in normal pregnancy. Obstet Gynecol 69:272–274, 1987.
106. Onyeije CI, Divon MY. The impact of maternal ketonuria on fetal test results in the setting of postterm pregnancy. Am J Obstet Gynecol 184:713–718, 2001.
107. Gilbert DL, Pyzik PL, Freeman JM. The ketogenic diet: Seizure control correlates better with serum beta-hydroxybutyrate than with urine ketones. J Child Neurol 15:787–790, 2000.
108. Hurlbut TA, Littenberg B. The diagnostic accuracy of rapid dipstick tests to predict urinary tract infection. Am J Clin Pathol 96:582–588, 1991.

109. Pels RJ, Bor DH, Woolhandler S, Himmelstein DU, Lawrence RS. Dipstick urinalysis screening of asymptomatic adults for urinary tract disorders. II. Bacteriuria. JAMA 262:1221–1224, 1989.
110. Bulloch B, Bausher JC, Pomerantz WJ, Connors JM, Mahabee-Gittens M, Dowd MD. Can urine clarity exclude the diagnosis of urinary tract infection? Pediatrics 106:E60, 2000.
111. Gorelick MH, Shaw KN. Screening tests for urinary tract infection in children: A meta-analysis. Pediatrics 104:E54, 1999.
112. Roberts KB. Practice parameter: The diagnosis, treatment, and evaluation of the initial urinary tract infection in febrile infants and young children. American Academy of Pediatrics, Committee on Quality Improvement, Subcommittee on Urinary Tract Infection. Pediatrics 103:843–852, 1999 (errata in: 103:1052, 1999; 104:118, 1999; 105:141, 2000).

12
Occult Blood

Martin Fleisher
Memorial Sloan-Kettering Cancer Center, New York, New York, U.S.A.

Ronald J. Schoengold
Beckman Coulter, Inc., Palo Alto, California, U.S.A.

INTRODUCTION

Occult bleeding refers to an unexpected presentation of blood in stool, urine, or other body fluids without visible evidence as to the origin of the bleeding. Rapid, inexpensive, and sensitive methods to detect occult blood are clinically important to help locate the source of bleeding and evaluate the significance of blood loss. The detection of blood in stool can suggest clinically relevant problems, especially in patients who present with unapparent anemia or other generalized indications of a possible gastrointestinal disease or disorder (1,2).

A positive occult blood test can be a useful finding in near-patient emergency situations, especially with patients who are unable to cooperate fully with their healthcare provider. These point-of-care tests (POCTs) are administered at the patient's bedside (3–5).

The principal application of the fecal occult blood test (FOBT), however, is to screen asymptomatic average-risk individuals for colorectal neoplasia (polyps and cancer). Patients with this condition are generally unaware that they are at risk or that they have the disease because it is often silent in its early stages. Such individuals are typically not motivated to accept screening without some form of medical intervention (6).

The FOBT methods used to conduct screening require both patient and physician involvement for the preparation of samples and their evaluation. These tests also fall within the definition of POCTs.

Occult blood POCTs are complimentary and necessary components in a quality healthcare system since they can rapidly deliver specific test results at or near the patient when the examining physician deems such information to be clinically important (6). Other examples of POCTs are blood chemistry, hematology, and coagulation tests. These tests are discussed elsewhere in the text. They are generally useful in helping to monitor the status of the patient prior to or following more extensive diagnostic workups and procedures.

There are many factors that have led to the increasing relevance of POCTs in certain clinical situations, including acute care and general wellness checkups. A good example is the FOBT where there may be a need for a rapid test result to determine the risk of performing more extensive procedures (6). Turnaround time for such tests, whether done in the physician's office, clinic, or hospital emergency room is short owing to the simplicity of the method, its reliability, and the minimal training needed by the operator to achieve accurate test results. The FOBT is categorized under the Clinical Laboratory Improvement Act of 1988 (CLIA'88) as a *waived* tests. A physician, nurse, or technician with only minimum training and adherence to simple quality control procedures can perform the FOBT reliably.

This chapter considers all of the currently available occult blood test procedures performed on feces, urine, and gastric fluid. Recommendations for the use of FOBTs in several clinical and near-patient settings are summarized. The chapter concludes with statements about the significance of screening for early detection of disease associated with a positive occult blood finding.

FECAL OCCULT BLOOD

Review of Methods and Procedures

The Dutch scientist J. Izaak Van Deen is credited with the earliest discovery, in 1864, that gum guaiac could be used to detect the presence of blood in feces and other body fluids (7). The concept of routinely using a fecal occult blood test in the pathology laboratory was proposed in 1901 by Boas who used a gum guaiac method to detect hidden blood in stool and named it "occult bleeding" (8,9). These observations that were documented over 100 yr ago, described the pseudoperoxidase activity of hemoglobin, which functions chemically as a catalyst, in the presence of guaiac (chromogen) and peroxide (oxidizing agent), to produce a color change. These tests were typically performed using an alcoholic extract of guaiac in a test tube, which has now been abandoned by the laboratory for technical reasons (10). Reagents were unstable and had to be prepared fresh for use. Raw materials were derived from natural resins (e.g., guaiac) and were difficult to standardize from batch to batch. In addition, suspending a small stool sample in a liquid medium greatly amplified the sensitivity of the tests, yielding extremely low specificities and positive predictive values for gastrointestinal pathology (3,11).

During this period, numerous other tests were developed that also relied on the ability of hemoglobin to oxidize a chromogenic substance to produce a color change. Such chromogens include ferrocyanide, 3-aminophthalic acid, hydrazide, *p*-phenylenediamine, chlorohydrate, pyramidone, aloin, phenolphthalein, dihydrochloride, malachite green, benzidine, and o-tolidine (9,10,12). Nearly all these methods have been replaced in clinical and laboratory practice with stable, highly standardized, paper tests or other solid phase tests.

This chapter discusses mainly qualitative tests to detect occult blood in feces, urine, and gastric fluid. The application of a quantitative ^{51}Cr method was described by early investigators before endoscopy was widely available as a diagnostic tool (13). These methods have also been used to estimate the normal, nonpathological, daily blood loss in the gut. These findings were used to establish cutoff levels for the current qualitative FOBTs (10,14).

A major use of the FOBT is to screen asymptomatic individuals for colorectal neoplasia (polyps and cancer) as part of their regular health checkups. Such testing requires the individual to prepare six separate tests at home, by applying two stool samples from each of three bowel movements to a test card over a period of several days. Test cards with stool samples applied are then returned to the laboratory for development and interpretation (15,16). Such tests are properly classified as point-of-care methods since their usefulness relies heavily on prompt sample preparation by the patient on the test device immediately after the evacuation of stool.

Fecal occult blood tests are also commonly performed at other point-of-care (outside the laboratory) settings by healthcare professionals, including physicians, nurses, technicians, and medical support personnel seeking immediate presumptive information about occult gastrointestinal bleeding. These tests are commonly done on single fecal samples obtained at the patient's bedside or during a digital rectal examination. Patients undergoing this mode of testing have no dietary preparation, making the results more difficult to interpret (5,17). A positive FOBT obtained in this manner is clinically useful in acute care settings to *rule in* the possibility of gastrointestinal bleeding. A single positive FOBT may warrant a more extensive follow-up evaluation. This FOBT method has lower sensitivity for gastrointestinal bleeding and must not be used as a substitute for colorectal cancer screening (15). But this decision rests with the examining physcian, who must judge the relative value of the findings in light of the patient's overall presentation. Unfortunately, this mode of FOBT has not been subjected to extensive clinical evaluation (15). The examining physician must, therefore, rely more on opinion and judgment in evaluating such patients. The physician must also explain the benefits and risks of this finding to the patient. Nevertheless, common sense dictates that a positive FOBT by any method should be regarded as a true positive and evaluated appropriately (12).

Consequently, to achieve reliable test results, emphasis must be placed on well-validated procedures for patient preparation, sample collection, processing test cards, reading and interpreting the tests, recording the information in the patient's records, and accurately and promptly reporting the results and their significance to the patient. The ultimate goal is for the treating physician to have timely, accurate data that will insure the highest standard of patient care for each clinical situation. Following well-established evidence-based methods when they are available, and applying them according to guidelines and recommendations from authoritative bodies, are the most useful approaches in clinical practice and have proven historically to best serve the needs of the patient (15). In the absence of highly validated methods, some level of testing may still be appropriate but more physician judgment must prevail (6,12).

Certain gastrointestinal (GI) diseases or disorders can manifest themselves as overt bleeding that may be acute and apparent or intermittent and unapparent. Although the FOBT may be useful in some of these situations, it is often a small part in determining the clinical status of the patient. This type of bleeding is not the subject of this chapter. The reader is referred to other source material to evaluate the medical usefulness of FOBT for these applications (6).

Chemical Methods

The best known and most widely accepted chemical fecal occult blood test method is the guaiac paper slide and hydrogen peroxide developer (18). The slide is manufactured by treating high-quality filter paper with guaiac reagent. Each slide also has a positive and negative quality control test area to ensure the functionality of the test. The positive control area is located away from the test sample area and contains a measured quantity of a hemoglobin-derived catalyst designed to mimic the reactivity of heme, hemin, hematin, or hemoglobin that may be present in the fecal sample. The developer solution is an aqueous/alcoholic mixture of hydrogen peroxide stabilized with sodium stannate (18,20) (Tables 1 and 2).

The slides and developer are packaged for use as single tests or triple tests (three tests on one card) for serial, three-day testing. Single slides are typically used in near-patient medical settings. Triple test cards (slides) are the preferred method for colorectal cancer screening in which the patient applies fecal samples over three days in the privacy of their home, then returns the slide to the laboratory. Slides are routinely batched for testing (development) and the results reported directly to the patient's physician. Clinical studies have shown that the laboratory can develop the test up to 14 days after the first fecal specimen was

Table 1 FOBT Screening Methods

Method	Analyte detected (probable source of bleeding)
Guaiac	Heme in feces based on peroxidase activity (entire GI tract)
Immunochemical	Intact hemoglobin (globin) in feces by ligand-binding assay (lower GI tract)
Heme-porphyrin	Heme-derived porphyrins in feces by fluorometric assay (entire GI tract)
Tetramethylbenzidine	Heme based on peroxidase activity in toilet bowl water (entire GI tract)

applied to the slide without significant loss of peroxidase (hemoglobin) reactivity (18,20,21). The guaiac slides and developer solution are highly stable and only require storage at room temperature (15–30°C), away from volatile chemicals such as oxidizing agents, to maintain their long shelf life.

The earliest fecal occult blood test slide was evaluated in clinical practice in 1967 (19). Commercial development of the concept continued and led to the front-back, catch-cover paper slide design that was introduced for professional medical use in the hospital, clinic, and physician office in 1970 (11). Since that time, it has received widespread acceptance, replacing the previous methods that required collection of a large fecal mass to be brought to the laboratory in containers for testing. Chemists and technicians had a natural aversion to testing large stool collections for occult blood, even when their laboratories were equipped with the most up-to-date hoods, room ventilation, and disposal systems to minimize odor and other hazards in handling of such specimens. The paper slide design greatly increased the number of tests routinely performed by minimizing the aesthetic problems associated with fecal testing.

The paper slide design was a very significant step forward in stool testing for the laboratory. It brought a higher level of standardization to fecal occult blood testing using stable guaiac and hydrogen peroxide reagents, consistently manufactured according to a precise formula. Importantly, the paper slide design established a new way to collect and transport stool samples, especially important when FOBT is used to screen for colorectal cancer (14,22).

The chromogen in the paper slide is gum guaiac, a natural resin comprised mainly of α- and β-guaiaconic acids (leuco dyes) extracted from the bark of the *Guaiacum officinale* shrub from the West Indies (8). The basic chemistry of the guaiac method is the oxidation of guaiac by hydrogen peroxide in the presence of a catalyst such as heme, hematin, hemoglobin, or other active substances that mimic the catalytic activity of hemoglobin products such as myoglobin or plant peroxidases. When this oxidative reaction occurs, a highly conjugated quinone structure forms and the visual color of the matrix changes from tan to blue. The

Table 2 Features of FOBTs

Type	Method	Sample	Endpoint
Chemical	Guaiac	Fecal smear on card	Blue color on or around fecal smear
	Tetramethylbenzidine	Flotation pad in toilet bowl	Blue-green color on flotation pad
	Heme-porphyrin	Weighed stool sample	Quantitative fluorometric result
Immunochemical	Antihemoglobin antibody	Fecal smear or liquid extract from fecal sample	Colored line on immunochromatographic test strip, latex or red cell agglutination, quantitative enzyme-linked immunosorbent assay (ELISA)

most reactive constituent of the natural guaiac product is β-guaiaconic acid. However, the reaction is very unstable in the absence of other constituents in the natural product. [Personal observations.] Consequently, attempts to purify the active constituents in gum guaiac have proved to be unsuitable for clinical applications (14) (Figure 1).

The guaiac slide test is a rapid, convenient, disposable qualitative test to detect occult bleeding. The lower threshold of daily blood loss associated with gastrointestinal pathology is 2–3 mL in 100–150 g of stool (22,23). This is equivalent to approximately 0.3 mg hemoglobin per gram of stool, assuming the hemoglobin was uniformly distributed in the stool. This is an estimate of the residual detectable blood and its degradation products (heme, hemin, and hemoglobin), and it takes into account that all substances that transit the bowel are degraded over a 24–48 hr period by naturally occurring digestive and bacterial enzymes. It is important to note that these estimates are subject to very wide variations due to the nonuniform way that blood from a lesion in the bowel distributes in the stool (14,22).

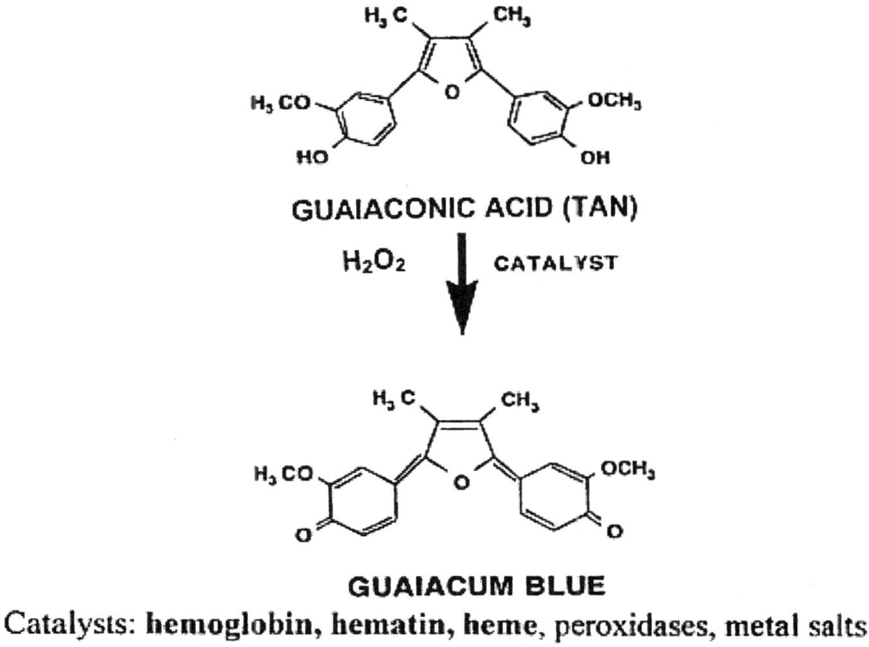

Figure 1 Chemistry of the guaiac test. Chemical representation of the conversion of guaiaconic acid from a reduced to an oxidized state in the presence of a catalyst.

The original guaiac method (Hemoccult, Beckman Coulter, Inc., Fullerton, CA) can detect a threshold level of fecal occult blood (0.3 mg hemoglobin/g stool) with an analytical sensitivity of about 50%. A more recently developed method (Hemoccult SENSA) incorporates a phenolic-type enhancing agent in the reagent formulation but does not alter the basic guaiac chemistry. This results in detecting a threshold level of fecal occult blood (0.3 mg hemoglobin/g stool) with an analytical sensitivity of about 75%. Thus, the newer method has slightly greater sensitivity for fecal occult blood and significantly better readability when compared with the original method. The main advantage of the newer method is better stabilization of the blue color that forms on the test without a significant loss of specificity in detecting hemoglobin products. Of course, as the level of hemoglobin in the fecal sample increases beyond the threshold quantity, the analytical sensitivity of both methods increases to a maximum of about 95% (18,23). These estimates of occult blood detection are based upon a significant number of clinical trials where the endpoints were the detection of clinical neoplastic disease (adenomas and cancers) by endoscopy, as a follow-up to a positive FOBT. The results of these trials vary widely based on demographical and biological variation normally found in the cohort (24–33). In vitro laboratory studies have also been done to validate these clinical findings. A further explanation of these variations is given later in this chapter.

Each manufacturer of guaiac slide tests provides specific instructions on the proper method of collecting a fecal sample. To achieve consistent test results, each manufacturer's instructions should always be closely adhered to. The following principles apply generally to all tests in this category. Each individual or serial test slide should be properly identified and have at least the patient's name and the date the fecal sample was applied to the test slide. Samples must be collected immediately after defecation to avoid degradation of blood, if present, by the biological action of the feces. Bacterial and digestive enzymes will degrade blood, if the stool is left at room temperature for several hours. It is best to sample each stool in two different locations to minimize the problems associated with the distribution of blood that may be present. Samples should be taken before the stool makes contact with the toilet bowl water, although this is not an absolute requirement. A proper sample consists of taking two small (pea size) aliquots of stool and applying each to the two windows of the test slide. This sampling method is repeated for three successive days or bowel movements. The fecal samples are always applied as *thin smears* to the "front" of the test card after opening the paper cover and exposing the two windows. Application of excess stool is unnecessary and can increase the rate of false positive results because of the added mass of sample being applied (Table 3).

After application of the stool samples, it is important to wait at least 3–5 min before attempting to develop the test, to permit the sample to penetrate into the treated paper. If a single sample is being tested in a near-patient setting, two

Table 3 Proper Collection of Stool Samples for FOBT

- Strictly adhere to manufacturer's instructions.
- Stool samples should be collected by the patient immediately following defecation.
- Patients must avoid straining to pass stool.
- Patients must follow specific dietary restrictions and other cautions for the periods indicated by the manufacturer.
- Small fecal samples should be taken from different locations of the passed stool.
- Contact of stool samples with toilet bowl water should be avoided or minimized.

Patients must return collected samples within the prescribed time period, usually 5–7 days after the first sample is collected.

drops of the alcoholic hydrogen peroxide developer are applied on the opposite side of the slide, after opening the serrated test side, as indicated. The two drops should be added in quick succession. At the same time, the technician should immediately begin to observe for the appearance of blue color for up to 1 min. A test is negative if no blue color is seen within 1 min. Some fecal samples contain substances that can rapidly degrade the blue color that forms. Consequently, it is important for the technician to observe for transient blue color before it fades. The manufacturer's instructions state that any blue color that appears on or at the edge of the original fecal smear is a positive test result. After developing and interpreting the test areas (two windows), the technician is instructed to add 1 drop of the developer to the Performance Monitor or control area of the slide. Once again, it is important to immediately begin observing the control area for the formation of a blue color in the positive (+) area and insure that no blue color forms in the negative (−) area. The control results should always be apparent within 10 sec of applying the developer solution. The control area (Performance Monitor) is designed to provide assurance to the operator or technician that the reagents are functioning correctly (18,20).

In addition to the best known products, Hemoccult and Hemoccult SENSA, several other tests are commonly found in the market (Table 4). They include Seracult and Seracult Plus (Propper Manufacturing Company, Inc.), ColoScreen and ColoScreen-ES (Helena Laboratories), HemaChek (Miles Laboratories), Hema-Screen (Immunostics), Quik-Cult (Laboratory Diagnostics/Cenogenics), and Hemaprompt (Aerscher).

In addition, there are two toilet bowl tests that are sold over-the-counter: ColoCare (Helena Laboratories) and EZ Detect (Biomerica, Inc.). The toilet bowl tests use a tetramethylbenzidine chromogenic material to qualitatively detect the presence of a catalyst (e.g., heme from hemoglobin) in toilet bowl water. These tests are designed to be placed into the toilet bowl immediately following defeca-

Table 4 Commercially Available FOBTs[a]

Commercial test name(s)	Manufacturer
Guaiac tests	
Hemoccult, Hemoccult II, Hemoccult SENSA, Hemoccult II SENSA	Beckman Coulter, Inc., Primary Care Diagnostics
Seracult, Seracult Plus	Propper Manufacturing Company, Inc.
ColoScreen, ColoScreen-ES	Helena Laboratories
Colo-Rectal, HemoFEC	Hoffman LaRoche, AG
Hema-Chek	Miles Laboratories
Quik-Cult	Laboratory Diagnostics/Cenogenics
Hemaprompt	Aerscher
EARLYSCREEN, HemaWipe, Hema-Slide, Instaccult	Medtek
Immunochemical tests	
Immudia HemSp	Fujirebio, Inc.
OC Hemodia	Eiken, Inc.
Hemolex	Orion Diagnostics
Mono-Haem	Chemicon International, Inc.
Inform, Inform OBT	Enterix Australia, Enterix US
Toilet bowl tests	
EZ Detect	Biomerica, Inc.
ColoCARE	Helena Laboratories

[a] The information provided is based on current published information from the manufacturers and is subject to change.

tion, observed by the patient for several minutes, and interpreted according to written instructions based on color and/or symbol changes that occur on the pad. The pad is then flushed away with the stool sample. To be clinically useful, there are several inherent problems with the method that still need to be resolved. The product is purchased over-the-counter, by the patient. Accordingly, there is no mechanism for insurance or medical reimbursement by government agencies. Such tests are not part of regular patient test regimens administered by healthcare systems. The tests are performed infrequently by patients who are over age 50 and may have vision problems, especially in the widely variable lighting conditions of bathrooms in the home. Test results reside with the patient who has discretion about sharing their personal findings, conjectures, and/or beliefs with their physician and healthcare provider. Any positive test findings reported to the physician present a dilemma in terms of the proper follow-up tests to further evaluate this situation. Patients often do not connect physical signs and symptoms with changes in their health until they progress to advanced stages. This leads to lack of involvement with preventive services that can detect significant diseases in their early stages (18).

Orthotoluidine Tablet Test (Hematest, Ames Co.) was an early test method in which the chromogen was formulated into a tablet. In practice, the tablet was placed on a small piece of filter paper on which a fecal sample had been applied. A hydrogen peroxide solution was added to the tablet and the paper observed for a color change for up to 2 min. This test has been replaced by less cumbersome, more reliable methods (10,11).

The bench guaiac test was used for forensic applications and in early investigation of fecal occult bleeding for clinical purposes. Culver (12) described the preparation of a saturated alcoholic solution of gum guaiac powder in which a small stool sample was immersed. Following the addition of a hydrogen peroxide solution, the operator observed for blue color in the solution. Green colors were often observed due to the natural content of colored substances in the stool. But the method instructed the user to disregard any color formation other than blue as insignificant. As discussed earlier, this procedure has been replaced by more reliable solid phase methods (10).

Early efforts to perfect a benzidine test for fecal occult blood applications were successful for a short period of time. However, once the carcinogenic properties of this chemical were described, the application of this laboratory method declined sharply.

Immunochemical Methods

The immunochemical fecal occult blood tests (IFOBTs) are designed to specifically detect the epitopes of human hemoglobin (Figure 2) using various ligand binding systems of capture antibodies, coupled with detector systems that vary widely (ELISA, latex agglutination, hemagglutination, immunochromatographic colloidal gold particles, immunochromatographic colored latex particles, etc.). The cost to manufacture such tests is generally higher than chemical tests, making them more expensive to purchase. The test methods usually require a minimum of two to three steps to perform, compared with one step for guaiac methods. Test reagents are less stable and may require storage at 2–8°C. The IFOBTs are more complex in terms of their chemistry and test platforms. With the proper selection of antibodies and other reagents, immunochemical tests have greater specificity than chemical methods despite their increased complexity (14,24,40) (Figure 3). Like the chemical tests, they are qualitative but can accommodate a level of semiquantitative output, if such results can be shown to be clinically relevant. This feature permits the establishment of different cutoff values for different populations or clinical settings that can have a direct impact on the cost of follow-up and diagnosis as to the source of gastrointestinal bleeding (18,40).

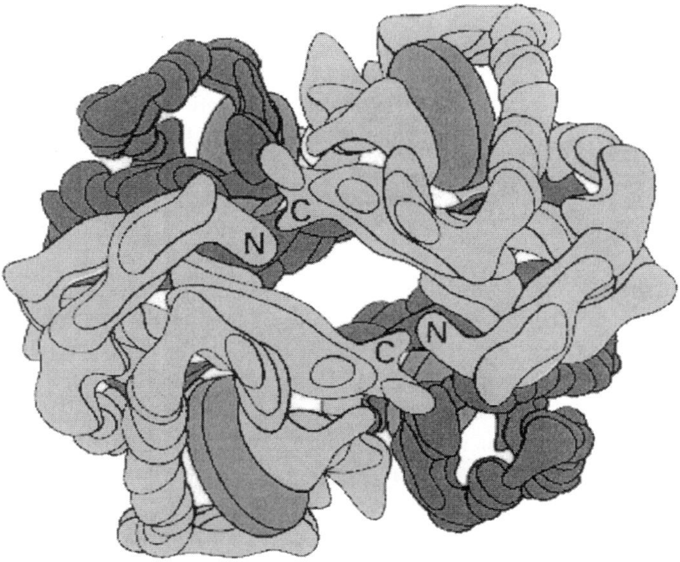

Figure 2 Hemoglobin. A three-dimensional representation of a hemoglobin molecule based on x-ray diffraction studies. The disc-shaped objects represent the heme groups, one for each of the four globulin chains (2 α chains and 2 β chains). Used with permission, © 1964 by Scientific American, Inc.

The IFOBTs are colon specific based on the general degradation patterns of the protein moieties of blood (hemoglobin) as it transits the GI tract. Globin is a labile protein that is rapidly degraded by bacterial and digestive enzymes normally present in the gastrointestinal tract. Thus, the higher the source of bleeding, the less likely it will be detected by an immunochemical FOBT.

Since there is no interference reported from ingestion of foods and medicines (i.e., no interference with lifestyle), such test methods are likely to gain wider acceptance from patients who are candidates for colorectal cancer (CRC) screening. This will improve the effectiveness of colorectal cancer screening and its consequent outcomes, since the level of patient acceptance of testing has the most significant influence on reducing the incidence and mortality from CRC (18).

The IFOBTs, however, are subject to the same biological variations associated with the biology of bleeding in the GI tract: nonuniform distribution of blood and intermittency of lesions that may bleed. It is important, therefore, to follow a strict protocol of testing multiple fecal samples to help overcome statistical bias. Since hemoglobin is stable in a dried fecal sample, on-slide fecal specimen

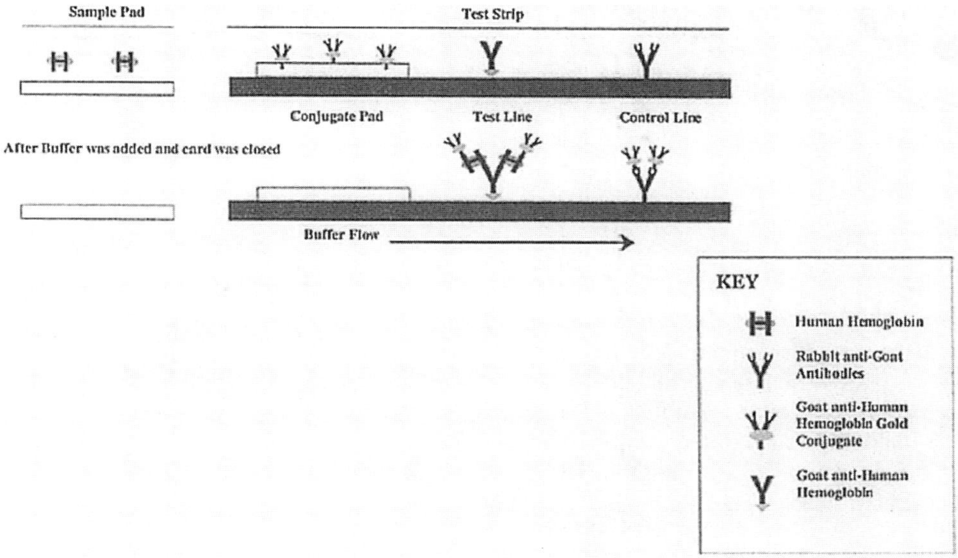

Figure 3 Principle of immunochemical FOBT. A diagrammatic representation of a sandwich assay in an immunochemical chromatographic format. Hemoglobin in a sample is recognized and binds to a particle-antibody conjugate, and is subsequently captured by an antihemoglobin antibody on a test strip, where it can be seen visually as a colored line.

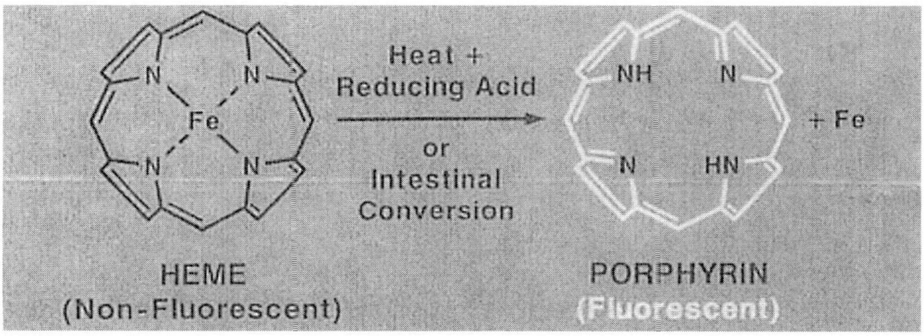

Figure 4 Biochemical basis for HemoQuant test. A diagrammatic representation of heme (nonfluorescent) before and after it has been degraded to porphyrin (fluorescent). The chemical characteristics of heme and porphyrin provide a means to differentiate the two molecules biochemically.

Table 5 Sensitivity of FOBT Methods

Derivative	Gastric	Proximal large bowel	Distal large bowel
Intact hemoglobin	−	+	++
Intact heme	+	+	++
Heme-derived porphyrins	+++	++	+

stability (for tests that use this method of sample collection) is the same as chemical methods—up to 14 days.

For quality control purposes, external controls in addition to on-board functional controls are required and are usually supplied as separate materials or products. This adds to the cost of testing.

The sensitivity of the IFOBT is approximately 0.15 mg Hb/g stool (about twice as sensitive as a guaiac test) (18) (Tables 5 and 6).

Heme-Porphyrin Method

A chemical laboratory method to degrade hemoglobin and intermediate breakdown products that may be found in the stool to porphyrins was described by Schwartz et al. (41). The HemoQuant assay method is a quantitative spectrofluorometric laboratory-based procedure that requires pretreatment of a precisely weighted amount of stool to degrade all hemoglobins and heme to porphyrins under a controlled set of laboratory conditions (34,41). The HemoQuant method is generally subject to dietary interference from ingested red meats, drugs that cause upper GI bleeding, and certain other heme-containing foods. These interferences can significantly affect test specificity, making it less useful in the clinical setting (18,34).

Significant efforts to simplify and apply this method for screening have been unsuccessful. The method is currently used in the research setting when

Table 6 Sensitivity of FOBT Methods for GI Bleeding

FOBT method	Intact hemoglobin	Heme-derived porphyrins	Intact heme
Guaiac	+	−	+
Heme-porphyrin	+	+	+
Immunochemical	+	−	−

there is need for semiquantitative measurement of heme-derived porphyrins in a stool sample (42) (Figure 4).

Interferences and Factors Affecting Test Results

Early analytical occult blood studies demonstrated that small quantities of blood are normally present in the stool due mainly to turnover of the colonic epithelium. Radioactive chromium (^{51}Cr-labeled erythrocytes) studies estimated normal blood loss in the stool at 0.5–1.5 mL per day (13,14). Several investigators report increased normal blood loss in the stool due to vigorous exercise, such as distance running (18). All test methods, including qualitative methods, therefore, must establish a cutoff value for the assay based on normal blood loss. This can cause a higher positivity rate that has no added clinical benefit.

Stool samples are inherently heterogeneous and can vary widely in their composition and consistency depending on the foods and drugs ingested, microflora, and general health status of the individual (35–37,39). The measurement of specific analytes in such samples is therefore subject to wide fluctuations unless the substance being measured is present in large amounts. This is typically not the case for occult blood (38) (Table 7).

The physical consistency (i.e., water content) of the stool sample can alter the sensitivity of some test methods, especially those done on paper cards containing dry reagents. In general, blood in stool samples with higher water content will be more easily detected, thus making the test appear to be more sensitive compared with blood in a hard, more formed stool.

The biology of stool formation in the colon, transit time, and the physical location of bleeding (i.e., cecum; ascending, transverse, descending, sigmoid colon; or rectum) can have a significant impact on how the blood is distributed in the sample. Blood from proximal lesions is generally distributed more uniformly than blood from distal lesions. Blood from distal lesions tends to accumulate more at the surface of the stool than the core.

Further complicating the ability to detect occult bleeding is the fact that many lesions, especially adenomas, bleed intermittently. Thus, when the stool is actually sampled can impact the clinical accuracy of the test (14,18).

Paper treated with guaiac reagent is subject to oxidation when exposed to air, ultraviolet (UV) light, or certain oxidizing chemicals. Occasionally, a light blue discoloration or haze is noticed on the test slide before the hydrogen peroxide developer is applied to initiate the reaction. This discoloration does not affect the accuracy or performance of the test if the manufacturer's instructions are followed. When the developer is added to the slide directly over the fecal smear, the blue background color rapidly migrates outward forming a blue ring at the edge of the wetted area. The paper immediately around the fecal smear is restored to its off-white tan color, leaving a clear area for observing blue color that forms

Table 7 Interfering Substances for FOBTs

Method-type substance	Interfering substance	Possible effect on test accuracy
Chemical-dietary	Red meats (e.g., beef, lamb)	Chemical false positive
	Very high peroxidase-containing raw vegetables (e.g., horseradish, turnip, radish)	Chemical false positive
	Excessive amounts of vitamin C enriched foods (e.g., fruit juices)	Chemical false positive
	Excessive amounts of alcoholic beverages	Clinical false positive due to in vivo bleeding
Chemical-drugs	Aspirin in excess of 325 mg daily	Clinical false positive due to in vivo bleeding
	Other nonsteroidal anti-inflammatory drugs (e.g., ibuprofen, indomethacin, naproxen)	Clinical false positive due to in vivo bleeding
	Corticosteroids, phenylbutazone, reserpine, antimetabolites, chemotherapeutics	Clinical false positive due to in vivo bleeding
	Topical antiseptics to anal area (e.g., povidone/iodine)	Chemical false positive
Immunochemical-dietary	None	None
Immunochemical-drugs	None reported in published literature	None

from the fecal smear. Any blue color that forms on or at the edge of the fecal smear is positive for occult blood.

Highly colored stools due to ingested substances can sometimes obscure or mask the blue color from a positive test. This occurs rarely (18).

Studies at several clinical centers have shown that insufficient holding time (in days) between fecal sample application to the test slide and its development can alter the accuracy of the test. Holding the card with dried fecal samples for 3 days permits peroxidase activity from fruits and vegetables to degrade naturally. Peroxidase activity from hemoglobins, animal and human, is inherently more stable. This biological characteristic increases the specificity of the test for blood (18,38).

Rehydration with a drop of water just before development with the alcoholic developer significantly increases the sensitivity of the test for all peroxidatively active materials, especially those from fruits and vegetables. This procedure is not recommended by the manufacturers since it significantly degrades the clinical specificity of the test (18).

Clinical Manifestations and Case Studies

Gastrointestinal lesions that produce lower GI bleeding are most commonly caused by polyps, carcinoma, colitis, diverticula, arteriovenous malformations, and hemorrhoids. In addition, bleeding from the upper GI tract (esophagus and stomach) may contribute to apparent lower GI bleeding.

Lower GI bleeding may be acute lasting for 2–3 days or chronic and intermittent. The FOBT is used to detect bleeding but if improperly performed could give little useful clinical information. For example, stool samples collected on the fingertip during a digital rectal examination, though useful in certain clinical situations, is not a colorectal cancer screening method. The recommended screening procedure for CRC requires that the patient collect two samples from three consecutive specimens (43–45). This approach is necessary because bleeding may be intermittent and thus may not be detected at the time of a single examination. Several studies have demonstrated the advantage of the three-sample protocol in detecting colorectal neoplasia. The American Cancer Society and the American Gastroenterological Association (AGA) recommend that a positive FOBT be followed up by a colonoscopy or if not practicable, a double contrast barium enema and flexible sigmoidoscopy (44). If a clinically relevant source of bleeding is not identified during visualization (colonoscopy), then a source of bleeding outside the large bowel should be considered.

Several randomized, controlled trials demonstrated the effectiveness of FOBT in mortality reduction (26–30). The largest reduction in mortality was in the Minnesota trial in which annual FOBT screening resulted in a 33% reduction in mortality over 18 years of follow-up.

Trials in the United States and Europe were shown to be consistent in terms of mortality reduction as a function of the type of FOBT and frequency of screening (26–28). It is well accepted that FOBT is an effective tool in screening for colorectal cancer. A recently published review related to colorectal cancer screening states, "There has been great debate as to which screening test is the best, but the best screening test is the one that gets done" (47).

Two case studies are presented to illustrate commonly observed clinical findings and problems that underscore the utility of occult blood detection.

Case 1: (Modified from Ransohoff and Sandler [21].) A healthy 50-year-old woman with no personal or family history of cancer presented to her primary care physician for a periodic health checkup. The only risk factor for colorectal cancer exhibited by the patient was her age. A FOBT was performed as part of the physical examination. The FOBT performed was the three-stool method, two samples each from three daily stools, serially collected and applied to a triple FOBT card. The stool specimens were collected by the patient at home, then returned to her physician for development and evaluation.

One of the three stool specimens gave a positive result. The patient was offered and accepted a follow-up colonoscopy that was successful in examining the entire colon to the cecum, to investigate a possible source of bleeding. The patient was advised that the probability of finding a colorectal cancer or large polyp ranges from 17–46% among those with a positive FOBT (21).

The FOBT is the most commonly performed screening test for colorectal cancer in the United States. The average-risk patient can be offered a choice of several screening tests for colorectal cancer including FOBT, FOBT with flexible sigmoidoscopy, or colonoscopy. But considering costs and risks of the procedure, patients often prefer FOBT, a noninvasive method. Annual FOBT has been demonstrated to be 90% effective in detecting colonic neoplasia when properly performed (25).

Case 2: A 68-year-old, apparently healthy male presented with cramping or steady abdominal pain associated with constipation. A digital rectal examination revealed no abnormalities. The patient was given a three-day FOBT that was completed within a week of the initial presentation. One of the FOBT cards gave a weak positive result, suggesting a trace amount of blood may have been present in the stool. A follow-up flexible sigmoidoscopy led to a diagnosis of acute diverticulitis. Diverticulitis occurs when pouches form within the colon and become infected. Initial follow-up treatment of the patient offered little relief of symptoms and since the patient was over age 50 a colonoscopy was performed. Careful examination of the colon revealed a stage 2 cancer in the ascending colon approximately 10 cm distal to the ileocecal junction. The ascending colon constitutes the upper third of the large bowel. The patient required a surgical resection and follow-up therapy that included chemotherapy and radiation treatment. Approximately 75% of stage 2 colorectal cancer patients are cured (47,48).

According to the statistics published by the American Cancer Society, colorectal cancer represents about 11% of all cancer deaths in the United States. However, if detected early, the cure rate of this cancer is 90%. Colon cancer typically begins in the inner lining of the colon or rectum and often, with time, may metastasize to surrounding tissue and lymph nodes. It should be stressed, as this case study typifies, that the simplest and cheapest test for colon cancer is a digital examination combined with a triple-slide FOBT (47,48).

Screening for Colorectal Cancer

A large number of worldwide authoritative bodies have endorsed evidence-based methods to screen for colorectal cancer, including the use of an annual FOBT. These recommendations have evolved over the past 25 yr, yet only a minority of those at risk are offered and accept screening as a part of their general health program. Low participation in screening is generally attributed to the failure of healthcare providers to offer testing, lack of patient understanding and acceptance, inadequate insurance and government reimbursement, lack of medical expertise and facilities to conduct proper follow-up of screening tests, and poor monitoring and reminder systems for patients who do not participate regularly in preventive healthcare programs. The strongest contributor to successful screening programs is an understanding of the disease and the benefits and risks of screening, and development of a cooperative relationship between the patient and physician (21,44,49) (Table 8).

Newer methods (e.g., characterization of stool DNA) are on the horizon but remain in the discovery and research mode.

Cost Effectiveness of FOBT Screening

The cost effectiveness of FOBT screening must take into consideration the cost of screening tests, follow-up testing of positive patients to determine a probable source of gastrointestinal bleeding, and the possible complications of follow-up endoscopy. The most significant contributor to these costs is the number (or percent) of positive screening tests. Positivity rates vary according to the FOBT method chosen. In general, chemical FOBTs have higher positivity rates than immunochemical methods. This occurs mainly because chemical FOBTs are more affected by dietary factors, especially in populations that regularly consume a diet of high peroxidase-containing foods. Positivity rates for chemical FOBTs are also affected by consumption of irritants (e.g., aspirin) that can cause incidental, nonpathological upper gastrointestinal bleeding, since the analyte being detected is heme. Immunochemical FOBTs are unaffected by diet and generally unaffected by upper gastrointestinal bleeding. The analyte being detected is a

Table 8 Recommended Screening Methods: Tests, Intervals, and Year Recommended[a]

Test	Preventive services task force	Gastrointestinal consortium	NCCN	ASCRS	ACG	ACS
Three-sample FOBT, alone	Yearly	Yearly	Yearly	Yearly	Yearly	Yearly
Three-sample FOBT, plus flexible sigmoidoscopy	Insufficient evidence	Yearly AND every 5 yr	Yearly AND every 5 yr	Yearly AND every 5 yr	Yearly AND every 5 yr	Yearly AND every 5 yr
Year recommended	1996	1997	1999	1999	2000	2001

[a] For average-risk individuals (>50 yr). (Modified from Refs. 28 and 51.)

fragile protein, globin, that is unlikely to survive intact as it transits from the upper to lower gastrointestinal tract and is evacuated in the stool (18,50).

Despite the risks, screening is a good use of medical resources when compared with other medical services and testing commonly in use. The cost effectiveness of screening with FOBTs for colorectal cancer compares favorably to screening for other significant pathological conditions, such as other cancers (e.g., breast, cervical, prostate). Studies have been done using various mathematical models and input assumptions that estimate the collective cost of FOBT screening to be in the range of $10,000–30,000 per life-year saved (18,50).

A critical consideration not discussed here is the cost of building a proper institutional infrastructure to conduct clinical follow-up of positive FOBT screening results. Estimates of the true cost effectiveness of FOBT screening must also take these factors into consideration.

Despite the barriers, successful screening programs have been developed that can serve as models to further advance screening to a broader base of at-risk individuals (49). Coupling these successes with ongoing research to find better screening and prevention strategies will significantly reduce the burden of colorectal cancer.

HEMATURIA AND HEMOGLOBINURIA

Overview

Hematuria is the presence of red blood cells in urine. Hemoglobinuria is defined as the presence of free hemoglobin in urine. Over the years, the methods for detecting red blood cells and hemoglobin in urine have advanced significantly. Historically, a clear red urine indicated hemoglobinuria, and was differentiated from so-called "smokey" red urine that indicated hematuria. Most urines containing red blood cells will also contain hemolyzed occult blood.

Hematuria is commonly detected in patients presenting with bladder cancer. Gross or microscopic blood is found in 80% of patients with bladder tumors (51). A test for hematuria is routinely performed as part of urinalysis. Cytological examination, along with a test for blood in urine, are noninvasive, harmless, and essential procedures that will demonstrate in situ or invasive carcinoma. Failure to use these easily performed tests can result in undue delay in the diagnosis of bladder cancer (52). Although the examination of urine for the presence of occult blood has been used as a screening test for bladder cancer, this could result in problems of clinical interpretation. A relatively large number of normal asymptomatic individuals ranging from 4–10% of the general population have detectable red blood cells in the urine (52). Thus, the high rate of false positive test results would limit the use of blood in urine as a screening test for cancer. Indeed, the microscopic hematuria test was shown to be inferior as a screening test for bladder cancer when compared with the Papanicolauo test, a screening test for cervical cancer.

Test Methods

The reagent test strip is the simplest and least expensive test for the presence of blood in urine. The test strip is impregnated with tetramethylbenzidine (TMB) and buffered organic peroxide. The pseudoperoxidase activity of hemoglobin or myoglobin (muscle hemoglobin) will catalyze the oxidation of TMB, causing the formation of a green to dark blue color. Although most positive reactions are caused by the presence of red blood cells in the urine, the strip test is more sensitive to hemoglobin. Red blood cells that do not lyse in urine will be detected in urine sediment. Urine specimens must be well mixed when testing for occult blood or false negative results will occur. Multistix (Bayer Inc., New Haven, CT) have an occult blood sensitivity of 0.015–0.062 mg/dL hemoglobin (equivalent to 5–20 Ery/μL).

Interferences and Factors Affecting Test Results

False positive test results will be obtained if urine is contaminated with strong oxidizing agents such as chlorine bleach or bacterial peroxidase activity associated with urinary tract infection. Blood as a contaminant from menstruation will also give a positive test strip result. Microscopic examination of the urine sediment will confirm the presence of red blood cells in urine specimens (51,52).

Clinical Manifestations

A positive test for occult blood indicates bleeding in the urinary tract that may occur in a variety of disorders, such as renal disease or dysfunction, infection, tumors, stone formation, or anticoagulant usage. Urinary occult blood is an early indicator of renal dysfunction that should not be overlooked or clinically underestimated. Hematuria may be the only indication of renal damage and is a typical finding in glomerular nephritis (51).

Hemoglobinuria may indicate significant intravascular hemolysis or hemolysis within the kidney or lower urinary tract. Free hemoglobin in urine may also indicate transfusion reaction, hemolytic anemia, or paroxysmal hemoglobinuria. In addition, certain poisons or severe burns may be the cause for hemoglobinuria.

OCCULT BLOOD IN GASTRIC FLUID

In testing for the presence of occult blood in gastric fluids, medical practitioners have erroneously relied upon products designed for fecal occult blood testing or

Table 9 Interfering Substances for Detecting Gastric Occult Blood

Substance	Analytical cutoff in gastric fluid	Effect on test accuracy
High peroxidase foods	>0.2 units peroxidase as HRP	False positive
Iron and copper salts	>0.02 M	False positive
Antacids		
Mylanta II	>2 mL/dL	False negative
Maalox Plus	>5 mL/dL	False negative
Alternagel	>10 mL/dL	False negative
Riopan Plus	>10 mL/dL	False negative
Ascorbic acid	>250 mL/dL	False negative

urinary heme detection (53). These methods are subject to interference from low pH of the sample, certain ingested medications, and metal ions that are frequently present at widely varying concentrations in gastric fluid. Gastroccult (Beckman Coulter, Inc., Fullerton, CA), the first product designed specifically to test gastric fluid for occult blood and pH (in the same test) was introduced in 1982. When compared with other occult blood tests, the sensitivity of the Gastroccult method proved to be more useful in a clinical setting, based on the cutoff of the test (9,10,16). Classical guaiac-based chemistry tests are insensitive for detecting occult blood at low pH (pH <3). The sensitivity of the Gastroccult test is 30–50 μg blood/dL of gastric fluid (based on a normal hemoglobin level), over a range of pH from 1 to 9 (Table 9).

The gastric occult blood test was developed for use in the hospital emergency and intensive care units. Gastroccult is a rapid guaiac-based slide test used primarily to detect occult gastric bleeding due to trauma or deteriorating gastric condition (e.g., stress ulcer syndrome). The test is specially formulated and has the ability to buffer for low pH to accurately detect occult blood under these conditions. Standard fecal occult blood tests (e.g., Hemoccult) are not suitable for use with gastric specimens (54–56).

SUMMARY AND CONCLUSIONS

Occult blood tests are rapid, inexpensive and useful tools commonly used in a variety of practice settings. Their principal use is as "rule in" test methods that lead the physician to choose specific diagnostic pathways in the evaluation of patients who may be bleeding. In screening situations, the direct involvement of the patient and physician to prepare and test samples in a timely manner defines another essential characteristic of point-of-care methods. In acute care settings, the necessity for rapid turnaround times established FOBTs as one of the earliest point-of-care methods in medical practice (6,18).

Although these tests began to be commercialized and standardized by medical device manufacturers more than 50 yr ago, they have survived the test of time. This can be attributed to their simplicity, speed, ease of use, and low cost for the value of information they provide. The mercurial rate of growth of point-of-care technologies will inevitably lead to new advancements, some of which will be costly to develop and justify for routine use in this setting. Biosensors, polarography, and miniaturization of devices that make them highly portable, are but a few examples of this trend. All of this has forced the clinicial laboratorian and clinician to reorganize their thinking in matters that relate to better understanding the performance characteristics of the products being offered, choosing the correct product in the appropriate medical setting and paying very close attention to connectivity and patient management.

The FOBT, urinary occult blood test, and, more recently, the gastric occult blood test were developed at a time that preceded the avalanche of point-of-care tests for glucose, therapeutic drugs, drugs of abuse, coagulation, and metabolites. The occult blood tests met an important clinical need even before the technology explosion and still survive because they are clinically useful. Occult blood methods retain a place in point-of-care testing and are likely to continue in that position in the future until they can be replaced by new technologies that provide the same quality of information without incurring substantially higher costs.

REFERENCES

1. American Gastroenterological Association. Medical position statement: Evaluation and management of occult and obscure gastrointestinal bleeding. Gastroenterology 118:197–200, 2000.
2. Rockey DC. Occult gastrointestinal bleeding. N Engl J Med 341:38–46, 1999.
3. Morris DW, Hansell JR, Ostrow JE, Lee CS, Weigand P. Reliability of chemical tests for fecal occult blood in hospitalized patients. Dig Dis 21:845–852, 1976.
4. Barrison IG, Primavesi J, Gilmore IT, Littlewood ER, Sharples A, Parkins RA. Screening for occult gastrointestinal bleeding in hospital patients. Proc R Soc Med 74:41–43, 1981.
5. Eisner MS, Lewis JH. Dianostic yield of positive fecal occult blood test found on digital rectal examination. Does the finger count? Arch Intern Med 151:2180–2184, 1991.
6. Zuckerman GR, Prakash C, Askin MP, Lewis BS. AGA technical review on the evaluation and management of occult and obscure gastrointestinal bleeding. Gastroenterology 118:201–221, 2000.
7. Van Deen J. Tinctura Guaijaci und ein Ozonträgu, als Reagens auf sehr geringe

Blutmengen, namentlich in medico-forensischen Fallen. Arch Holländ beitr Natura Heilk 3:228–231, 1864.
8. Boas I. Uber okkulte Magenblutungen o. Dtsch Med Wochenschr 27:315–317, 1901.
9. Boas I. Die Phenophthalinprobe als Reagen auf okkulte Blutungen des magendarmkanals. Dtsch Med Wochenschr 37:63–64, 1911.
10. Irons GV, Kirsner JB. Routine chemical tests of the stool for occult blood: An evaluation. Am J Med Sci 249:247–260, 1965.
11. Ostrow DJ, Mulvaney CA, Hansell JR, Rhodes RS. Sensitivity and reproducibility of chemical tests for fecal occult blood with an emphasis on false-positive reactions. Am J Dig Dis 18:930–940, 1973.
12. Culver PJ. Examination of the stool. In: Page LB, Culver PJ (eds). A Syllabus of Laboratory Examinations in Clinical Diagnosis. Rev. Ed. Harvard University Press, Cambridge, MA, pp 377–378, 1961.
13. Ebaugh EG, Clemens T, Rodnar G, Peterson RE. Quantitative measurement of gastrointestinal blood loss. Am J Med 25:169–181, 1958.
14. Young GP, St John DJB. Selecting an occult blood test for use as a screening tool for large bowel cancer. Front Gastrointest Res 18:135–156, 1991.
15. Winawer SJ, Fletcher RH, Miller L, Godlee F, Stolar M, et al. Colorectal cancer screening: Clinical guidelines and rationale. Gastroenterology 112:594–642, 1997.
16. Ransohoff DF, Lang CA. Screening for colorectal cancer with the fecal occult blood test: A background paper. Ann Intern Med 126:811–822, 1997.
17. Sharma VK, Komanduri S, Nayyar S, Headly A, Modlinger P, Metz DC, Verghese VJ, Wanahita A, Go MF, Howden CW. An audit of the utility of in-patient fecal occult blood testing. Am J Gastroenterol 96:1256–1260, 2001.
18. Rozen P, Young GP, Levin B, Spann SJ. Colorectal cancer in clinical practice: Prevention, early detection and management. Martin Dunitz, London, 2002, pp 77–99, 115–129.
19. Greegor DH. Diagnosis of large-bowel cancer in the asymptomatic patient. JAMA 201:943–945, 1967.
20. Ransohoff DF, Lang CA. Suggested technique for fecal occult blood testing and interpretation in colorectal cancer screening. Ann Intern Med 126:808–810, 1997.
21. Ransohoff DF, Sandler RS. Screening for colorectal cancer. N Engl J Med 346:40–44, 2002.
22. McRae FA, St John DJB. Relationship between patterns of bleeding and Hemoccult sensitivity in patients with colorectal cancers or adenomas. Gastroenterology 82: 891–898, 1982.
23. Petty MT, Deacon MC, Alexeyeff MA, St John DJB, Young GP. Readability and sensitivity of a new faecal occult blood test in a hospital ward environment. Med J Aust 156:420–423, 1992.
24. Allison JE, Tekawa JS, Ransom LJ, Adrian AL. A comparison of fecal occult blood tests for colorectal cancer screening. N Engl J Med 334:144–159, 1996.
25. Church TR, Ederer F, Mandel JS. Fecal occult blood screening in the Minnesota study: Sensitivity of the screening test. J Nat Cancer Inst 89:1440–1448, 1997.
26. Hardcastle JD, Chamberlain JO, Robinson MHE, Moss SM, Amar SS, et al. Randomised controlled trial of faecal-occult-blood screening for colorectal cancer. Lancet 348:1472–1477, 1996.

27. Kronborg O, Fenger C, Olsen J, Jorgensen OD, Sondergaard O. Randomised study of screening for colorectal cancer with faecal-occult blood test. Lancet 348:1467–1471, 1996.
28. Jorgensen OD, Kronborg O, Fenger C. A randomised study of screening for colorectal cancer using faecal occult blood testing: Results after 13 years and seven biennial screening rounds. Gut 50:29–32, 2002.
29. Mandel JS, Bond JH, Church TR, Snover DC, Bradley GM, et al. Reducing mortality from colorectal cancer by screening for fecal occult blood. N Engl J Med 328:1365–1371, 1993.
30. Mandel JS, Church TR, Bond JH, Ederer F, Geisser MS, et al. The effect of fecal occult-blood screening on the incidence of colorectal cancer. N Engl J Med 343: 1603–1607, 2000.
31. Lang CA, Ransohoff DF. What can we conclude from the randomized controlled trials of fecal occult blood test screening? Eur J Gastroenterol Hepatol 10:199–204, 1998.
32. Rennert G, Rennert HS, Miron E, Peterburg Y. Population colorectal cancer screening with fecal occult blood test. Cancer Epidemiol Biomarkers Prevent 10:1165–1168, 2001.
33. Levin B, Hess K, Johnson C. Screening for colorectal cancer: A comparison of 3 fecal occult blood tests. Arch Intern Med 157:970–976, 1997.
34. St John DJB, Young GP, McHutchinson JG, Deacon MC, Alexeyeff MA. Comparison of the specificity and sensitivity of Hemoccult and HemoQuant in screening for colorectal neoplasia. Ann Intern Med 117:376–382, 1992.
35. Anderson GD, Yuellig TR, Krone RE. An investigation into the effects of oral iron supplementation on in vivo Hemoccult stool testing. Am J Gastroenterol 85:558–561, 1990.
36. Feinberg EJ, Steinberg WM, Banks BL, Henry JP. How long to abstain from eating red meat before fecal occult blood tests. Ann Intern Med 113:403–404, 1990.
37. Fleisher M. Problems and pitfalls in fecal occult blood testing. Primary Care Cancer 29–35, 1988.
38. Sinatra M, St John DJB, Young GP. Interference of plant peroxidases with guaiac-based fecal occult blood tests is avoidable. Clin Chem 45:123–126, 1999.
39. Rozen P, Knaani J. Samuel Z. Eliminating the need for dietary restrictions when using a sensitive guaiac fecal occult blood test. Dig Dis Sci 44:756–760, 1999.
40. Rozen P, Knaani J, Samuel Z. Comparative screening with a sensitive guaiac and specific immunochemical occult blood test with an endoscopy study. Cancer 89:46–52, 2000.
41. Schwartz S, Dahl J, Ellefson M, Ahlquist DA. The HemoQuant test: A specific and quantitative assay of heme (hemoglobin) in feces and other materials. Clin Chem 29:2061–2067, 1983.
42. Ahlquist DA, McGill DB, Schwartz S, Taylor WF, Owen RA. Fecal blood levels in health and disease. A study using HemoQuant. N Engl J Med 312:1422–1428, 1985.
43. Byers T, Levin B, Rothenberger D, Dodd GD, et al. American Cancer Society guidelines for screening and surveillance for early detection of colorectal polyps and cancer: Update 1997. CA 47:154–160, 1997.

44. Smith RA, Cokkinides V, von Eschenback AC, Levin B, et al. American Cancer Society guidelines for the early detection of cancer. CA 52:8, 2002
45. Fletcher RH, Colditz GA, Pawlson LG, Richman H, Rosenthal D, Salber PR. Screening for colorectal cancer: The business case. Am J Manag Care 8(6):531–538, 2002.
46. Guidelines for colorectal cancer screening and surveillance. Gastrointest Endosc 51: 777–782, 2000.
47. Winawer SJ. A quarter century of colorectal cancer screening: Progress and prospects. J Clin Oncol 19(suppl):6s–12s, 2001.
48. American Cancer Society. Colorectal Cancer Profiler [http://www.cancer.org]. February 5, 2002.
49. Paaso B. Community-based colorectal cancer screening: An essential part of wellness for asymptomatic patients. Point of Care 2002 1:20–27, 2002.
50. Tengs TO, Adams ME, Pliskin JS, Safran DG, Siegel JE, Weinstein MC, Graham JD. Five hundred life-saving interventions and their cost-effectiveness. Risk Anal 15:369–390, 1995.
51. Rowland RG, Garrett RA. Tumors of the urinary bladder. In: Conn HF, Conn RB (eds). Current Diagnosis. Saunders, Philadelphia, 1980, p 824.
52. Koss LG. Evaluation of hematuria (letter). JAMA 247:1274, 1982.
53. Rosenthal P, Thompson J, Singh M. Detection of occult blood in gastric juice. J Clin Gastroenterol 6:119–121, 1984.
54. Derrida S, Nury B, Slama R, Marois F, Moreau R, et al. Occult gastrointestinal bleeding in high-risk intensive care unit patients receiving antacid prophylaxis: Frequency and significance. Crit Care Med 17:122–125, 1989.
55. Eisenberg P. Monitoring gastric pH to prevent stress ulcer syndrome. Focus Crit Care 17:316–322, 1990.
56. Holman JS, Shwed JA. Influence of sucralfate on the detection of occult blood in simulated gastric fluid by two screening tests. Clin Pharm 11:625–627, 1992.

13
Hemoglobin and Coagulation

Gregory A. Nuttall and Paula Santrach
Mayo Clinic, Rochester, Minnesota, U.S.A.

INTRODUCTION

Over the last decade, point-of-care testing (POCT) has grown from a novelty to an accepted and commonly used tool in patient care. Assessment of coagulation is the second most common category of POCT performed in the United States, impacting both inpatients and outpatients in multiple medical situations and settings. Applications include assessment of hemostasis, diagnosis of abnormalities, monitoring of anticoagulation therapy, and guidance of transfusion therapy. Multiple outcome studies have been performed to assess the utility of this testing from both clinical and resource perspectives.

It is projected that by the year 2010 there will be large deficiencies in the American blood supply secondary to the aging of the American population (1). The National Blood Data Resource Center, in its *1998 Nationwide Blood Collection and Utilization Survey*, noted an alarming trend of decreasing numbers of blood donations and increasing numbers of blood transfusions (2). A large percentage of allogeneic blood is given to patients in the operating room, especially to cardiac surgery patients (3,4), with 20% of blood transfusion being thought to be inappropriate (5). Elective surgical procedures have already been delayed at many institutions throughout the United States due to shortages of blood products.

As will be shown below, use of point-of-care testing of hemoglobin and coagulation in transfusion algorithms is able to reduce blood transfusions. There have been multiple consensus conferences and specialty society task forces convened to publish recommendations for the transfusion of different blood components. These include those by the National Institutes of Health, the American College of Obstetricians and Gynecologists, the American Association of Blood

Banks, the American College of Physicians, the College of American Pathologists, and the American Society of Anesthesiologists. The most recent published recommendations for the transfusion of different blood components are the practice guidelines for blood component therapy reported by the American Society of Anesthesiologists task force on blood component therapy published in 1996 (6). All of these consensus conferences and specialty society task forces have advocated the use of coagulation tests to guide non–red blood cell and red blood cell transfusions, yet this still may not be commonly done. A major reason these tests are not done is the time it takes for the test results to become available. Point-of-care testing of hemoglobin and coagulation allows rapid test results to be available for clinical decision making.

Point-of-care testing of hemoglobin and coagulation is most useful in certain patient populations. These patient populations generally fall into those patients at high risk for transfusion, cardiac surgery, and liver transplant, and patients requiring anticoagulation therapy. This chapter is divided based upon those patient populations.

PREANALYTICAL ISSUES IN POINT-OF-CARE COAGULATION TESTING

Prior to the actual analysis, a number of factors can affect the results of coagulation testing. Such issues are critical for both test operators and clinicians to understand for accurate testing and interpretation. With POCT, the impact may be greater due to small sample sizes, alternative collection techniques, and a lack of familiarity with potential problems. The possible causes of variability in coagulation test results are as follows:

1. Biologic Variation

Patient-related factors can significantly influence test results: ongoing illness can alter the patient's baseline hemostatic function; patients with liver disease may appear hypocoaguable; and cancer can induce a hypercoaguable state. Acute illness can also have an impact. Both diet and medications can influence hemostasis, which is particularly important in patients on anticoagulation therapy with warfarin.

2. Sample Variation

In the laboratory, citrated plasma is the specimen of choice for most coagulation-based testing. However, in POCT, fresh or citrated whole blood is much more commonly used. Fresh blood requires rapid initiation of testing for accuracy.

With citrated samples, the volume of specimen in relation to the amount of citrate present in the collection tube is very important; significant alterations in the blood/anticoagulant ratio can markedly affect results. Results from whole blood specimens are often different from those when plasma samples are tested. Collection techniques also play an important role: capillary specimens are subject to technique variability; specimens collected from indwelling catheters may be contaminated by flush solution; and difficulty with venous or arterial collection may result in premature activation of the coagulation system. Sample size is also important in relation to the amount of reagent in the test cartridge. Specimens that are too large or too small can produce inaccurate results.

3. Reagent and Instrument Variation

Different reagents may be used to perform the same test and these reagents may have varying sensitivities to factor deficiency and anticoagulant effect. Furthermore, each reagent–instrument combination can produce somewhat different results and standardization is typically not possible. As a result, tests from POCT and from the laboratory do not match. Therefore, clinical decision points must be validated for the test method to be used. Providers must be aware of the appropriate decision points and maintain consistency in testing (POCT or laboratory) in order to avoid confusion.

4. Nontraditional Test Operators

With POCT, test operators are typically physicians, nurses, perfusionists, and other allied healthcare personnel who are not familiar with the impact of preanalytical variables. With multiple operators, there may also be significant variations in technique, particularly if testing is infrequent. Therefore, training and ongoing competency assessment of test operators is crucial.

PATIENTS REQUIRING HEART SURGERY ANDCARDIOPULMONARY BYPASS

Excessive bleeding following cardiopulmonary bypass (CPB) is one of the most common complications of cardiac surgery, which has important health and economic consequences (5,7). Bleeding following cardiac surgery can have multiple etiologies (8). Extracorporeal circulation and heparinization may induce many abnormalities in the coagulation system, including thrombocytopenia (9), platelet dysfunction (10,11), coagulation factor deficiencies (12), residual heparin following protamine administration (13), and fibrinolysis (14). Insufficient surgical hemostasis also is an important cause of bleeding following CPB. The multifactorial nature of coagulation disorders following CPB complicates the decision of what therapeutic treatment is needed. The absence or delay of available laboratory data further complicates the decision of what therapeutic treatment is needed. Therefore, the treatment of excessive bleeding following CPB is often nonspecific and constitutes the transfusion of multiple types of blood products simultaneously (e.g., additional protamine, platelet concentrates and fresh frozen plasma and possibly cryoprecipitate).

Inappropriate use of blood products in cardiac surgical patients has important adverse health and economic consequences, and national practice guidelines have been published (5,15–17). Excessive bleeding following CPB remains an important cause of patient morbidity and increased mortality and hospital costs in those patients who require surgical re-exploration of the thorax for excessive bleeding (18,19). Excessive hemorrhage results in the transfusion of allogeneic blood products, which may expose the patient to additional risks (AIDS, hepatitis, and transfusion reactions) (20,21) and increased expense. There is large variability among institutions in transfusion behavior for cardiac surgery patients (3,4). Educational outreach has improved transfusion practice in surgery, and the decision to transfuse blood should be made with relevant laboratory data (16,22).

The cardiac surgical patient population is a large user of allogeneic blood transfusions. It has been estimated that in the year 2000, approximately 500,000 patients in the United States would undergo cardiac surgery employing CPB (23). The majority of these patients (65–75%) would be transfused with allogeneic blood (3). Between 10 and 20% of the approximately 12 million units of red blood cells transfused in the United States annually are to cardiac surgical patients at a direct societal cost of 0.2–0.4 billion dollars (1,24). About 50% of the over 7 million units of platelets transfused annually are to patients undergoing cardiac surgery (25). The use of platelet transfusion continues to grow, placing accelerated demands on the banked blood supply (26). Despite advances in clinical and laboratory sciences over the past three decades, approximately 47% of platelets, 32% of fresh frozen plasma, and 15% of red blood cells are inappropriately transfused (5). Clinicians are limited in their ability to predict excessive bleeding following CPB and identify patients who will require blood transfusion.

Anticoagulation

Heparin

Systemic anticoagulation is required for CPB to prevent thrombus formation within the cardiopulmonary bypass pump. Unfractionated heparin is the preferred anticoagulant. Inhibition of thrombin and clot formation during cardiopulmonary bypass is the foremost function of heparin anticoagulation for CPB. Unfractionated heparin is composed of a heterogenous group of polysaccharides. A unique pentosaccharide sequence of heparin interacts with the serine protease enzyme antithrombin III (ATIII) (27). The interaction of heparin with ATIII enhances the anticoagulant activity of ATIII. The activated ATIII binds to thrombin (factor II), factor IX, and factor X and inhibits their activity. Thrombin is the key element in the coagulation amplification process, resulting in fibrin generation as well as activation of platelets and fibrinolysis. Despite heparin therapy during CPB, thrombin is continuously generated during CPB (28). Thrombin formation stimulates consumption of hemostatic components that increase the risk of coagulopathy, excessive bleeding, and perioperative allogeneic blood transfusion.

In 1975, Bull et al. (29,30) introduced the activated clotting time (ACT) as a simple and safe point-of-care method for anticoagulation monitoring of unfractionated heparin therapy during CPB. A baseline ACT is measured. Following heparin administration, usually intravenous 300 units/kg, an ACT is obtained to determine if anticoagulation is adequate for commencement of CPB. Additional heparin is given to maintain the ACT at or above a certain value during CPB, usually 450 sec. Culliford et al. along with others have shown that factors other than plasma heparin concentration have an influence on the ACT during CPB. These other factors are principally hypothermia and hemodilution (31). Because the ACT prolongation during cardiopulmonary bypass could be partially attributed to these and other factors, some have suggested directed monitoring of blood heparin concentration during CPB.

The credibility of the "safe" ACT for anticoagulation during CPB was challenged when Young et al. (32) demonstrated the presence of fibrin monomer in animals with "safe" ACT values during CPB even though clot was not identified in the CPB circuit. This has been confirmed recently (33). Inadequate anticoagulation even on a subclinical level increases the likelihood of coagulopathy after CPB (28). Subsequently, the merits of the ACT versus heparin concentration to monitor the adequacy of anticoagulation during CPB in relation to bleeding and transfusion are important considerations.

The Hepcon (Medtronic Blood Management, Parker, CO) is a point-of-care monitoring device that generates both ACT and an accurate whole blood heparin concentration measurement via an automated protamine titration method (31). In 1990, Gravlee et al. (34) compared standard heparin dosing and ACT monitoring to heparin dosing with heparin concentration using the Hepcon in a randomized trial of 21 cardiac surgical patients. Patients managed with heparin concentration received the largest amount of heparin and had the highest postoperative blood loss. But in a subsequent study of 63 adults undergoing cardiac surgery, Gravlee et al. (35) concluded that heparin dosing and heparin concentration monitoring did not significantly influence postoperative blood loss or transfusion requirements. In 1995, Jobes et al. (36) found the 24-hr mediastinal chest tube drainage (MCTD) and transfusion requirements were less in the heparin concentration group concluding that it was responsible for improved hemostasis in cardiac surgical patients. However, heparin concentration monitoring only identifies the amount of heparin in the blood, but it does not reflect the extent of anticoagulation (28). As noted above, the anticoagulant activity of heparin is mediated by ATIII. Patients can develop an acquired ATIII deficiency through prior heparin, nitroglycerin, or intraaortic balloon pump use (37). Patients also can rarely have a genetic deficiency of ATIII. In all these patients, heparin concentration may not reflect the extent of anticoagulation.

Currently, it is possible to determine a patient's "in vivo thrombin activity" by performing a heparin dose response (HDR) to identify a *specific* heparin concentration that will achieve "adequate anticoagulation." Despotis et al. (38) randomized 254 patients requiring CPB to either a fixed dose of 250 units/kg of heparin or a treatment group with an initial heparin dose based on an automated HDR and heparin concentration. The heparin concentration group had significantly lower fresh frozen plasma (FFP) and platelet transfusions than control patients but the first 8- and 24-hr MCTD in the intensive care unit (ICU) was similar. Control patients had indirect evidence of increased clotting factor consumption.

Hirudin

Heparin-induced thrombocytopenia with thrombosis (HITT) type II is a life-threatening complication of heparin therapy that most often occurs after 5–10 days of exposure to heparin (39). It is produced by an antiheparin immunoglobulin (Ig)G in plasma that binds to repeating antigenic determinants of heparin and to the platelet surface epitopes, heparin bound to platelet factor 4 (PF4) (40). After antiheparin IgG binding to the heparin-PF4 complex, the platelets become activated and aggregate. The platelets are progressively consumed in the formation of disseminated thromboses and embolism, which can result in limb and organ ischemia (41).

The incidence of HITT type II in cardiac surgery patients is estimated to be 1.3% (42). The appearance of antibodies, platelet factor 4 complex ELISA, is more frequent (43). If HITT type II develops after cardiac surgery, 51% of patients develop thromboembolic complications with a lethality of 37% (42). Therefore, heparin administration in any form should be avoided in patients with documented HITT type II.

This is a big problem for patients with HITT type II being prepared for cardiac surgery with CPB. Systemic anticoagulation is required for CPB and heparin is the preferred anticoagulant. The U.S. Food and Drug Administration (FDA) has approved recombinant hirudin (Lepirudin) for anticoagulation in patients with documented HITT type II. Hirudin is an extremely potent and specific inhibitor of thrombin, which is a small protein (65 amino acids) originally isolated from the salivary glands of the medicinal leech but now produced by genetic engineering methods (44).

Hirudin can be used as the anticoagulant for CPB, but the appropriate dose to be given and how the anticoagulant effect of hirudin should be monitored are not fully standardized.

Suggested hirudin dosing for CPB has been devised by Koster et al. (39) and shown to be effective:

- 0.25 mg/kg hirudin bolus prior to CPB
- 0.20 mg/kg in CPB pump prime
- continuous infusion 0.5 mg/min following bolus and throughout CPB

There also is an effective point-of-care test to measure hirudin levels during CPB based upon the FDA-approved coagulation device called the Thrombolytic Assessment System (TAS). The test cartridge for the TAS that measures hirudin levels is the ecarin clotting time (ECT) (39). The ECT cartridge has recently received a humane device exemption (HDE) from the FDA (HDE—h9900012). Prior to CPB, an in-vitro titration of hirudin using the patient's blood should be performed to develop a titration curve for the ECT test's response to various hirudin concentrations.

The ECT results are available in 5 min. Koster et al. (45) reported on 57 patients with HITT type II who underwent cardiopulmonary bypass using hirudin and the ECT point-of-care test. All the patients did well except for four patients who had renal insufficiency and developed excessive bleeding and three patients who died of complications unrelated to the perioperative anticoagulation management.

Hemostasis Following Cardiopulmonary Bypass

As noted above, there are multiple possible causes for excessive bleeding following cardiac surgery with CPB. The use of cardiopulmonary bypass and heparinization may induce many abnormalities in the coagulation system. Insufficient surgical hemostasis also is an important cause of bleeding following CPB. The absence or delay of available laboratory data further complicates the decision of what therapeutic treatment is needed. Therefore, the treatment of excessive bleeding following CPB is often nonspecific and constitutes the transfusion of multiple types of blood products simultaneously (e.g., additional protamine, platelet concentrates and fresh frozen plasma and possibly cryoprecipitate).

There have been several prospective randomized studies that have documented a reduction in the use of allogeneic blood transfusions in cardiac surgery patients with the institution of point-of-care coagulation test–based transfusion algorithms. Despotis et al. (46) found that using the routine coagulation test, platelet count, with a whole blood point-of-care prothrombin time (PT) and activated partial thromboplastin time (aPTT) from a Biotrack 512 coagulation monitor to guide therapy and treatment of microvascular (nonsurgical) bleeding was effective in reducing allogeneic blood product transfusion. In the above randomized and controlled study, cardiac surgical patients determined to have "microvascular" bleeding at the cessation of CPB were assigned to algorithm driven ($n = 30$) or standard ($n = 36$) transfusion therapy. The algorithm to guide transfusion therapy utilized platelet counts <50,000, 50,000–100,000, and >100,000 to guide platelet transfusion therapy, and PT and APTT values greater than 1.5 or 1.8 times control to guide fresh frozen plasma (FFP) transfusion. The algorithm treatment patients received fewer allogeneic hemostatic blood component units ($p = 0.008$) and had fewer total donor exposures ($p = 0.007$) during the entire hospitalization period. They also documented a reduction in blood loss in the ICU following the use of the algorithm in the operating room compared with the standard therapy group. They found that the more directed transfusion therapy may have resulted in less dilution of needed blood factors by unnecessary transfusions, which resulted in reduced bleeding in the ICU.

A prospective randomized study by Shore-Lesserson et al. (47) found a reduction in chest-tube blood loss and transfusion requirements in the ICU for patients whose blood transfusions were guided by a thromboelastograph (TEG)-based algorithm compared with those patients whose blood transfusions were guided by standard coagulation tests in the operating room. There were no differences in blood transfusion requirements in the operating room. The TEG is a viscoelastic test that measures the change in the physical properties of whole blood with clot formation. The TEG assesses clot function from the time of initial clot formation with fibrin formation and platelet aggregation until clot lysis. The entire life of the clot is reflected in a gross manner, without clear delineation of the individual inputs of each component of the coagulation system. The strength of the clot is reflected on the recording as a symmetric deviation from the centerline and standard parameters may be measured from the recording. The five parameters most frequently discussed in the literature are, R, $R+K$, *alpha*, *MA*, and A_{60}. The R value is the time from sample placement until initial pen deflection, and the $R+K$ is the time from initial sample placement until the pen is deflected 20 mm. *Alpha* is the angle formed by the tangent of the tracing's amplitude at the initial pen deflection. The *MA* is the maximal amplitude of the deflection, and the A_{60} is the amplitude of the tracing 60 min following the *MA*. The five TEG parameters are not independent variables. They are interdependent, and a change in one aspect of the coagulation system frequently effects many of the variables. The two most important variables affecting clot strength, and the subsequent *MA* of the TEG tracing, are the fibrinogen concentration and the platelet function and count. There are several activators, such as tissue factor and celite, that are sometimes added to the whole blood to speed the time to TEG results.

A retrospective study by Spiess et al. (48) found that after institution of TEG-guided coagulation studies in the perioperative period, there was a significant reduction in number of blood transfusions and the incidence of mediastinal re-exploration for hemorrhage in cardiac surgery patients.

Nuttall et al. (49) performed a randomized prospective trial of allogeneic blood use comparing standard transfusion practice with a new transfusion algorithm in 92 adult patients with excessive bleeding following CPB. At enrollment, the participants were randomized to one of two groups: a control group (clinical judgment) group and an algorithm group. Once it was determined on clinical grounds that the patient was bleeding excessively, their transfusion therapy was determined by their group designation. There were no differences between the groups in demographic or surgical variables. The algorithm group had transfusion therapy guided by the 512-coagulation monitor PT and aPTT, platelet count, TEG *MA*, and fibrinogen concentration. The algorithm group received less allogeneic fresh frozen plasma in the operating room (OR) following CPB median (range) 0 (0, 7) units than the control group 3 (0, 10) units ($p = 0.0002$). The median (range) platelet transfusions in the OR following CPB was 4 (0, 12) in the algorithm group compared with 6 (0, 18) units in the control group ($p = 0.0001$). Blood loss in the ICU was significantly less in the algorithm group. The control group also had a significantly greater incidence of surgical re-exploration of the mediastinum for bleeding.

LIVER TRANSPLANT PATIENTS

Liver transplant has become an important therapy for patients with end-stage liver disease. Massive blood loss associated with the liver transplantation is a major clinical problem with the procedure (50). End-stage liver disease is associated with almost complete disarray of the procoagulant and anticoagulant proteins. The liver produces most of the blood coagulation factor proteins, and deficiencies of these factors in patients in end-stage liver disease results in prolonged prothrombin times and activated partial thromboplastin times (51). End-stage liver disease patients also frequently have thrombocytopenia secondary to gastrointestinal bleeding, malnutrition, and splenomegaly. Despite aggressive medical management, it is frequently impossible to normalize hemostasis prior to liver transplantation. Most liver transplant patients also have numerous collateral vessels and portal hypertension along with capillary fragility that result in large difficulties in surgical hemostasis. This population's bleeding problems are further complicated by dilutional coagulopathy secondary to massive blood transfusion with hypofibrinogenemia and thrombocytopenia. Fibrinolysis develops in the majority of patients during the anhepatic phase of the surgery and increases on reperfusion of the homograph liver, resulting in consumption of coagulation factors.

The severe coagulopathy associated with liver transplantation is usually treated with a combination of drug and blood transfusion therapy (52). This drug and blood transfusion therapy is guided by clinical coagulation test monitoring of coagulation at many institutions. The type of clinical coagulation monitoring used is controversial. Many institutions use coagulation profiles consisting of PT, aPTT, fibrinogen level, fibrinogen degradation products (FDP), and platelet count. At other centers, TEG is used. Despite the severe abnormalities associated with end-stage liver disease documented above, the results of extensive preoperative coagulation tests, such as the PT, aPTT, fibrinogen level, FDP, antithrombin III concentrations, thrombin time, and platelet count, have not been found to have predictive value for intraoperative bleeding. There is evidence that use of coagulation tests intraoperatively to guide transfusion and drug therapy is useful.

Kang et al. (53) performed a prospective observational study of 66 consecutive patients undergoing liver transplants who were monitored by TEG and analytic coagulation profile. The analytic coagulation profile consisted of PT; aPTT; thrombin time; reptilase lysis; factor levels for I, II, V, VII, VIII, IX, X, XI, and XII; fibrin degradation product level; euglobulin lysis time; and platelet count. There was a significant correlation between the TEG *R* time and aPTT, the TEG *MA* with the platelet count and fibrinogen concentration, and the TEG whole blood lysis time with euglobulin lysis time. They compared the transfusion requirements of TEG-monitored patients in their study with patients who were unmonitored prior to their study. They noted that those patients in the TEG-monitored group received less red blood cells, 17 ± 12.5 units, than the nonmonitored group, 26.7 ± 23.8 units ($p < 0.05$). The TEG-monitored group also received significantly less fresh frozen plasma and total fluids infused (both $p < 0.05$) than the unmonitored group. A confounding factor was that the monitored group received significantly greater amounts of platelet and cryoprecipitate transfusions than the unmonitored group and there was no difference in total number of different blood transfusions between the groups.

Plevak et al. (54) reported a prospective randomized trial of 49 liver transplant patients comparing TEG-guided versus "conventional" guided transfusion therapy for the first 24 hr after liver transplantation. The conventional laboratory tests consisted of PT, aPTT, fibrinogen, and platelet count. They found statistically significant reductions in fresh frozen plasma, cryoprecipitate, and total donor exposures to blood products with the use of TEG transfusion guidance. They also noted a statistically significant reduction in cost associated with TEG transfusion guidance. Larger prospective randomized trials of POCT coagulation used to guide transfusion therapy in this population would be useful. There is evidence that excessive transfusion of blood products to liver transplant patients results in lower patient survival rates (55).

Isovolemic Hemodilution

Acute isovolemic hemodilution involves the acute intraoperative withdrawal of blood with simultaneous infusion of crystalloid or colloid to achieve isovolemic filling of the heart. This blood is then stored and re-infused during the large blood loss part of the operation. The purpose of acute isovolemic hemodilution is to reduce transfusion of allogeneic red blood cells by decreasing the hemoglobin content of the blood shed during the surgical procedure. The use of acute isovolemic hemodilution is controversial and it is relatively underutilized.

Acute isovolemic hemodilution has been used successfully to decrease the number of allogeneic blood transfusions in cardiac, vascular, hepatic, spinal, and prostate surgery (56,57). The average blood savings have been between 1.5 to 3.5 units or 500–1200 mL of allogeneic blood transfusions. Use of POCT hemoglobin monitoring is very useful to accomplish acute isovolemic hemodilution, to prevent excessively low hematocrits, and to fine-tune the volume of blood withdrawn.

TRAUMA PATIENTS

Severe trauma is frequently associated with large, rapid losses of blood through hemorrhage. Infusions of crystalloid or colloid solutions are usually used as first-line agents to achieve isovolemic filling of the heart. Red blood cell infusions are also frequently needed to maintain hemoglobin concentrations for oxygen transport. Hemostasis may be compromised secondary to the large volumes of fluid and red blood cells infused, lack of primary hemostasis from bleeding vessels, hypothermia, and concomitant disease states. Therefore, infusions of non–red blood cell blood products are also frequent. A system for rapid interrogation of the patient's hemoglobin and coagulation function would be very useful and POCT hemoglobin and coagulation tests would be very useful in this population. Unfortunately, there are very few studies in this patient population.

PATIENTS UNDERGOING CARDIAC CATHETERIZATION

Cardiac catheterization requires systemic anticoagulation to prevent intracoronary thrombosis during the procedure. The standard anticoagulant is unfractionated heparin and monitoring is done at the point of care utilizing the activated clotting time (ACT). Because the procedures tend to be shorter than cardiopulmonary bypass and there is no extracorporeal circuit, less intense anticoagulation is acceptable. The optimal level of heparinization is somewhat controversial. In most circumstances, an initial bolus of heparin (10,000 units or 100 units/kg) is followed by an infusion to keep the ACT >300 sec (58,59). Protection against postprocedural ischemia seems to be optimal with an ACT of 350–375 sec according to a recent study (60). However, other investigators have had success with only a 2500 unit bolus and an average ACT of 185 seconds (61). Regardless of which protocol is selected, the decision points should be validated for the particular ACT test system in use as the results may vary depending on the nature of the reagent (kaolin versus celite) and the instrument (60,62,63).

At the conclusion of the procedure, protamine reversal is usually not performed. The femoral sheath is left in place until anticoagulation has diminished as indicated by an ACT of <180 sec. Femoral hematomas may still occur because the standard ACT is not sensitive to low levels of heparin (<1 unit/mL). So some investigators have utilized either a point-of-care aPTT or an ACT modified to be more heparin sensitive. Another important aspect of hemostasis assessment in cardiac catheterization patients is platelet function. For many years, aspirin therapy has been used as a means to inhibit platelet function and thereby prevent acute coronary thrombosis. Newer agents, such as ticlopidine and clopidogrel, are also effective in this regard. Another class of therapeutics, the platelet glycoprotein IIb/IIIa inhibitors (abciximab, eptifibatide, and tirofiban), is now being used routinely to prevent recurrent ischemic events after percutaneous coronary revascularization with or without stent placement. Glycoprotein IIb/IIIa is the platelet receptor for fibrinogen; receptor blockade prevents the binding of fibrinogen and thus clot formation beyond initial platelet aggregation. Although these agents have been shown to be effective (64,65), questions remain about the degree of inhibition that is required for a good clinical outcome with minimal risk of hemorrhagic events (66). A number of platelet function tests have been studied, but their clinical utility has not been firmly established. The Platelet Function Analyzer (PFA-100) (Dade Behring, Miami, FL) is an in vitro simulation of the bleeding time; it uses high shear rates of whole blood through an aperture coated with collagen and other agonists to stimulate clotting. This test is significantly prolonged during IIb/IIIa inhibition therapy, but may be too sensitive for routine use (67,68). The Clot Signature Analyzer (CSA) (Xylum Corp., San Diego, CA) also tries to replicate the bleeding time through a different methodology. Although it too is responsive to inhibitor agents (69), the CSA is not FDA-cleared for clinical use. The Rapid Platelet Function Assay (RPFA Ultegra) (Accumetrics Inc., San Diego, CA) is the most widely studied test method. This assay directly measures platelet agglutination resulting from activation of the IIb/IIIa receptors and shows a dose-dependent decrease in agglutination during inhibitor therapy (69,70). The results of this assay correlate highly with both standard platelet aggregation tests ($r = 0.98$) and the percentage of unblocked glycoprotein IIb/IIIa ($r = 0.96$) (71). Recently, Steinhubl et al. (72) have shown that the level of platelet function inhibition varies both among patients and by agent used. Tirofiban and eptifibatide demonstrate a different inhibition profile as compared with abciximab. Their work suggests that the degree of platelet inhibition, as measured by the RPFA at 10 min after the start of therapy, is significantly associated with the likelihood of a major cardiac adverse event within 7 days of the catheterization procedure.

The challenge with assessment of platelet inhibition therapy is the complexity of platelet function and the multiplicity of tests, both currently available and in development, that try to reflect such complexity. There may be no single test that is universally helpful. More likely, specific therapies and tests will need to be matched to best determine the clinical utility under various clinical situations. Much work remains to be done.

PATIENTS UNDERGOING HEMODIALYSIS

Hemodialysis for acute and chronic renal failure requires anticoagulation in order to prevent clotting of the extracorporeal circuit during the procedure. However, the balance between thrombosis and hemorrhage during anticoagulation can be challenging in these patients. Uremia typically results in an underlying coagulopathy that appears related to platelet dysfunction. Risk of thrombosis, particularly of the vascular access, is also significant. The choice of anticoagulant and the subsequent monitoring strategy depends on the nature of the dialysis technique used and the patient's underlying medical condition, particularly in regard to their risk of hemorrhage.

The most common choice of anticoagulant is unfractionated heparin, administered as a bolus followed by a continuous infusion or as intermittent dosing. This therapy is typically monitored using the activated clotting time; one source suggests that adequate anticoagulation is achieved when the ACT is prolonged 140–180% of the baseline (73). The prolongation may be reduced to 125–150% for patients at increased risk of hemorrhage. The ACT test systems do vary in their sensitivity to heparin and the formulation of their reagents for dialysis applications. Monitoring has also been performed with a POC aPTT method showing good correlation with the laboratory aPTT and using a 1.5–3.5 time prolongation compared with baseline (74). Harenberg et al. (75) utilized a whole blood clotting assay for anti-Xa activity to monitor heparin anticoagulation during dialysis. No matter what monitoring method is chosen, the circuit is also routinely assessed for clinical evidence of clotting.

Patients with an increased risk of hemorrhage may require an alternative anticoagulation protocol for hemodialysis. High-flow-rate hemodialysis has been performed without any anticoagulation. Low doses of unfractionated heparin or regional citrate anticoagulation may also be employed. Both low-molecular-weight heparins (enoxaparin, etc.) (76) and heparinoids (danaparoid) (77) can be used; these drugs are typically given as a single bolus dose prior to the procedure and may be monitored using an anti-Xa assay or by observation of clot formation in the circuit. Recently, there have been reports of the use of lepirudin as a dialysis anticoagulant in patients with heparin-induced thrombocytopenia (78–80).

PATIENTS WITH OR AT RISK OF THROMBOEMBOLIC DISEASE

Anticoagulation is the primary therapy for patients with venous thrombosis or embolism. Patients are initially given a bolus of unfractionated heparin followed by a continuous infusion. Heparin is used because of its rapid onset of action and studies have shown that patients have a lower risk of recurrence if they reach a therapeutic level of anticoagulation quickly (81). On the other hand, excessive dosing can result in a significant risk of hemorrhage. Furthermore, patients vary in their responsiveness to heparin, and heparin preparations differ in their effect, which adds to the complexity of this therapy.

There are two approaches to heparin dosing. Traditionally, patients have been given a fixed bolus of heparin (5–10,000 units) and a standard continuous infusion. Periodic aPTT measurements are used for monitoring and dose adjustments; the goal is an aPTT ratio (patient value/normal control value) of at least 1.5. Recently, weight-based nomograms have become more widely used. Under these protocols, the bolus and infusion doses are determined by the patient's weight. A very specific algorithm for dose adjustment based on aPTT results is also used. Multiple studies have shown better patient outcomes with the nomogram approach as compared with a fixed dosing schedule (82–90): the time to a therapeutic level was shorter, the risk of thrombotic recurrence was decreased, and the risk of hemorrhage was the same.

The potential problem with these algorithms is the use of the aPTT result to guide therapy. It is well known that aPTT reagents differ significantly in their responsiveness to heparin; thus, two different assays may give different aPTT results for the same patient sample. The algorithms typically have very specific aPTT ranges for therapeutic action, which is applicable to the authors' institution but may not be relevant for other facilities. Thus, each program must confirm the clinical decision points based on their own aPTT test system since no standardization is available. Because of these problems with the aPTT, some investigators recommend that heparin levels be measured instead (91,92). Either anti-Xa or protamine titration methods may be used, but again, they do not give the same results. The therapeutic range for the anti-Xa method is 0.3–0.7 units/mL; for the protamine titration assay, it is 0.2–0.4 units/mL (93).

What is the role of point-of-care testing in heparin monitoring for thromboembolic disease? Point-of-care devices that measure the aPTT exist and are subject to the same variability in terms of responsiveness to heparin. Therefore, validation of dosing algorithms should be performed for these devices and one method should be consistently used for dosing decisions to avoid confusion (94). One study compared the use of point-of-care aPTT results versus those from the laboratory in 33 patients undergoing active heparinization (95). The time from test completion to dose adjustment and the time to achievement of therapeutic aPTTs were both significantly decreased with point-of-care testing (14.5 min versus 3.0 hr, $p < 0.001$ and 8.2 versus 18.1 hr, $p < 0.005$, respectively). Similarly improved intermediate outcomes have been seen in multicenter trials as well (96,97).

Long-term anticoagulation for patients at risk of thromboembolism is accomplished with warfarin therapy. Since its mechanism of action is the antagonism of vitamin K, patients on warfarin have significantly decreased levels of factors II, VII, IX, and X. This effect is best monitored by measurement of the prothrombin time. As with other coagulation test reagents, the thromboplastins for the PT have variable sensitivities to decreases in the vitamin K-dependent factors. To overcome these differences, each reagent preparation is compared with a known reference reagent and an International Sensitivity Index (ISI) is determined. The ISI is then used in the following formula to calculate the International Normalized Ratio (INR):

$$\text{INR} = (\text{patient PT/mean normal PT})^{\text{ISI}}$$

Thus, for each patient, the PT result is converted to an INR result, which is intended to be comparable among different reagents. The INR has become the standard for monitoring of warfarin anticoagulation.

Although the INR is intended to standardize results across different reagent–instrument systems, it is by no means perfect. Measurement of the INR is less accurate in patients at the start of warfarin treatment; it was designed primarily for use during stable, long-term anticoagulation. The INR may also be inaccurate when reagents with high ISIs are used or when the ISI has not been calculated correctly by the manufacturer. The inability of the INR to eliminate method-based differences in results has been documented by Davis et al. (98). Another study (99) compared the INR results from three different laboratories and two POC devices in 41 patients. Although correlations coefficients were high, the results from one laboratory and one POC device were significantly different from the others. They estimated that a change of therapy might result just because of these intermethod differences, 10–30% of the time. Therefore, intermethod variability continues to exist and consistent use of a single method to monitor the patient over time is highly recommended.

Warfarin anticoagulation is indicated for patients with venous thromboembolism and artificial heart valves. It is also given to prevent thrombosis and embolism in patients with acute myocardial infarction, valvular heart disease, and atrial fibrillation. The therapeutic range for the INR is typically 2.0–3.0 with higher levels for patients with mechanical heart valves (INR 2.5–3.5) (100). Time spent in this therapeutic range is an important indicator of patient outcome. In patients with atrial fibrillation, the risk of stroke significantly increases below an INR of 2; the odds ratio for stroke is 3.3 at an INR of 1.5 according to one study (101). On the other hand, Hylek and Singer (102) have shown that the risk of intracranial hemorrhage dramatically rises above an INR of 4. Other outcome measures include the rates of both thromboembolic and bleeding events.

Usual care of patients on warfarin involves periodic visits (monthly or so) to their primary physicians who measure the INR and make dosage decisions on the basis of the test result and the patient's condition. Consideration of the patient's diet, medications, and concurrent illnesses is an important aspect of the decision-making process as each can significantly affect the INR. Although this practice model is common, the use of specialized anticoagulation clinics is becoming more widely accepted (103–107). In this model, the patient is seen periodically by a team of providers (physicians, nurses, and pharmacists) who specialize in anticoagulation therapy. The INR testing is performed rapidly either by the laboratory or with a point-of-care device; dosing advice is given to the patient during the clinic visit. This specialized approach has resulted in better patient outcomes as measured by time spent in the therapeutic range and by the incidence of adverse events (104–108); significant cost savings have also been realized in some studies (105–107,109).

Improved outcomes have also been documented in multiple studies evaluating the clinical utility of patient self-testing for the INR. Currently, there are at least two point-of-care instruments for measuring the INR that are cleared of home use. In this practice model, the patient performs the INR test at home, often on a weekly basis. In some programs, the patients are given algorithms to follow for dose adjustments; for other programs, the results are reported to the healthcare provider who then advises the patient. Patients are still seen in the clinic setting but on a less frequent basis. For most patients, their INRs are more often in the therapeutic range and their complication rate is lower. In six randomized control trials (110–115), the time spent in the therapeutic range significantly increased by 6–24%. Carefully selected patients have been shown to be competent in test performance and in algorithm-guided decision making (116–118). Although patient self-management tends to increase the cost of medical care, the cost to the patient is lower resulting in less overall cost (119). And when the rate of adverse events is considered, patient self-management appears to be cost saving. Given these positive outcomes, the Center for Medicare and Medicaid Services in the

United States has recently decided to provide reimbursement for this approach in patients with mechanical heart valves.

Short-term prophylaxis for thromboembolism is administered to at-risk patients after certain surgical procedures such as hip replacement. Subcutaneous heparin and low-molecular-weight heparins are typically utilized in these situations; ongoing monitoring is usually not performed. Patients with heparin-induced thrombocytopenia and thrombosis, as described previously, are anticoagulated with hirudin. In these circumstances, the aPTT is used to monitor therapy.

CONCLUSION

Point-of-care coagulation testing has numerous applications in patient care, predominantly in the cardiovascular arena. Also, in many cases, outcome studies have been able to document clinical utility despite increased test costs. At the same time, these tests are subject to more variability due to methodological differences, preanalytic specimen collection/handling, and nontraditional operators. Therefore, validation of test performance, clinical decision points, and operator competency are crucial to the effective implementation of these tests.

REFERENCES

1. Vamvakas EC, Taswell HF. Epidemiology of blood transfusion. Transfusion 34: 464–470, 1994.
2. National Blood Data Resource Center. Blood collections continue to decline. American Association of Blood Banks, Bethesda, 1999, p 9.
3. Goodnough LT, Johnston MF, Toy PT. The variability of transfusion practice in coronary artery bypass surgery. Transfusion Medicine Academic Award Group. JAMA 265:86–90, 1991.
4. Stover EP, Siegel LC, Parks R, Levin J, Body SC, Maddi R, D'Ambra MN, Mangano DT, Spiess BD. Variability in transfusion practice for coronary artery bypass surgery persists despite national consensus guidelines: A 24-institution study. Institutions of the Multicenter Study of Perioperative Ischemia Research Group. Anesthesiology 88:327–333, 1998.
5. Goodnough LT, Soegiarso RW, Birkmeyer JD, Welch HG. Economic impact of inappropriate blood transfusions in coronary artery bypass graft surgery. Am J Med 94:509–514, 1993.
6. American Society of Anesthesiologists Task Force on Blood Component Therapy. Practice guidelines for blood component therapy. Anesthesiology 84:732–747, 1996.
7. Munoz JJ, Birkmeyer NJ, Birkmeyer JD, O'Connor GT, Dacey LJ. Is epsilon-

aminocaproic acid as effective as aprotinin in reducing bleeding with cardiac surgery? A meta-analysis. Circulation 99:81–89, 1999.

8. Bick RL. Hemostasis defects associated with cardiac surgery, prosthetic devices, and other extracorporeal circuits. Semin Thromb Hemost 11:249–280, 1985.
9. Palanzo DA, Zarro DL, Manley NJ, Montesano RM, Quinn M, Gustafson PA. Effect on surface coating on platelet count drop during cardiopulmonary bypass. Perfusion 14:195–200, 1999.
10. Campbell FW. The contribution of platelet dysfunction to postbypass bleeding. J Cardiothorac Vasc Anesth 5(suppl 1):8–12, 1991.
11. Parolari A, Guarnieri D, Alamanni F, Toscano T, Tantalo V, Gherli T, Colli S, Foieni F, Franze V, Stanghellini M, Gianotti GA, Biglioli P, Tremoli E. Platelet function and anesthetics in cardiac surgery: An in vitro and ex vivo study. Anesth Analg 89:26–31, 1999.
12. Despotis GJ, Joist JH, Goodnough LT. Monitoring of hemostasis in cardiac surgical patients: Impact of point-of-care testing on blood loss and transfusion outcomes. Clin Chem 43:1684–1696, 1997.
13. LaDuca FM, Zucker ML, Walker CE. Assessing heparin neutralization following cardiac surgery: Sensitivity of thrombin time based assays versus protamine titration methods. Perfusion 14:181–187, 1999.
14. Slaughter TF, Faghih F, Greenberg CS, Leslie JB, Sladen RN. The effects of epsilon-aminocaproic acid on fibrinolysis and thrombin generation during cardiac surgery. Anesth Analg 85:1221–1226, 1997.
15. Welch HG, Meehan KR, Goodnough LT. Prudent strategies for elective red blood cell transfusion. Ann Intern Med 116:393–402, 1992.
16. Goodnough LT, Johnston MF, Ramsey G, Sayers MH, Eisenstadt RS, Anderson KC, Rutman RC, Silberstein LE. Guidelines for transfusion support in patients undergoing coronary artery bypass grafting. Transfusion Practices Committee of the American Association of Blood Banks. Ann Thorac Surg 50:675–683, 1990.
17. American College of Physicians. Practice strategies for elective red blood cell transfusion. Ann Intern Med 116:403–406, 1992.
18. Moulton MJ, Creswell LL, Mackey ME, Cox JL, Rosenbloom M. Reexploration for bleeding is a risk factor for adverse outcomes after cardiac operations. J Thorac Cardiovasc Surg 111:1037–1046, 1996.
19. Rady MY, Ryan T, Starr NJ. Perioperative determinants of morbidity and mortality in elderly patients undergoing cardiac surgery. Crit Care Med 26:225–235, 1998.
20. Schreiber GB, Busch MP, Kleinman SH, Korelitz JJ. The risk of transfusion-transmitted viral infections. The Retrovirus Epidemiology Donor Study. N Engl J Med 334:1685–1690, 1996.
21. Lackritz EM, Satten GA, Aberle-Grasse J, Dodd RY, Raimondi VP, Janssen RS, Lewis WF, Notari EP, Peterson LR. Estimated risk of transmission of the human immunodeficiency virus by screened blood in the United States. N Engl J Med 333: 1721–1725, 1995.
22. Soumerai SB, Salem-Schatz S, Avorn J, Casteris CS, Ross-Degnan D, Popovsky MA. A controlled trial of educational outreach to improve blood transfusion practice. JAMA 270:961–966, 1993.

23. Edwards FH, Clark RE, Schwartz M. Coronary artery bypass grafting: The Society of Thoracic Surgeons National Database experience. Ann Thorac Surg 57:12–19, 1994.
24. Klein HG. Oxygen carriers and transfusion medicine. Artif Cells Blood Subtit Immobil Biotechnol 22:123–135, 1994.
25. Wallace EL, Surgenor DM, Hao HS, An J, Chapman RH, Churchill WH. Collection and transfusion of blood and blood components in the United States, 1989. Transfusion 33:139–144, 1993.
26. Wallace EL, Churchill WH, Surgenor DM, An J, Cho G, McGurk S, Murphy L. Collection and transfusion of blood and blood components in the United States, 1992. Transfusion 35:802–812, 1995.
27. Hirsh J. Heparin. N Engl J Med 324:1565–1574, 1991.
28. Despotis GJ, Gravlee G, Filos K, Levy J. Anticoagulation monitoring during cardiac surgery: A review of current and emerging techniques. Anesthesiology 91: 1122–1151, 1999.
29. Bull BS, Korpman RA, Huse WM, Briggs BD. Heparin therapy during extracorporeal circulation. I. Problems inherent in existing heparin protocols. J Thorac Cardiovasc Surg 69:674–684, 1975.
30. Bull BS, Huse WM, Brauer FS, Korpman RA. Heparin therapy during extracorporeal circulation. II The use of a dose-response curve to individualize heparin and protamine dosage. J Thorac Cardiovasc Surg 69:685–689, 1975.
31. Despotis GJ, Summerfield AL, Joist JH, Goodnough LT, Santoro SA, Spitznagel E, Cox JL, Lappas DG. Comparison of activated coagulation time and whole blood heparin measurements with laboratory plasma anti-Xa heparin concentration in patients having cardiac operations. J Thorac Cardiovasc Surg 108:1076–1082, 1994.
32. Young JA, Kisker CT, Doty DB. Adequate anticoagulation during cardiopulmonary bypass determined by activated clotting time and the appearance of fibrin monomer. Ann Thorac Surg 26:231–240, 1978.
33. Slaughter TF, LeBleu TH, Douglas Jr JM, Leslie JB, Parker JK, Greenberg CS. Characterization of prothrombin activation during cardiac surgery by hemostatic molecular markers. Anesthesiology 80:520–526, 1994.
34. Gravlee GP, Haddon WS, Rothberger HK, Mills SA, Rogers AT, Bean VE, Buss DH, Prough DS, Cordell AR. Heparin dosing and monitoring for cardiopulmonary bypass. A comparison of techniques with measurement of subclinical plasma coagulation. J Thorac Cardiovasc Surg 99:518–527, 1990.
35. Gravlee G, Rogers A, Dudas L, Taylor R, Roy R, Case L, Triscott M, Brown C, Mark L, Cordell A. Heparin management protocol for cardiopulmonary bypass influences postoperative heparin rebound but not bleeding. Anesthesiology 76:393–401, 1992.
36. Jobes DR, Aitken GL, Shaffer GW. Increased accuracy and precision of heparin and protamine dosing reduces blood loss and transfusion in patients undergoing primary cardiac operations. J Thorac Cardiovasc Surg 110:35–45, 1995.
37. Staples MH, Dunton RF, Karlson KJ, Leonardi HK, Berger RL. Heparin resistance after preoperative heparin therapy or intra-aortic balloon pumping. Ann Thorac Surg 57:1211–1216, 1994.
38. Despotis G, Joist J, Hogue Jr C, Alsoufiev A, Kater K, Goodnough L, Santoro S,

Spitznagel E, Rosenblum M, Lappas D. The impact of heparin concentration and activated clotting time monitoring on blood conservation. A prospective, randomized evaluation in patients undergoing cardiac operation. J Thorac Cardiovasc Surg 110:46–54, 1995.
39. Koster A, Kuppe H, Hetzer R, Sodian R, Crystal GJ, Mertzlufft F. Emergent cardiopulmonary bypass in five patients with heparin-induced thrombocytopenia type II employing recombinant hirudin. Anesthesiology 89:777–780, 1998.
40. Insler SR, Kraenzler EJ, Bartholomew JR, Kottke-Marchant K, Lytle B, Starr NJ. Thrombosis during the use of the heparinoid Organon 10172 in a patient with heparin-induced thrombocytopenia. Anesthesiology 86:495–498, 1997.
41. Ballard JO. Anticoagulant-induced thrombosis. JAMA 282:310–312, 1999.
42. Walls JT, Curtis JJ, Silver D, Boley TM. Heparin-induced thrombocytopenia in patients who undergo open heart surgery. Surgery 108:686–692; discussion 692–683, 1990.
43. Bauer TL, Arepally G, Konkle BA, Mestichelli B, Shapiro SS, Cines DB, Poncz M, McNulty S, Amiral J, Hauck WW, Edie RN, Mannion JD. Prevalence of heparin-associated antibodies without thrombosis in patients undergoing cardiopulmonary bypass surgery. Circulation 95:1242–1246, 1997.
44. Johnson PH. Hirudin: Clinical potential of a thrombin inhibitor. Annu Rev Med 45:165–177, 1994.
45. Koster A, Hansen R, Kuppe H, Hetzer R, Crystal GJ, Mertzlufft F. Recombinant hirudin as an alternative for anticoagulation during cardiopulmonary bypass in patients with heparin-induced thrombocytopenia type II: A 1-year experience in 57 patients. J Cardiothorac Vasc Anesth 14:243–248, 2000.
46. Despotis GJ, Grishaber JE, Goodnough LT. The effect of an intraoperative treatment algorithm on physicians' transfusion practice in cardiac surgery. Transfusion 34:290–296, 1994.
47. Shore-Lesserson L, Manspeizer H, DePerio M, Francis S, Vela-Cantos F, Ergin M. Thromboelastography-guided transfusion algorithm reduces transfusions in complex cardiac surgery. Anesth Analg 88:312–319, 1999.
48. Spiess BD, Gillies BS, Chandler W, Verrier E. Changes in transfusion therapy and reexploration rate after institution of a blood management program in cardiac surgical patients. J Cardiothor Vasc Anesth 9:168–173, 1995.
49. Nuttall GA, Oliver WC, Santrach PJ, Bryant S, Dearani JA, Schaff HV, Ereth MH. Efficacy of a simple intraoperative transfusion algorithm for nonerythrocyte component utilization after cardiopulmonary bypass. Anesthesiology 94:773–781; discussion 775A–776A, 2001.
50. Kang Y. Thromboelastography in liver transplantation. Semin Thromb Hemost 21: 34–44, 1995.
51. Everson GT. A hepatologist's perspective on the management of coagulation disorders before liver transplantation. Liver Transpl Surg 3:646–652, 1997.
52. Kang Y. Coagulation and liver transplantation: Current concepts. Liver Transplant Surg 3:465–467, 1997.
53. Kang YG, Martin DJ, Marquez J, Lewis JH, Bontempo FA, Shaw BW, Starzl TE, Winter PM. Intraoperative changes in blood coagulation and thrombelastographic monitoring in liver transplantation. Anesth Analg 64:888–896, 1985.

54. Plevak D, Divertie G, Carton E, Bowie EJ, Rettke S, Taswell H, Wiesner R, Krom R. Blood product transfusion therapy after liver transplantation: Comparison of the thromboelastogram and conventional coagulation studies. Transplant Proc 25:1838, 1993.
55. Palomo Sanchez JC, Jimenez C, Moreno Gonzalez E, Garcia I, Palma F, Loinaz C, Gonzalez Ghamorro A. Effects of intraoperative blood transfusion on postoperative complications and survival after orthotopic liver transplantation. Hepatogastroenterology 45:1026–1033, 1998.
56. Spahn DR, Leone BJ, Reves JG, Pasch T. Cardiovascular and coronary physiology of acute isovolemic hemodilution: A review of non–oxygen-carrying and oxygen-carrying solutions. Anesth Analg 78:1000–1021, 1994.
57. Nuttall GA, Oliver WC, Ereth MH, Santrach PJ, Bryant SC, Orszulak TA, Schaff HV. Comparison of blood-conservation strategies in cardiac surgery patients at high risk for bleeding. Anesthesiology 92:674–682, 2000.
58. Ferguson JJ, Dohmen P, Wilson JM, Vaughn WK, Khoshnevis R, Kmonicek P, McKinney AA, Plachetka JR. Results of a national survey on anticoagulation for PTCA. J Invasive Cardiol 7:136–141, 1995.
59. Klein LW, Agarwal JB. When we "act" on ACT levels: Activated clotting time measurements to guide heparin administration during and after interventional procedures. Cathet Cardiovasc Diagn 37:154–157, 1996.
60. Chew DP, Bhatt DL, Lincoff M, Moliterno DJ, Brener SJ, Wolski KE, Topol EJ. Defining the optimal activated clotting time during percutaneous coronary intervention: Aggregate results from 6 randomized, controlled trials. Circulation 103:961–966, 2001.
61. Kaluski E, Krakover R, Cotter G, Hendler A, Zyssman I, Milovanov O, Blatt A, Zimmerman E, Goldstein E, Nahman V, Vered Z. Minimal heparinization in coronary angioplasty—how much heparin is really warranted? Am J Cardiol 85:953–956, 2000.
62. Bowers J, Ferguson JJ. The use of activated clotting times to monitor heparin therapy during and after interventional procedures. Clin Cardiol 17:357–361, 1994.
63. Popma JJ, Prpic R, Lansky AJ, Piana R. Heparin dosing in patients undergoing coronary intervention. Am J Cardiol 82:19P–24P, 1998.
64. EPIC Investigators. Use of a monoclonal antibody directed against the platelet glycoprotein IIb/IIIa receptor in high risk coronary angioplasty. N Engl J Med 330: 956–961, 1994.
65. EPIC Investigators. Platelet glycoprotein IIb/IIIa receptor blockade and low dose heparin during percutaneous coronary revascularization. N Engl J Med 336:1689–1696, 1997.
66. Harrington RA, Kleiman NS, Granger CB, Ohman EM, Berkowitz SD. Relation between inhibition of platelet aggregation and clinical outcomes. Am Heart J 136: S43–S50, 1998.
67. Hezard N, Metz D, Nazeyrollas P, Droulle C, Elaerts J, Potron G, Nguyen P. Use of the PFA-100 apparatus to assess platelet function in patients undergoing PTCA during and after infusion of c7E3 Fab in the presence of other antiplatelet agents. Thromb Haemost 83:540–544, 2000.
68. Madan M, Berkowitz SD, Christie DJ, Jennings LK, Smit AC, Sigmon KN, Glazer

S, Tcheng JE. Rapid assessment of glycoprotein IIb/IIIa blockade with the platelet function analyzer (PFA-100) during percutaneous coronary intervention. Am Heart J 141:226–233, 2001.

69. Simon D, Liu C, Ganz P, Kirshenbaum J, Piana R, Rogers C, Selwyn A, Popma J. Cathet A comparative study of light transmission aggregometry and automated bedside platelet function assays in patients undergoing percutaneous coronary intervention and receiving abciximab, eptifibatide, or tirofiban. Cardiovasc Intervent 52: 425–432, 2001.
70. Kereiakes DJ, Broderick TM, Roth EM, Whang D, Shimshak T, Runyon JP, Hattemer C, Schneider J, Lacock P, Mueller M, Abbottsmith CW. Time course, magnitude, and consistency of platelet inhibition by abcizimab, tirofiban, or eptifibatide in patients with unstable angina pectoris undergoing percutaneous coronary intervention. Am J Cardiol 84:391–395, 1999.
71. Li CKN, Hoffmann TJ, Hsieh PY, Malik S, Watson W. Xylum CSA: Automated system for assessing hemostasis in simulated vascular flow. Clin Chem 43:1788–1790, 1997.
72. Steinhubl S, Talley J, Braden G, Tcheng J, Casterella P, Moliterno D, Navetta F, Berger P, Popma JJ, Dangas G, Gallo R, Sane D, Saucedo J, Jia G, Lincoff A, Theroux P, Holmes D, Teirstein P, Kereiakes DJ. Point-of-care measured platelet inhibition correlates with a reduced risk of an adverse cardiac event after percutaneous coronary intervention: Results of the GOLD (AU-Assessing Ultegra) multicenter study. Circulation 103:2572–2578, 2001.
73. Ward R, Aronoff G. In: Henrich W, ed. Principles and Practice of Dialysis. Williams & Wilkins, Baltimore, 1999, pp 70–78.
74. Eiswirth G, Walch S, Bommer J. New bedside test for monitoring anticoagulation during hemodialysis. Artif Organs 22:346–352, 1998.
75. Harenberg J, Haaf B, Dempfle C, Stehle G, Heene D. Monitoring of heparins in haemodialysis using an anti–factor-Xa-specific whole-blood clotting assay. Nephrol Dial Transplant 10:217–222, 1995.
76. Saltissi D, Morgan C, Westhuyzen J, Healy H. Comparison of low-molecular-weight heparin (enoxaparin sodium) and standard unfractionated heparin for haemodialysis anticoagulation. Nephrol Dial Transplant 14:2698–2703, 1999.
77. Neuhaus T, Goetschel P, Schmugge M, Leumann E. Heparin-induced thrombocytopenia type II on hemodialysis: Switch to danaparoid. Pediatr Nephrol 14:713–716, 2000.
78. Dager W, White R. Use of lepirudin in patients with heparin-induced thrombocytopenia and renal failure requiring hemodialysis. Ann Pharmacother 35:885–890, 2001.
79. Bucha E, Nowak G, Czerwinski R, Thieler H. R-hirudin as anticoagulant in regular hemodialysis therapy: Finding of therapeutic R-hirudin blood/plasma concentrations and respective dosages. Clin Appl Thromb Hemost 5:164–170, 1999.
80. Fischer K, Van de Loo A, Bohler J. Recombinant hirudin (lepirudin) as anticoagulant in intensive care patients treated with continuous hemodialysis. Kidney Int 72(suppl):S46–S50, 1999.
81. Hull RD, Raskob GE, Brant RF, Pineo GF. Relation between the time to achieve the lower limit of the aPTT therapeutic range and recurrent venous thromboembo-

lism during heparin treatment for deep vein thrombosis. Arch Intern Med 157: 2562–2568, 1997.
82. Raschke RA, Reilly BM, Guidry JR, Fontana JR, Srinivas S. The weight-based heparin dosing nomogram compared with a "standard care" normogram. A randomized controlled trial. Ann Intern Med 119:874–881, 1993.
83. Shalansky KF, FitzGerald JM, Sunderji R, Traboulay SJ, O'Malley B, McCarron BI, Naiman S. Comparison of a weight-based heparin nomogram with traditional heparin dosing to achieve therapeutic anticoagulation. Pharmacotherapy 16:1076–1084, 1996.
84. Mungall D, Lord M, Cason S, Treadwell P, Williams D, Tedrick D. Developing and testing a system to improve the quality of heparin anticoagulation in patients with acute cardiac syndromes. Am J Cardiol 82:574–579, 1998.
85. Brown G, Dodek P. An evaluation of empiric vs. nomogram-based dosing of heparin in an intensive care unit. Crit Care Med 25:1534–1538, 1997.
86. Cruickshank MK, Levine MN, Hirsh J, Roberts R, Siguenza M. A standard heparin nomogram for the management of heparin therapy. Arch Intern Med 151:333–337, 1991.
87. Hollingsworth JA, Rowe BH, Brisebois FJ, Thompson PR, Fabris LM. The successful application of a heparin nomogram in a community hospital. Arch Intern Med 155:2095–2100, 1995.
88. Gunnarsson PS, Sawyer WT, Montague D, Williams ML, Dupuis RE, Caiola SM. Appropriate use of heparin. Empiric vs nomogram-based dosing. Arch Intern Med 155:526–532, 1995.
89. Paradiso-Hardy FL, Cheung B, Geerts WH. Evaluation of an intravenous heparin nomogram in a coronary care unit. Can J Cardiol 12:802–808, 1996.
90. Elliott CG, Hiltunen SJ, Suchyta M, Hull RD, Raskob GE, Pineo GF, Jensen RL, Yeates S, Kitterman N. Physician-guided treatment compared with a heparin protocol for deep vein thrombosis. Arch Intern Med 154:999–1004, 1994.
91. Baker BA, Adelman MD, Smith PA, Osborn JC. Inability of the activated partial thromboplastin time to predict heparin levels. Time to reassess guidelines for heparin assays. Arch Intern Med 157:2475–2479, 1997.
92. Levine MN, Hirsh J, Gent M, Turpie AG, Cruickshank M, Weitz J, Anderson D, Johnson M. A randomized trial comparing activated thromboplastin time with heparin assay in patients with acute venous thromboembolism requiring large daily doses of heparin. Arch Intern Med 154:49–56, 1994.
93. Olson JD, Arkin CF, Brandt JT, Cunningham MT, Giles A, Koepke JA, Witte DL. College of American Pathologists Conference XXXI on laboratory monitoring of anticoagulant therapy: Laboratory monitoring of unfractionated heparin therapy. Arch Pathol Lab Med 122:782–798, 1998.
94. Werner M, Gallagher J, Ballo M, Karcher D. Effect of analytic uncertainty of conventional and point-of-care assays of activated partial thromboplastin time on clinical decisions in heparin therapy. Am J Clin Pathol 102:237–241, 1994.
95. Becker R, Cyr J, Corrao J, Ball S. Bedside coagulation monitoring in heparin-treated patients with active thromboembolic disease: A coronary care unit experience. Am Heart J 128:719–723, 1994.
96. Becker RC, Ball SP, Eisenberg P, Borzak S, Held AC, Spencer F, Voyce SJ, Jesse

R, Hendel R, Ma Y, Hurley T, Hebert J. Antithrombotic Therapy Consortium Investigators. A randomized, multicenter trial of weight-adjusted intravenous heparin dose titration and point-of-care coagulation monitoring in hospitalized patients with active thromboembolic disease. Am Heart J 137:59–71, 1999.
97. Zabel KM, Granger CB, Becker RC, Bovill EG, Hirsh J, Aylward PE, Topol EJ, Califf RM. Use of bedside activated partial thromboplastin time monitor to adjust heparin dosing after thrombolysis for acute myocardial infarction: Results of GUSTO-I. Global Utilization of Streptokinase and TPA for Occluded Coronary Arteries. Am Heart J 136:868–876, 1998.
98. Davis KD, Danielson CFM, May LS, Han Z-Q. Use of different thromboplastin reagents causes greater variability in international normalized ration results than prolonged room temperature storage of specimens. Arch Pathol Lab Med 122:972–977, 1998.
99. Finck K, Doetkott C, Miller D. Clinical impact of interlaboratory variation in international normalized ratio determinations. Am J Health Syst Pharm 58:684–688, 2001.
100. Hirsh J, Dalen J, Anderson D, Poller L, Bussey H, Ansell J, Deykin D. Oral anticoagulants: Mechanism of action, clinical effectiveness, and optimal therapeutic range. Chest 119:8S–21S, 2001.
101. Hylek E, Skates S, Sheehan M, Singer D. An analysis of the lowest effective intensity of prophylactic anticoagulation for patients with nonrheumatic atrial fibrillation. N Engl J Med 335:540–546, 1996.
102. Hylek E, Singer D. Risk factors for intracranial hemorrhage in outpatients taking warfarin. Ann Intern Med 120:897–902, 1994.
103. Ansell JE, Hamke AK, Holden A, Knapic N. Cost effectiveness of monitorin warfarin therapy using standard versus capillary prothrombin times. Am J Clin Pathol 91:587–589, 1989.
104. Ansell JE, Hughes R. Evolving models of warfarin management: Anticoagulation clinics, patient self-monitoring, and patient self-management. Am Heart J 132: 1095–1100, 1996.
105. Chiquette E, Amato MG, Bussey HI. Comparison of an anticoagulation clinic with usual medical care: Anticoagulation control, patient outcomes, and health care costs. Arch Intern Med 158:1641–1647, 1998.
106. Fitzmaurice DA, Hobbs FDR, Murray ET. Primary care anticoagulant clinic management using computerized decision support and near patient International Normalized Ratio (INR) testing: Routine data from a practice nurse-led clinic. Fam Pract 15:144–146, 1998.
107. Gray DR, Garabedian-Ruffalo SM, Chretien SD. Cost-justification of a clinical pharmacist-managed anticoagulation clinic. Drug Intell Clin Pharm 19:575–580, 1985.
108. Conte RR, Kehoe WA, Nielson N, Lodhia H. Nine-year experience with a pharmacist-managed anticoagulation clinic. Am J Hosp Pharm 43:2460–2464, 1986.
109. Ansell J, Holden A, Knapic N. Patient self-management of oral anticoagulation guided by capillary (fingerstick) whole blood prothrombin times. Arch Intern Med 149:2509–2511, 1989.
110. White R, McCurdy S, von Marensdorff H, Woodruff DJ, Leftgoff L. Home pro-

thrombin time monitoring after the initiation of warfarin therapy. A randomized, prospective study. Ann Intern Med 111:730–737, 1989.
111. Sawicki PT. Working Group for the Study of Patient Self-Management of Oral Anticoagulation. A structured teaching and self-management program for patients receiving oral anticoagulation: A randomized controlled trial. Anticoagulation. JAMA 281:145–150, 1999.
112. Beyth R, Quinn L, Landefeld C. A multicomponent intervention to prevent major bleeding complications in older patients receiving warfarin. A randomized, controlled trial. Ann Intern Med 133:687–695, 2000.
113. Cromheecke ME, Levi M, Colly LP, de Mol BJM, Prins MH, Hutten BA, Mak R, Keyzers KJC, Buller HR. Oral anticoagulation self-management and management by a specialist anticoagulation clinic: A randomised cross-over comparison. Lancet 356:97–102, 2000.
114. Watzke HH, Forberg E, Svolba G, Jimenez-Boj E, Krinninger B. A prospective controlled trial comparing weekly self-testing and self-dosing with the standard management of patients on stable oral anticoagulation. Thromb Res 83:661–665, 2000.
115. Kortke H, Korfer R. International normalized ration self-management after mechanical heart valve replacement: Is an early start advantageous? Ann Thorac Surg 72:44–48, 2001.
116. Oral Anticoagulation Monitoring Study Group. Prothrombin measurement using a patient self-testing system. Am J Clin Pathol 115:280–287, 2001.
117. Oral Anticoagulation Monitoring Study Group. Point-of-care prothrombin time measurement for professional and patient self-testing use: A multicenter clinical experience. Am J Clin Pathol 115:288–296, 2001.
118. Ansell JE, Patel N, Ostrovsky D, Nozzolillo E, Peterson AM, Fish L. Long-term patient self-management of oral anticoagulation. Arch Intern Med 155:2185–2189, 1995.
119. Lafata JE, Martin SA, Kaatz S, Ward RE. Anticoagulation clinics and patient self-testing for patients on chronic warfarin therapy: A cost-effectiveness analysis. J Thromb Thrombolysis 9:S13–S19, 2000.

14

Point-of-Care Testing for Biochemical Markers of Acute Coronary Syndromes

Robert H. Christenson and Hassan M. E. Azzazy El-Badawy
University of Maryland School of Medicine, Baltimore, Maryland, U.S.A.

INTRODUCTION

Heart disease is the world's leading cause of mortality, accounting for approximately 500,000 deaths per year in the United States alone (1). Currently, cardiovascular disease affects nearly 70 million Americans, and each year an estimated 8 million patients present acutely to Emergency Departments (ED) with symptoms suspicious of ischemic heart disease (2). About 5 million patients will be admitted to medical centers, of which 1.1 million patients are diagnosed as having myocardial infarction (MI). The remaining three million patients are released from the ED, but of these about 30,000 (1%) are misdiagnosed and will likely have adverse outcomes (3). These misdiagnosed patients account for the largest source of malpractice dollars awarded in Emergency Medicine (2,3). The overall yearly financial burden of heart disease in the United States is believed to exceed 10 billion dollars.

Biochemical markers of cardiac injury play an essential role in the diagnosis, prognosis, monitoring, and risk stratification of suspected heart attack patients, and have become a central part of therapeutic and interventional guidelines for clinicians. For these reasons, cardiac marker measurements have become a ubiquitous service available at all medical centers having urgent care areas. Although cardiac markers have traditionally been performed exclusively in the central laboratory, over the past 25 years availability of cardiac marker measurements has evolved from once-per-day batches (weekdays only); to several batches per day, seven days a week; and finally to immediate availability. More recently, point-of-care testing (POCT) for cardiac markers has been driven by the time-critical clinical need for immediate cardiac marker testing, to provide timely patient risk stratification, disposition, expedite appropriate treatment, and improve outcomes.

PATHOPHYSIOLOGY OF ACUTE CORONARY SYNDROMES AND HEART FAILURE

Coronary Artery Atherogenesis

Rupture of unstable coronary plaques and the resulting thrombus formation are the causal pathologies underlying MI (4). Coronary artery plaques result from atherogenesis, which as indicated in Figure 1 begins early in life when lipid-rich deposits containing macrophages and T-lymphocytes exist in the aorta shortly after birth and increase with age. By early adulthood, fatty streaks are present in a large proportion of individuals as demonstrated by autopsy studies of young Korean War casualties (5). With increasing age, expanding lesions become more numerous and may affect normal laminar blood flow. The lesions contain smooth muscle cells that form a fibrous plaque. In more advanced lesions, the fibrous plaque can become vascularized, and the size of the lipid-rich core increases depending on anatomical location and a number of genetic and lifestyle risk factors including: age, gender, family history, blood pressure, smoking habit, and blood lipid concentrations (6). Comorbidities, including diabetes mellitus and the metabolic syndrome, are also recognized as important risk factors (6). Recently, the inflammatory process has been recognized as an important component of atherogenesis (7). Infectious disease may also play a role in atherogenesis, however the nature of this effect is poorly understood at present.

Acute Coronary Syndromes: A Continuum of Disease

Figure 1 indicates that plaques may become unstable and rupture at any age, causing the common pathophysiological feature of the "acute coronary syndromes," a continuum of ischemic disease ranging from unstable angina, associated with reversible myocardial cell injury, to frank MI with large areas of necrosis. Rupture of an atherogenic fibrous plaque in a focal segment of an epicardial coronary artery exposes subendothelial proteins, such as collagen and von Willebrand factor (vWF), to circulation leading to adhesion of platelets having surface receptors for these proteins. This interaction triggers a change in the platelet's shape from disk to stellate. The enzyme thrombin is generated on the membrane of activated platelets from circulating prothrombin. Thrombin converts fibrinogen to fibrin that will form polymers that make up the framework of a thrombus,

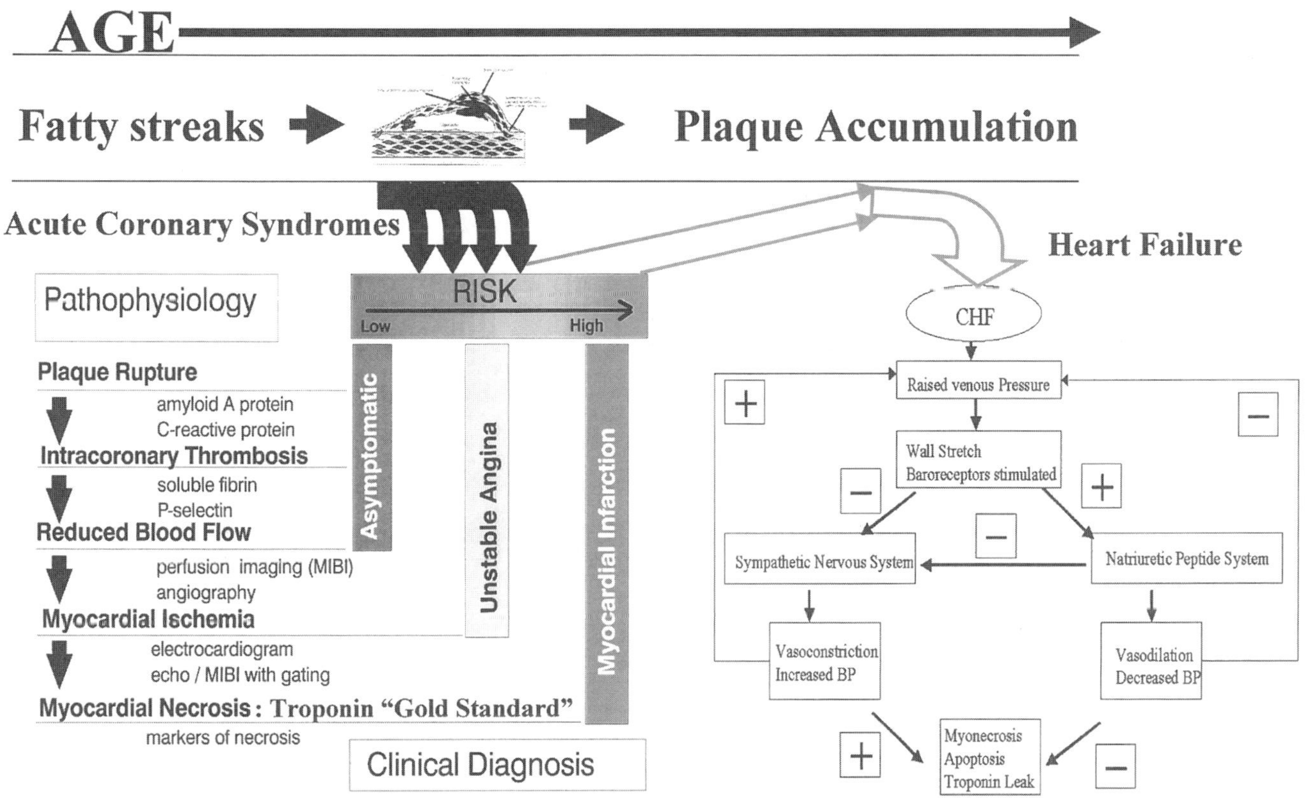

Figure 1 Cardiac injury: the big picture. This diagram summarizes the pathophysiology of acute coronary syndromes (ACS) and congestive heart failure (CHF). Accumulation of fatty streaks lead to the formation of plaques that upon rupture lead to ACS (left). Necrosis caused by myocardial infarction may cause CHF (right).

trapping platelets and red and white blood cells. Because fibrinogen and vWF are multivalent, they bind to multiple activated platelets, leading to their aggregation.

Stable angina usually involves stable plaques resulting from years of atherosclerotic deposition in coronary arteries; these plaques are usually subocclusive and are not typically unstable. Clinical symptoms of stable angina occur when the oxygen demand of heart tissue cannot be adequately supplied by the coronary artery blood flow and is characterized by transient episodes of chest pain precipitated by exercise or increased activity; the pain is usually resolved with rest or nitroglycerin. Unstable angina pectoris is principally defined as chest pain occurring at rest. In unstable angina, the plaque has ruptured, causing platelet aggregation and activation of the coagulation systems, resulting in the formation of a platelet-rich thrombus (white thrombus). A thrombus rich in fibrin and erythrocytes (red thrombus) may evolve and extend up- or downstream in the artery. Extensive local thrombosis rich in platelets will result in episodic flow-limiting coronary stenosis and myocardial ischemia associated symptomatically with unstable angina or with necrosis that characterizes non–Q wave MI (Figure 2). If the plaque ruptures and thrombosis is extensive and rich in fibrin, the coronary artery may fully occlude and result in Q wave MI (see Figure 2). In unstable angina patients, spontaneous ischemia results from reductions in coronary blood flow caused by atherosclerotic plaque combined with thrombosis and vasoconstriction. However, it is unclear why disruption of a particular plaque leads to occlusive thrombus in some cases but not others. If oxygen is not restored to the myocardium within 10–15 min, myocyte cell death and loss of membrane integrity occur. Infarct size and location are important in determining the clinical course and prognosis of an acute MI.

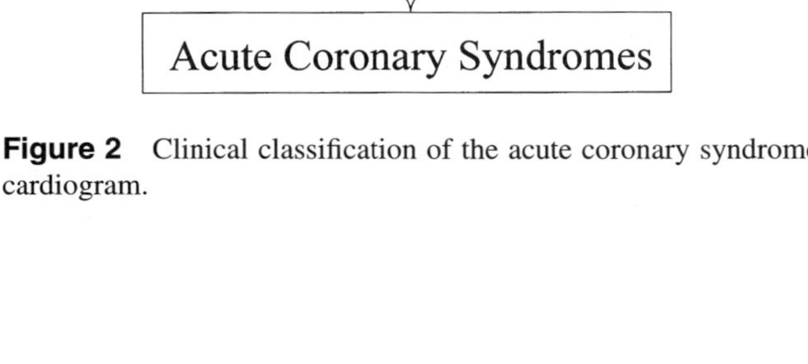

Figure 2 Clinical classification of the acute coronary syndromes based on the electrocardiogram.

Myocardial Infarction Interventions

Figure 2 indicates that acute coronary syndrome patients can be grouped by their electrocardiograph (ECG) findings. The ECG is important for guiding therapy because patients having ST elevation generally have thrombus that is rich in fibrin. For this reason, early fibrinolytic therapy using intravenous streptokinase or tissue plasminogen activator is efficacious in ST elevation patients. In contrast, patients with non–ST elevation MI (see Figure 2) generally have clots that are platelet rich. Therefore, therapies in non–ST elevation patients are aimed at inhibiting platelet aggregation. A change in the conformation of the glycoprotein (GP) IIb/IIIa receptor is the final step in platelet aggregation and has been a primary therapeutic target of inhibition.

The goal of mechanical and therapeutic interventions for acute coronary syndrome patients is to reduce morbidity and mortality by opening the occluded artery, thereby limiting infarct size and controlling complications. Because half of MI deaths occur within 1 hr of symptom onset, and the effectiveness of reperfusion strategies depends on early intervention, it is crucial to identify high-risk cardiac patients rapidly so that lifesaving treatment can be initiated. Nitroglycerin is given to relax smooth muscles, leading to vasodilatation. Aspirin, considered to be the standard of care in all MI patients, inhibits platelet aggregation by irreversibly blocking the action of cyclo-oxygenase. Heparin acts at multiple sites in the coagulation cascade to inhibit the clot formation.

Mechanical intervention usually consists of cardiac catheterization and percutaneous coronary intervention (PCI) or angioplasty, to remove the obstruction(s). Along with PCI, placement of a stent(s) to sustain patency is also very common. Usually, medications to inhibit platelet aggregation are administered to these patients to help prevent reocclusion. Point-of-care testing for biochemical markers is particularly important for determining the care and improving the outcome of non–ST elevation patients.

Heart Failure

Heart failure is a common health problem in the United States with 400,000–700,000 new cases each year. The disease occurs in 1.5% of the population and its prevalence can increase up to 20% in individuals over age 70. The key to treatment of heart failure is early intervention, since administration of therapeutic agents such as angiotensin-converting enzyme (ACE) inhibitors and beta-blockers have been shown to improve survival. Clinically, the New York Heart Association has established four classes of heart failure according to criteria listed in Table 1.

Heart failure is defined by the inability of the heart to generate adequate cardiac output to meet the demands of the metabolizing tissues. It may be precipi-

Table 1 New York Heart Association (NYHA) Classification of Heart Failure

Class I.	No limitation of physical activity. No shortness of breath, fatigue, or heart palpitations with ordinary physical activity.
Class II.	Slight limitation of activity. Shortness of breath, fatigue, or heart palpitations with ordinary physical activity, but patients are comfortable at rest.
Class III.	Marked limitation of activity. Shortness of breath, fatigue, or heart palpitations with less than ordinary physical activity, but patients are comfortable at rest.
Class IV.	Severe to complete limitation of activity. Shortness of breath, fatigue, or heart palpitations with any physical exertion and symptoms appear even at rest.

tated by a variety of causes, including pulmonary embolism, infection, thyrotoxicosis, arrhythmias, and MI. As indicated in Figure 1, symptoms of heart failure occur when the balance between the sympathetic and natriuretic mechanisms is disrupted, leading to fluid overload. Fluid overload and increased filling pressure causes stretching of heart tissue and release of B-type natriuretic peptide (BNP), a hormone that induces excretion of sodium and obligate water by the renal tubules. The severity of clinical symptoms associated with congestive heart failure (CHF) are simultaneous with left ventricular enlargement, elevated filling pressures, and increased systolic wall stress. Cellular changes revealed by examination of the failing heart include disorganization of myofibrils, enlarged sarcoplasmic reticulum, intracytoplasmic vacuoles, and disruption of the plasma membrane. These cellular changes typically result in extensive damage, multiple micronecrotic foci, and loss of myocytes. The interstitial changes in the myocardium are associated with extensive fibrosis and edema, and reduced capillary density that lead to chronic hypoxia and promote myocyte injury and death.

BIOCHEMICAL TOOLS FOR MONITORING HEART PATHOPHYSIOLOGY

General

Characteristics of the Ideal Cardiac Marker

The ideal marker has absolute cardiac specificity and does not exist in other tissues under normal or pathological conditions and allows a reliable, highly specific diagnosis of myocardial injury in the presence of other conditions. The marker must have high diagnostic sensitivity, i.e., have high concentration in myocardial tissue and low concentration in circulation. The ideal marker must be able to differentiate between reversible (ischemia) and irreversible (necrosis) damage such as may occur in angina and myocarditis. In MI, the marker should permit monitoring of reperfusion, detection of reocclusion, estimation of infarct size, and should allow both early and late diagnosis. The marker must be stable, appear in blood immediately following a clinical event, and then remain in circulation long enough to allow detection of cell death in patients who present late. Rapid whole blood measurement that is easy to perform, quantitative, and cost effective should be available for the marker. Unfortunately, a single marker that satisfies all these characteristics does not exist, so use of a profile of cardiac markers is necessary to cover all potential uses.

Quantitative versus Qualitative Data

The assessment of myocardial necrosis, acute cardiac ischemia, and presence/absence of heart failure all utilize cutpoints that are, in essence, a qualitative binary approach. These cutpoints provide a context in which qualitative testing for cardiac markers is feasible. A potential advantage of qualitative testing is realized for troponin. Because values for the various quantitative assays may vary by 30-fold, use of a qualitative assay may avoid discord between POC and main laboratory assays. However, there is overall general agreement that quantitative assays are a desirable characteristic, particularly for monitoring the release (rise) and clearance (fall) of cardiac markers. Other applications, such as risk stratification, reperfusion assessment, and prognosis, all require continuous (numerical) data.

Serial Sampling

Biochemical markers indicating myocardial necrosis require serial sampling to optimize diagnostic performance (8,9). Markers of ischemia and heart failure may require serial monitoring because their concentrations change rapidly in response to clinical events and they have a relatively short half-life in blood. It is critically important to place cardiac markers in the temporal context of clinical symptoms and signs. This is a substantial advantage for POCT, where availability of the biochemical marker is in the time frame when caregivers are focusing on the individual patient, particularly in the ED. This is because POCT saves physician time, allows high-risk patients to be treated more rapidly, and allows low-risk patients to be released in more timely fashion.

Markers of Early Myocardial Ischemia

Background

The release of currently available myocardial markers into circulation is believed to require tissue necrosis, whereas the assessment of cardiac ischemia before or

Table 2 Biochemical Markers of the Acute Coronary Syndromes

Biochemical marker	Point-of-care test available?	Molecular weight, g/mole	Cardiac specific?	Advantage	Disadvantage	Duration of elevation	Diagnostic performance and comments
Myocardial ischemia markers							
Ischemia modified albumin	Not at present	65,000	Unknown	Biochemical marker would be helpful because myocardial ischemia is difficult to diagnose	No ischemia "gold standard," agreed reference clinical standard, or biochemical test for myocardial ischemia	Preliminary data suggests 6–8 hr	Clinical trials pending
Glycogen phosphorylase-BB	No	177,000	Yes +++	Biochemical marker would be helpful because myocardial ischemia is a difficult diagnosis	Inability to reproduce initial results	8 hr	Initial data promising, but unable to be reproduced
Myocardial necrosis markers[a]							
Myoglobin	Yes	18,000	No	High sensitivity and negative predictive value Useful for early detection of MI and reperfusion	Low specificity in presence of skeletal muscle injury and with renal insufficiency Rapid clearance after necrosis	12–24 hr	2–6 hr after presentation: Sensitivity: 90% (CI[b]: 88–93%) Specificity: 86% (CI: 85–87%) Negative predictive value: 96%

CK-MB, mass assays	Yes	85,000	Yes +++	Ability to detect reinfarction Large clinical experience Previous "gold standard" for myocardial necrosis	Lowered specificity in skeletal muscle injury	24–36 hr	Two serial values above 99th percentile of control reference population in the setting of ischemia is benchmark for myocardial necrosis
Cardiac troponin T	Yes	37,000	Yes ++++	Tool for risk stratification Detection of MI up to 2 wk High specificity for cardiac tissue	Not an early marker of myocardial necrosis Limited ability to detect reinfarction	10–14 days	A single value above 99th percentile of control reference population is surrogate of myocardial necrosis in setting of myocardial ischemia
Cardiac troponin I	Yes	23,500	Yes ++++	Tool for risk stratification Detection of MI up to 7 days High specificity for cardiac tissue	Not an early marker of myocardial necrosis No analytical reference standards Limited ability to detect reinfarction	4–7 days	A single value above 99th percentile of control reference population is surrogate of myocardial necrosis in setting of myocardial ischemia

[a] Time of first increase for the markers are 1–3 hr for myoglobin, 4–6 hr for CK-MB mass, 3–4 hr for cardiac troponin T, and 4–6 hr for cardiac troponin I.
[b] CI = 95% confidence interval.

in the absence of cell death is almost always an important component of clinical decision making for the suspected acute coronary syndrome patient. However, the diagnosis of cardiac ischemia is extremely difficult and lacks a "gold standard"; there is no set of reference criteria or guidelines for cardiac ischemia. Therefore, detection of cardiac ischemia depends on individual physician gestalt based on clinical assessment and imperfect tools, including the ECG, echocardiography, and imaging studies (10). A sensitive biochemical marker of ischemia would be clinically useful, particularly if available at the point of care.

Glycogen Phosphorylase-BB

Initial data for the marker glycogen phosphorylase-BB were encouraging (11), but others have been unable to confirm these results.

Ischemia Modified Albumin

A biochemical marker termed "ischemia modified albumin" (IMA) has been identified that results from changes to the N-terminus of albumin caused by ischemia (12). The basis of this marker is that the low pH resulting from ischemia causes two biochemical events: a structural modification to the N-terminus of albumin, and release of copper from the protein ceruloplasmin, which binds with high affinity to the N-terminus of the intact albumin. A test for IMA monitors the binding between serum albumin and the transition metal cobalt (13). This assay, termed the Albumin Cobalt Binding (ACB™) Test (Ischemia Technologies, Inc., Denver, CO), is based on observations that the binding of cobalt is reduced in serum from acute coronary syndrome patients (12). This decreased binding reflects ischemic changes to the N-terminus of albumin, the binding site for transition metals such as cobalt, and the blocking of binding sites by copper released from ceruloplasmin. Other information regarding IMA and myocardial ischemia is listed in Table 2.

Markers of Myocardial Infarction

Myoglobin

Table 2 shows characteristics of myoglobin, a heme protein that is located in the cytoplasm of both cardiac and skeletal muscle cells (14). Myoglobin is the earliest appearing biochemical marker that is routinely available for assessment of the acute coronary syndrome patient. Myoglobin's characteristic early and robust rise is due to its relatively small molecular size and high concentration in heart tissue; myoglobin's rapid peak and return to normal is due to fast renal clearance. Meta-analysis has shown that the clinical sensitivity of myoglobin exceeds 90% with serial sampling at presentation and then 2–6 hr later (15). However, because myoglobin's amino acid sequence is the same in both cardiac and skeletal muscle, clinical specificity is compromised due to increased values with skeletal muscle injury. Also, patients with renal insufficiency have elevated myoglobin levels due to decreased clearance. There are a number of studies that have examined the negative predictive value (NPV) of myoglobin, finding satisfactory high values in the range of 96% when chest pain onset is acute. Therefore, the role for myoglobin in testing guidelines focuses on early clinical sensitivity and NPV, with rapid availability of results. Not all clinicians are convinced that myoglobin measurements contribute significantly to the assessment of acute coronary syndrome patients. However, evidence from the CHECKMATE study clearly indicates that myoglobin significantly contributes to other markers for predicting outcome (16). To optimize clinical utility, myoglobin results must be available within 30 min of the request. The major method used for myoglobin measurement is two-site immunoassay.

Creatine Kinase-MB Isoenzyme

Creatine kinase (CK) is an enzyme located in the cytoplasm of all striated muscle cells where it catalyzes the phosphorylation/dephosphorylation of creatine/creatine phosphate. Cytoplasmic CK is dimeric, composed of M and/or B subunits that associate to form CK-MM, CK-MB, and CK-BB isoenzymes. In patients having significant myocardial disease, the CK-MB isoenzyme comprises approximately 20% of the total CK in this tissue. The CK-MB is diagnostically sensitive for myocardial injury, however skeletal muscle has higher total CK activity per gram of tissue that may be comprised of up to 3% CK-MB. This potentiates compromised diagnostic specificity, particularly in patients with concomitant myocardial and skeletal muscle injury. To confer greater cardiac specificity to CK-MB measurements, a CK-MB "index" is frequently calculated according to the following equation:

$$\text{CK-MB index} = 100\% \ (\text{CK-MB}/\text{total-CK})$$

Some authors suggest that CK-MB index values exceeding 2.5% are associated with a myocardial source of the MB isoenzyme; however, a recent review shows that the index is reportedly as low as 2% and as high as 5% depending on the variability of both the numerator and denominator (5). The CK-MB mass assays were considered the "gold standard" for MI diagnosis through the 1980s until about 1995, having a sensitivity of 96.8% (95% CI: 95–98%) and specificity of 89.6% (95% CI: 87–92%) (17). Although CK-MB has lost its "gold standard" status to troponins (see Table 2), CK-MB mass measurement is still a sound tool useful in the evaluation of MI (9).

The first rise in CK-MB after MI occurs 4–6 hr after onset of symptoms, but serial sampling over a period of 8–12 hr is required for high sensitivity (14).

Thus, despite excellent clinical performance, CK-MB is not an early marker and tissue specificity may be an issue.

The POCT methods utilize two-site immunoassays, or so called "mass" assays. The CK-MB mass assays are automated, highly sensitive (<1 μg/L) and specific and have a rapid turnaround time (as low as 7 min). These methods require the use of CK-MB calibrators, for which there is no clearly agreed-upon reference standard; however, mass assays agree relatively well. Recently, the American Association for Clinical Chemistry proposed a recombinant CK-MB material for standardization of CK-MB mass assays (18).

Proteins of the Troponin Complex

Figure 3 shows that the troponin complex is located on the thin filament of striated muscle and consists of three subunits. The three-member troponin complex is essential for muscle contraction; Troponin T (TnT) is a binding protein, which attaches the troponin complex to tropomyosin. Troponin I (TnI) modulates the interaction of actin and myosin by acting as an inhibitor of the troponin-tropomyosin regulatory complex that confers calcium sensitivity to actomyosin ATPase activity. Troponin C (TnC) is the calcium-binding subunit of the troponin complex. Different isoforms are found in cardiac and skeletal muscle for both TnT and TnI muscle; the cardiac forms are designated cTnT and cTnI, respectively. The cTnT and cTnI have different amino acid sequences from the isoforms in

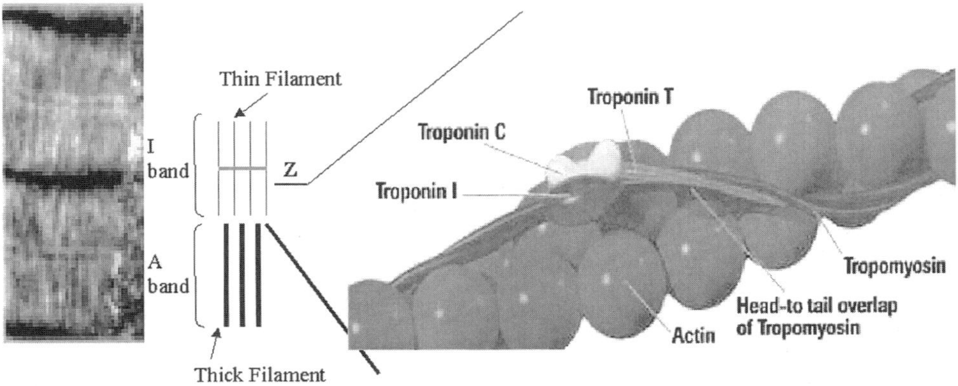

Figure 3 Structure of troponin complex. (Left) Electron micrograph of cardiac muscle; (right) schematic diagram of troponin complex. Troponin mediates calcium activation of striated muscle contraction. Troponin T binds the troponin complex to tropomyosin strand. Troponin C contains four calcium-binding sites and regulates contraction. Troponin I inhibits actomyosin ATPase.

skeletal muscle because they are encoded by separate genes. These amino acid differences allow production of antibodies that specifically recognize the cardiac forms. Because TnC has an identical amino acid sequence in both skeletal and cardiac tissues, it has no potential as a cardiac specific marker.

As indicated in Table 2, cTnT and cTnI are markers of cardiac necrosis and require several hours to rise above detectable limits after onset of acute ischemia. For this reason, troponin is not an early marker of necrosis and sampling for diagnostic use with high sensitivity and specificity requires specimen collection at patient presentation, at 6–9 hr, and at 12–24 hr if clinical suspicion is high and earlier results were negative (9). Table 2 indicates that elevation of both cTnI and cTnT after necrosis is prolonged; this allows these markers to be utilized for diagnosis many days after MI has occurred. The tradeoff is that the precise pattern of troponin release is somewhat unpredictable, so cTnT and cTnI are not useful for assessing reocclusion or for infarct sizing (see "Reocclusion (Reinfarction)" section).

Although the nature of the troponin complex released after myocardial injury is not fully characterized, several reports suggest that a large portion of TnI enters circulation as TnC-cTnT-cTnI and cTnI-TnC complexes, with only a small portion of TnI circulating in a free form (19). Several studies have examined the degradation of the troponins both inside the cell and in circulation (20). The release forms of cTnI and cTnI degradation in circulation after MI are incompletely understood at present.

Standardization of cTnI assays is a substantial issue in laboratory medicine. This problem is complicated because there are both systematic (reference value) and assay-specific (antibody) issues. Systematic issues take the form of value assignment for a reference material; assay-specific differences result because different cTnI epitopes are targeted by the various assays. This situation is far less for cTnT because all of the commercial assays are produced by a single manufacturer. At present there can be a 30-fold difference between cTnI assays, which may be resolved, in part, by defining a reference material (21).

Markers of Heart Failure

B-Type Natriuretic Peptide

B-type (or brain) natriuretic peptide (BNP) is a 32-amino-acid polypeptide containing a 17-amino-acid ring structure common to all natriuretic peptides (22). The BNP functions as a cardiac hormone secreted from the cardiac ventricles as an "emergency" measure against ventricular overload and pressure volume expansion. It shows great potential as an aid in the diagnosis of heart failure. Such a marker is needed because clinical symptoms and physical findings are considered insensitive for making an accurate heart failure diagnosis and for discriminating heart failure from other conditions. Also, echocardiography, the benchmark for diagnosing left ventricular dysfunction is expensive, may not always reflect an acute condition, and is not easily accessible.

B-type natriuretic peptide is a component of the natriuretic peptide system that is stimulated by a rise in venous pressure caused when insufficient amounts of blood are pumped to the body. The natriuretic system works by secreting several different peptides in response to wall stretch resulting from the increased volume; two important peptides are atrial natriuretic peptide (ANP), which is released in response to increased atrial wall stress, and BNP, which is secreted in response to ventricular dilation. As illustrated in Figure 1, activation of the natriuretic system results in vasodilatation, sodium excretion, and diuresis, thus lowering blood volume and blood pressure. Compared with ANP, BNP has emerged as a superior marker for heart failure and left ventricular dysfunction since its production is rapidly activated at the gene level, BNP has a longer half-life, and it is more sensitive to left ventricular dysfunction (23,24).

CLINICAL APPLICATION OF CARDIAC MARKERS

Measurement of cardiac markers, alone and in combination, is a standard of care for the assessment, diagnosis, monitoring, risk stratification, prognosis, and guidance of therapy for patients within the continuum of acute coronary syndromes (see Figure 1). Presently available biochemical markers indicate necrosis, and cTnT and cTnI have become surrogates for cell death (9). However, markers of other processes fundamental to the acute coronary syndromes would also be useful. Plaque instability/disruption and platelet activation are common physiological features in the acute coronary syndromes; therefore, markers reflecting plaque stability and activated or "angry" platelets would have great clinical potential. Inflammation markers such as C-reactive protein have demonstrated use for assessment of long-term risk, but also may have a role in assessing the suspected acute coronary syndrome patient. Ischemia is the central physiological process; initial data on IMA are promising, and testing for acute cardiac ischemia would also have an important role in clinical settings. The evidence for markers of cardiac necrosis, including myoglobin, CK-MB, and troponin, is well established (8,9,14) and utilization of these markers is the focus of this section.

Assessment of Cardiac Ischemia

Conditions for altering albumin's amino terminus region, and therefore albumin cobalt binding, can occur within minutes of an ischemic event due to induced endothelial and extracellular hypoxia, acidosis, free radical injury, and sodium and calcium pump disruptions (25,26). Although there is no agreed-upon reference for assessing myocardial ischemia, IMA testing may add useful information into clinical acumen, imaging techniques, and stress testing.

Diagnosis of Myocardial Infarction

For over 20 yr prior to the year 2000, the definition and diagnosis of MI were based on modified World Health Organization (WHO) criteria in which patients must meet at least two of three conditions (27): typical symptoms of ischemia, a diagnostic ECG, and a characteristic rise and fall in "enzymes," later interpreted as CK-MB. There were a number of issues with these MI criteria; although symptoms are generally what cause patients to seek care, typical clinical signs of ischemia are absent in one-third of patients (28). The ECG, as indicated in Figure 2, is essential for assessment and classification of acute coronary syndrome patients. However, only 45% of patients who are eventually diagnosed as having MI present with a diagnostic ECG (14). Also, when the WHO criteria were defined in 1979, "enzyme" biochemical markers included total CK activity, lactate dehydrogenase (LDH), and aspartate transaminase (AST). In the years after the definition of WHO criteria, a typical rise and fall in CK-MB became the accepted benchmark from the 1980s to ~1995 (14). An update in MI definition was needed since entering "the era of troponin."

Development of sensitive and specific assays for CK-MB mass, cTnT, cTnI, and myoglobin, as well as evolution of precise imaging technologies, have prompted re-evaluation of the established MI definition by a joint committee of the European Society of Cardiology (ESC) and the American College of Cardiology (ACC) (9). The resulting ESC/ACC consensus presented a new definition of myocardial necrosis in which elevations of the troponins or CK-MB are the cornerstone. Biochemical criteria for detecting myocardial necrosis in the setting of myocardial ischemia are (9):

1. Maximal concentration of cTnT or cTnI exceeding the 99th percentile of a reference control group on at least one occasion during the first 24 hr.
2. "Maximal" value of CK-MB exceeding the 99th percentile of the values for a reference control group on two successive samples, or maximal value exceeding twice the upper limit of normal for the specific institution on one occasion during the first 24 hr.

Further the ESC/ACC committee recommended that imprecision, coefficient of variation (CV), at the marker cutpoint should be ≤10%.

The following criteria satisfy the diagnosis of acute, evolving, or recent MI:

Typical rise and gradual fall (troponin) or more rapid rise and fall (CK-MB) of biochemical markers of myocardial necrosis with at least one of the following:

a. ischemic symptoms
b. development of pathologic Q waves on the ECG
c. ECG changes indicative of ischemia (ST segment elevation or depression)
d. coronary artery intervention (e.g., coronary angioplasty)

These new criteria are particularly significant because many patients who were previously diagnosed as having severe stable or unstable angina will now have the diagnosis of MI, with all the associated sociological, epidemiological, financial, and other implications. The incidence of MI will increase by an estimated 15–30%, which translates into about 100,000–200,000 more MI cases each year, as a result of this redefinition.

Importantly, the ESC/ACC report stressed the importance of serial sampling for cardiac markers, recommending sampling upon presentation, at 6–9 hr, and again at 12–24 hr if the earlier samples were negative and the clinical index of suspicion is high (9).

A clinical setting where POCT for cardiac markers may have an important role is for monitoring myocardial cell death in the setting of percutaneous coronary intervention. As stated in the previous section, a rise in troponin or CK-MB during angioplasty indicates MI and an increased risk of future cardiac events. Infarcts can be detected with serial monitoring before the procedure, at 6–8 hr, and at 24 hr (9).

Reocclusion (Reinfarction)

Reocclusion occurs in up to 10–20% of MI patients and is an important determinant of early and late morbidity and mortality (29). Criteria commonly used to identify recurrent MI include prolonged chest pain, new ECG changes, and biochemical markers. Because cTnT and cTnI have an extended half-life in blood and their time course is somewhat unpredictable, markers with a shorter, more predictable time-course such as CK-MB are utilized to more clearly indicate timing of the clinical event.

The rapid turnaround offered by POC measurements could develop into an important component of care for these patients because benefits from the interventional options for reocclusion are time sensitive.

Noninvasive Assessment of Reperfusion

As discussed earlier, ST elevation or new left bundle branch block on the ECG guides the use of reperfusion therapy that includes "clot busting" thrombolytic drugs such as streptokinase and tissue plasminogen activator. The "gold standard" for assessing the success of reperfusion therapy is angiography using the following grading scale from the Thrombolysis in Myocardial Infarction (TIMI) Trial (30):

TIMI 0: No anterograde flow beyond the point of occlusion
TIMI 1: Penetration without perfusion
TIMI 2: Partial perfusion
TIMI 3: Complete perfusion

Successful reperfusion is defined as TIMI 2 or 3 flow in some studies, but success for optimizing outcome is usually considered establishment of TIMI 3 flow in the infarcted artery (31).

Thrombolytic therapy is successful in achieving TIMI 3 patency in only 60–70% of patients (30). Because cardiac catheterization is invasive, expensive, and is not available at every medical center, strategies that include biochemical markers have been developed to assist clinicians in determining patients whose infarct-related artery patency remains suboptimal, and who may benefit from immediate, alternative interventions. A model that combines clinical variables with myoglobin and CK-MB data in samples collected just before thrombolytic therapy, and then at 60 and 90 min later shows substantial promise (32,33). Myoglobin, due to its rapid "washout" after thrombolysis, CK-MB, and perhaps also troponin may be important for reperfusion monitoring (33). Point-of-care testing will be critical for monitoring the success of reperfusion because a rapid turnaround time is needed to determine if thrombolysis has not been successful, so that alternate care strategies, such as PCI or coronary artery bypass surgery, may be considered to fully "open the artery" and improve outcome.

Risk Stratification

The discovery that cTnT and cTnI predict increased risk for an adverse outcome in acute coronary syndrome patients must be considered one of the most important findings in laboratory medicine over the past decade. A number of outcome studies demonstrating this increased risk have been analyzed in systematic reviews. One meta-analysis that included results of 2847 unstable angina patients showed that a positive cTnT was associated with a 2.7-fold (95% CI: 2.1–3.4) increased risk for either MI or death by 42 days (34). For positive cTnI results, this meta-analysis (34) yielded a cumulative odds ratio (OR) of 4.2 (95% CI: 2.7–6.4) in 1901 patients. A separate systematic review examined the association of positive cTnT or cTnI with 30-day death or MI in a total of 18,982 acute coronary syndrome patients from 21 studies (35). This larger analysis indicated that positive troponin indicated greater risk with a cumulative OR of 3.44 (95% CI: 2.94–4.03). This study (35) also examined troponin results based on ECG findings; a positive troponin in ST elevation patients was associated with a 2.86-fold (95% CI: 2.35–3.47) increased risk of 30-day death or MI; in the non–ST elevation group, risk of death or MI was increased 4.93-fold (95% CI: 3.77–6.45). Further, a study that examined troponin and mortality or MI at 1 yr also found a higher risk profile for troponin positive patients at this endpoint (36). The consistent message is that troponin positive acute coronary syndrome patients are at three- to fivefold increased risk of death or MI in the 30–40 days following the index event, and that this higher risk extends to longer times.

Timing of sampling for troponin measurement is important for risk stratification. Although troponin measurement at presentation provides the most information, measurements must be performed in samples collected at 8–16 hr because this strategy shows a significant improvement in the ability to risk stratify (36). Also, sampling at presentation and then 8–16 hr later helps to avoid possible methodological differences among troponin assays.

This strong evidence for risk stratification indicates that testing for cTnT and cTnI are appropriate for triage and decisions relating to hospital admission and perhaps interventions, such as PCI (37,38). Development of POC assays for cTnT and cTnI have facilitated delivery of this important information, so that caregivers can appropriately stratify high-risk patients. Most importantly, clinical management and guidance of therapy for acute coronary syndrome patients based on risk stratification by biochemical markers "is an idea whose time has come" (39).

Guidance of Therapy and Intervention

The strong evidence that positive troponin measurements translate to increased risk in acute coronary syndrome patients has led to guidelines for unstable angina and non–ST elevation that designate troponin positive patients as high risk. These patients should receive medications such as aspirin, beta-blockers, nitrates, and either an early invasive or early conservative strategy of care (37,38). This translation of troponin positivity to increased risk has been confluent with development of novel therapeutics targeting platelet physiology. These therapeutics are aimed at improving the outcome of acute coronary syndrome patients, particularly those having unstable angina and non–ST elevation MI. Because these drugs are frequently expensive and definitive benefit is difficult to demonstrate, directing therapy at high-risk patients identified with biochemical markers is a logical extension of knowledge.

Identifying patients with unstable coronary artery disease who may benefit from low-molecular-weight (LMW) heparin by use of cTnT measurements was examined in the FRISC study (40). In patient groups having positive cTnT ($\geq$0.1 ng/mL), those receiving placebo had a significantly higher incidence of death and/or MI compared with patients randomized to LMW heparin. On the other hand, patient groups that were cTnT negative ($<$0.1 ng/mL) were both at low risk and showed no difference in outcome whether they received placebo or LMW heparin.

An important focus in cardiovascular therapeutics has been development of agents that are antagonists for the platelet GP IIb/IIIa receptor. These agents inhibit conformational changes in the GP IIb/IIIa receptor, which is the final step in platelet activation. Blockage of this receptor prevents platelets from becoming activated (angry) and potentiating thrombosis. The CAPTURE study included unstable angina patients who were randomized to receive either the GP IIb/IIIa receptor inhibitor abciximab or placebo (41). Patients for whom cTnT was negative (<0.1 ng/mL) showed a similar low incidence of death or MI in both in-hospital and on 6-mo follow-up whether they received placebo or the GP IIb/IIIa inhibitor. Consistent with risk stratification data, patients receiving placebo who were cTnT positive had a significantly higher rate of adverse events. Importantly, however, the cTnT positive patients who received the GP IIb/IIIa inhibitor had a significantly lower rate of death or MI, which was similar to the cTnT negative groups. Thus, cTnT measurements identified a high-risk group that benefited from administration of the drug. Another GP IIb/IIIa inhibitor, tirofiban, was examined in the PRISM study (42). This randomized trial also showed that cTnI and cTnT reliably identified high-risk patients who benefited from treatment. Finally, the PARAGON B study examined the association between troponin concentrations and a third GP IIb/IIIa inhibitor termed lamifiban (43). PARAGON B also found that cTnT identified patients who had better outcomes with drug treatment. Together these GP IIb/IIIa inhibitor studies included over 4500 patients and served to validate utilization of troponin for identification of high-risk individuals and guidance of GP IIb/IIIa inhibitor therapy. These compelling data have prompted inclusion of troponin positivity into guidelines for identification and clinical management of high-risk unstable angina patients (37) and also for guiding management of patients with acute MI (38).

Point-of-care testing for biochemical markers will be driven by the improvement in outcome attributed to earlier intervention with cardiac catheterization and PCI or GP IIb/IIIa inhibitors. Findings of the EARLY trial also indicate that the sooner appropriate patients receive GP IIb/IIIa inhibitors, the better their outcome (M. Roe, personal communication). For this reason, the National Heart Attack Alert Program has designated that time from order to availability time (turnaround time) for cardiac markers should be 30 min, and that this time should become a quality indicator. Point-of-care testing for cardiac markers will become essential at most institutions to meet this criterion.

Prognosis (Infarct Sizing)

Assessing myocardial cell death after prolonged ischemia is a semiquantitative system according to the following four pathological classifications (9):

1. Microscopic, with focal necrosis
2. Small, <10% of the left ventricle
3. Medium, 10–30% of the left ventricle
4. Large, >30% of the left ventricle

However, clinically and for use in clinical trials where short-term mortality is relatively low, the use of biochemical marker curves for prognostication and predicting outcomes is most appropriate (9). Since the 1970s, investigators have studied the use of markers for quantifying (sizing) myocardial necrosis (44,45), reasoning that the greater the extent of cardiac cell death, the worse the prognosis. The general approach has involved serially measuring markers in blood over hours and days after the clinical event and then mathematically modeling the release profile. By integrating the area of the time-release curve, calculating peak concentration, etc., it was possible to determine the quantity of myocardial tissue that was injured irreversibly.

Biochemical markers including α-hydroxybutyrate dehydrogenase, myoglobin, total CK, and CK-MB have been used for infarct sizing and prognosis. Tradeoffs in sample timing and predictability of release have favored use of total CK and CK-MB, and their association with outcomes is well established (46,47). Infarct size correlates closely with mortality as well as other prognostic indexes such as cardiac failure, ventricular function, and arrhythmia (48). Peak CK-MB value has been found to significantly correlate with 5-yr outcome (49). In the setting of PCI, measured elevations in CK-MB have demonstrated a strong association with outcomes (50).

Point-of-care testing of cardiac markers, mainly CK-MB, may be performed in the intensive care unit, or in the postintervention areas to provide clinicians with timely prognostic information.

Heart Failure

Differentiating heart failure, i.e., impaired pump function with reduced cardiac output and subsequent venous congestion, from other causes of dyspnea is crucial in patients presenting to the ED with acute shortness of breath (51). The mean BNP blood levels in patients with heart failure were shown to be significantly higher ($p < 0.001$) than in patients without heart failure (52). At a blood concentration of 80 pg/ml, BNP was able to accurately predict the presence of heart failure (95%); lower levels had a high negative predictive value of 98% (51).

The increased awareness and clinical significance of BNP have led to development of a POC assay to rapidly identify and assess the severity of heart failure. This assay allows caregivers to determine whether patients with suspected heart failure need to be further evaluated by invasive, resource intensive procedures such as echocardiography and radionuclear ventriculography. The body of evidence for clinical use of BNP as a potential marker for sensitive and specific assessment and monitoring of heart failure patients is growing rapidly.

SPECIFIC POC ASSAYS FOR CARDIAC MARKERS

Immunoassay is the common analytic strategy for POC measurement of cardiac markers. Although the assay principles are similar to central laboratory testing, POC devices and technologies have been modified to simplify performance, reduce the chance of operator error, use a whole blood sample matrix, provide faster results, and streamline quality control (QC)/quality assurance (QA) processes. There are two general platform types that support POCT: small benchtop analyzers and handheld devices. These devices are designed for simple operation, but are actually complex systems that perform several tasks, such as separating cells from plasma, apportioning the proper amount of sample, reading analyte signal, data processing, and system interface. The following is a description of the available POC technologies for measurement of cardiac markers displayed in Table 3.

Roche Cardiac T® and Roche Cardiac™ M Tests

As displayed in Figure 4, cTnT and myoglobin tests are available in separate rapid assay formats termed Roche Cardiac T and Roche Cardiac M, respectively (Roche Diagnostics Corporation, Indianapolis, IN). Both these assays are about the size of a standard Band-Aid, and utilize immunochromatography with two antibodies that bind to different molecular epitopes in a single-step "sandwich" immunoassay format. One of the antibodies is biotinylated, to facilitate capture with polystreptavidin, and the second is conjugated to gold particles for detection. The cTnT assay uses the same pair of anti-cTnT antibodies that are used for measurement with Roche's Elecsys® laboratory system. This facilitates harmonization between POC and central lab results.

Measurements are initiated by addition of heparinized whole blood to the sample well. Capillary action combined with filtration separates cellular constituents from the plasma, which solubilizes the antibodies and other reagents. The two antibodies form a sandwich complex with any cTnT or myoglobin present. The sandwich complex migrates with plasma along the test strip by capillary action until it reaches polystreptavidin, which is immobilized in a thin line across the read window of the test strips. At this point the polystreptavidin captures the biotinylated end of any immune sandwiches, serving to concentrate the complexes. Further flow of plasma through the read window carries unreacted anti-cTnT or antimyoglobin antibodies conjugated with gold particles past the polystreptavidin read window, where they combine with a fragment of cTnT or myoglobin bound to an anchor protein immobilized in the QC test line (see Fig-

Table 3 Characteristics of Currently Available Cardiac POC Assays

Device	Cardiac marker	Suggested cutoff	Manufacturer's claim	Time (min)	Specimen (type and volume)
Roche Cardiac T Rapid Assay	cTnT	0.1 ng/mL[a]	Myocardial damage is detected	12	150 μL heparin whole blood
Roche Cardiac M Rapid Assay	Myoglobin	Male: 76 ng/mL Female: 64 ng/mL	Above normal range	8	150 μL heparin whole blood
Cardiac STATus device (Spectral Diagnostics)[b]	CK-MB Myoglobin cTnI	5 ng/mL (Abbott method) 50 ng/mL (Behring Diagnostics method) 1.5 ng/mL (Dade Stratus method)	Aid in the diagnosis of cardiac ischemia	15	200 μL serum or heparinized whole blood or plasma
Alpha Dx POINT-OF-NEED System (First Medical)	Total CK mass CK-MB RI (%) Myoglobin cTnI	190 ng/mL 7.0 ng/mL 5.0 100 ng/mL 0.40 ng/mL	Aid in the diagnosis of AMI	18	1.5 mL EDTA whole blood or serum
Stratus CS STAT Fluorometric Analyzer (Dade Behring, Inc.)	CK-MB Myoglobin cTnI	3.5 ng/mL Male: 98 ng/mL Female: 56 ng/mL 0.06 ng/mL	All markers: Aid in the diagnosis of AMI cTnI: Risk stratification	14 min to first result, 4 min for each additional result	Whole blood (lithium or sodium heparin): 3 mL Plasma (lithium or sodium heparin): 200 μL for first test, 100 μL for each additional test on the same run
Triage Cardiac Panel (Biosite Diagnostics)	CK-MB Myoglobin cTnI	10.0 ng/mL 170.0 ng/mL 1.0 ng/mL	Aid in the diagnosis of MI	~15	250 μL heparinized whole blood or plasma
Triage BNP	BNP	100 pg/mL	Aid in the diagnosis of CHF	~15	250 μL EDTA whole blood or plasma
Myoglobin (Response Biomedical)[c]	Myoglobin	—	—	—	Heparinized whole blood or plasma

[a] Values <0.05 ng/mL indicate negative TnT; values between 0.05 and <0.1 ng/mL indicate low TnT and test should be repeated within 1 hr with a fresh blood sample; values between 0.1 and 2.0 ng/mL indicate myocardial damage; values >2.0 ng/mL indicate massive myocardial damage.
[b] This assay yields qualitative results. [c] This assay is not commercially available at time of publication.

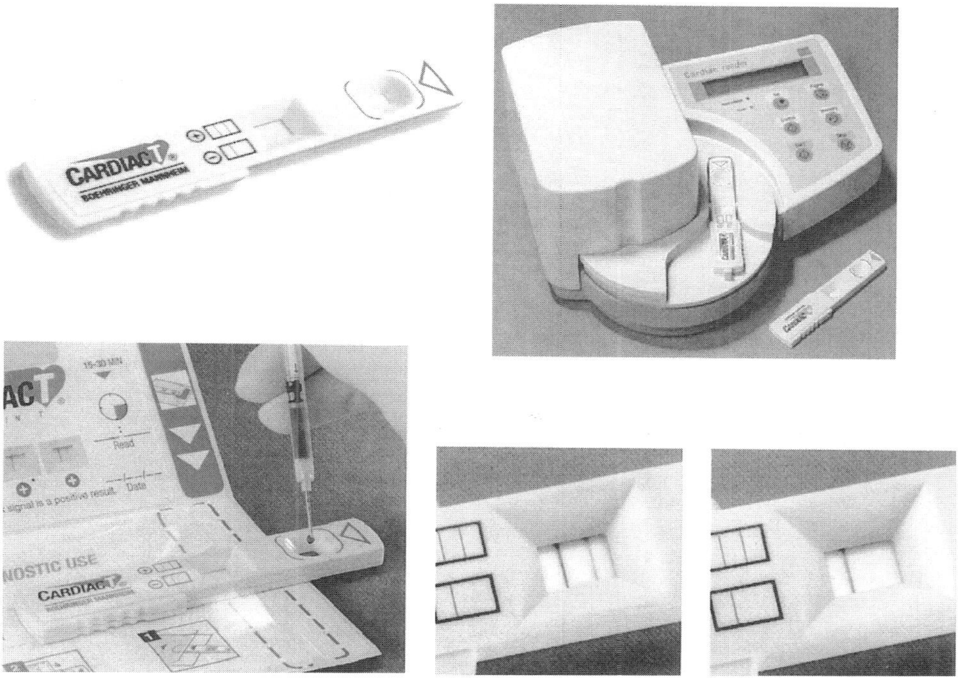

Figure 4 Cardiac T rapid assay (top left) and reader (top right). The rapid assay is dosed with 150 μl of venous blood using the syringe provided (bottom left). Results (bottom right) appear within 15 min; two lines indicate a positive result (myocardial damage), whereas one line indicates a negative result (no detectable cTnT). (Courtesy of Roche Diagnostics.)

ure 4). The concentrated gold particles produce a reddish purple line(s) that is interpreted visually for qualitative tests (CARDIAC T only), or quantified by the Roche CARDIAC™ Reader, a device about the size of a Frisbee. As indicated in Figure 4, the on-board positive QC test line is integral to each rapid assay strip and must be formed for the test result to be valid. The intensity and rate at which the colored line develops is directly proportional to the concentration of cTnT or myoglobin in the blood.

For quantitative results, the CARDIAC Reader uses a specific calibration for each lot of assay test strips that is designed to match serum cTnT or myoglobin measurements on the Elecsys immunoassay analyzer. At a minimum, a positive and negative QC must be run with each new lot number of rapid assay strips or when irregularities in storage conditions are suspected.

Cardiac STATus™ Device

As shown in Figure 5, the STATus assay system (Spectral Diagnostics Inc., Toronto, Canada) uses chromatographic solid-phase immunoassay technology to provide qualitative results for a testing panel that includes myoglobin, CK-MB mass, and cTnI. A second device for qualitative measurement of cTnI is also available. The devices measure $3^1/_2 \times 1^1/_2 \times {}^1/_2$ inches.

Heparinized whole blood, heparinized plasma, or serum specimens may be used. After initial separation of the plasma fraction from the cellular blood components by a glass fiber fleece, the migrating plasma dissolves a buffer and solubilizes the reagent antibodies. The myoglobin, CK-MB, or cTnI analyte in the patient sample reacts with dye-labeled antibodies that are analyte specific. The [dye-labeled antibody/analyte] complexes migrate by immunochromatography to

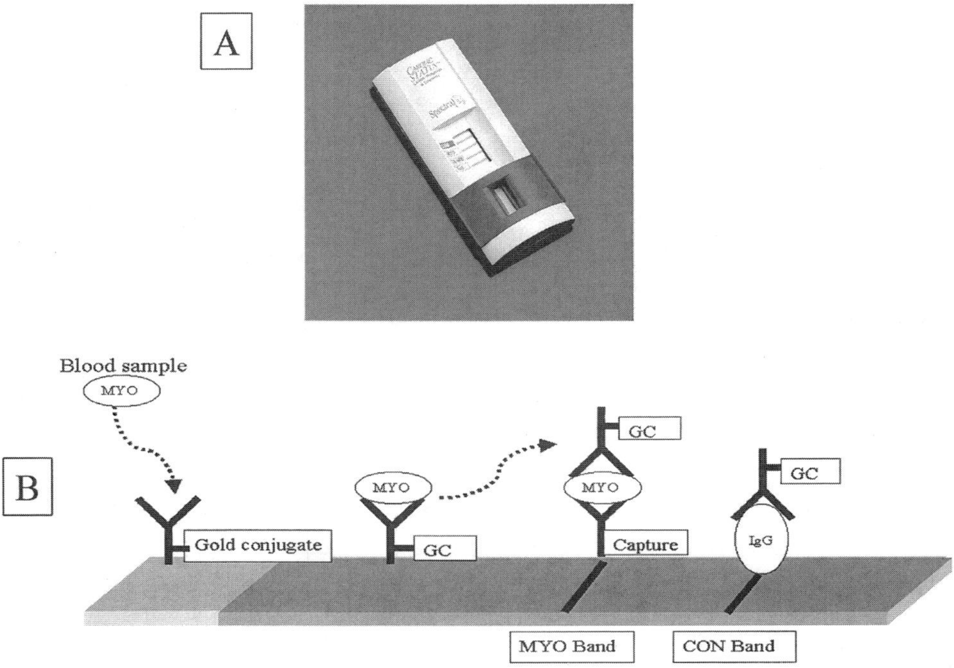

Figure 5 (A) Cardiac STATus device. The device provides qualitative results for cTnI, myoglobin, and CK-MB in whole blood, plasma, or serum without instrumentation. (Courtesy Spectral Diagnostics.) (B) Schematic of the STATus technology illustrating binding of antigen (myo) with conjugated antibody, migration of this complex in the device, and immobilization by capture antibody.

the detection zone, where capture antibodies directed at different epitopes on the myoglobin, CK-MB, or cTnI molecules immobilize the complexes at different positions, each in line formation. Unbound labeled antibodies migrate out of the test area and are later captured by solid-phase anti-IgG antibodies in the control "CON" area, forming a fourth QC line shown in Figure 5. The appearance of the control line confirms proper performance of the device, including unimpeded plasma flow. A similar strategy is used for the cTnI device; however, two lines are present for a positive test, one for cTnI and one for the control. If a band is present only in the "CON" area, the test result is read as negative. If no band is present in the "CON" area, the test should be considered invalid and another device must be run, regardless of the presence or absence of a band in the test area.

The STATus system has been classified as moderately complex under CLIA regulations. At a minimum, performance of liquid positive and negative control specimens is necessary with each shipment of reagents. It is important to note that confirmation of any positive CK-MB, myoglobin, or cTnI results by a quantitative laboratory assay is not required.

Triage® System for Cardiac and B-Type Natriuretic Peptide Measurement

Figure 6 indicates that the Triage Cardiac system (Biosite Diagnostics Inc., San Diego, CA) consists of two basic components, a wafer-shaped test cartridge that

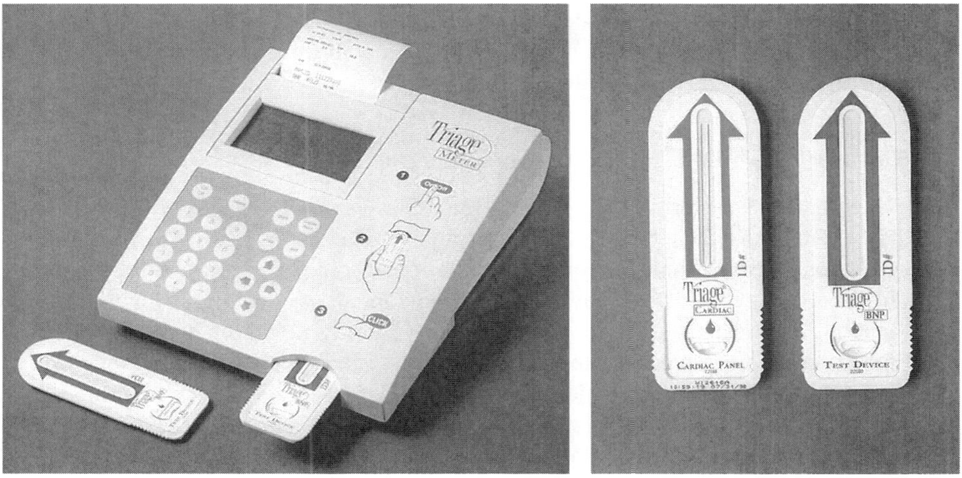

Figure 6 The Triage Meter (left) and Triage Cardiac Panel and BNP immunoassay test cartridges (right). (Courtesy of Biosite Diagnostics.)

contains all necessary analytic reagents and the Triage Meter that is about the size of a telephone. The system provides for quantitative measurement of a cardiac marker panel including myoglobin, CK-MB, and cTnI. Analytes are quantified simultaneously in respective one-step "sandwich" immunoassays using immunochromatography with fluorescence detection.

After dosing the cartridge with heparinized whole blood or plasma, the plasma and cellular constituents are separated by filtration. The plasma phase is delivered to areas on the cartridge containing dried immunoassay reagents specific for myoglobin, cTnI, or CK-MB measurement. During incubation, the reaction mixture flows down a microcapillary and comes in contact with immobilized antibodies, directed at different myoglobin, CK-MB, or cTnI epitopes, that are oriented as different lines for each analyte in the detection zone. The binding of analyte labeled with fluorescent reagents in these zones is measured by a fluorometer in the Triage Meter and is directly proportional to the concentration of the analytes being tested. The signal for each cardiac marker is compared with its specific analytical curve, allowing quantitative measurement. Each of the myoglobin, cTnI, and CK-MB immunoassays has internal quality control zones to ensure their validity and accuracy.

The Triage BNP test is also a fluorescence immunoassay for the quantitative measurement in whole blood and plasma specimens. The principles of BNP measurement are the same as for other markers only a specific cocktail of BNP antibodies is utilized.

Results for the Triage system can be printed and are stored in the meter memory for downloading to a laboratory information system. The system has been classified as moderately complex under CLIA regulations. At a minimum, performance of liquid positive and negative control specimens is necessary with each shipment of reagents or every 30 days.

Stratus® CS STAT Fluorometric Analyzer

The Stratus CS system (Dade Behring Inc., Glasgow, DE) displayed in Figure 7 is 18″ high by 27″ wide by 22″ deep in size. The Stratus CS uses two-site sandwich immunoassay technology and fluorometric detection in a solid-phase radial partition chromatography format for random access quantitative measurement of CK-MB mass, myoglobin, and cTnI in lithium and sodium heparin whole blood or plasma samples. The test system employs monoclonal capture antibodies conjugated to dendrimers, which are polymers composed of polyamine groups characterized by uniformity in size and shape. Compared with earlier technology, dendrimers enhance presentation and functionality of the immobilized antibody on the system's solid phase, resulting in more efficient antigen capture. The cTnI-specific antibodies are identical to those used on the Dimension® system so there

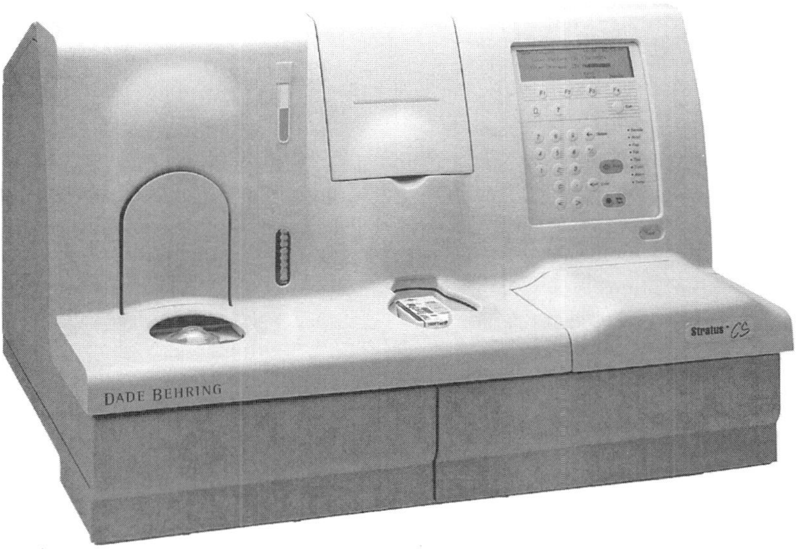

Figure 7 The Stratus CS STAT fluorometric analyzer is a whole blood analyzer that is capable of running single tests in fully automated mode. Tests available on this system are cTnI, myoglobin, and CK-MB. (Courtesy of Dade Behring.)

is analytical harmony between the POC and central laboratory systems. Also, the Stratus CS and Dimension antibodies bind both free and complexed cTnI.

The Stratus CS analyzer uses on-board centrifugation to separate plasma from whole blood prior to the analytic phase; alternatively, heparinized plasma can be analyzed. During measurement, plasma is automatically pipetted onto the solid phase where it reacts with an immobilized monoclonal antibody, linked to dendrimer, which recognizes a distinct epitope on the myoglobin, CK-MB, or cTnI analyte. Following incubation, a second monoclonal antibody, conjugated to alkaline phosphatase, which recognizes a different antigenic site on the analyte, is pipetted onto the reaction zone. Detection and removal of unbound conjugated antibody are accomplished simultaneously by addition of the enzyme substrate and wash solution. Front surface fluorometry of the 4-methylumbelliferone enzyme product is used for quantitation.

Quality control requires the processing of a daily System Check (electronic QC) that interrogates the system's optical detection, temperature, mechanical alignment, and fluid delivery components. Two levels of liquid controls are only required after each calibration, with each new shipment of reagents, when indicated by troubleshooting or part replacement procedures, and whenever the system performance needs to be checked.

Alpha Dx™ POINT-OF-NEED™ System™

Figure 8 shows the Alpha Dx POINT-OF-NEED system (First Medical, Mountain View, CA), a platform that integrates automated solid-phase sandwich immunoassay technology with fluorescence detection. In comparison with a typical sandwich fluorescent immunoassay, the Alpha Dx POINT-OF-NEED system utilizes three antibodies: a fluorescein-labeled antibody, a solid-phase capture antibody directed at a different epitope, and a fluorescent-labeled (Cy5) antifluorescein monoclonal antibody that is conjugated to dextran. The three antibody system increases signal amplification and enhances assay sensitivity.

In addition to the Alpha Dx POINT-OF-NEED analyzer, the system includes a calibration diskette, Safe-T-Coupler™ unit for direct tube sampling, and a fluid cassette. The system uses an EDTA whole blood sample to quantitatively measure a profile of cardiac markers that includes myoglobin, total CK mass, CK-MB mass, and cTnI. The Safe-T-Coupler unit is used to load a primary blood collection tube into the analyzer, where a small aliquot of the sample is metered from a standard phlebotomy tube into the system's test disk (see Figure 8). The test disk consists of four fluidically connected chambers: one for sample (or control) introduction, containing the fluorescein-labeled antibodies to the analytes; a second chamber for reaction, containing analyte-specific capture antibodies; a third for the fluorescent-labeled anti-fluorescein dextran conjugate for detection, and a fourth wash chamber. Small magnetically activated stainless steel balls in the sample and label chambers facilitate reagent rehydration and mixing; the disk is spun to move fluids through the chambers. Each disk has three sets, or "zones" of fluidic chambers. One zone is used for the test sample and the others are for two levels of on-board quality control. Each disk also contains a waste ring and a hematocrit chamber where packed cell volume is measured and used to convert the measured whole blood sample data to matched serum results. In all assays, fluorescence intensity is proportional to the amount of bound label and consequently to analyte concentration in the sample or control.

A calibration diskette contains all lot-specific calibration and quality control information. Biohazard waste and assay fluids are contained within the test disk and Safe-T-Coupler unit. As stated above, the test disk has two levels of controls built-in that are processed in parallel with each patient sample and therefore there is no need for external QC protocols. The system automatically calculates the relative index of CK-MB and CK. The software includes quality control display and management, display of temporal patient data, and other enhancements.

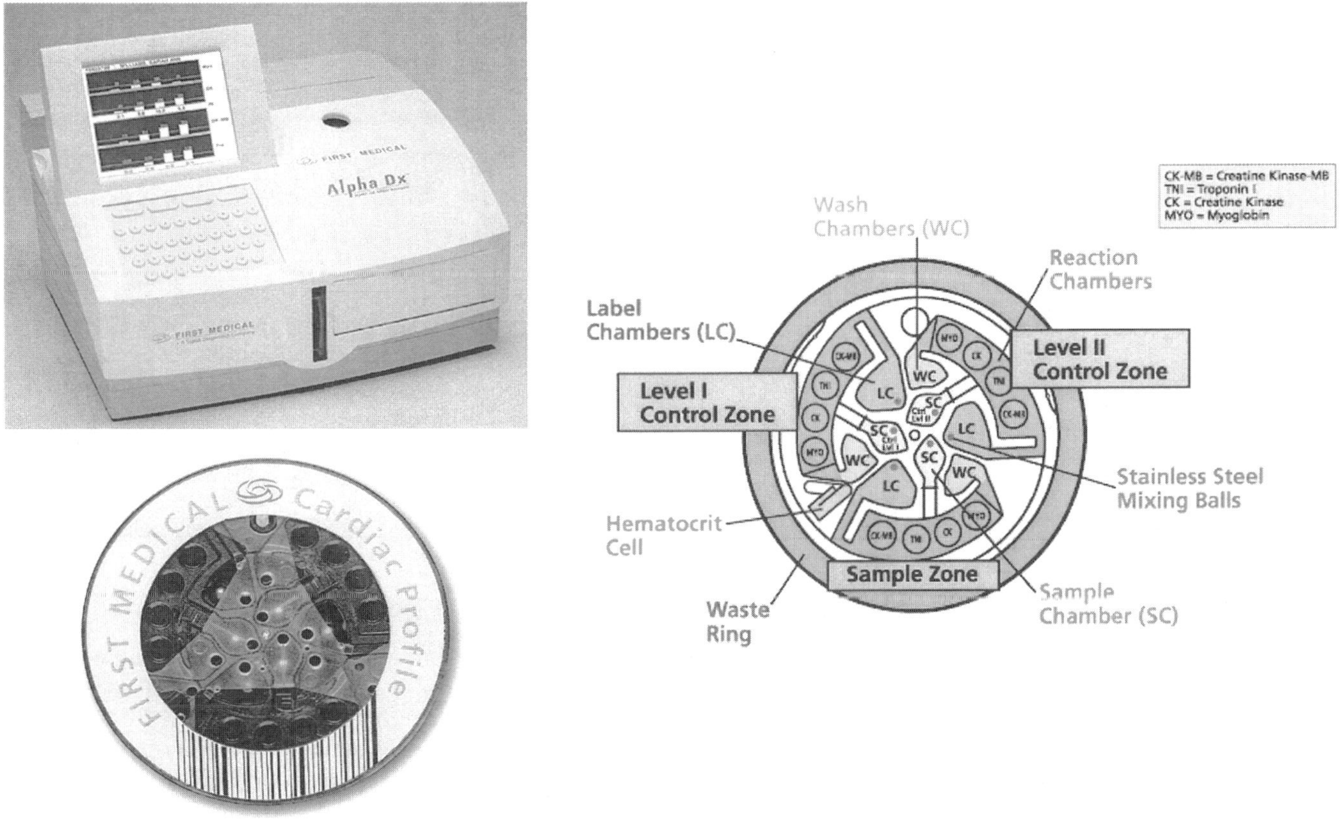

Figure 8 Alpha Dx analyzer (top left) and cardiac panel test disk (bottom left). Details of cardiac profile test disk (right) showing three zones (one sample and two controls), different chambers (for sample, reaction, label, and wash), waste ring, and hematocrit cell (Courtesy of First Medical.)

RAMP™ Cardiac Marker Testing

Figure 9 shows the Rapid Analyte Measurement Platform (RAMP) (Response Biomedical Inc., Burnaby, BC, Canada), which uses immunochromatography and fluorescently dyed latex for quantification of myoglobin and other cardiac markers. The system uses either heparinized whole blood or plasma samples; samples are pipetted into the well of a test cartridge, then inserted into the RAMP reader. Once inserted, the liquid sample is drawn by capillary action along the membrane

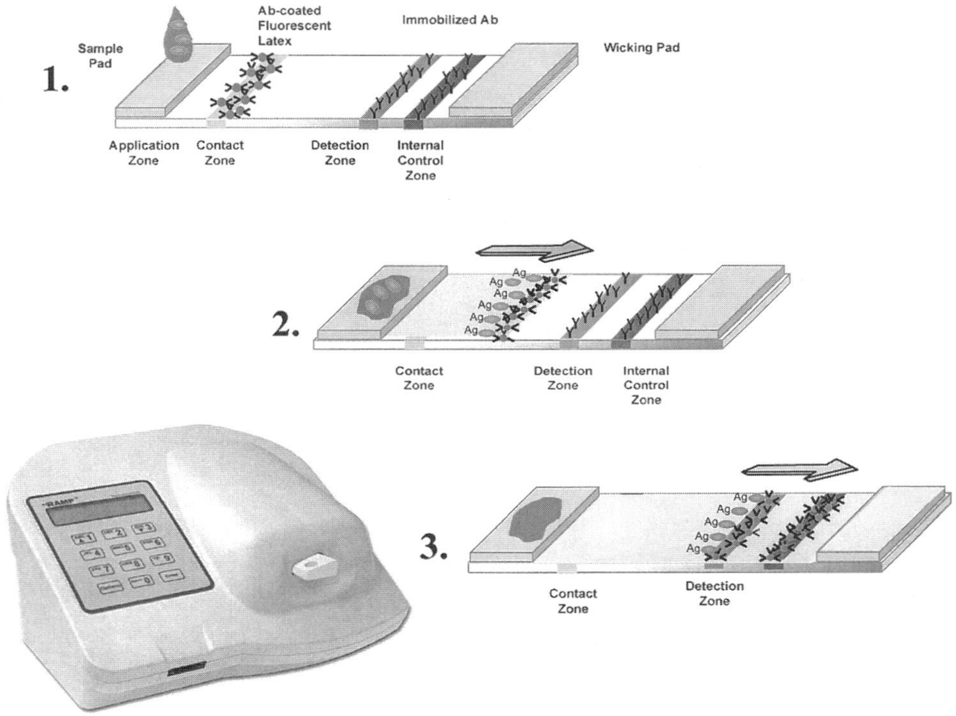

Figure 9 The RAMP system (bottom left) promises quantitative results with the ease use of immunoassay. The RAMP cartridge accommodates an analyte-specific test strip. Step 1: A liquid sample is added to the application zone at one end of the RAMP cartridge and migrates along the membrane by capillary action and passes through the contact zone. Step 2: When the liquid sample migrates through the contact zone, antibody-coated fluorescent latex particles are carried along the membrane strip by capillary flow. The target analyte in the sample binds covalently to the antibodies on the latex. Step 3: The amount of latex particles immobilized in the detection zone is directly related to the concentration of target analyte in the sample. (Courtesy of Response Biomedical.)

through the contact zone where it comes into contact with the fluorescent-labeled antibody-coated latex particles.

When the liquid migrates through the contact zone, the latex particles are mobilized and carried along the membrane strip (see Figure 9). The particles are labeled with a mouse monoclonal antibody against analyte such as myoglobin. In the contact zone, analyte (myoglobin) present in the sample binds covalently to the antibody on the test latex particles. Sample fluid matrix, latex particles bound to analyte (myoglobin), and unbound particles move together by capillary action along the strip to the detection and internal standard zones (see Figure 9). The detection zone is embedded with a second immobilized antianalyte (antimyoglobin) antibody. Migrating analyte–latex particle complexes are captured by the immobilized antibody and concentrated in the detection zone. The quantity of latex particles immobilized in the detection zone is directly related to the concentration of analyte (myoglobin) in the sample (see Figure 9). Past the detection zone is the internal standard zone; this area is embedded with immobilized antimouse immunoglobulin (Ig) from goat. Some of the remaining antibody-coated latex particles are immobilized in this zone. The RAMP system has a single channel scanning fluorometer that measures the amount of fluorescence emitted by the complexes bound on the detection and internal standard zones. For quantitation, the reader calculates a ratio between the two readings. The scanning also allows background subtraction and numerous QC checks of the assay. The internal standard both corrects for membrane variability and provides an internal validation of the assay. Results are complete within 8–15 min, depending on which assay is being run, and appears on an LCD readout. The result can also be stored, printed, or downloaded to a laboratory or hospital information system.

Cardiac Markers: Why POCT?

Addressing clinically focused questions is essential for achieving clinically relevant answers. The following are clinically based questions that focus on issues relevant to POCT for cardiac markers.

Question 1. Is troponin important for identification of patients at increased risk of adverse outcomes?

Troponin results are definitely needed for appropriate risk stratification of patients suspected of acute coronary syndromes. Meta-analyses (34,35) provide strong and compelling evidence and the ACC/AHA Task Force issued practice guidelines for the management of patients with unstable angina and non–ST segment elevation MI (37). For early risk stratification, these ACC/AHA recommendations state that "biomarkers of cardiac injury should be measured in all patients who present with chest discomfort consistent with acute coronary syndromes. A cardiac-specific troponin is the preferred marker . . . it should be measured in all patients. In patients with negative cardiac markers within 6 hours of the onset of pain, another sample should be drawn in the 6- to 12-hour time frame (e.g., at 9 hours) after the onset of symptoms."

Question 2. Is turnaround time ("vein-to-brain" or order-to-availability time) of biochemical markers (troponin) related to outcome for high-risk patients?

Studies have demonstrated that earlier treatment of high-risk acute coronary syndrome patients with GP IIb/IIIa inhibitors improves clinically important outcomes (53). Also, early intervention with PCI improves outcomes (50). Practice guidelines list positive biomarker (troponin) results as important, evidence-based determinants of high risk (37,38). For these reasons, the National Heart Attack Alert Program (NHAAP) has listed a "vein-to-brain" time of 30 min as a goal, and that order-to-availability time for biochemical markers should be a quality indicator for clinical care.

Question 3. Does POCT of biochemical markers improve availability ("vein-to-brain") time?

Two studies comparing central laboratory versus POCT have shown that POCT markedly improved availability of troponin results by 8-fold (median of 128 versus 15 min) (54) and 3.5-fold (72 versus 20 min) (55). Transport time and need for centrifugation and processing are key components that delay availability of data with centralized laboratory testing. If the laboratory component exceeds 25% of the decision time, then POCT testing should be implemented (55). According to the NHAAP goal of 30 minutes, this translates to a total in-laboratory time of 7.5 minutes.

Question 4. Which cardiac markers should be included in POCT? Does the availability of POCT for cardiac markers affect the outcome and management of patients with suspected acute coronary ischemia?

Evidence answering this critical question was presented in the CHECKMATE study (16). This study of 1005 chest pain patients without ST segment elevation was designed to prospectively evaluate the ability of quantitative bedside measurement of a three-member panel including myoglobin, CK-MB, and cTnI (My-MB-cTnI); a two-member panel (MB-cTnI); and the local laboratory strategy for risk stratification of outcomes 30-day death and MI. With sampling at 0, 3, 6, 9–12, and 24 hr, the My-MB-cTnI and MB-cTnI strategies identified positive patients earlier than the local laboratory strategy. Thus, use of a multimarker panel enables earlier treatment or intervention compared with the local laboratory strategy. Importantly, the My-MB-cTnI panel discriminated 30-day death better than either the MB-cTnI, or local laboratory strategies (16). The My-MB-cTnI panel also performed better than a My-cTnI profile (L. Kristin Newby, personal communication). The My-MB-cTnI panel identified positive patients earlier, provided better risk stratification for mortality, and is therefore the panel of choice for assessing chest pain patients arriving in the ED with suspected non–ST elevation acute coronary syndromes.

CONCLUSIONS

Point-of-care testing based on important clinical outcomes is justified. Qualitative and quantitative POCT devices are now available for myoglobin, CK-MB, cTnI, cTnT, and BNP. These assays use anticoagulated whole blood and have total analysis times <20 min. Eliminating transport of samples to the central laboratory, centrifugation, and processing enables an order-to-availability time of 30 min. The POC tests provide diagnostic performance that is similar to that of the central laboratory cardiac assays. Currently, most POC tests measure a panel of cardiac markers with complementary diagnostic information. Harmony between values for the central laboratory and POCT site remains an important issue.

We are in a new era for identifying and treating patients within the spectrum of acute coronary syndromes. In the early 1990s, when it became clear that reducing time-to-treatment of ST elevation patients with thrombolytic therapy led to better outcomes, the NHAAP made the recommendation that physicians treat all patients within 30 min of arrival in the ED and began the very successful "4 Ds" initiative (56):

- The first "D" stands for door (patient presentation)
- The second "D" signifies data (obtain ECG, blood pressure, etc.)
- The third "D" is for decision (synthesis of information to determine treatment plan)
- The fourth "D" is administration of drug (thrombolytics to appropriate patients)

Over the past decade, knowledge has increased regarding non–ST elevation acute coronary syndrome physiology. Parallel advances have been made in therapeutics and development of better biochemical markers (troponin). These advances have initiated a new era and expanded the second of the "4Ds" (data) to include troponin, and the fourth "D" (drug) to include administration of GP IIb/IIIa inhibitors and LMW heparin to high-risk patients.

As with any POCT program, success of implementing POC cardiac markers depends on cooperation among the clinical staff, i.e., physicians and nurses, hospital administrators, laboratorians, and manufacturers. It seems clear that responsibility for POCT must reside with the laboratory where involvement must include the selection of POCT devices, education, training, maintenance, and implementation of a quality assurance program with appropriate monitors. Proper implementation of POCT provides the laboratorian with an excellent opportunity to work with clinicians and improve the outcomes of patients with acute coronary syndromes—the world's most lethal killer.

REFERENCES

1. American Heart Association. 2001 Heart and Stroke Statistical Update. American Heart Association, Dallas, TX, 2000.
2. Storrow AB, Gibler WB. Chest pain centers: Diagnosis of acute coronary syndromes. Ann Emerg Med 35:449–461, 2000.
3. Rusnak RA, Stair TO, Hansen K, Fastow JS. Litigation against the emergency physician: Common features in cases of missed myocardial infarction. Ann Emerg Med 18:1029–1034, 1989.
4. Weissberg PL. Atherosclerosis involves more than just lipids: Plaque dynamics. E Heart J Supplements 1(suppl T):T13–T18, 1999.
5. Keffer JH. Myocardial markers of injury. Evolution and insights. Am J Clin Pathol 105:305–320, 1996.
6. Executive Summary of the Third Report of the National Cholesterol Education Program (NCEP) Expert Panel on Detection, Evaluation and Treatment of High Blood Cholesterol in Adults (Adult Treatment Panel III). JAMA 285:2486–2497, 2001.
7. Danesh J, Collins R, Appleby P, Peto R. Association of fibrinogen, C-reactive protein, albumin, or leukocyte count with coronary heart disease: Meta-analyses of prospective studies. JAMA 279:1477–1482, 1998.
8. Balk EM, Ioannidis JP, Salem D, Chew PW, Lau J. Accuracy of biomarkers to diagnose acute cardiac ischemia in the emergency department: A meta analysis. Ann Emerg Med 37:478–494, 2001.
9. Myocardial infarction redefined—a consensus document of The Joint European Society of Cardiology/American College of Cardiology Committee for the redefinition of myocardial infarction. J Am Coll Cardiol 36:959–969, 2000.
10. Ioannidis JP, Salem D, Chew PW, Lau J. Accuracy of imaging technologies in the diagnosis of acute cardiac ischemia in the emergency department: A meta analysis. Ann Emerg Med 37:471–477, 2001.
11. Rabitzsch G, Mair J, Lechleitner P, Noll F, Hofmann U, Krause EG, Dienstl F, Puschendorf B. Immunoenzymometric assay of human glycogen phosphorylase isoenzyme BB in diagnosis of ischemic myocardial injury. Clin Chem 41:966–978, 1995.

12. Chan B, Dodsworth N, Woodrow J, Tucker A, Harris R. Site-specific N-terminal autodegradation of human serum albumin. Eur J Biochem 227:524–528, 1995.
13. Christenson RH, Duh SH, Sanhai WR, Wu AH, Holtman V, Painter P, Branham E, Apple FS, Murakami M, Morris DL. Characteristics of an albumin cobalt binding test for assessment of acute coronary syndrome patients: A multicenter study. Clin Chem 47:464–470, 2001.
14. Christenson RH, Azzazy HME. Biochemical markers of acute coronary syndromes. Clin Chem 44:1855–1864, 1998.
15. Christenson RH, Duh SH. Evidence based approach to practice guides and decision thresholds for cardiac markers. Scand J Clin Lab Invest 59(suppl):90–102, 1999.
16. Newby LK, Storrow AB, Gibler WB, Garvey JL, Tucker JF, Kaplan AL, Schreiber DH, Tuttle RH, McNulty SE, Ohman EM. Bedside multimarker testing for risk stratification in chest pain units: The chest pain evaluation by creatine kinase-MB, myoglobin and troponin I (CHECKMATE) study. Circulation 103:1832–1837, 2001.
17. Wu AH, Lane PL. Meta-analysis in clinical chemistry: Validation of cardiac troponin T as a marker for ischemic heart diseases. Clin Chem 41:1228–1233, 1995.
18. Christenson RH, Vaidya H, Landt Y, Bauer RS, Green SF, Apple FS, Jacob A, Magneson GR, Nag S, Wu AH, Azzazy HME. Standardization of creatine kinase-MB (CK-MB) mass assays: The use of recombinant CK-MB as a reference material. Clin Chem 45:1414–1423, 1999.
19. Wu AH, Feng YJ, Moore R, Apple FS, McPherson PH, Buechler KF, Bodor GS. Characterization of cardiac troponin subunit release into serum after acute myocardial infarction and comparison of assays for troponin T and I. American Association for Clinical Chemistry Subcommittee on cTnI Standardization. Clin Chem 44:1198–1208, 1998.
20. Labugger R, Organ L, Collier C, Atar D, Van Eyk JE. Extensive troponin I and T modification detected in serum from patients with acute myocardial infarction. Circulation 102:1221–1226, 2000.
21. Christenson RH, Duh SH, Apple FS, Bodor GS, Bunk DM, Dalluge J, Panteghini M, Potter JD, Welch MJ, Wu AH, Kahn SE. Standardization of cardiac troponin I assays: Round robin of ten candidate reference materials. Clin Chem 47:431–437, 2001.
22. Mair J, Friedl W, Thomas S, Puschendorf B. Natriuretic peptides in assessment of left-ventricular dysfunction. Scand J Clin Lab Invest 59(suppl):132–142, 1999.
23. Yoshimura M, Yasue H, Okumura K, Ogawa H, Jougasaki M, Mukoyama M, Nakao K, Imura H. Different secretion patterns of atrial natriuretic peptide and brain natriuretic peptide in patients with congestive heart failure. Circulation 87:464–469, 1993.
24. Selvais P, Donckier J, Robert A, Laloux F, Van Liden F, Ketelslegers S, Rousseau M. Cardiac natriuretic peptides for diagnosis and risk stratification in heart failure: Influences of left ventricular dysfunction and coronary artery disease on cardiac hormonal activation. Eur J Clin Invest 28:636–642, 1998.
25. Cobbe SM, Poole-Wilson PA. The time of onset and severity of acidosis in myocardial ischaemia. J Mol Cell Cardiol 12:745–760, 1980.
26. Berenshtein E, Mayer B, Goldberg C, Kitrossky K, Chevion M. Patterns of mobiliza-

tion of copper and iron following myocardial ischemia: Possible predictive criteria for tissue injury. J Mol Cell Cardiol 29:3025–3034, 1997.
27. Nomenclature and criteria for diagnosis of ischemic heart disease. Report of the Joint International Society and Federation of Cardiology/World Health Organization Task Force on standardization of clinical nomenclature. Circulation 59:607–609, 1979.
28. Canto JG, Shlipak MG, Rogers WJ, Malmgren JA, Frederick PD, Lambrew CT, Ornato JP, Barron HV, Kiefe CI. Prevalence, clinical characteristics and mortality among patients with myocardial infarction presenting without chest pain. JAMA 283:3223–3229, 2000.
29. Weisman HF, Healy B. Myocardial infarct expansion, infarct extension and reinfarction: Pathophysiologic concepts. Prog Cardiovasc Dis 2:73–110, 1987.
30. The Thrombolysis in Myocardial Infarction (TIMI) Trial. Phase I Findings. TIMI Group Study. N Engl J Med 312:932–936, 1985.
31. Anderson JL, Karagounis LA, Becker LC, Sorensen SG, Menlove RL. TIMI perfusion grade 3 but not grade 2 results in improved outcome after thrombolysis for myocardial infarction. Ventriculographic, enzymatic and electrocardiographic evidence from the TEAM-3 Study. Circulation 87:1829–1839, 1993.
32. Christenson RH, Ohman EM, Topol EJ, Peck S, Newby LK, Duh SH, Kereiakes DJ, Worley SJ, Alosozana GL, Wall TC, Califf RM. Assessment of coronary reperfusion after thrombolysis with a model combining myoglobin, creatine kinase-MB and clinical variables. TAMI-7 Study Group. Thrombolysis and Angioplasty in Myocardial Infarction-7. Circulation 96:1776–1782, 1997.
33. Apple FS. Biochemical markers of thrombolytic success. IFCC Committee on Standardization of Markers of Cardiac Damage. Scand J Clin Lab Invest 59(suppl):60–66, 1999.
34. Olatidoye AG, Wu AH, Feng YJ, Waters D. Prognostic role of troponin T versus troponin I in unstable angina pectoris for cardiac events with meta-analysis comparing published studies. Am J Cardiol 81:1405–1410, 1998.
35. Ottani F, Galvani M, Nicolini FA, Ferrini D, Pozzati A, Di Pasquale G, Jaffe AS. Elevated cardiac troponin levels predict the risk of adverse outcome in patients with acute coronary syndromes. Am Heart J 140:917–927, 2000.
36. Newby LK, Christenson RH, Ohman EM, Armstrong PW, Thompson TD, Lee KL, Hamm CW, Katus HA, Cianciolo C, Granger CB, Topol EJ, Califf RM. Value of serial troponin T measures for early and late risk stratification in patients with acute coronary syndromes. The GUSTO-IIa Investigators. Circulation 98:1853–1859, 1998.
37. Braunwald E, Antman EM, Beasley JW, Califf RM, Cheitlin MD, Hochman JS, Jones RH, Kereiakes D, Kupersmith J, Levin TN, Pepine CJ, Schaeffer JW, Smith EE III, Steward DE, Theroux P, Gibbons RJ, Alpert JS, Eagle KA, Faxon DP, Fuster V, Gardner TJ, Gregoratos G, Russell RO, Smith SC Jr. ACC/AHA guidelines for the management of patients with unstable angina and non–ST-segment elevation myocardial infarction: Executive summary and recommendations. A report of the American College of Cardiology/American Heart Association Task Force on practice guidelines (Committee on the Management of Patients with Unstable Angina). Circulation 102:1193–1209, 2000.

38. Ryan TJ, Antman EM, Brooks NH, Califf RM, Hillis LD, Hiratzka LF, Rapaport E, Riegel B, Russell RO, Smith EE III, Weaver WD, Gibbons RJ, Alpert JS, Eagle KA, Gardner TJ, Garson A Jr, Gregoratos G, Ryan TJ, Smith SC Jr. ACC/AHA guidelines for the management of patients with acute myocardial infarction. A report of the American College of Cardiology/American Heart Association Task Force on Practice Guidelines (Committee on Management of Acute Myocardial Infarction). J Am Coll Cardiol 34:890–911, 1999.
39. Roberts R, Fromm RE. Management of acute coronary syndromes based on risk stratification by biochemical markers: An idea whose time has come. Circulation 98:1831–1833, 1998.
40. Lindahl B, Venge P, Wallentin L. Troponin T identifies patients with unstable coronary artery disease who benefit from long-term antithrombotic protection. Fragmin in Unstable Coronary Artery Disease (FRISC) Study Group. J Am Coll Cardiol 29: 43–48, 1997.
41. Hamm CW, Heeschen C, Goldmann B, Vahanian A, Adgey J, Miguel CM, Rutsch W, Berger J, Kootstra J, Simoons ML. Benefit of abciximab in patients with refractory unstable angina in relation to serum troponin T levels. c7E3 Fab Antiplatelet Therapy in Unstable Refractory Angina (CAPTURE) Study Investigators. N Engl J Med 340:1623–1629, 1999.
42. Heeschen C, Hamm CW, Goldmann B, Deu A, Langenbrink L, White HD. Troponin concentrations for stratification of patients with acute coronary syndromes in relation to therapeutic efficacy of tirofiban. PRISM Study Investigators. Platelet Receptor Inhibition in Ischemic Syndrome Management. Lancet 354:1757–1762, 1999.
43. Newby LK, Ohman EM, Christenson RH, Moliterno DJ, Harrington RA, White HD, Armstrong PW, Van De Werf F, Pfisterer M, Hasselblad V, Califf RM, Topol EJ. Benefit of glycoprotein IIb/IIIa inhibition in patients with acute coronary syndromes and troponin T-positive status: The PARAGON-B troponin T substudy. Circulation 103:2891–2896, 2001.
44. Shell WE, Kjekshus JK, Sobel BE. Quantitative assessment of the extent of myocardial infarction in the conscious dog by means of analysis of serial changes in serum creatine phosphokinase activity. J Clin Invest 50:2614–2625, 1971.
45. Roberts R, Henry PD, Sobel BE. An improved basis for enzymatic estimation of infarct size. Circulation 52:743–754, 1975.
46. Grande P, Hansen BF, Christiansen C, Naestoft J. Estimation of acute myocardial infarct size in man by serum CK-MB measurements. Circulation 65:756–764, 1982.
47. Ottani F, Galvani M, Ferrini D, Sorbello F, Limonetti P, Pantoli D, Rusticali F. Prodromal angina limits infarct size. A role for ischemic proconditioning. Circulation 91:291–297, 1995.
48. Christenson RH, Vollmer RT, Ohman EM, Peck S, Thompson TD, Duh SH, Ellis SG, Newby LK, Topol EJ, Califf RM. Relation of temporal creatine kinase-MB release and outcome after thrombolytic therapy for acute myocardial infarction. TAMI Study Group. Am J Cardiol 85:543–547, 2000.
49. Bahr RD, Leino EV, Christenson RH. Prodromal unstable angina in acute myocardial infarction: Prognostic value of short- and long-term outcome and predictor of infarct size. Am Heart J 140:126–133, 2000.
50. Tardiff BE, Califf RM, Tcheng JE, Lincoff AM, Sigmon KN, Harrington RA, Ma-

haffey KW, Ohman EM, Teirstein PS, Blankenship JC, Kitt MM, Topol EJ. Clinical outcomes after detection of elevated cardiac enzymes in patients undergoing percutaneous intervention. IMPACT-II Investigators. Integrilin (eptifibatide) to Minimize Platelet Aggregation and Coronary Thrombosis-II. J Am Coll Cardiol 33:88–96, 1999.
51. Dao Q, Krishnaswamy P, Kazanegra R, Harrison A, Amirnovin R, Lenert L, Clopton P, Alberto J, Hlavin P, Maisel AS. Utility of B-type natriuretic peptide in the diagnosis of congestive heart failure in an urgent-care setting. J Am Coll Cardiol 37:379–385, 2001.
52. Clerico A, Iervasi G, Del Chicca MG, Emdin M, Maffei S, Nannipieri M, Sabatino L, Forini F, Manfredi C, Donato L. Circulating levels of cardiac natriuretic peptides (ANP and BNP) measured highly sensitive and specific immunoradiometric assays in normal subjects in patients with different degrees of heart failure. J Endocrinol Invest 21:170–179, 1998.
53. Bhatt DL, Topol EJ. Current role of platelet glycoprotein IIb/IIIa inhibitors in acute coronary syndromes. JAMA 284:1549–1558, 2000.
54. Sanhai WR, Bahr R, Wentz C, Christenson RH. Bedside cardiac markers: Tracking time, bedside/lab results and cardiac troponin I+ patients. Clin Chem 46(suppl): A86, 2000.
55. Collinson PO. The need for a point of care testing: An evidence based appraisal. Scand J Clin Lab Invest 59(suppl):67–73, 1999.
56. Emergency Department: Rapid identification and treatment of patients with acute myocardial infarction. National Heart Attack Alert Program Coordinating Committee, 60 Minutes to Treatment Working Group. Ann Emerg Med 23:311–329, 1994.

15

Intraoperative Parathyroid Hormone

Lori J. Sokoll
Johns Hopkins Medical Institutions, Baltimore, Maryland, U.S.A.

INTRODUCTION

Compared with other topics in this book examining tests used at the point-of-care such as glucose, urinalysis, occult blood, hemoglobin, cardiac markers, drugs of abuse, etc., parathyroid hormone (PTH), may appear out of place. However, the definition of point-of-care testing has expanded considerably and thus, as a result, so have the number and diversity of tests available. Point-of-care testing no longer refers only to critical-care-type tests performed using a handheld device but to any test or diagnostic procedure performed near or at the point of patient care regardless of test type, methodology, or device characteristics. Thus, PTH, although not in the category of waived tests, yet analyzed in a rapid fashion in the operating and angiography suites, can be included in the rapidly growing list of point-of-care tests (1).

The function of PTH is to regulate the extracellular calcium concentration. Measurement of serum intact PTH concentrations is used in the differential diagnosis of hypercalcemia and for the investigation of suspected parathyroid disease. Modifications to intact PTH assays now allow assays to be performed rapidly with results available in 15 min or less. Due to the availability of the rapid intact PTH assay and the short half-life of PTH, the utility of the intact PTH assay has been expanded to allow for real-time testing during parathyroid surgery. Intraoperative monitoring of intact PTH concentrations provides an indication of the success of surgical removal of hyperfunctioning parathyroid glands and aids in identifying multiglandular disease. This chapter discusses the implementation of PTH as an aid to monitor parathyroid function in patients undergoing parathyroidectomy and its impact on patient and financial outcomes.

BACKGROUND

Parathyroid Hormone Metabolism

Parathyroid hormone is an 84-amino-acid molecule produced in the parathyroid glands. The parathyroid glands, typically four in number, are located in the neck region on or near the thyroid gland, although they can also be found in ectopic locations including in the thymus or in the posterior mediastinum. Parathyroid hormone secretion from the parathyroid glands is regulated by the concentration of the biologically active ionized (free) calcium in the blood or extracellular fluid. Binding of ionized calcium to calcium-sensing receptors affects intracellular calcium levels, which in turn regulates PTH synthesis and secretion (2,3).

Biological activity of the PTH molecule resides in the amino terminal portion of the molecule. The intact, biologically active PTH molecule as well as inactive PTH fragments are secreted into the circulation from the parathyroid glands. These fragments are primarily midmolecule and carboxy terminal fragments. Parathyroid hormone fragments are also generated by the peripheral metabolism of the intact molecule, which takes place in the liver and kidneys. Primary circulating PTH forms consist of the intact, midmolecule and carboxy terminal fragments. Biologically active N-terminal fragments do not appear to enter the circulation in a significant quantity. The intact molecule has a half-life of less than 5 min, while PTH fragments have half-lives 10-fold higher. Therefore, the majority of the circulating forms of PTH, 75–95%, are the inactive fragments. Inactive fragments are dependent upon glomerular filtration for clearance and may be elevated in patients with renal disease (2,3).

The function of PTH is to regulate the extracellular calcium concentration. Parathyroid hormone acts in kidney and bone to: (1) increase calcium transport or reabsorption in the distal tubules, (2) decrease reabsorption of phosphate in the proximal tubules, (3) induce the 1α-hydroxylase enzyme to produce $1,25(OH)_2$ vitamin D (active form of the vitamin) resulting in increased intestinal absorption of calcium and phosphate, and (4) increase bone resorption with chronic exposure to PTH. These actions result in increased serum calcium concentrations and decreased serum phosphate concentrations, while urine phosphate and often urine calcium concentrations are increased. In kidney and bone, PTH binds to PTH receptors on cell membranes with effects mediated through the actions of cyclic adenosine monophosphate (cAMP).

Disease States

Measurement of parathyroid hormone is useful in the diagnosis of parathyroid disease and in the differential diagnosis of hypercalcemia and hypocalcemia. Hypercalcemia can be attributed to a number of causes including parathyroid disease, malignancy, vitamin D abnormality, high bone turnover, and renal failure (4,5). Approximately 90% of hypercalcemia cases can be attributed to hyperparathyroidism and malignancies. Primary hyperparathyroidism is the most common disease of the parathyroids and results from increased secretion of PTH. Hypercalcemia results from the direct and indirect actions of PTH mobilizing calcium from bone, conserving calcium by reducing its renal excretion, and increasing the absorption of calcium in the gut.

Primary hyperparathyroidism has been estimated to have a prevalence of 0.1% overall and 1% in patients over age 60, with a peak incidence of the disease between the third and fifth decades of life. There is a predominance of the disease in women with a ratio of 2 : 1 or 3 : 1. The apparent incidence increased substantially in the late 1960s and early 1970s as a result of developments in clinical diagnostics, specifically the introduction of automated chemistry analyzers for measuring serum total calcium concentrations. With the development of this disease occurring in middle age and the aging of the population, it is expected that it will become increasingly common in the years to come.

In primary hyperparathyroidism, the majority of abnormalities (80%) are attributed to a single adenoma or hyperfunctioning gland with three normal parathyroid glands. Approximately 15% of patients have four-gland hyperplasia usually associated with hereditary syndromes such as multiple endocrine neoplasia (MEN) with the remainder attributed to multiple adenomas or parathyroid carcinoma. Parathyroid carcinoma is extremely rare however, accounting for less than 1% of primary hyperparathyroid cases.

The clinical presentation of primary hyperparathyroidism is often vague and greater than 80% of patients are, in fact, asymptomatic or show only mild symptoms (4–6). Renal, bone, neuromuscular, and gastrointestinal (GI) disturbances are much less common now that diagnoses are made much earlier, most notably due to abnormal total serum calcium concentrations present during routine physical exams. The classical presentation of primary hyperparathyroidism includes renal and bone disease caused by kidney stones and osteitis fibrosa cystica, respectively. These long-term diseases are rarely observed, however, because primary hyperparathyroidism is typically detected prior to their development. Symptoms are related to the rate in the rise of serum calcium concentrations as well as the absolute serum concentration. The diagnosis of primary hyperparathyroidism can be made from serum measurements of total calcium and intact PTH. Hypophosphatemia as well as an increased excretion of urinary calcium may also be observed.

Treatment of individuals with primary hyperparathyroidism having symptomatic hypercalcemia usually requires surgical intervention, while implementation of this treatment modality in asymptomatic cases is less clear. Other options for these individuals include medical management and surveillance. Guidelines, developed from a National Institutes of Health (NIH) consensus conference, and recommendations on the management of patients with asymptomatic hyperparathyroidism have been published (6,7). The surgical success rate for hyperparathyroidism is reported to be 90–95%, with a low mortality, minimal morbidity, and low recurrence rates (4). However, in some cases, persistent hypercalcemia or permanent hypoparathyroidism may result. Recurrent hypercalcemia most often results from residual hyperfunctioning parathyroid tissue attributable to an unrecognized or inaccessible adenoma, insufficient excision of hyperplastic tissue, or difficulty in distinguishing adenomatous and hyperplastic parathyroid tissue histopathologically. Re-exploration can be problematic due to fibrosis and scarring, and has a higher complication rate and lower success rate than initial surgeries. Therefore, a number of approaches to monitor parathyroidectomy success were developed. However, use of intraoperative biochemical measurements of serum total or ionized calcium, phosphorus, and urinary cAMP did not prove to change concentration rapidly enough to be clinically useful and DNA histograms, tissue density determinations, and intracellular fat measurements have not been widely accepted (8).

In 1988, the use of PTH was proposed as an intraoperative monitor with the discovery that a highly sensitive intact PTH assay could be modified to obtain results in a short amount of time (9). Parathyroid hormone is a useful measure because PTH is only produced in parathyroid glands and the intact 84-residue molecule has a half-life of less than 5 min. In addition, secretion of PTH is suppressed in normal parathyroid glands after the removal of all hyperfunctioning tissue and, therefore, PTH concentrations should decline rapidly shortly after all hypersecreting parathyroid tissue has been removed (10). However, the utility of intact PTH and successful implementation was only realized a number of years later when assays were developed with greatly shortened incubation times and nonradioactive labels.

Intact Parathyroid Hormone Measurement

Traditional Assays

The first assays for PTH were developed over 30 yr ago. These radioimmunoassays used bovine PTH as standards and as immunogenic material for antibody production (11). With the availability of synthetic human PTH peptides, assays were subsequently developed with polyclonal antibodies developed against N-terminal (1–34), midmolecule (44–68), or C-terminal (53–84) regions. The sensitivities and specificities of these assays were affected by low concentrations of intact PTH, heterogeneity of circulating fragments, and high concentrations of inactive fragments. In the late 1980s, immunometric sandwich assays utilizing two antibodies were developed for intact PTH (12). In this type of assay, one antibody is attached to a solid support while the other functions as the signal antibody that may have a radioactive, chemiluminescent, or other label. During incubation, antibodies generated against two distinct epitopes on the molecule form a sandwich with the antigen in the specimen. Following washing to remove components not bound to the solid phase, quantitation takes place. In contrast to radioimmunoassays (RIAs), antibodies are present in excess allowing capture of all immunoreactive molecules. The signal is therefore directly proportional to the concentration of analyte present. Sandwich assays will therefore measure the intact PTH molecule and will not measure C-terminal fragments; however, measurement of other fragments is not precluded (13). The immunometric approach is therefore advantageous because of its ability to measure the biologically active intact PTH molecule and also due to the improved ability of PTH measurements using this assay to discriminate between primary hyperparathyroidism and hypercalcemia of malignancy. Intact PTH assays have now evolved from manual assays with radioactive labels to luminescent-based assays available on a number of automated immunoassay platforms.

Rapid, Intraoperative Assays

Descriptions. The first rapid or intraoperative assay was reported in 1988 by the same group that developed the Intact PTH Immunoradiometric assay (IRMA). They modified a commercialized version of the assay and reduced the assay incubation time from 22 hr to 15 min although the resulting limit of detection of the assay was 25 pg/mL compared with 1 pg/mL for the original assay (9). Several other quick assays were subsequently developed with incubation times ranging from 10–30 min utilizing either serum, plasma, or whole blood, resulting in turnaround times of up to 1 hr (14–16). Increased incubation temperatures, introduction of continuous shaking, and alterations in sample and reagent volumes were employed to expedite the antibody–antigen interactions. The majority of these assays were limited in their usefulness due to long turnaround times, with results obtained when the patient was already in the recovery room, and decreased analytical sensitivity compared with the full-length assay. Finally, widespread adoption of these quick assays was limited in part to the radioactive tracer in the assay, which imposed difficulties in performing assays in or in close proximity to the operating suite due to safety concerns and radioactive waste disposal issues. In addition, the short half-life of iodine-125 (^{125}I) decreased the shelf life of kits containing an ^{125}I-labeled signal antibody (17).

Subsequently, in the mid-1990s immunochemiluminometric (ICMA) assays for intact PTH were introduced. The ability to modify these methods for use intraoperatively eliminated disadvantages inherent to the IRMA methods and modifications to both a commercial assay (17–20) and an in-house method (21) were reported. Currently, there are three PTH assays for use intraoperatively that have been cleared for marketing by the U.S. Food and Drug Administration (FDA) (Table 1). All three assays can use EDTA plasma as a specimen type to eliminate clotting time required for serum and have results available in 15 min or less.

The first intraoperative assay, the QuiCk-IntraOperative Intact PTH assay, was commercialized by Nichols Institute Diagnostics (San Juan Capistrano, CA) in the mid-1990s. In this procedure, blood is drawn from the patient and transferred to an EDTA-containing vacutainer tube (i.e., 3 mL) and gently mixed. Aliquots of 700 μL of blood are pipetted into two microcentrifuge tubes and centrifuged for 30 sec at 6400 rpm (QuiCk-Pak MicroCentrifuge). Two hundred μL of plasma are then pipetted into two 12 × 75-mm glass tubes and 100 μL of the acridinium-labeled signal antibody and the capture antibody–coated polystyrene bead are added. Tubes are then incubated at 45°C for 7 min while shaking at 400 rpm in a heater shaker apparatus (QuiCk-Pak Kinetic Enhancer). Following incubation, beads are washed three times with 2 mL of saline. Beads are transferred to clean 12 × 75 tubes and counted for 2 sec in a luminometer. The chemiluminescent reaction occurs when the acridinium ester is treated with hydrogen peroxide and sodium hydroxide. The concentration of intact PTH in the sample is directly proportional to the amount of light produced and the PTH concentration determined from the standard curve stored in the luminometer (QuiCk-Pak Quantifier). The total time to perform this assay, including specimen processing, is approximately 12–14 min. Approximately 1 hr of technician time prior to the surgery is required to perform instrument performance checks, to generate the assay standard curve, and to run quality control material. A cart that can be transported into or adjacent to the operating suite holds the instrumentation required for the assay (microcentrifuge, heater shaker apparatus, bead washer, and luminometer) and provides a small work-area. In contrast to the other two commercially available assays, the QuiCk-IntraOperative Intact PTH assay is packaged for individual patient use.

The reference range for this assay is 10–65 pg/mL with an analytical sensitivity defined by the manufacturer of 6 pg/mL. Achieving a sensitivity of 1 pg/mL, similar to the Nichols IRMA or Advantage assays is not required for the application of monitoring parathyroid surgery. Intra-assay coefficients of variation (CVs) for the assay are 9.4, 8.0, and 10.7%, at concentrations of 29.1, 162.4, and 883.5 pg/mL, respectively. Despite the modifications of the rapid PTH assay, PTH results by this assay correlate well with those obtained using the standard-length assays (20,21) with a slope of 1.03 by linear regression analysis and a

Table 1 Characteristics of Intraoperative Intact Parathyroid Hormone Assays

Assay	QuiCk-IntraOperative Intact PTH	*Turbo* Intact PTH	STAT-IO-I-PTH
Manufacturer	Nichols Institute Diagnostics	Diagnostic Products Corporation	Future Diagnostics
Platform	Single-well luminometer	IMMULITE	Strip luminometer
Automated system	No	Yes	No
Assay design	Chemiluminescent immunometric/coated bead	Chemiluminescent enzyme immunometric/coated bead	Chemiluminescent immunometric/microtiter strips with accusphere
Specimen type	EDTA plasma	EDTA plasma, serum	EDTA plasma, serum
Specimen volume (assay)	200 µL	100 µL	100 µL
Incubation time	7 min	10 min	5 min
Time to result	~15 min	15 min	~10 min
Incubation conditions	Shake 400 rpm @ 45°C	Intermittent agitation @ 37°C	Shake 1400 rpm @ room temperature
Measuring range	6–1250 pg/mL	4–2500 pg/mL	6–2500 pg/mL
Standard curve	Each assay	Readjust every 2 wk	Each assay
Intra-assay precision[a]	9.4% (29.1 pg/mL) 8.0% (162 pg/mL)	6.7% (49 pg/mL) 6.5% (247 pg/mL)	10.7% (41 pg/mL) 4.9% (255 pg/mL)
Reference range	10–65 pg/mL	12–72 pg/mL	10–65 pg/mL

[a] Manufacturer's specifications.

correlation coefficient of 0.99 in comparison with the Nichols Chemiluminescence Intact PTH kit.

A second rapid PTH assay was subsequently introduced by Diagnostic Products Corporation (Los Angeles, CA) on the IMMULITE analyzer. The IMMULITE is a completely automated benchtop instrument. The *Turbo* Intact PTH assay is a modified version of the chemiluminescent sandwich IMMULITE Intact PTH assay with a calibration stability of 2 wk. The assay uses 100 μL of specimen for analysis with 250 μL required volume in the sample cup. The patient sample is incubated in the test unit with a polyclonal goat anti-PTH (44-84) antibody–coated bead and an alkaline phosphatase conjugated polyclonal anti-PTH (1-34) antibody at 37°C with intermittent agitation for 6 min. Unbound conjugate is then removed by a centrifugal wash. Substrate, a phosphate ester of adamantyl dioxetane, is added and incubated for 4 min. Emission of light proportional to the intact PTH concentration, resulting from hydrolysis of the substrate by alkaline phosphatase, is detected by the luminometer.

As reported by the manufacturer, this assay has a reportable range of 4–2500 pg/mL with a reference range of 12–72 pg/mL. Intra-assay precision ranges from 5.7–12% over the range of 13–1252 pg/mL. Comparison to the IMMULITE Intact PTH assay in 93 specimens resulted in a regression equation of $Y = 1.03X - 17.2$ pg/mL. Although the instrument and controlling PC could theoretically be transported to the operating room, and in fact an IMMULITE *TurboCart* has recently been introduced by the manufacturer, the size of the analyzer makes it more suitable for a satellite or a central laboratory location in conjunction with specimen transport by pneumatic tube or messenger (22). Specimens cannot be analyzed for non-*Turbo* assays while *Turbo* assays are running.

The QuiCk-IntraOperative Intact PTH assay and IMMULITE *Turbo* Intact PTH assay have been compared both analytically and clinically in two studies (23,24). In one study, specimens were analyzed on the same day in the operating room with the Nichols assay and in the central laboratory with the Diagnostic Products Corporation assay. Regression equations were IMMULITE *Turbo* PTH = 1.57 (Nichols PTH) − 18.17 pg/mL ($r = 0.96$) for all specimens ($n = 79$) and IMMULITE *Turbo* PTH = 1.38 (Nichols PTH) − 4.66 pg/mL ($r = 0.95$) for specimens with PTH concentrations less than 300 pg/mL ($n = 67$). In the second study, a comparison of the two assays in 36 paired samples resulted in a regression equation of IMMULITE *Turbo* PTH = 1.71 (Nichols PTH) − 33.34 pg/mL ($r = 0.84$). In the 26 patients evaluated by both assays in the two studies, there was 100% diagnostic agreement between both assays.

The most recent intraoperative PTH assay is the STAT-IntraOperative-Intact-PTH (STAT-IO-I-PTH) kit from Future Diagnostics (San Clemente, CA) which was FDA cleared in 2000. This chemilumiescent immunometric sandwich assay utilizes microtiter strips with accusphere technology with all system modules (centrifuge, shaker, washer, and reader) contained in a compact mobile cart. The solid phase of the assay is a microtiter strip plate consisting of 48 wells that is coated with a polyclonal goat anti-PTH (39-84) antibody. Plasma or serum specimens (150 μL), as well as standards and controls, are first transferred into noncoated microtiter strips in duplicate. Using an eight-channel pipette, 100 μL of sample is transferred to the coated strips and incubated while shaking for 5 min in the STAT-Shake. The detector antibody, an isoluminol-labeled polycolonal goat anti-PTH (1-34) antibody lyophilized in an accusphere, is contained in each well. The strip holder is placed in the STAT-Wash and washed three times with 500 μL solution and then the strips are loaded into the STAT-Read where activators containing sodium hydroxide and hydrogen peroxide are added in order to oxidize the isoluminol resulting in emitted light. Strips are counted for 3 sec with Relative Light Units directly proportional to the intact PTH concentration. A data reduction program in the Stat-Read generates a standard curve and calculates unknown specimen values. Results are available with this assay in 10–12 min.

The STAT-IO-I-PTH has a sensitivity of 6 pg/mL and utilizes six standards over the range of 0–1500 pg/mL. Intra-assay precision was reported in the package insert as 10.7, 9.8, 4.9, and 6.2% at intact PTH concentrations of 41, 77, 255, and 540 pg/mL, respectively. Sixty-seven samples measured with the STAT-IO-I-PTH assay and a commercially available ICMA assay resulted in a linear regression equation of $Y = 0.99X - 1.3$ pg/mL ($r = 0.98$). A reference range of 10–65 pg/mL with calcium values between 8.8 and 10.5 mg/dL has been established by the manufacturer.

Utilization. In 2001, the College of American Pathologists surveyed participants of their Special Ligand Proficiency Survey regarding intraoperative PTH testing. The response rate to the questionnaire was 86% with 320 participants out of 372 who submitted PTH results responding. Twenty-nine percent ($n = 92$) of 320 respondents reported performing intraoperative testing at their institution with 47% using the Diagnostic Products Corp. (DPC) IMMULITE *Turbo* assay and 33% using the Nichols Institute Diagnostics (Nichols) QuiCk-IntraOperative Intact PTH assay (Figure 1). The remainder of respondents reported using other assays, which may represent home-brew or commercial PTH assays modified in-house. Despite the use of these assays as intraoperative monitors, the majority of respondents (77%) perform testing in the central laboratory or a satellite laboratory and not in the operating suite (see Figure 1). Intraoperative PTH testing is performed for all parathyroid surgeries in 32% of hospitals, greater than 50% of surgeries in 31% of hospitals, and less than 50% of surgeries in 30% of hospitals. The frequency of testing ranged from 1–20 surgeries per month, with 55% of respondents performing testing four or fewer times a month and, 80% performing testing six or fewer times per month.

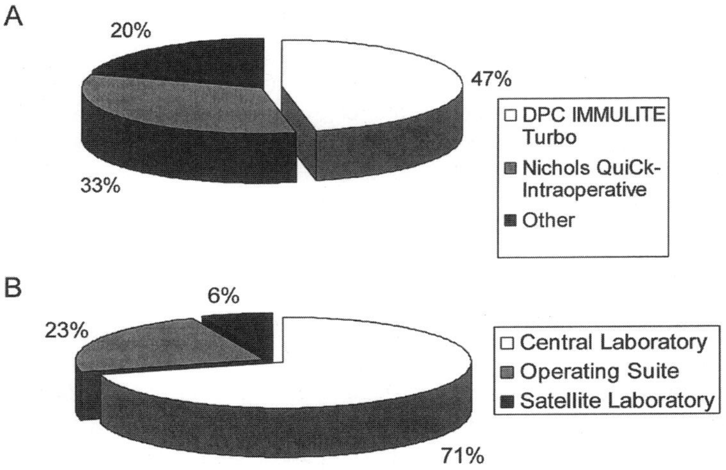

Figure 1 Methods (A) and locations (B) of intraoperative intact PTH testing in 92 sites performing intraoperative PTH (2001 College of American Pathologists survey).

Patient Sampling Procedures. During the surgical procedure, specimens are drawn from a peripheral venous line at the start of the operation, prior to gland removal, and at timed intervals following parathyroid gland excision (Table 2). Alternatively, specimens may be drawn from vessels in the neck. In concert with the 3–5 min half-life of the intact PTH molecule, a 50% decrease in intact PTH concentration is expected 5 min postexcision if all hypersecreting parathyroid tissue has been removed (17). If PTH concentrations fall to expected levels, further exploration is unnecessary. If PTH concentrations do not fall adequately, then the surgeon must look further for additional abnormal gland(s).

Table 2 Intraoperative Intact Parathyroid Hormone Procedures

Laboratory		
	Standard curve generated or master curve adjusted (if required)	
	Quality control analyzed	
Patient/operating room		
	Specimens drawn and analyzed	
		Start operation
		Timed intervals following excision(s)
	Results interpreted by surgeon	
		50% Drop expected within 5–10 min if all hypersecreting tissue removed
		Further exploration if PTH concentrations do not fall to expected levels

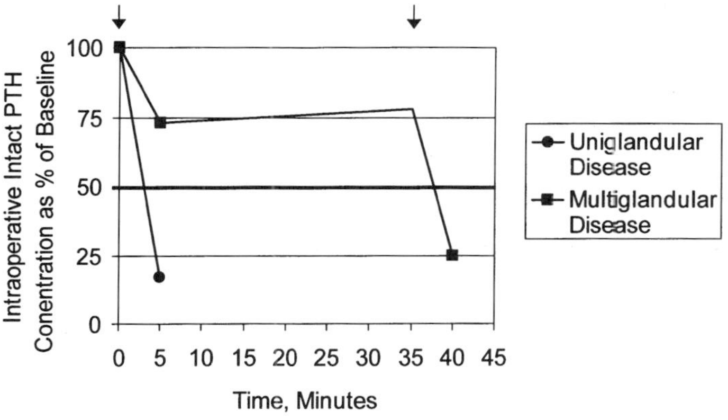

Figure 2 Example of possible changes in intact PTH concentrations in patients with uniglandular or multiglandular disease undergoing surgery for primary hyperparathyroidism. Arrows indicate time of parathyroid gland resection.

Figure 2 illustrates the use of the rapid PTH assay during parathyroid surgery. In a patient with uniglandular disease, the intact PTH concentration declines greater than 50% compared with baseline levels 5 min after removal of an abnormal parathyroid gland, indicating that the patient has been cured. In another patient, there is not a significant drop in PTH concentrations into the PTH reference range when an abnormal gland was removed. Therefore further exploration was required. A second abnormal gland was located and excised. At this point, the PTH concentration fell to 25% of baseline confirming that multiglandular disease was present.

INTRAOPERATIVE INTACT PARATHYROID HORMONE CLINICAL UTILITY AND APPLICATIONS

As discussed above, the first reported rapid assay, developed in 1988, was a modification of an intact PTH IRMA assay (9). In a small group of patients (n = 12) undergoing neck exploration for clinically suspected and biochemically proven primary hyperparathyroidism, intact PTH was measured prior to and 15 and 30 min following excision of a single parathyroid adenoma. At 15 min, all patients exhibited a decline in intact PTH values to 40% of baseline, with a mean decline of 22%. The authors concluded that the assay could complement the judgment and skill of the surgeon to determine surgical care, providing guidance regarding the scope of neck exploration. They also described the rapid PTH assay as a “biochemical frozen section.” Similar to this initial study, the vast majority of studies have shown the rapid PTH assay to have promise as an adjunct to parathyroid surgery, although several very early studies, in which assays were not performed in real-time, did not find the assay advantageous (8,14,25).

The evolution of the rapid PTH assay into a technique used in clinical practice today is generally credited to endocrine surgeon George Irvin from the University of Miami School of Medicine. Irvin and colleagues have been responsible for the development and clinical testing of rapid assays with both radioactive (16,26) and nonradioactive formats (17,18). In one of the first studies to show the clinical utility of a nonradioactively formatted assay, a modified ICMA with a 7-min incubation time was utilized in or adjacent to the operating room in 16 patients undergoing parathyroidectomy for primary hyperparathyroidism. Specimens were drawn prior to anesthesia, prior to gland excision, and 5 and 10 min following gland excision. Sensitivity and specificity of the assay were determined to be 94 and 100%, respectively, using a guideline of a decrease in PTH concentration of more than 50% at the 5-min time point as a predictor of postoperative normocalcemia (17).

Since the introduction of commercial assays for intraoperative intact PTH, the clinical utility of the assay in primary hyperparathyroidism has been examined in several large series of patients (27–29). Garner and Leight (28) reported their experience with intraoperative intact PTH in 130 patients with primary hyperparathyroidism operated on by one surgeon. In these patients, baseline specimens were drawn after the patient was anesthetized and upon identification of an adenomatous parathyroid gland, but prior to excision, and at 5 and 10 min postexcision with additional samples obtained if needed. The QuiCk-IntraOperative Intact PTH assay was used in this study. In 120 of the cases, the 10-min sample was the final sample while in the 10 other patients, additional specimens were required. In the 120 patients, PTH decreased an average of 69.2 ± 1.1% (SEM) and 77.4 ± 0.8% (SEM) at 5 and 10 min postexcision of the adenoma or hyperplastic glands from the higher baseline, respectively. The two baselines were very similar on average (171.3 vs. 177.1 pg/mL). In 96.2% (125/130) of cases, the rapid PTH assay predicted the postoperative outcome, including two of five patients with multiglandular disease. Of the five remaining cases, three were false positives and two false negatives. The authors concluded the assay may provide valuable information, but should be combined with other clinical information as well as the judgment of the experienced surgeon.

Gordon et al. (29) determined that the intraoperative intact PTH assay was accurate from a study they performed in 72 patients undergoing bilateral neck exploration for primary hyperparathyroidism. The Nichols assay was used to analyze specimens drawn before skin incision and at 5, 10, and 20 min postexcision with a 50% decrease from baseline at 10 min indicative of curative excision. The surgeons did not use assay results to guide extent of exploration or tissue resection, and the accuracy of the assay in identifying uniglandular versus multiglandular disease was based on gross morphology. Of the 72 patients, 76% had uniglandular and 24% had multiglandular disease, with an 89% accuracy rate in predicting the disease state. The authors noted their incidence of multiglandular disease was higher than had previously been reported. These results were considered, at worst, comparable to conventional parathyroidectomy with, hypothetically, 6% of patients undergoing unnecessary extended exploration and 6% requiring reoperation for unidentified multiglandular disease.

The largest series of consecutive cases evaluating the clinical utility of the intraoperative PTH assay was a study of 200 cases reported in 2000 from The Johns Hopkins Hospital (27). The QuiCk-IntraOperative Intact PTH was utilized on-site in the operating suite with a 50% decline in PTH concentration from baseline indicative of successful gland removal. In addition to the baseline specimen drawn prior to exploration, all patients had specimens drawn at 5–10 min post–gland resection although the number and frequency of draws depended upon surgical technique used and experience gained with the assay over the 2 yr of this study. All patients were operated on by one endocrine surgeon. Of the 200 parathyroidectomies, 189 patients had primary hyperparthyroidism (94%) with 26 reoperative cases, 11 had secondary/tertiary hyperparathyroidism (6%) with 1 reoperative case, and 5 had incomplete or discontinued assay results or an undetermined outcome. Of the non-reoperative primary hyperparathyroid cases, 91% had uniglandular disease and 9% had multiglandular disease. Out of the 195 cases using intraoperative testing with complete results and defined clinical outcomes, the overall accuracy of the assay in predicting surgical success was 88% using the criterion of a 50% decrease at 5–10 min and 97% including the subset of patients with a delayed declines in PTH (>10 min). Six cases were false negative, in which patients were normocalcemic although a 50% decrease in PTH concentrations was not achieved, and the judgment of the surgeon that these patients were cured proved to be correct. In these patients, declines were just above the 50% guideline and were attributed to low baseline concentrations and suspected tumor manipulation causing initially increased values postresection. Sampling location, such as from neck veins, and factors affecting PTH clearance are other considerations.

As illustrated in the previous study, a role exists for intraoperative PTH not just in initial surgical intervention for primary hyperparathyroidism. The assay also has proven utility in surgery for secondary/tertiary hyperparathyroidism (20,27), reoperative cases (27,30,31), multiple endocrine neoplasia type 1 (MEN 1) (32), and parathyroid cancer (33). Clary et al. (20) studied the use of intraoperative PTH monitoring in 13 consecutive patients with secondary hyperparathyroidism undergoing either total or subtotal parathyroidectomy. Intact PTH concentrations in these patients decreased an average of 65% compared with a baseline value when measured with a modified ICMA assay 5 min following excision of the last gland or segment. Following the operation, all patients had improved symptoms, and PTH concentrations at early follow-up were below intraoperative levels. Irvin et al. (30) compared patients who underwent reoperative parathyroidectomy for failed surgery or recurrent disease prior to and after introduction of the intraoperative assay. Using a postoperative calcium concentration of less than 10.2 mg/dL as an outcome measure, they found the success rate of the surgery increased from 76 to 94% when intraoperative PTH assays were employed to facilitate localization and confirm excision. Tonelli et al. (32) examined the use intraoperative PTH measurements in 16 patients with MEN 1–associated primary hyperparathyroidism undergoing subtotal or total parathyroidectomy and found it to be a valuable adjunct in the diagnosis of multiglandular involvement and the prediction of surgical treatment, as PTH concentrations were on average 23% of baseline values following removal of the last gland with no persistent or recurrent disease on follow-up. Finally, a patient with parathyroid carcinoma from a series of 100 consecutive patients undergoing surgery over a 38-mo period was normocalcemic and disease-free following surgery in which PTH concentrations decreased 60 and 68% at 5 and 10 min, respectively, after excision of the affected gland (33).

In addition to use of the rapid PTH assay intraoperatively as a guide in parathyroid surgery, the assay been shown to have value in localizing abnormal parathyroid tissue both in the operating and angiography suites (34–37). Patients undergoing repeat exploration for primary hyperparathyroidism have a higher failure and complication rate due to difficulties related to fibrosis and scarring. Therefore, prior to surgery, studies to localize abnormal tissue are performed using noninvasive imaging techniques such as sestamibi scans often in combination with single photon emission computed tomography (SPECT), ultrasonography, computed tomography (CT), and magnetic resonance imaging (MRI) scans. In some cases, however, these scans will be discordant or uninformative, and it is recommended that these patients undergo an invasive localization procedure consisting of selective angiography combined with venous sampling for PTH. In the past, samples were collected from catheterized veins in the neck and mediastinum, transported to the laboratory, and analyzed in batch. Results would be matched to sampling location in order to compare values and locate a venous gradient. With the advent of the rapid assay, specimens could be analyzed in real time and would allow the angiographer to obtain additional specimens when a potentially significant venous gradient is detected. The first case report describing the use of this technique was reported in 2000 (34) where it was noted that angiographic localization may prove to be the most beneficial application of the rapid/intraoperative PTH assay.

Alternatively, the rapid assay has been used in the operating suite for venous localization (35). Surgeons may sample veins on both sides of the neck to locate the hyperfunctioning gland or may sample following stimulation by local massage to identify glands not located visually or upon palpation, particularly in an ectopic location. Another novel application of the intraoperative assay is in parathyroid aspiration as an alternative to frozen section analysis to confirm the identification of removed tissue as parathyroid. It was shown that when parathyroid glands were aspirated with a syringe, placed in saline, centrifuged, and measured using an intraoperative PTH assay, values greater than 1500 pg/mL were indicative of tissue diagnosis (37).

OUTCOMES

Outcomes have been defined as the result of an intervention, and many medical outcomes specifically may result in economic, operational, and service benefits to the hospital and hospital staff as well as provide health and humanistic benefits to the patient (38,39). As shown in Table 3, the implementation of intraoperative PTH testing has resulted in significant medical outcomes benefitting the patient, surgeon, and institution.

The most significant consequence of the introduction of intraoperative PTH analysis has been the change in approach to parathyroid surgery. In the traditional surgical approach, bilateral neck exploration takes place under general anesthesia whereby the surgeon visualizes all parathyroid glands and excises grossly enlarged glands. With innovations such as improved preoperative imaging with sestamibi and SPECT, intraoperative PTH measurement, and the ability to perform surgery with local or regional anesthesia in an outpatient setting, a unilateral approach is possible (40,41). Although bilateral neck exploration is a highly suc-

Table 3 Benefits of Intraoperative Intact Parathyroid Hormone Testing[a]

Patient
Allows minimally invasive surgical approach including:
Local or regional anesthesia
Outpatient procedure
Decreased exploration
Smaller incision, better cosmetic results, and less pain
Improved surgical success rate
Less morbidity
Physician
Provides a functional result of parathyroid resection
Helps identify multiglandular disease
Financial
Decreased OR time and associated fees
Decreased use of frozen sections
Decreased length of stay

[a] In some instances, in conjunction with other techniques.

cessful procedure, modified procedures, including the use of intraoperative PTH assays, have allowed the surgeon to reduce incision size and extent of neck exploration as well as minimize costs, such as operating room times, frozen section use, and hospital lengths of stay (18,19,42,44–46).

In what he termed as "a new approach to parathyroidectomy," Irvin et al. (18) described in 1994 the combined the use of ^{99m}Tc sestamibi (MIBI) scintigraphy with quick intact PTH measurements in 18 patients with primary hyperparathyroid disease. Tumors were localized with the MIBI nuclear scan preoperatively and the operation terminated when the identified gland was removed; the rapid PTH assay was used to confirm the removal of all hyperfunctioning tissue. In this series of 18 patients, 16 patients with positive scintigraphy had successful surgeries confirmed by quick PTH measurements, while two patients had mediastinal tumors that could not be resected with this approach. The combination of these two techniques predicted a return to normal calcium concentrations and the average operating time was shorter (36 vs. 90 min) compared with patients who had parathyroidectomy without localization and PTH monitoring.

Two years later (43), these two techniques were evaluated for the ability to provide parathyroidectomy on an outpatient or ambulatory basis. Of 85 consecutive patients with primary hyperaparathyroidism, 57 were offered outpatient parathyroidectomy based on medical and social concerns. In 56 of 57 patients, intraoperative PTH concentrations declined an average of 80% at 10 min postexcision and one patient had a delayed decline. The average procedure time was 52 min with minimal neck dissection. Minimal postoperative complications and normal serum calcium concentrations at 7-mo follow-up confirmed the safety of the ambulatory approach. It was expected that cost savings would result from this procedural approach as the ambulatory setting charges were subsequently determined to be 39% less than an overnight procedure. In long-term studies, use of the surgical approach combining localization with PTH monitoring has significantly decreased the operative failure rate at that institution from 6 to 1.5%, eliminated the most common causes of parathyroidectomy failure (48), and shown that the incidence of recurrent hyperfunctioning did not change with limited parathyroidectomy compared with bilateral neck exploration (40).

Several studies have directly compared the impact of directed, concise surgeries with PTH use to conventional surgical procedures (19,42,44,47,49). Miccoli et al. (44) performed a prospective randomized study comparing conventional surgery with bilateral exploration and frozen section tissue analysis in 18 patients with primary hyperparathyroidism to video-assisted surgery with intraoperative PTH measurements performed in 20 patients. Two patients in the video-assisted group underwent surgery using locoregional anesthesia while the remainder of all patients had general anesthesia. At 6 mo following surgery, all patients were normocalcemic regardless of surgical approach. Operative time was significantly shorter in the second group (57 vs. 70 min) as was the postoperative inactivity period (12 vs. 16 days). Patient satisfaction regarding cosmetic result (esthetics of scar) was assessed by questionnaire at 1, 3 and 6 mo following surgery. Satisfaction was significantly greater in the experimental group who had barely visible scars at 6 mo. These patients also experienced significantly less pain in the postoperative period.

In a recent study (49), concise parathyroidectomy with both preoperative imaging and intraoperative PTH analysis using the IMMULITE *Turbo* assay in a group of 49 patients was compared with a historical control group of 55 patients. Compared with the control group, the experimental group had significantly more unilateral neck explorations (65 vs. 0%), greater use of local anesthesia (33 vs. 0%), fewer frozen sections (1.4 vs. 2.5), and increased same day discharge (17 vs. 0). In another study comparing two approaches to selective unilateral exploration for sporadic primary hyperparathyroidism (19), the use of concise parathyroidectomy with added sestamibi-SPECT and intraoperative PTH assays resulted in a significantly decreased length of stay from 1.90 to 1.07 days compared with an intraoperative palpation method and increased unilateral explorations (63% vs. 41%). Perioperative costs were not affected and mean operating time was slightly lower. The group with imaging and intraoperative PTH also tended to have fewer operative failures and less morbidity.

At our institution, an outpatient, minimally invasive technique was adopted that consists of preoperative sestamibi-SPECT imaging, surgeon-administered local or regional anesthesia, exploration through small incisions of 1–4 cm, and intraoperative PTH measurements at 5–10 min after parathyroid resection (42). This technique was used in 33 consecutive patients with primary hyperparathyroidism and compared with 184 consecutive patients who underwent bilateral exploration with general anesthesia. Thirty of the patients had resection of a single adenoma under regional anesthesia with 26 as an outpatient procedure. Three patients were converted to general anesthesia for bilateral exploration and determined to have multiglandular disease. These three patients were hospitalized overnight. The minimally invasive parathyroidectomy (MIP) patients and bilateral parathyroid exploration patients were similar with respect to age, preoperative calcium and parathyroid hormone levels, cause of primary hyperparathyroidism, and weight of resected glands. Patient outcomes were also similar with respect to cure rate and morbidity. However, significant reductions were observed with the new procedure in both hospital lengths of stay and total hospital charges. Length of stay with the minimally invasive procedure was 0.3 ± 0.2 (mean ± SEM) days compared with 1.8 ± 0.1 days with the standard procedure, while average hospital charges were reduced to \$3174 ± 386 from \$6328 ± 292. Reduced charges were attributed to shortened operative time and length of hospital stay.

This series has recently been expanded with a report on the outcomes of

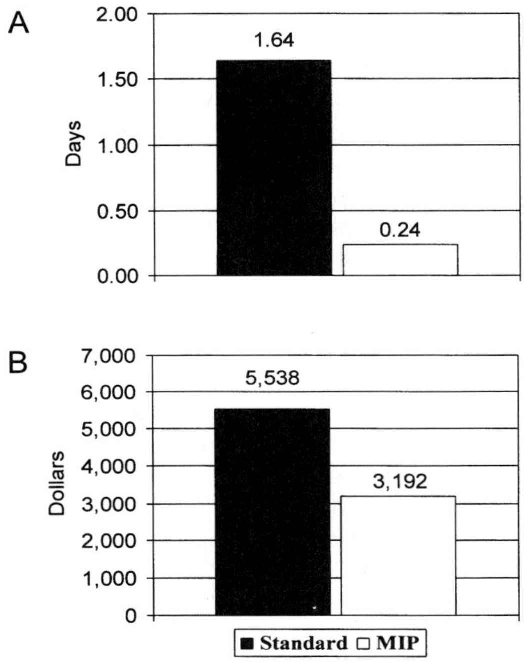

Figure 3 Comparison of outcomes (A, length of hospital stay; B, total hospital charges) between patients undergoing surgery for primary hyperparathyroidism by a single surgeon by either standard bilateral cervical exploration (standard) or minimally invasive parathyroidectomy (MIP). (From Ref. 47.)

656 consecutive parathyroid explorations by a single surgeon over an 11-yr period (47). Of the 656 patients explored for primary hyperparathyroidism, 61% were performed employing the standard technique and 39% were selected for MIP. The success rate for the entire series was 98% with no significant differences between the two techniques. As shown in Figure 3, the MIP technique was associated with approximately a 50% reduction in operating time and total hospital charges, and a seven-fold reduction in length of hospital stay.

LIMITATIONS

Despite the improved outcomes achieved using rapid PTH measurements as a monitor of parathyroid surgery, there are limitations to the use and implementation of the assay. One is that it is not intended to replace the experience of the surgeon since clinical judgment is required in interpreting assay values in light of the patient's condition. For example, postexcision values may be close to, but not meet the 50% guideline as a result of low baseline levels, tumor manipulation, sampling location, or altered PTH clearance. In addition, technologists and OR staff need to work together to ensure specimens are free from interferences and are not diluted with IV fluids. Another limitation is the potential impact on the laboratory. Despite the fact that intraoperative PTH testing may result in overall cost savings to the institution as well as benefit the patient and patient charges per result have been reported to be equivalent to a frozen section analysis (44,45), reagent and labor costs to the laboratory are important considerations. Although it is difficult to quote exact pricing, intraoperative PTH testing is in general more expensive than conventional PTH testing with type of assay (i.e., manual vs. automated), equipment required, volume of testing, and assay packaging contributing to costs. For example, the Nichols QuiCk-IntraOperative Intact PTH assay is packaged for individual patient use. In addition, labor costs would be greater to provide a dedicated technologist to perform the assay on site as opposed to the central laboratory where the technologist would not be limited to PTH testing, however turnaround times and the ability to interact with the surgical team to ensure specimen integrity may be compromised. Although a financial advantage to using IMMULITE *Turbo* reagents has been suggested (49), in another report intraoperative testing was preferred due to the improved turnaround times despite costs for the IMMULITE system that were half of the QuiCK-Pak system (24).

SUMMARY

Since the first suggestion of the utility of intraoperative PTH measurements as an adjunct to parathyroid surgery over a decade ago and commercialization of assays approximately 5 yr ago, use of the assay is now routine in many institutions (28) and considered a standard of care, contributing to a shift in the surgical treatment of primary hyperparathyroidism to MIP (47). Although not a typical point-of-care test, the use of intraoperative PTH testing has illustrated how incorporation of this laboratory test into patient management has contributed to significant medical and financial outcomes, benefiting the patient, surgeon and hospital staff, and the hospital as a whole.

REFERENCES

1. Sokoll LJ, Udelsman R, Chan DW. Intraoperative parathyroid hormone measurement. Diagn Endocrinol Metab 17:295–302, 1999.

2. Endres DB, Rude RK. Mineral and bone metabolism. In: Burtis CA, Ashwood ER, eds. Tietz Textbook of Clinical Chemistry. 3rd ed. Saunders, Philadelphia, 1999, pp 1395–1457.
3. Kronenberg HM, Bringhurst FR, Segre GV, Potts JT Jr. Parathyroid biosynthesis and metabolism. In: Bilezikian JP, Levine MA, Marcus R, eds. The Parathyroids. Raven Press, New York, 1994, pp 125–137.
4. Potts JT Jr. Diseases of the parathyroid gland and other hyper- and hypocalcemic disorders. In: Isselbacher KJ, Braunwald E, Wilson JD, Martin JB, Fauci AS, Kasper DL, eds. Harrison's Principles of Internal Medicine. 13th ed. McGraw-Hill, New York, 1994, pp 2151–2171.
5. Bilezikian JP, Silverberg SJ, Gartenberg F, Kim T-S, Jacobs TP, Siris ES, Shane E. Clinical presentation of primary hyperparathyroidism. In: Bilezikian JP, Levine MA, Marcus R, eds. The Parathyroids. Raven Press, New York, 1994, pp 457–469.
6. Bilezikian JP. Primary hyperparathyroidism. When to observe and when to operate. Endocrinol Metab Clin North Am 29:465–478, 2000.
7. Consensus Development Conference panel. Diagnosis and management of asymptomatic primary hyperparathyroidism: Consensus development conference statement. Ann Intern Med 114:593–597, 1991.
8. McHenry CR, Pollard A, Walfish PG, Rosen IB. Intraoperative parathormone level measurement of hyperparathyroidism. Surgery 108:801–808, 1990.
9. Nussbaum SR, Thompson AR, Hutcheson KA, Gaz RD, Wang C-A. Intraoperative measurement of parathyroid hormone in the surgical management of hyperparathyroidism. Surgery 104:1121–1127, 1988.
10. Brasier AR, Wang C-A, Nussbaum SR. Recovery of parathyroid hormone secretion after parathyroid adenomectomy. J Clin Endocrinol Metab 66:495–500, 1988.
11. Nussbaum SR, Potts JT Jr. Advances in immunoassays for parathyroid hormone. In: Bilezikian JP, Levine MA, Marcus R, eds. The Parathyroids. Raven Press, New York, 1994, pp 157–169.
12. Nussbaum SR, Zahradnik RJ, Lavigne JR, et al. Highly sensitive two-site immunoradiometric assay of parathyrin, and its clinical utility in evaluating patients with hypercalcemia. Clin Chem 33:1364–1367, 1997.
13. Colford JW, Salvati M, Sokoll LJ, Levine MA. Isolation and characterization of PTH fragments reported in intact PTH assays from serum. Clin Chem 43:S189, 1997.
14. Proye CAG, Goropoulos A, Carnaille B, Vix M, Quievreux JL, Couplet-Lebon G, Racadot A. Usefulness and limits of quick intraoperative measurements of intact (1-84) parathyroid hormone in the surgical management of hyperparathyroidism: Sequential measurements in patients with multiglandular disease. Surgery 110: 1035–1042, 1991.
15. Ryan MF, Jones SR, Barnes AD. Modification to a commercial immunoradiometric assay permitting intraoperative monitoring of parathyroid hormone levels. Ann Clin Biochem 27:65–68, 1990.
16. Irvin GL III, Dembrow VD, Prudhomme DL. Operative monitoring of parathyroid gland hyperfunction. Am J Surg 162:299–302, 1991.
17. Irvin GL III, Deserio GT III. A new, practical intraoperative parathyroid hormone assay. Am J Surg 168:466–468, 1994.

18. Irvin GL III, Prudhomme DL, Deserio GT, Sfakianakis G, Chandarlapaty SKC. A new approach to parathyroidectomy. Ann Surg 5:574–581, 1994.
19. Carty SE, Worsey MJ, Virji MA, Brown MA, Watson CG. Concise parathyroidectomy: The impact of preoperative SPECT ^{99m}Tc sestamibi scanning and intraoperative parathormone assay. Surgery 122:1107–1116, 1997.
20. Clary BM, Garner SC, Leight GS Jr. Intraoperative parathyroid hormone monitoring during parathyroidectomy for secondary hyperparathyroidism. Surgery 122:1034–1039, 1997.
21. Kao PC, van Heerden JA, Taylor RL. Intraoperative monitoring of parathyroid procedures by a 15-minute parathyroid hormone immunochemiluminometric assay. Mayo Clin Proc 69:532–537, 1994.
22. Wenk RE, Efron G, Madamba L. Central laboratory analyses of intact PTH using intraoperative samples. Lab Med 31:158–161, 2000.
23. Sokoll LJ, Udelsman R, Bruzek DJ, Wallerson G, Drew H, Dunn W, Evans L, Terry C, Chan DW. Evaluation of the IMMULITE *Turbo* Intact PTH assay in an intraoperative setting (abstr). Clin Chem 46(suppl):A124, 2000.
24. Wians FH Jr, Balko JA, Hsu RM, Byrd W, Snyder WH III. Intraoperative vs central laboratory PTH testing during parathyroidectomy surgery. Lab Med 31:616–21, 2000.
25. Tan P, Wilkinson H, Leveson SH. Limited role for intraoperative intact PTH measurement in parathyroid surgery. Ann R Coll Surg Engl 77:28–30, 1995.
26. Irvin GL, Dembrow VD, Prudhomme DL. Clinical usefulness of an intraoperative "quick parathyroid hormone" assay. Surgery 114:1019–1023, 1993.
27. Sokoll LJ, Drew H, Udelsman R. Intraoperative parathyroid hormone analysis: A study of 200 cases. Clin Chem 46:1262–1268, 2000.
28. Garner SC, Leight GS Jr. Initial experience with intraoperative PTH determinations in the surgical management of 130 consecutive cases of primary hyperparathyroidism. Surgery 126:1132–1138, 1999.
29. Gordon LL, Snyder WH III, Wians F Jr, Nwariaku F, Kim LT. The validity of quick intraoperative parathyroid hormone assay: An evaluation in seventy-two patients based on gross morphologic criteria. Surgery 126:1030–1035, 1999.
30. Irvin GL, Molinari AS, Figueroa C, Carneiro DM. Improved success rate in reoperative parathyroidectomy with intraoperative PTH assay. Ann Surg 229:874–878, 1999.
31. Dackiw APB, Sussman JJ, Fritsche HA, Delpassand ES, Stanford P, Hoff A, Gagel RF. Relative contributions of technetium Tc-99m sestamibi scintigraphy, intraoperative gamma probe detection, and the rapid parathyroid hormone assay to the surgical management of hyperparathyroidism. Arch Surg 135:550–557, 2000.
32. Tonelli F, Spini S, Tommasi M, Gabbriella G, Amorosi A, Brocchi A, Brandi ML. Intraoperative parathormone measurement in patients with multiple endocrine neoplasia type I syndrome and hyperparathyroidism. World J Surg 24:556–563, 2000.
33. Mandell DL, Genden EM, Mechanick JI, Bergman DA, Diamond EJ, Urken ML. The influence of intraoperative parathyroid hormone monitoring on the surgical management of hyperparathyroidism. Arch Otolaryngol Head Neck Surg 127:821–827, 2001.
34. Udelsman R, Osterman F, Sokoll LJ, Drew H, Levine MA, Chan DW. Rapid para-

thyroid hormone measurement during venous localization. Clin Chim Acta 295:193–198, 2000.

35. Saharay M, Farooqui A, Farrow S, Fahie-Wilson M, Brown A. Intra-operative parathyroid hormone assay for simplified localization of parathyroid adenomas. J R Soc Med 89:261–364, 1996.
36. Irvin GL. Presidential address: Chasin' hormones. Surgery 126:993–997, 1999.
37. Perrier ND, Ituarte P, Kikuchi S, Siperstein AE, Duh QY, Clark OH, Gielow R, Hamill T. Intraoperative parathyroid aspiration and parathyroid hormone assay as an alternative to frozen section for tissue identification. World J Surg 24:1319–1322, 2000.
38. Price CP. Evidence-based laboratory medicine: Supporting decision-making. Clin Chem 46:1041–1050, 2000.
39. Orfield K. Increasing the laboratorian's role in assessing patient outcomes. Lab Med 31:16–21, 2000.
40. Carneiro DM, Irvin GL. Late parathyroid function after successful parathyroidectomy guided by intraoperative hormone assay (QPTH) compared with the standard bilateral neck exploration. Surgery 128:925–929, 2000.
41. Sosa JA, Zeiger MA. Surgery for hyperparathyroidism. Trends Endocrinol Metab 10:72–75, 1999.
42. Chen H, Sokoll L, Udelsman R. Outpatient minimally invasive parathyroidectomy: A combination of sestamibi-SPECT localization, cervical block anaesthesia, and intraoperative parathyroid hormone assay. Surgery 126:1016–1022, 1999.
43. Irvin GL, Sfakianakis G, Yeung L, et al. Ambulatory parathyroidectomy for primary hyperparathyroidism. Arch Surg 131:1074–1078, 1996.
44. Miccoli P, Bendinelli C, Berti P, Vignali E, Pinchera A, Marcocci C. Video-assisted versus conventional parathyroidectomy in primary hyperparathyroidism: A prospective randomized study. Surgery 126:1117–1122, 1999.
45. Sofferman RA, Standage J, Tang ME. Minimal-access parathyroid surgery using intraoperative parathyroid hormone assay. Laryngoscope 108:1497–1503, 1998.
46. Udelsman R, Donovan PI, Sokoll LJ. One hundred consecutive minimally invasive parathyroid explorations. Ann Surg 232:331–339, 2000.
47. Udelsman R. 656 Consecutive explorations for primary hyperparathyroidism. Ann Surg 235:665–670, 2002.
48. Boggs JE, Irvin GL, Carneiro DM, Molinari AS. The evolution of parathyroidectomy failures. Surgery 126:998–1003, 1999.
49. Johnson LR, Doherty G, Lairmore T, Moley JF, Brunt LM, Koenig J, Scott MG. Evaluation of the performance and clinical impact of a rapid intraoperative parathyroid hormone assay in conjunction with preoperative imaging and concise parathyroidectomy. Clin Chem 47:919–925, 2001.

16

Rationale for Point-of-Care Testing (POCT) for Drugs of Abuse and Ethyl Alcohol

Alan H. B. Wu
Hartford Hospital, Hartford, Connecticut, U.S.A.

INTRODUCTION

There are two major arenas where testing for drugs of abuse in urine and ethyl alcohol in blood are important. In the emergency department (ED), patients who present with various "toxidromes" are candidates for drug testing. A toxidrome is a collection of clinical signs and symptoms that may be indicative of intoxication by a drug or substance (1). Table 1 lists the common toxidromes and the drugs that can be responsible for producing the toxidrome. Drug tests with a rapid turnaround time (TAT) can be very important in the triage and management of intoxicated or overdosed patients. For many toxidromes, there are antagonists that can be given to reverse the toxic effect of the culprit substance. Therapy with other drugs, such as the benzodiazepines, may be helpful to prevent known side effects of an intoxicant, such as the prevention of seizures. Proper acute therapy and management may be important in reducing the morbidity and mortality of the affected patient. For drugs-of-abuse testing of ED patients, urine is the specimen of choice. Serum, breath, and saliva are useful for ethyl alcohol testing.

The forensic or medicolegal field is the other major area where drug testing is prevalent. In general, the need for rapid turnaround time is more for logistic rather than clinical reasons. In the medical examiner's office, drug testing is important in determining the cause of death. Because it is more important in this situation for tests to be more accurate than timely, there is little need for rapid drug testing.

Table 1 Clinical Toxidromes

Toxidrome	Symptoms	Compounds
Cholinergic	Hypersecretory	Organophosphates
Anticholinergic	Flush, dry, warm	Tricyclic antidepressants, antihistamines
Sympathetic	Stimulation	Amphetamines, PCP, monoamine oxidase inhibitors
Opiates	Coma, slow respiration, pinpoint pupils	Opiates, propoxyphene
Sedative-hypnotic	Depression	Barbiturates, benzodiazepines, ethyl alcohol
Hallucinogenic	Delirium	Cocaine, phencyclidine, marijuana, LSD

Workplace urine drug testing has become an important strategy for many corporations in their attempts to reduce drug use among their employees. Drug testing is mandated for all employees of the U.S. federal government, armed forces, and those who are employed in "public safety–sensitive" positions, such as the transportation industry. Workers could be tested before they are considered for employment, at random intervals, for licensure, in situations where there may be probably cause for drug use, and after accidents and mishaps. Federal drug testing currently consists of collecting urine and sending it to certified laboratories for screening and confirmation analysis. The turnaround time for screening results by immunoassay is typically 12–24 hr, with results of confirmation testing by gas chromatography/mass spectrometry (GC/MS) available within 48 hr. While this strategy is also used for testing within the private sector, more and more corporations are conducting the screening test at the point of care. For individuals who produce a negative immunoassay screen result, the sample does not need to be sent for further confirmation analysis, and the employee can immediately return to duty.

DRUG TESTING AND POINT-OF-CARE DEVICES

There are many analytical methods for drugs-of-abuse testing in urine or serum. Procedures that test for the presence of a wide range of drugs include thin-layer chromatography, liquid chromatography, and gas chromatography/mass spectrometry. As the procedures or instrumentation are substantial, none of these procedures are amendable for testing at the bedside. In the central laboratory, immunoassays loaded onto automated chemistry analyzers are the most widely used technique for testing patients from the emergency department. Immunoassays are not comprehensive, as they are targeted against specific drugs or classes of drugs. Essentially all POCT devices are based on immunochromatography whereby the drug or drug classes of interest move through the device by capillary action and are captured and detected through the use of specific antibodies. There are several different designs, depending on the intended use. Most do not require pretreatment steps, the addition of reagents, or washing steps. There are single "dipstick-like" devices, which requires a small quantity of urine to be pipetted or dipped directly to the sampling area. Multiple-analyte devices either have a sampling area or are designed such that they can be directly inserted into a urine cup for sampling. There are also devices whereby the immunochromatography test is built into the urine collection cup itself. In the case of TesTcup® (Roche Diagnostics, Brandenberg, NJ), the cap is turned one direction to seal the sample for transportation, or turned in the opposite direction to enable the flow of urine to the test area (2). A thorough review of the commercially available POCT devices has recently been published (3) and is beyond the scope of this chapter.

There are also several approaches that can be taken for the POCT of ethyl alcohol. Breath alcohol analyzers have been used for many years in conjunction with traffic law enforcement and are becoming more prevalent in emergency departments. Breath alcohol testing is currently exempt by the Clinical Laboratory Improvement Act of 1988, because a breath sample is not separately collected and tested. More recently, POCT of saliva for ethyl alcohol has been developed. The STC device (Bethlehem, PA) uses a mouth swab that is transferred to a device that quantitatively measures the ethyl alcohol concentration with the alcohol dehydrogenase assay (4). Unlike urine, the ethyl alcohol concentration in breath and saliva can be directly correlated to blood concentrations. This may be useful to determine if a patient is impaired by the presence of alcohol, an assessment that cannot be made with urine drug testing. There are currently no whole blood, serum, or plasma POCT devices for ethyl alcohol. In addition, there are no POCT assays for the other volatile and nonvolatile alcohols, such as methyl alcohol, isopropyl alcohol, ethylene glycol, and propylene glycol. Due to the infrequent need for such testing, it is unlikely that POCT testing for these "toxic" alcohols will be available.

ADVERSE EFFECTS FOR SELECTED DRUGS OF ABUSE

As a rationale for conducting clinical outcomes studies, a discussion on the toxicities and attributes of immunoassays for selected drugs of abuse is necessary and provided below.

Cocaine

Cocaine is a naturally occurring stimulant derived from the leaves of the *Erythroxylon coca* shrub. It was first isolated in 1855 and was initially used as an anesthetic. Cocaine is abused by intravenous injection or nasal insufflation of the hydrochloride salt, or smoking of the free base of cocaine. The toxic effects of this drug result from the direct stimulation to the cardiovascular and central nervous systems (CNS). It acts by interfering with sodium channels, blocking the reuptake of norepinephrine and dopamine at neuronal synaptic junctions, and inhibits the release of other nerotransmitters such as gamma-aminobutyric acid (GABA). Cocaine is principally metabolized in the liver in roughly equal amounts to benzoylecgonine and ecgonine methyl ester, which are inactive metabolites that are excreted into the urine. Patients with a cocaine overdose present with agitated behavior, altered mental status, and confusion. The cardiovascular effects include tachycardia, ventricular arrhythmias, and hypertension that can result in acute coronary syndromes, seizures, stroke, and rhabdomyolysis. Chronic use can also potentiate pulmonary disease. Patients in the ED who present with cocaine toxicities can be treated with benzodiazepines, such as diazepam, which augment the effect of GABA at the central nervous system receptor sites. Immunoassays for cocaine are directed toward the benzoylecgonine metabolite, with little cross-reactivity toward cocaine as the free drug. Urine remains positive for cocaine metabolites for 2–3 days after use.

Opiates

The opiates are a family of drugs that have a common chemical structure. Many are derived from the poppy plant *Papaver somniferum.* Codeine and morphine are widely prescribed for pain control and as a medication for the common cold. Oral administration is used for outpatient prescription use and intravenous (IV) administration for inpatient, hospital use. Heroin was also used as a narcotic but, due to its toxicity, it has been removed from any legitimate medical use. The major metabolite of both codeine and heroin is morphine. Prior to the production of morphine, heroin also produces a short-lived intermediate metabolite, 6-monoacetylmorphine. The semisynthetic opiates include hydrocodone, hydromorphone, oxycodone, and oxymorphone, and the synthetic opiates include methadone, propoxyphene, and meperidine. Opioids, the general term applied to all substances with morphine-like properties, bind to specific central nervous system receptors and mimic the natural effects of endorphins and enkephalins. This has led to the widespread abuse of this drug. The opiates are addictive and abrupt disuse can lead to significant withdrawal symptoms.

The toxic effects of opiate overdoses include respiratory depression, pinpoint pupils, hypotension, and cyanosis. Coma and death can result from severe intoxications. The toxic effects are aggravated by the presence of other CNS depressive drugs such as alcohol, hypnotics, or sedatives. The best therapy for opioid overdoses is the administration of an opiate antagonist. Naloxone is a synthetic antagonist that binds to opiate receptors but does not itself have agonistic properties. It also does not produce positive results on opiate immunoassays (5). The drug is short acting, however, and a return to opioid symptoms can occur after the naloxone is cleared. Naltrexone is a longer acting antagonist to reversibly block the effects of opiates. Immunoassays for opiates are directed toward morphine and codeine. They have a fair degree of cross-reactivity to hydromorphone, a low cross-reactivity toward oxycodone, and no cross-reactivity toward methadone, propoxyphene, meperidine, or fentanyl. A separate immunoassay is available for methadone and propoxyphene. Immunoassays for 6-monoacetylmorphine are being developed for central laboratory use, particularly for workplace drug testing. Whether they become incorporated into a POCT device remains to be seen.

Amphetamines

The amphetamines are a family of drugs that have central nervous system stimulant activity, anorectic, and sympathomimetic properties. The *l*-isomers of amphetamine, methamphetamine, methylenedioxyamphetamine (MDA), and methylenedioxymethamphetamine (MDMA) are stimulants that are listed as controlled substances by the Drug Enforcement Agency. Methamphetamine and MDMA metabolize to amphetamine and MDA, respectively. Ephedrine, pseudoephedrine, deoxyephedrine, phenylpropanolamine, phenylamine, phenfluramine, and phentermine are among the sympathomimetic drugs and substances in this class. Some of these medications are prescribed for weight reduction. These drugs are typically given as oral medications. The amines stimulate the sympathetic nervous system and act by inhibiting the reuptake of catecholamines in neurons and inhibit monoamine oxidases that catabolize the neurotransmitters.

Toxic concentrations of amphetamines can produce seizures, intracranial hemorrhage, tachycardia, hyperthermia, rhabdomyolysis, and muscular rigidity. Patients can be agitated, combative and exhibit aggressive behavior. Benzodiazepines can be used to treat many of the presenting symptoms. Hyperthermia can be treated with aggressive external cooling. Fluid hydration may be necessary in patients who are hypotensive due to catecholamine depletion. There are two types of immunoassays for amphetamines. The class assay has significant cross-reactivity toward most of these amines, while the monoclonal amphetamine assay is directed toward true *l*-amphetamine isomers and its congeners. The former assay is more useful in a clinical toxicology environment, while the latter assay is used for workplace drug testing.

Hallucinogens

The hallucinogens include, among others, marijuana (tetrahydrocannabinol, THC), lysergic acid diethylamide (LSD), and phencyclidine (PCP). While THC has a high prevalence in the U.S. population, it does not contribute to major acute symptoms. Thus, the utility of measuring urine for THC metabolites in the ED setting is of questionable value. Lysergic acid diethylamide can produce hallucinations and widely hysterical behavior. However, there are no POCT assays currently available for LSD. Phencyclidine is highly toxic, and produces symptoms of combativeness, agitation, hypertension, respiratory depression, and seizures. The prevalence of PCP use in the U.S. is very low. Point-of-care testing devices are available for THC and PCP but were developed more for on-site workplace drug testing use. It is unlikely to be used for widespread screening of ED patients.

Barbiturates and Benzodiazepines

The barbiturates and benzodiazepines are a family of depressants and hypnotics. The barbiturates are derived from barbituric acid. Ultra-short- and short-acting barbiturates are used as an aid for sleeping. Longer acting barbiturates are used as sedatives, hypnotics, and for seizure control. The toxic effects of barbiturates include depression of the respiratory center and CNS, slurred speech, lethargy, incoordination, hypothermia, and impaired thinking. Respiratory depression should be treated with intubation and mechanical ventilation. Gastric lavage or activated charcoal can be used to treat overdoses.

Most benzodiazepines also are derived from a common chemical structure. They are used as anxiolytic agents, anticonvulsants, muscle relaxants, sedation, and for the treatment of alcohol withdrawal. Toxic manifestations include ataxia, drowsiness, slurred speech, respiratory and cardiac depression. Many of the benzodiazepines produce a temporary memory loss. As such, flunitrazepam is illicitly used as a "date rape" drug. Benzodiazepine overdoses can be treated with flumazenil, a benzodiazepine antagonist.

The immunoassays for barbiturates are directed toward the central barbituric structure and have reasonable sensitivity toward most of the family of barbiturate drugs. Immunoassays for benzodiazepines are directed toward oxazepam, the principal metabolite for many of the drugs in this family. However, some drugs, such as lorazepam and clonazepam are not metabolized to oxazepam and are not excreted in high concentrations as free drugs. When these drugs are present, false negative urine drug testing results can occur using some commercial immunoassays (6).

Ethyl Alcohol

Together with nicotine and caffeine, ethyl alcohol is among the most commonly used drugs in the world. The concentration of ethyl alcohol ranges from 3–6% in beer and malt liquors, 9–12% in wine and wine coolers, and 20–60% in distilled beverages. Ethyl alcohol is metabolized in the liver by alcohol dehydrogenase and alcohol oxidase to acetaldehyde and acetic acid, respectively. Unlike most drugs that are eliminated under first-order kinetics (i.e., the rate dependent on concentration), ethyl alcohol is metabolized under zero-order kinetics (i.e., the rate independent on concentration) at about 15–20 mg/dL/hr.

Low blood alcohol concentrations are associated with euphoria and stimulation. However, higher concentrations depress the central nervous system and can lead to confusion, disorientation, muscle incoordination, ataxia, loss of consciousness, coma, and death. Patients intoxicated with ethyl alcohol should be treated with intravenous glucose, as hypoglycemia is a frequent complication, maintenance of body temperature if hypothermic, and maintenance of airway and respiration. If patients present with an alcoholic ketosis, correction of the metabolic acidosis is appropriate with bicarbonate infusion.

POTENTIAL POINT-OF-CARE TESTING OUTCOMES STUDIES FOR DRUGS OF ABUSE

Outcome studies for the use of POCT have traditionally focused on demonstrating that the implementation of such testing improves the clinical outcomes of the tested patients. This might include reductions in death rate, frequency of medical complications, hospital or unit length of stay, or overall costs (beyond the laboratory's); an improvement in the management efficiencies for providing these results; or a perceived higher quality of care, as assessed by patient satisfaction surveys. In reference to POCT for drugs of abuse and alcohol, while there have been many studies to compare the analytical performance of POCT versus laboratory-based analysis, there have been no studies to date that have documented improvements in clinical or economic outcome measures. Thus, in the absence of these data, the following protocols are potential POCT outcomes studies that could be conducted to determine the clinical impact of various POCT assays for drugs of abuse, the therapy for overdoses, and the effects on overall patient costs.

POCT versus the Central Laboratory for ED Patients

Possibly the most useful application of POCT is to determine if improved outcomes are produced for bedside testing for ED patients, as compared with toxicology testing conducted by the central laboratory. The POCT might be justified if the testing improved the efficiency of ED patient triage, as documented by a reduction in the average ED length of stay for these patients. Alternatively, if POCT reduces the time needed to administer an appropriate antagonist or countermeasure, there may be a reduction in the number of adverse effects suffered by the patient (e.g., number of seizures or frequency of withdrawal symptoms) or a faster patient recovery rate (e.g., time for patients to regain consciousness). As some antidotes, such as fomepizol for ethylene glycol exposure are expensive (7), POCT may also enable a reduced utilization of countermeasures by first identifying the patients who would benefit from the antidote in question. All of these potential outcomes presume that use of POCT within the ED reduces the assay turnaround times for results, e.g., from typically 1–2 hr for testing in the central laboratory to 15–20 min for POCT. If the analysis showed that these outcomes measures are not significantly better for POCT relative to the central laboratory, one would conclude that the faster TAT achieved for POCT would not justify the additional costs to implement this service.

Figure 1 illustrates one potential clinical trial that could be conducted to test these hypotheses. The study group consists of patients who have signs and symptoms of opiate abuse (e.g., miosis, respiratory depression, etc.). Testing for opiates is then randomized to POCT and the central laboratory. The results of this test are reported back to the attending ED physicians. If a patient is positive for opiates, the appropriate therapy is to administer an opiate antagonist, such as naloxone. The time between ordering the drug test and the administration of the antagonist is recorded along with the ED length of stay (LOS) for all patients in the study group. If the ED physicians are waiting for results of the opiate test before proceeding to therapy, POCT may result in a shorter time to drug treatment and resolution of clinical symptoms. On the other hand, many ED physicians may elect to administer naloxone on the basis of the clinical presentation alone

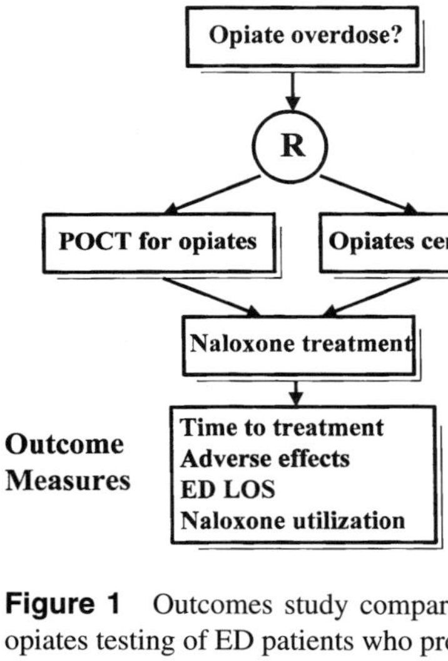

Figure 1 Outcomes study comparing POCT versus the central laboratory for urinary opiates testing of ED patients who present with signs and symptoms of opiate intoxication or overdose. R = randomization.

(i.e., without the opiate test result), and a faster turnaround time for urine drug testing would be unnecessary. Treating without a confirmed diagnosis of opiate use is a relatively common practice as naloxone is inexpensive and has minimal side effects. Under these conditions, it would be important to document how many non–opioid-intoxicated patients inappropriately received naloxone, and if this produced delays in determining the actual cause of the symptoms. If POCT results are made available in a more timely fashion, ED physicians might wait for opiate results before administering naloxone.

POCT in Screening for Specific Diseases

There are some drugs of abuse whose toxic effects potentiate pre-existing diseases. As such, their presence and influence might not be as obvious as other drugs that are the primary reason for the clinical presentation. One example is cocaine, which has been shown to produce chest pain that is similar in nature and scope as for patients with acute coronary syndromes. Drug testing in this population may be useful to screen for one possible etiology of ED patients who present with acute chest pain.

Figure 2 illustrates a clinical trial involving chest pain patients and cocaine testing. The study is randomized to patients for cocaine testing versus no cocaine testing. Although central laboratory testing could be conducted for cocaine, the turnaround time for reporting results of 1–2 hr may not be useful for emergent triaging decisions. This trial would be most effectively conducted in a population where there is a high prevalence for cocaine use, such as in an inner-city medical

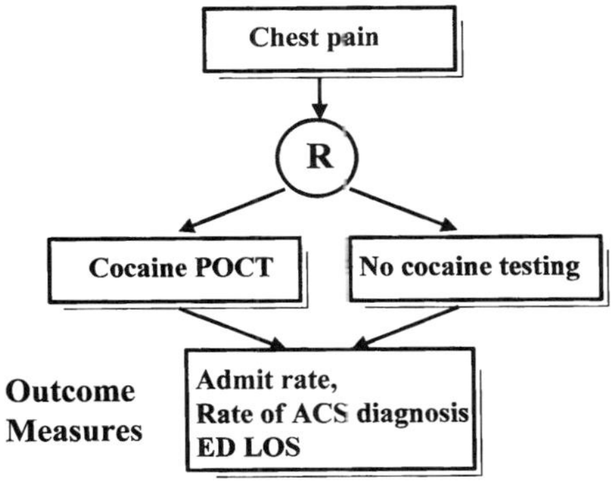

Figure 2 Outcomes study to determine the effectiveness of POCT versus no testing for urinary cocaine of ED patients who present with chest pain. R = randomization, ACS = acute coronary syndromes.

center. The outcome measures for this trial include the ED LOS, admission rate, and the number of patients with a diagnosis of acute myocardial infarction or angina pectoris. If patients who are positive for cocaine metabolites are associated with a higher admission rate or diagnosis of acute coronary syndromes, this information could be added as an additional risk factor.

The incidence of cocaine positive results in a group of chest pain patients presenting to the ED has been documented in a multicenter trial. In the report of Feldman et al. (8), the incidence of patients presenting with cocaine-associated complaints was 293 of 10,689 patients (2.7%) from 10 institutions. The incidence of acute coronary syndromes at 2% was extremely low. In the study of Kushman et al. (9), a 30-day follow-up of 171 patients with cocaine-associated chest pain was performed. There was only one case of major adverse clinical effects (death, acute myocardial infarction). In a study of stroke in women, the use of cocaine or amphetamine was identified as a risk factor, with an adjusted odds ratio of 7.0 (95% confidence interval 2.8–17.9) (10).

In these studies, no drug testing was performed to identify the patients involved. A higher incidence of cocaine use is likely to be uncovered if actual testing is conducted, because self-reporting of drug use is largely unreliable (11,12). There have been no prospective studies conducted on how a positive cocaine result might affect clinical practice for chest pain patients or stroke. However, based on the studies published thus far, it does not appear that screening for cocaine or amphetamine use in chest pain patients will justify implementation of POCT.

The notion that the concentration of cocaine and cocaine metabolites in *blood* may correlate better than urine testing was tested in patients presenting to an ED with chest pain (13). There was no statistical correlation between the concentration of cocaine or metabolites to the severity of clinical symptoms, disposition, need for treatment, or clinical outcomes. Screening plasma of patients for cocaine and amphetamine use was also not justified in determining the cause in ED patients who present with seizures. There were no cases of amphetamine positive results and only 14 of 248 (5.6%) patients positive for cocaine (14). If there had been a positive finding in either of these studies, a quantitative POCT assay using a device reader for cocaine could have been justified.

Effectiveness of POCT for Ethyl Alcohol Testing

Patients who present with acute trauma due to motor vehicle accidents are often tested for the presence of ethyl alcohol. Testing is conducted to determine if ethyl alcohol contributes to or is responsible for the patient's presenting signs and symptoms. The typical effects of this drug include slowed reflexes, slurred speech, confusion, muscular incoordination, ataxia, and a reduced level or complete loss of consciousness (15). Unfortunately, the results of ethyl alcohol testing

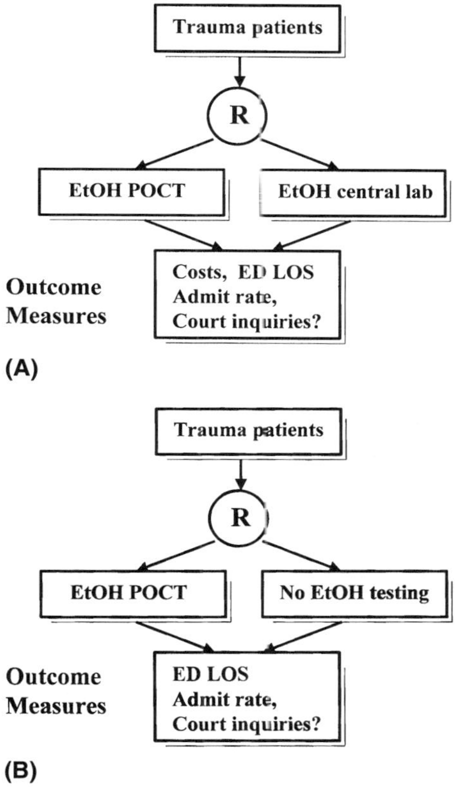

Figure 3 (A) Outcomes study to determine the effectiveness of POCT for breath or salivary alcohol (EtOH) versus the central laboratory for ED trauma patients. (B) Outcomes study to determine the effectiveness of POCT for breath or salivary alcohol versus no testing for trauma patients. R = randomization.

are sometimes used for legal proceedings. Figure 3(A) illustrates a potential clinical study that compares ED bedside testing, such as with a breath alcohol meter or saliva POCT device, with results from the central laboratory using serum or plasma. It is presumed that the reporting TAT for the POCT approach would be superior to the central laboratory, where an additional centrifugation step to separate the erythrocytes is required prior to analysis. The outcomes measures include costs, ED length of stay, and the admission rate. If results of POCT for ethyl alcohol are not recorded in the final medical record, the number of inquiries by law enforcement officers could also be tracked and used as an outcome measure; if alcohol testing results are not transmitted to the medical record, such data cannot be subpoenaed. Unfortunately, not listing test results makes billing for this test impossible. If ED physicians are waiting for the results of ethyl alcohol before triaging the patient to the appropriate level of care, then POCT may offer an advantage. It is unclear what effect rapid ethyl alcohol test results would have on therapeutic decisions, as death by direct alcohol overdose is uncommon. Thus the need for performing any POC alcohol testing in this clinical context can be questioned. The study shown in Figure 3(B) addresses some potential outcomes measures of POCT versus no testing. Obviously the latter course would be the most cost effective.

Effectiveness of Screening High-Risk Patients in an Outpatient Environment

Point-of-care testing for drugs of abuse may have advantages when used in a primary care setting relative to the testing of samples that are packaged and sent to a reference laboratory. The POCT results can be used by the primary care physician to make therapeutic and management decisions while the patient is still in the office. For example, a patient who presents with chest pain could be tested for cocaine. A positive result might prompt the physician to admit the patient for possible cardiac disease complications (as opposed to a noncardiac cause of the symptoms). Asthma is another potential complication of a cocaine user. Rome et al. (16) studied the impact of cocaine use on patients presenting to the ED with asthma and concluded that the severity of asthma exacerbation was worsened in patients positive for cocaine. Figure 4 shows a potential clinical outcomes study for asthma patients in an outpatient asthma or respiratory disease clinic. Subjects

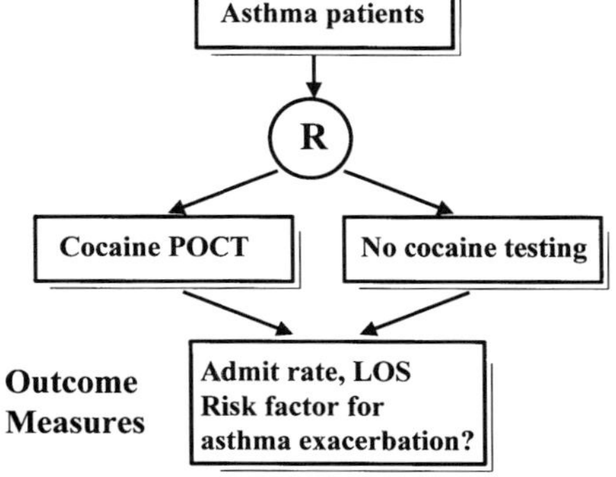

Figure 4 Outcomes study to determine the effectiveness of POCT versus no testing for urinary cocaine in asthma patients in an outpatient setting. R = randomization.

are randomized to testing or no testing for cocaine metabolites in urine. Outcomes measures include an assessment of the severity of symptoms, need for hospitalization, and the length of stay for hospitalized patients. Point-of-care testing for cocaine may be justified if it prospectively correlated to a higher frequency of asthma exacerbations.

Clinical Trial for Workplace Drug Testing

Immunoassays for drugs of abuse are the standard screening tests for workplace drug testing. There is much interest in performing on-site testing so that negative results of screens can be made immediately known to employers. When urine is tested for pre-employment purposes, an individual who has no drugs in their urine can be immediately offered a position. Individuals who are tested because of a work-related incident or accident or those who exhibit behavior suspicious of drug use can also be tested and return to work with a negative result. Although the costs for POCT devices are higher than the incremental reagents costs for central laboratory testing, on-site POCT is justified by not having to pay for delivery costs, maintaining chain-of-custody documentation, and providing a result that can be used without delays.

There have been several experimental programs that have evaluated the utility of on-site testing for drugs of abuse in the workplace. The U.S. Postal Service has conducted a pilot program using the Roche TesTcup (17). Recently, some states (e.g., Maryland and Georgia) have enacted legislation permitting on-site testing in the workplace environment. It is likely that the Substance Abuse and Mental Health Services Administration will soon allow on-site drug testing for federal employees.

Despite the interest in POCT, there have been no randomized outcomes studies that have directly compared on-site testing versus the central toxicology laboratory. Figure 5 illustrates a protocol that could be used. A sample is randomized to be tested by POCT versus sending it to the central laboratory. In the U.S. Postal Service trial, only the specimens screened positive by the POCT device were sent to the central laboratory for confirmation analysis. To determine if the POCT produced false negative results relative to automated immunoassays, all samples conducted by the on-site device must be sent to the toxicology laboratory for retesting. If the false positive rate for POCT is high, additional expenses will be necessary to retest this sample by the toxicology laboratory. If the false negative rate for POCT is high, there may be some employees who escape detection. Because the endpoint of POCT devices is visual, the accuracy of urine specimen containing drugs at or near the cutoff concentration is likely to be more of a problem than with instrument-based immunoassays. Studies have shown that the accuracy of POCT is variable depending on the manufacturer of the device and the drug tested on that device (18,19).

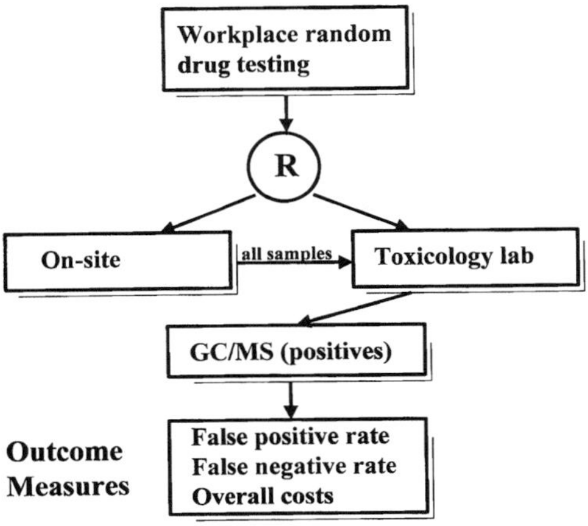

Figure 5 Outcomes study to determine the effectiveness of POCT versus reference toxicology laboratory for workplace drug testing. Samples positive by either approach are subsequently tested at a reference toxicology laboratory by gas chromatography/mass spectrometry (GC/MS) analysis. R = randomization.

SUMMARY

Urine drug testing is clearly big business for the in vitro diagnostics industry. The incidence of drug abuse in the United States is not diminishing, despite the implementation of workplace drug testing programs. The high prevalence of drugs in the United States and the western world makes it a clinical problem as well. In most cases, POCT will increase the costs for providing drug testing results when compared with the central laboratory, because most chemistry divisions have instrumentation that accommodate immunoassay drug testing. However, there may be clinical benefits of a faster turnaround times that outweigh the additional costs for POCT. These outcomes studies remain to be demonstrated in "evidence-based" studies. It may be possible that improvements in POCT technologies may be necessary, e.g., for tricyclic antidepressants or a wider menu or specimen types, to increase the utility of POCT.

REFERENCES

1. Mofenson HC, Caraccio TR. Toxidromes. Comp Ther 11:46–52, 1985.
2. Taylor EH, Oertli EH, Wolfgang JW, Mueller E. Accuracy of five on-site immunoassay drugs-of-abuse testing devices. J Anal Toxicol 23:119–124, 1999.

3. Wu AHB. Point-of-care testing for drugs of abuse. In: Shaw LM, ed. The Clinical Toxicology Laboratory. Contemporary Practice of Poisoning Evaluation. American Association of Clinical Chemistry Press, Washington, DC, 2001.
4. Bates ME, Martin CS. Immediate, quantitative estimation of blood alcohol concentration from saliva. J Stud Alcohol 58:531–538, 1997.
5. Storrow AB, Wians FH Jr, Mikkelsen SL, Norton J. Does naloxone cause a positive urine opiate screen? Ann Emerg Med 24:1151–1153, 1994.
6. Meatherall R. Benzodiazepine screening using EMIT II and TDx: Urine hydrolysis pretreatment required. J Anal Toxicol 18:385–390, 1994.
7. Brent J, McMartin K, Phillips S, Burkhart KK, Donovan JW, Wells M, Kulig K. Fomepizole for the treatment of ethylene glycol poisoning. Methylpyrazole for Toxic Alcohols Study Group. N Engl J Med 450:832–838, 1999.
8. Feldman JA, Fish SS, Beshansky JR, Griffith JL, Woolard RH, Selker HP. Acute cardiac ischemia in patients with cocaine-associated complaints: Results of a multicenter trial. Ann Emerg Med 35:469–476, 2000.
9. Kushman SO, Storrow AB, Liu T, Gibler WB. Cocaine-associated chest pain in a chest pain center. Am J Cardiol 85:394–396, 2000.
10. Petitti DB, Sidney S, Quesenberry C, Bernstein A. Stroke and cocaine or amphetamine use. Epidemiol 9:596–600, 1998.
11. Hollander JE, Brooks DE, Valentine SM. Assessment of cocaine use in patients with chest pain syndromes. Arch Intern Med 158:62–66, 1998.
12. Markovic N, Ness RB, Cefilli D, Grisso JA, Stahmer S, Shaw LM. Substance use measures among women in early pregnancy. Am J Obstet Gynecol 183:627–632, 2000.
13. Blaho K, Logan B, Winbery S, Park L, Schwilke E. Blood cocaine and metabolite concentrations, clinical findings, and outcome of patients presenting to an ED. Am J Emerg Med 18:593–598, 2000.
14. Steele MT, Westdorp EJ, Garza AG, Ma OJ, Roberts DK, Watson WA. Screening for stimulant use in adult emergency department seizure patients. J Toxicol Clin Toxicol 38:609–613, 2000.
15. Dubowski KM. Alcohol determination in the clinical laboratory. Am J Clin Pathol 74:747–750, 1980.
16. Rome LA, Lippmann ML, Dalsey WC, Taggart P, Pomerantz S. Prevalence of cocaine use and its impact on asthma exacerbation in an urban population. Chest 117:1324–1329, 2000.
17. Postal Service to trial onsite testing of all new employees. Drug Det Report 8:65–66, 1998.
18. Williams RH, Maggiore JA, Shah SM, Erickson TB, Negrusz A. Cocaine and its major metabolites in plasma and urine samples from patients in an urban emergency medicine setting. J Anal Toxicol 24:478–481, 2000.

17

Reproductive Testing: Ovulation and Pregnancy

David G. Grenache and Ann M. Gronowski
Washington University School of Medicine, St. Louis, Missouri, U.S.A.

INTRODUCTION

The use of point-of-care testing (POCT) for fertility or reproduction-related markers is limited to only a few types of tests. These include urine-based biochemical tests and bioelectric measurements for predicting ovulation, and urine-based testing for detecting pregnancy. This chapter examines the utility of these tests for predicting ovulation, timing insemination, timing postcoital tests, and detecting pregnancy.

PREDICTING OVULATION

The accurate prediction of ovulation is a key factor in reproductive evaluation and it is especially important for timing intercourse during clinical infertility treatment. The window for successful oocyte fertilization is brief and the introduction of sperm into the female reproductive tract within 2 days prior to ovulation is associated with the highest probability of conception (1). Although the exact time of ovulation is impossible to predict, it is generally accepted that it occurs between 32 and 38 hr after the luteinizing hormone (LH) surge is detected in the plasma (2). The LH is rapidly cleared from the plasma into the urine and the length of time for this clearance has been reported to be between 0 and 4 hr (3). Detection of LH in the urine is an indication that ovulation is approaching and identifies the beginning of peak fertility.

Other detectable changes in female physiology, such as changes in the quantity and viscosity of cervical mucus, can also be used to predict ovulation. Following menses, the glands of the endocervix secrete a small amount of viscous mucus, which increases dramatically in volume and becomes more watery and elastic during the later half of the follicular phase (4). Indeed, semiquantitative measurements of cervical mucus are perhaps the oldest of the methods used to predict pending ovulation and they are the basis for the Insler method of monitoring the menstrual cycle (5). Changes in basal body temperature (BBT) have also been used to monitor ovulation. There is a 0.5°F increase in body temperature coincident with the increase in serum progesterone following ovulation (6). Although this is a reliable and inexpensive method to detect ovulation, it is purely retrospective and does not predict the onset of ovulation.

Urine LH Tests

Urine LH testing is an easy and convenient method for predicting ovulation, and perfectly suited for POCT. The first home ovulation prediction kit, Ovustick, was marketed in 1984 by Monoclonal Antibodies, Inc. and took approximately 1 hr to perform (2). Since then, home ovulation kits have become easier to perform and have gained immense popularity. Since 1977, 34 over-the-counter devices have been given U.S. Food and Drug Administration (FDA) approval for the detection of urinary LH. A list of some of the kits currently available in the United States is given in Table 1. These kits generally consist of a number of tests that are either in-stream sticks (placed directly in the urine stream) or multistep tests. Testing begins several days before expected ovulation, depending on the average length of the woman's menstrual cycle, and continues once daily until a positive result is obtained. According to the test manufacturers, a positive test indicates that ovulation is likely to occur in the next 24–36 hr. The concentration of LH that produces a positive result is usually set above 35 or 40 mIU/mL to avoid detection of the low concentrations of LH that are normally present in the urine.

Since the introduction of home LH testing, various studies have evaluated the accuracy of these kits for predicting ovulation (Table 2) (3,7–12). Unfortunately, most of these studies were done in the late 1980s and early 1990s and many of the commercially available kits have changed since that time. In general, however, they do address the question of whether home measurement of urine LH can detect ovulation. All of the studies in Table 2 demonstrated excellent sensitivity (99–100%), indicating that LH in the urine is readily detectable in patients with confirmed ovulation. In studies that identified anovulatory women (7,8,12), the LH kits also showed excellent specificity (100%) with the exception of one (25%) (12). The populations included in each of these studies were varied. While some included only spontaneously ovulating women (3,9,12), others in-

Table 1 Commercial Kits Currently Available in the United States for Predicting Ovulation by Measuring Urinary Hormones[a]

Brand name	Manufacturer	Type	No. of tests in kit	Test time (min)	Analytes detected	Detection limit[b]	Diagnostic sensitivity (%)[b]
ClearPlan Easy	Unipath Diagnostics Co. (Bedford, UK)	In-stream	5	3	LH	>30 mIU/mL LH	99
Ovukit	Quidel Corp. (San Diego, CA)	Multistep	9	60	LH	35 mIU/mL LH	96
OvuQuick OneStep	Quidel Corp. (San Diego, CA)	One-step	6 or 9	3	LH	40 mIU/mL LH	>99
OvuQuick Self-test	Quidel Corp. (San Diego, CA)	Multistep	6 or 9	4	LH	40 mIU/mL LH	92 94
First Response	Carter-Wallace, Inc. (New York, NY)	In-stream	5	5	LH	NA[c]	98.5
ClearPlan Easy Fertility Monitor	Unipath Ltd. (Bedford, UK)	In-stream	20 or 30	5	LH and estrogen-3-glucoronide	>30 mIU/mL LH >20 ng/mL E3G	NA

[a] Partial list.
[b] According to manufacturer.
[c] NA = not available.

Table 2 Comparisons of Previous Studies of In-Home Urine LH Kits to Predict Ovulation

Reference	Assay kit and manufacturer	Timing of assay	Sensitivity[a]	Specificity[b]	Predictive value[c]	Method of confirming ovulation
Corson, 1986 (7)	Ovutime (Ortho Pharmaceutical Corp., Raritan, NJ) or OvuSTICK (Monoclonal Antibodies, Inc., Mountainview, CA)	Twice daily (midmorning and evening)	73/74 (99%)	4/4 (100%)	46/64 (72%)	BBT[d]
Elkind-Hirsch et al., 1986 (8)	OvuSTICK (Monoclonal Antibodies, Inc., Mountainview, CA)	Twice daily (midday and evening)	53/53 (100%)	22/22 (100%)	Not determined	Ultrasound and BBT
Vermesh et al., 1987 (11)	First Response (Carter-Wallace, Inc., New York, NY) OvuSTICK (Monoclonal Antibodies, Inc., Mountainview, CA)	Twice daily (first and late morning)	30/30 (100%) 24/24 (100%)	0/0 0/0	28/30 (93%) 24/24 (100%)	Transvaginal ultrasound
Lloyd et al., 1989 (9)	Q-test (Clay Adams, Parsippany, NJ)	Once daily (first morning)	33/33 (100%)	0/0	30/33 (91%)	Transvaginal ultrasound
Gudgeon et al., 1990 (10)	ClearPlan (Unipath Ltd., Bedford, UK)	Twice daily (first morning and evening, when possible)	118/118 (100%)	0/0	AM 58/65 (89%) PM 50/53 (94%) Both 47/49 (96%)	Serum LH, BBT, and cervical mucus scoring
Miller et al., 1996 (3)	Ovuquick (Quidel Corp., San Diego, CA)	Once daily (evening)	26/26 (100%)	0/0	24/26 (92%)	Transvaginal ultrasound
Guermandi et al., 2001 (12)	ClearPlan (Unipath Ltd., Bedford, UK)	Twice daily (first morning and early evening)	97/97 (100%)	1/4 (25%)	88/101 (87%)	Transvaginal ultrasound

[a] Numerator = number of patients who were LH positive, denominator = number of patients with confirmed ovulation.
[b] Numerator = number of patients who were LH negative, denominator = number of patients without confirmed ovulation.
[c] Defined as the detection of the urine LH surge within 48 hr prior to ovulation.
[d] BBT = basal body temperature.

cluded both normal cycling women and those being treated for fertility problems with medication for ovulation induction (7,8,10,11).

The ability of these tests to *detect* ovulation appears to be extremely accurate but their ability to *predict* ovulation may not be absolute (see Table 2, predictive value). Two studies, each of which used ultrasonographic imaging of the ovarian follicle to determine the day of ovulation, identified a urinary LH surge occurring after ovulation in approximately 9% of women (3,9). Another study reported that 3% of women enrolled in a donor insemination program demonstrated a urine LH surge 2 days after a peak serum LH (10). The reason why a LH surge would be detected postovulation is not entirely clear and it is likely that the standard used to confirm ovulation plays a significant role. For example, if ultrasonographic imaging of the ovary has falsely revealed a decrease in follicular size, the standard to which the surge is compared to is obviously flawed. The true "gold standard" for detecting ovulation is considered to be a rise in serum progesterone (6). However, this does not occur until several days after ovulation and aids little in determining the exact time of ovulation, but rather that ovulation did occur. This needs to be taken into consideration when interpreting the efficiency of these test kits.

Nonetheless, the detection of urinary LH appears to be a very reliable indicator of ovulation and, in at least one study, it has been demonstrated to be diagnostically superior to alternate methods (13). In this 1989 report, the authors evaluated tests used to predict ovulation, including serum LH, serum estradiol, cervical mucus scores, follicular size, BBT, and vaginal electrical impedance. The detection of urinary LH demonstrated the highest positive predictive value (90% in stimulated ovulations, 83% in spontaneous) and negative predictive value (96% in both stimulated and spontaneous ovulations) compared with all other methods tested (13).

There appears to be a diurnal rhythm associated with the LH surge in plasma and evidence suggests that it is most likely to occur in the early morning hours (2,14). This could potentially have an effect on the sensitivity of urinary LH tests if the user tests on the day of the LH surge but prior to its occurrence. It has been suggested that increasing the frequency of testing would increase the efficiency of LH surge detection. Although this question has been examined, the data are inconsistent. One study reported a detection frequency of 87% with the use of one first-morning specimen that increased to 99% when either a midday or an evening specimen was added (9). However, other studies have found no significant difference in LH surge detection when testing was done either once or twice per day (10,15). Increased frequency of testing may indeed result in optimal detection efficiency, however, in most cases, it is probably not necessary and is certainly more costly as well as inconvenient for the patient.

Urine LH and E3G Tests

A recent addition to the repertoire of POCT is a fertility monitor that simultaneously detects both LH and estrone-3-glucoronide (E3G), a metabolite of estradiol, in the urine. Estradiol is synthesized and released by the preovulatory follicle in increasingly higher concentrations as the menstrual cycle progresses toward ovulation. The addition of E3G to the monitoring system is designed to allow women to identify days of low, high, and peak fertility as E3G slowly rises, reaches its peak, and then declines.

The ClearplanEasy® Fertility Monitor (CPFM) (Unipath Diagnostics Co., Bedford, UK) is a complete system that consists of a handheld monitor and disposable, one-step, urine test sticks for detecting both LH and E3G. A testing cycle is initiated by pressing a button on the monitor to indicate the start of menses. The monitor will then prompt the user to do a test. Inserting the dipstick into the monitor after sampling allows the monitor to optically measure the intensity of the reaction areas on the dipstick and report one of three levels of fertility. When both hormones are at their baseline concentrations, "low fertility" is reported. When elevated concentrations of E3G are detected past a threshold (between 20 and 30 ng/mL), the monitor indicates the beginning of a "high fertility" period. Detection of the LH surge results in a change from high to "peak fertility," which will be displayed on the day of the LH surge and for the next day before returning to low fertility. The peak fertility indicator specifies that ovulation should occur within 24 hr. The need to distinguish high from peak fertility may not be of great concern to women with regular menstrual cycles, who could use less expensive urine LH kits to identify peak fertility. However, the use of a more expensive monitor may be of interest to women who have irregular cycles.

In a study performed to assess the ability of the monitor to predict ovulation and determine the fertile period in a population of 53 healthy women, the monitor identified high fertility for at least 7 days in 63.5% of 150 cycles (16). The detection of urinary E3G by the dipstick paralleled the corresponding increase of serum estradiol. Of 149 ultrasound-confirmed ovulations, peak fertility was identified 2 days prior to ovulation in 91% and three days prior in 97% of cycles (16). Ovulation did not occur in any cycle prior to the monitor identifying peak fertility, which is notable because intercourse after the day of ovulation is significantly less likely to result in pregnancy (1).

The same technology used by the CPFM is incorporated into the Persona® system for contraception. Also manufactured by Unipath Diagnostics Co., Persona is not FDA approved but it is marketed and available for use in the UK as being effective in preventing pregnancy when used as a guide to abstain from coitus as the only method of contraception. A study done to evaluate the efficacy of this system reported an effectiveness of 93.8% when used with abstinence on the fertile days as determined by the system (17).

Nonurine Tests for Predicting Ovulation

A novel prototype device called the Ovulon Fertility Monitor has recently been developed as an aid to predict and detect ovulation (Conception Technology, Inc., Fort Collins, CO). It has not been widely tested but it has received marketing approval from the FDA. The device consists of a handheld monitor and a carbonaceous probe that is inserted into the vagina to measure changes in electrical admittance (1/impedence) in the cervical mucus. The cervical tissues respond to changes in the plasma steroid hormone fluctuations during the menstrual cycle. The electrical changes that occur in the mucus may be due to redox reactions involving mucus glycoproteins (18).

The Ovulon monitor is capable of producing a profile with three distinct markers that forecast changes in fertility. The first marker (OL), a long-term predictive peak, occurs 5–7 days before ovulation, while a short-term peak (OS) occurs 1 day before ovulation (O). The final marker, a nadir of electrical admittance, indicates the day of ovulation (Figure 1).

A pilot study that compared the performance of the monitor with urine LH tests identified significant correlations between the LH surge and the short-term predictive peak ($r = 0.84$, $p \leq 0.01$) and between the urine LH surge and the nadir ($r = 0.84$, $p \leq 0.01$) (18). In 95% of the cycles, the nadir occurred after the detection of the LH surge. The authors readily admit that a major limitation of their study was its absence of a method to confirm ovulation. However, the results of the preliminary study are intriguing.

Similarly, the Cue™ Ovulation Monitor (Zetek, Inc., Aurora, CO) is a handheld electronic device that is used to predict and confirm ovulation by measuring salivary and vaginal electrical resistance. Either an oral or a vaginal electrode is used to detect changes in the ionic content of salivary or vaginal mucus induced by rising concentrations of blood estrogen. A peak signal from the salivary electrode was observed 5–6 days prior to the serum LH surge and a vaginal nadir occurred on the day of the LH surge in 12 subjects with normal ovulatory cycles ($n = 17$) (19). Similar results were observed in another, slightly larger study of 32 cycles from 23 subjects (20). These results suggest that the Cue Ovulation Monitor can define the start and end of the fertile period and, therefore, can be used for natural forms of birth control. One study of the device's potential for natural birth control found that the fertile period it predicted was significantly shorter (9 days) then the one predicted by examining the physical characteristics of vaginal mucus (11 days) (21). To be effective at preventing pregnancy, however, the device must be able to predict ovulation at least 5 days prior to its occurrence (as sperm can survive in the female reproductive tract for up to 5 days) and identify the end of the fertile period 1–2 days after ovulation. In a study of 22 normal menstrual cycles (13 women), no salivary signal was detected in two cycles and was detected only 4 days prior to ovulation in two cycles (22).

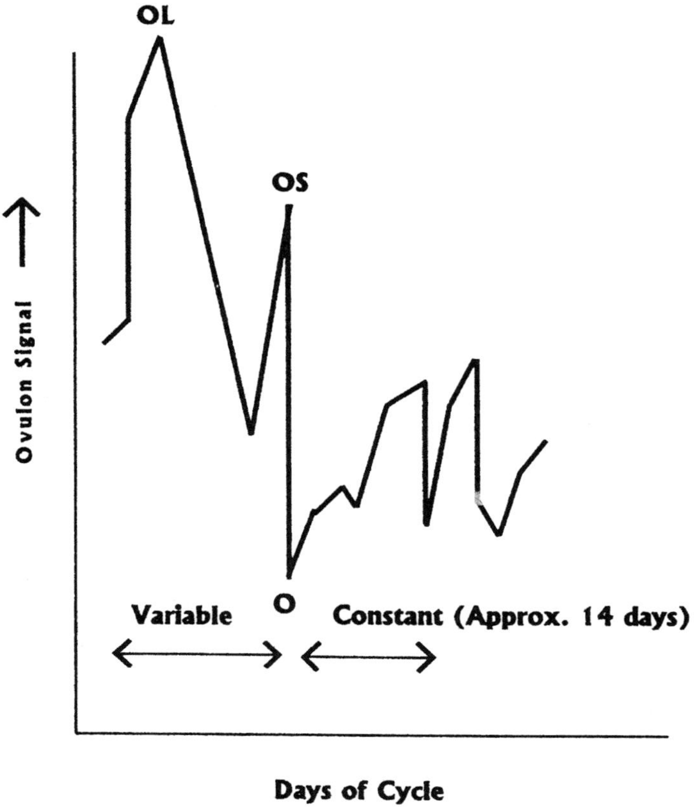

Figure 1 Ovulon Fertility Monitor profile forecasting changes in fertility. OL = Long-term Ovulon predictor occurring 5–7 days prior to ovulation; OS = short-term Ovulon predictor occurring the day before ovulation; O = nadir following the OS peak, indicating the day of ovulation. (From Ref. 18.)

Additionally, the device indicated a vaginal nadir at or before the day of ovulation in three cycles (22). Women engaging in unprotected intercourse during those days would be at potentially more risk for conception. Currently, the FDA has only allowed the Cue Ovulation Monitor to be marketed as a method to predict ovulation, not as a guide to abstain from coitus to prevent conception.

The PSC™ Fertility Monitor (Pheromone Sciences Corp., Calgary, Alberta, Canada) is another novel device that monitors changes in sweat electrolytes as a predictor of ovulation. It has been approved for marketing in Canada and underwent a multicenter clinical trial in the United States in 2001. According to limited information provided by the manufacturer, the appliance contains ion-selective electrodes and a microprocessor housed within a wristwatch-like device that is worn for at least 6 hr a day. Changes in sweat ion ratios occur as a result of the downward spike of plasma estrogen in the days preceding ovulation. These changes are then used to predict the fertile state of the wearer as not fertile, fertile, or ovulating. A pilot trial of the device was completed in Toronto, in which the monitor predicted ovulation within 2 days of actual ovulation in 76% of spontaneously ovulating women (manufacturer's claim).

These types of fertility monitors offer unique methods of ovulation detection, although their diagnostic efficiency is as of yet unclear. Additional prospective studies are needed to support these preliminary findings. If found to be comparable, then these monitors may have broad appeal, particularly due to the fact that the devices are reusable rather than disposable.

TIMING OF INSEMINATION

Discussed so far in this chapter has been the ability of various in-home devices to detect and predict ovulation. A major, unanswered question is whether these devices actually improve pregnancy rates in the general population of normal cycling women. Remarkably, studies of this kind have not been reported. What have been reported are analyses of in-home test kits to improve pregnancy rates following timed artificial insemination.

Artificial insemination (AI) is frequently sought as a treatment for infertility. Because the survival period of the oocyte is much less than that of spermatozoa, timing of AI is of considerable importance and should be done during the 24-hr period preceding ovulation. The use of basal body temperature, cervical mucus score, and cycle averaging have all been used to time AI, but they are plagued by inaccuracy in identifying the day of ovulation (2).

In theory, rates of conception following timed insemination should be increased with a reliable predictor of ovulation. Despite a variety of studies that have examined this application of urine LH testing, the results are far from conclusive. While the use of urine LH testing decreased the number of fertility clinic visits (15,23), some studies indicated that there was no difference among monthly fecundity (conceptions/cycle) or cumulative conception rates. One reported a monthly fecundity rate of 6.5% ($n = 123$ cycles) for patients whose insemination with cryopreserved semen was timed by both BBT and cervical mucus scoring and a rate of 8.1% ($n = 111$ cycles) for patients whose insemination was timed with urine LH testing alone (23). Another study, which timed insemination of fresh semen with BBT and cervical mucus scoring in all patients, but included urine LH testing in some women, reported monthly fecundity rates of 11% ($n = 331$ cycles) in those patients without urine LH testing and 13% ($n = 76$ cycles) in patients who used urine LH tests (24). It is noteworthy to point out that both of these studies compared urine LH testing with BBT and cervical mucus scoring, which are imprecise methods of ovulation prediction. Although both studies indicated that the differences in fecundity were not statistically significant, the results suggest that considerably larger study groups might prove otherwise.

The combination of urine LH testing with transvaginal sonography (TVS) has been shown to be effective in timing donor insemination. A study in which patients reported to a fertility clinic on the day of their first positive urine LH test for TVS and Insler mucus scoring showed that insemination was timed correctly and ovulation occurred during the 24-hr period following insemination in 100% ($n = 20$) of cycles (25). Reliance on only the urine LH results and mucus scores would have resulted in correctly timed inseminations in only 75% of patients (25). Although the study was not randomized and conception was not included in the outcomes, the authors did report an apparent increase in monthly fecundity using this combined method. They state that during the 6 mo prior to this study, in which timing of insemination was based on urine LH testing combined with Insler scoring, the monthly fecundity was 5%. The addition of TVS increased this rate to 9% (25).

Despite the positive reports, the use of urine LH tests has also been implicated in reduced pregnancy rates and increased frustration for patients seeking fertility treatments (26,27). In one study in which patients chose either laboratory or home urine LH testing to time insemination with cryopreserved semen, pregnancy rates were significantly reduced in home-tested (3.4%) compared with laboratory-tested cycles (12.7%) (26). Laboratory analysis performed on previously frozen aliquots of home-tested urine specimens revealed that insemination was performed on a day other than the first day of the LH surge in 28% of cycles ($n = 140$) (26). The authors suggest that insemination was more likely to be performed on an incorrect day in patients with a higher baseline of urine LH despite the fact that none of these patients were taking any antiestrogens (26). A comparison of urine LH baselines between the correctly and incorrectly timed patients revealed 5% of correctly timed patients with a baseline >2.0 IU/mmol creatinine compared with 25% in the incorrectly timed group (26). Not considered by the study are the different analytical sensitivities of the two urine LH assays. Home testers selected from one of three semiquantitative urine LH kits, while the laboratory used a quantitative kit that expressed LH concentration as units of LH per millimole of creatinine. Also, 33% of home testers indicated that they would have liked further assistance in performing and interpreting the urine test despite having received detailed verbal and written instructions (26). The possibility that incorrect test utilization rather than failure of the tests themselves resulted in the decreased pregnancy rate between the two groups should be considered.

Similarly, a 3-yr retrospective study examined clinical pregnancy rates in patients who received timed intrauterine insemination (with cryopreserved donor sperm) based upon either home urine LH testing or laboratory serum LH testing. The pregnancy rate per insemination was significantly higher for serum-monitored cycles at 18% ($n = 1119$) compared with urine-monitored cycles at 13.7% ($n = 346$) (27). As shown in Figure 2, the cumulative viable pregnancy rate was also significantly higher after nine serum-monitored cycles (70.2%) compared with nine urine-monitored cycles (54.8%) (27). In both groups, patient age, infertility factors, parity, and sperm parameters were similar, although the groups were not randomized and patients were allowed to choose either home or laboratory testing. Curiously, patients were advised that serum testing was likely the more accurate of the two methods thereby introducing an automatic bias into the subject populations. The authors make a point to state that subject interpretation of test results was not implicated as a contributing factor for the decreased fecundity in patients who used self-testing, something that is often mentioned in other studies as a very possible contributing factor.

A prospective study of 113 patients that compared the use of BBT graphs and urine LH tests for scheduling donor insemination with cryopreserved sperm demonstrated higher fecundity in the BBT group (28). However, in the BBT

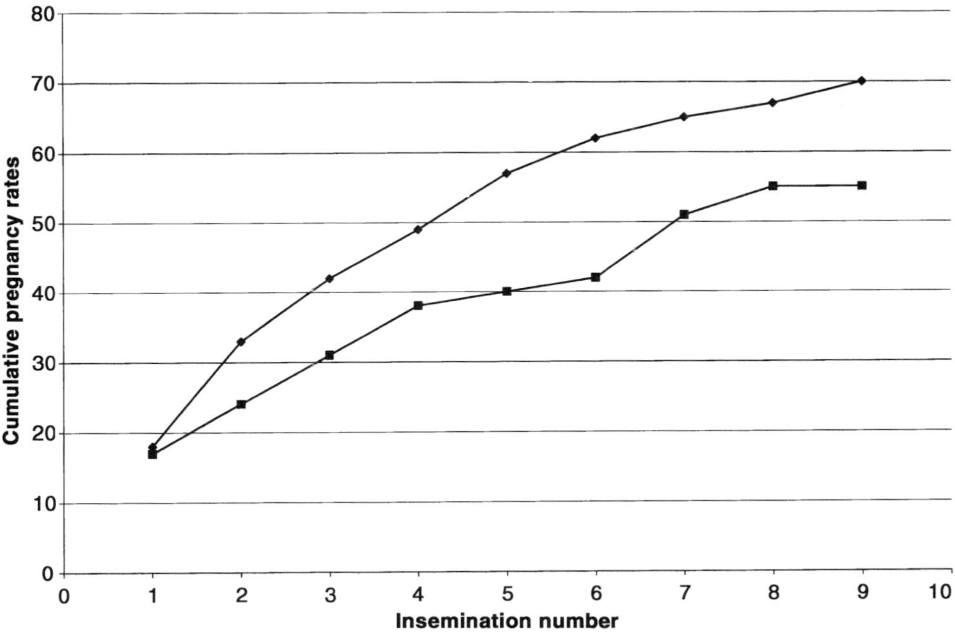

Figure 2 Cumulative clinical pregnancy rates. ◆ = Serum cycles; ■ = urine cycles. (From Ref. 27.)

group, two inseminations were scheduled based upon a physician's interpretation of each patient's BBT chart, while those in the LH group received a single insemination on the day following a positive test. The fecundity rate in the BBT group was 13% compared with 6% in the LH group (28). An obvious explanation for this disparity is the different number of inseminations provided to each group. The authors indicate that although patients in the BBT group were scheduled to have two inseminations per cycle, 31% of the patients cancelled the second inseminations due to a temperature rise one day before the insemination date. This resulted in an average of only 1.69 inseminations per cycle in the BBT group. Furthermore, 29.6% of patients in the BBT group attained pregnancy in a cycle in which only one insemination was performed, suggesting that the increased fecundity rate in the BBT group was not exclusively due to an increased number of inseminations (28). The increased pregnancy rate in the BBT group was also reported to be less expensive. Although patients in this group spent more for inseminations ($1536 vs. 1211), the cost per pregnancy was considerably less ($3997 vs. 6212) (28).

Two studies that have questioned the usefulness of urine LH testing to time insemination reported that urine LH testing did not improve conception rates (29,30). The first, a prospective study in which all patients received two inseminations timed by either BBT charts ($n = 26$) or urine LH tests ($n = 27$), reported a monthly fecundity of 4 and 7%, respectively (29). Again, this difference was not significant, however the authors determined that 378 patients would actually be required in each arm of the trial to demonstrate a significant difference assuming a similar patient population (29).

The second study retrospectively compared the use of BBT charts, serum LH, urine LH, and the Insler cervical mucus score for timing of insemination with cryopreserved semen. There were no significant differences in monthly fecundity among timing techniques in 418 patients, each of whom received two inseminations per cycle (30). As shown in Figure 3, the cumulative probability of conception after six cycles was 31% with BBT charts, 32% with urine LH, 34% with serum LH, and 37% with cervical mucus scoring (30).

Some have speculated that the timing of insemination may be of more importance using intrauterine insemination than it is for intracervical insemination (31). In intracervical insemination, the cervical mucus acts as a reservoir slowly releasing the sperm into the reproductive tract over time, a function lost by the use of intrauterine insemination (2). Further studies are required to support this theory.

TIMING OF THE POSTCOITAL TEST

The postcoital test (PCT) is commonly performed in the evaluation of infertile couples to assess the interaction between cervical mucus and sperm. An abnor-

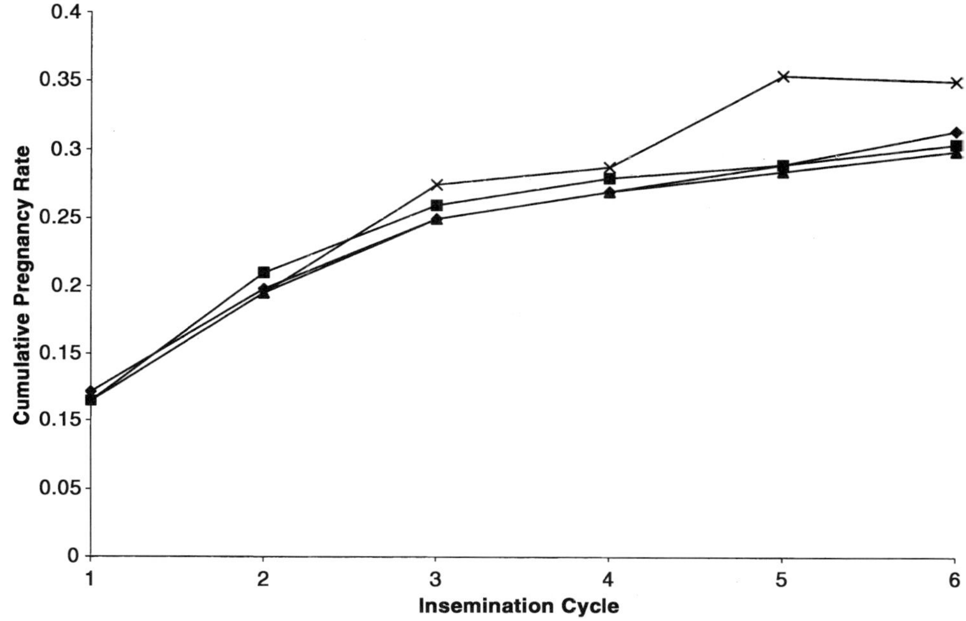

Figure 3 Cumulative probability plots of each timing regimen through six cycles. ◆ = Serum LH; ■ = urinary dipstick; ▲ = BBT charts; × = CM scoring. All pregnancy rates not significantly different ($p > 0.05$). (From Ref. 30.)

mality in this interaction is believed to be present in 10–15% of infertile couples (32). The test is usually performed 8–12 hr after coitus and consists of the aspiration of mucus from the cervix, which is then examined microscopically to see if live sperm are penetrating the mucus and to assess the amount of movement. If the sperm are all moving well the test is considered normal. The timing of the PCT is critical and should be performed in the immediate preovulatory period when the positive effect of serum estradiol on the cervical mucus-producing glands is greatest. During this period, large amounts of thin, clear, acellular cervical mucus are produced and sperm movement through the mucus is uncomplicated. Performing the PCT either too early or too late results in low scores indicating poor mucus quality.

Maximal mucus scores occur at the time of the detection of the urine LH surge (33) and some have advocated the use of urine LH tests to time the performance of the PCT. A randomized study of 37 patients concluded that PCT scores were not significantly different when timed with urine LH tests as compared with BBT (32). The PCT was scored on a scale of 0–9 taking into account the number of progressively motile sperm, percentage of motility, and activity grade. The mean PCT score for patients who used urine LH tests to time the PCT was 4.4 ± 3.1, while those using BBT to time the PCT had a mean score of 4.8 ± 3.6 (32). These findings are not surprising. While the BBT is an inaccurate prospective predictor of the precise day of ovulation, it does perform well as an indicator of the day of ovulation ±2 days. Clearly, acceptable timing of the PCT can be achieved with this degree of accuracy using the BBT.

DETECTING PREGNANCY

Since 1977, the FDA has approved 142 over-the-counter devices for detecting urine human chorionic gonadotropin (hCG). This constitutes 32% of all over-the-counter devices approved. Approximately 33% of women in a 1988 survey had used home hCG kits for detecting pregnancy (34). Today, these devices are routinely used in hospitals, emergency units, and doctors' offices, and they can be found in virtually every corner drugstore in the United States. Despite these facts, relatively few quality studies have examined the performance or impact of these POC tests. The remainder of this chapter summarizes the data that are available.

A list of some of the over-the-counter hCG kits currently available in the United States is given in Table 3. These kits make up one of the fastest growing segments of the home diagnostic testing market (35); therefore, it is difficult to account for all available tests. The concentration of hCG detected by these kits ranges from 15–100 IU/L, and according to their manufacturers, they are able to detect pregnancy as early as the first day of a missed menstrual period. One kit (First Response Early Result) even claims detection as early as three days prior to the expected onset of menses.

A 1998 meta-analysis of the diagnostic efficiency of POCT hCG tests by Bastien et al. (35), provides a nice history of hCG testing in the United States. Their analysis included five studies published from 1976–1989 and included a total of 16 home pregnancy test kits. The sensitivities and specificities of these kits ranged from 51.7–100% (Table 4). Interestingly, the authors found that the accuracy of home tests was greatly affected by their users. The kits demonstrated poor sensitivity when used in studies by women evaluating their own samples (sensitivity 0.75; 95% confidence interval 0.64–0.85) when compared with studies in which volunteers performed the tests (sensitivity 0.91; 95% confidence interval 0.84–0.96) (35). The test effectiveness score (a measure of the discriminatory power of the test, with higher scores implying greater effectiveness) was 2.75 (range, 2.3–3.2) for studies in which subjects were volunteers but 0.82 (range, 0.4–1.2) for studies with actual patients (Figure 4). One explanation for the low sensitivity in women who tested their own urine may be that they obtained their urine samples before the recommended number of days after their missed

Table 3 Commercial Kits Currently Available in the United States for Detecting Urinary hCG[a]

Brand name	Manufacturer	Type	Test time (min)	Detection limit (IU/L)[b]	Accuracy (%)[b]
LifeSign 1 Midstream	Geodesic Meditech, Inc. (Del Mar, CA)	In-stream	3	15	99
AimStick	Craig Medical Distribution, Inc. (Vista, CA)	One-step	3	20	99
First Response Early Result	Carter-Wallace, Inc. (New York, NY)	In-stream	3	25[c]	99
Equate	LifeCare Medical Int. Corp. (Philadelphia, PA)	In-stream	3–10	25	99.9
e.p.t.	Warner-Lambert Consumer Division of Pfiser (Morris Plains, NJ)	In-stream	3	40	99
ClearBlue Easy	Unipath Ltd. (Bedford, UK)	In-stream	1	50	>99
ClearPlan Easy	Unipath Ltd. (Bedford, UK)	In-stream	1	50	>99
Walgreens, Target, and RiteAid	Inverness Medical, Inc. (Waltham, MA)	In-stream	10	50	99
First Response One Step	Carter-Wallace, Inc. (New York, NY)	In-stream	2	100	99

[a] Partial list.

[b] According to manufacturer.

[c] Not available from manufacturer. Value obtained at URL www.fertilityplus.org/faq/htp.htm.

Table 4 Diagnostic Characteristics of Kits by Study

Source	Year	Type of kit	Sensitivity (%)	Specificity (%)	Effectiveness test score (95% CI)[a]
Baker et al. (49)	1976	Ova II	52.6	51.9	0.09 (−0.5 to 0.7)
Arends and Uldall (50)	1977	Predictor	97	96	3.4 (2.6 to 4.2)
Doshi (38)	1986	Answer	78	64	1.0 (0.4 to 1.6)
		Daisy 2	82	64	1.1 (0.3 to 1.9)
		e.p.t.	82	75	1.1 (0.5 to 1.7)
Hicks and Iosefsohn (51)	1989	e.p.t. plus	90	92	2.5 (1.9 to 3.1)
		Advance	86	91	2.2 (1.6 to 2.8)
Latman and Bruot (39)	1989	Fact	100	93.5	3.7 (2.1 to 5.3)
		e.p.t. plus	94.6	100	3.6 (2.1 to 5.2)
		Answer 2	100	93.5	3.6 (2.0 to 5.2)
		First Response	92.9	100	3.3 (1.8 to 4.9)
		Advance	91.2	100	3.3 (1.8 to 4.8)
		e.p.t.	88.2	100	3.2 (1.7 to 4.7)
		Predictor	100	76.7	2.9 (1.4 to 4.4)
		Daisy 2	97.5	60.5	2.0 (1.1 to 3.0)
		Acu to test	51.7	88.9	1.3 (0.5 to 2.1)

[a] CI indicates confidence interval.
Source: Ref. 35.

menstrual period. Collection may have occurred during the time in which the concentration of urine hCG is below the detectable limit of the test kits (35). Another likely reason is operator error resulting from failure to read or follow the test instructions (35). In order to increase the sensitivity of consumer-performed tests, the authors suggest that women wait at least 2 wk after a missed period before performing the test and they encourage manufacturers of POCT hCG kits to publish results of trials in actual patients prior to marketing their products. A home pregnancy kit that demonstrates a low sensitivity is a potential public health risk. False negative results can delay appropriate prenatal care and are likely to provide a false sense of security in the patient who could potentially engage in activities that put the fetus at risk (36).

A study of 11 POCT hCG tests sold in France also revealed a lower sensitivity than the one stated by the manufacturer when performed by laypersons (37). Although nearly all the negative specimens were correctly interpreted, 53% of urine specimens with hCG concentrations at the detection limit and 39% of specimens with twice the detection limit were considered negative (37). The main reason for the low sensitivity was determined to be the users' difficulty in interpreting the instructions.

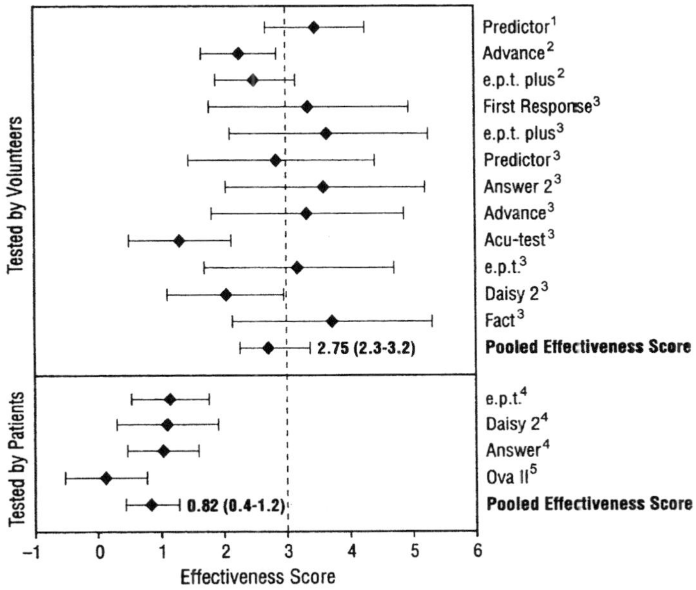

Figure 4 Effectiveness scores for the home pregnancy test kits according to whether the kits were tested by patients or volunteers. The dashed line indicates that an effectiveness score of 3.0 would yield results for pregnant women that are 3 SDs away from those of a population of nonpregnant women. [1]Ref. 50; [2]Ref. 51; [3]Ref. 39; [4]Ref. 38; [5]Ref. 49. (From Ref. 35.)

Other earlier studies reported similar results. An evaluation of three hCG kits with 109 women whose menses were between 6 and 20 days late found test accuracies to be lower (60–85.7%) than those reported by the manufacturers (98–99%) (38). Another study of nine hCG kits, using normal male urine spiked with varied concentrations of hCG, reported accuracies that ranged from 70–97% (39). The problems involved with laypersons performing home pregnancy tests is discussed further by Hicks (36).

A large-molecular-weight variant of hCG, called hyperglycosylated hCG (H-hCG), contains a high content of branched oligosaccharides. It is the principal form of hCG produced in the week following implantation (40) and may represent the predominant immunoreactive protein in serum and urine shortly after conception (41). The ability of in-home tests to detect this early form of hCG was recently investigated (42). Fifteen widely available hCG kits were tested using normal male urine spiked with either regular hCG or H-hCG at concentrations ranging from 6.3–50 IU/L. While all 15 kits were able to detect regular hCG at a concentration of 50 IU/L, 4 of the 15 (27%) failed to detect H-hCG at the same concentration (42). At a concentration of 25 IU/L, 1 of the 15 (7%) did not detect the regular hCG standard and 7 of the 15 (47%) did not detect the H-hCG standard (42). Because users of in-home hCG tests are likely to perform the test at a time when H-hCG is most abundant, the authors suggest that it may be important that these assays detect this glycosylated form of the hormone.

Surprisingly, very few studies have been published in reference to the accuracy of rapid qualitative hCG tests marketed to and used by clinical laboratories. One study from 1990 evaluated three in-laboratory kits (Tandem Icon II, Hybritech, Inc.; Novoclone Target, Novo Industries; Abbott Test Pack, Abbott Laboratories) and reported accuracies that ranged from 74–92% for urine and 72–92% for serum (43). The Novoclone Target assay failed to detect hCG in urine specimens collected from two patients who had serum hCG concentrations of 65,000 and 72,000 IU/L (43). The authors had no explanation for these false negatives. An even older report, from 1986, investigated eight hCG tests of varying methodologies and reported accuracies ranging from 89–99% (44). This study identified the high-dose hook effect as the potential cause of some false negative results. The high-dose hook effect (also known as a prozone effect) occurs in one-step sandwich assays when antigen excess prevents sandwich formation and causes falsely low values (45,46). Indeed, others have also reported a hook effect when testing urine with a high hCG concentration with qualitative hCG tests (47). Both false positive and false negative results have been reported due to elevated protein concentrations (44,48) and blood in the urine (44).

SUMMARY

The introduction of rapid, qualitative fertility tests has undeniably changed the home healthcare market. Women seeking answers to their fertility status need go no further than their local drugstore. Using the appropriate devices, they should be able to identify their most fertile period and detect a resulting pregnancy without visiting a physician's office.

The majority of devices used to predict ovulation continue to be immunoassays for detecting the urinary LH surge. While it is clear that these tests accurately detect the hormone, what is less certain is their ability to deliver what they are marketed for: an increased chance for conception. To our knowledge, no studies have been published investigating this issue with normal cycling women who are not seeking fertility treatment. This is remarkable considering that these devices are marketed to exactly that population of consumers. Nonurine tests for predicting ovulation are few in number and most have not yet received approval for marketing from the FDA.

Urine hCG tests make up the largest segment of over-the-counter testing devices and are marketed as being sensitive enough to detect hCG on the day of the missed menstrual period or even sooner. Surprisingly, this issue has also not been addressed in published studies. While the devices are analytically capable of detecting small quantities of the hormone, the diagnostic performance as stated by their manufacturers has not been scrutinized.

A common remark in many of the studies is regarding inability of consumers to follow the instructions provided with the devices and to properly perform the test. If the consumer is unable or unwilling to follow the instructions then even the most sensitive tests are likely to perform poorly. Package inserts must be absolutely specific in their instructions and consumers should be counseled to follow them explicitly.

Point-of-care testing as it applies to fertility testing is deceptively simple. Current test methodologies are well defined in concept but their application to conception and pregnancy is not always straightforward. Further studies are required in order to answer some of the most fundamental questions regarding the increased probability for conception and the detection of pregnancy.

REFERENCES

1. Wilcox AJ, Weinberg CR, Baird DB. Timing of sexual intercourse in relation to ovulation. N Engl J Med 333:1517–1521, 1995.
2. Corsan GH, Ghazi D, Kemmann E. Home urinary luteinizing hormone immunoassays: Clinical applications. Fertil Steril 53:591–601, 1990.
3. Miller PB, Soules MR. The usefulness of a urinary LH kit for ovulation prediction during menstrual cycles of normal women. Obstet Gynecol 87:13–17, 1996.
4. Carr BR. Disorders of the ovaries and the female reproductive tract. In: Wilson JD, Foster DW, Kronenberg HM, Larsen PR, eds. Williams' Textbook of Endocrinology. Saunders, Philadelphia, 1998, pp 751–817.
5. Insler V, Melmed H, Eichenbrenner I, Serr DM, Lunenfeld B. The cervical score: A simple semiquantitative method for monitoring of the menstrual cycle. J Gynaecol Obstet 10:223–228, 1972.
6. Gronowski AM, Landau-Levine M. Reproductive endocrine function. In: Burtis CA, Ashwood ER, eds. Tietz Textbook of Clinical Chemistry. Saunders, Philadelphia, 1999, pp 1601–1641.
7. Corson SL. Self-prediction of ovulation using a urinary luteinizing hormone test. J Reprod Med 31:760–763, 1986.
8. Elkind-Hirsch K, Goldzieher JW, Gibbons WE, Besch PK. Evaluation of the ovuSTICK urinary luteinizing hormone kit in normal and stimulated menstrual cycles. Obstet Gynecol 67:450–453, 1986.
9. Lloyd R, Coulam CB. The accuracy of urinary luteinizing hormone testing in predicting ovulation. Am J Obstet Gynecol 160:1370–1375, 1989.
10. Gudgeon K, Leader L, Howard B. Evaluation of the accuracy of the home ovula-

tion detection kit, ClearPlan, at predicting ovulation. Med J Aust 152:344–349, 2001.
11. Vermesh M, Kletzky OA, Davajan V, Israel R. Monitoring techniques to predict and detect ovulation. Fertil Steril 47:259–264, 1987.
12. Guermandi E, Vegetti W, Bianchi MM, Uglietti A, Ragni G, Crosignani P. Reliability of ovulation tests in infertile women. Obstet Gynecol 97:92–96, 2001.
13. Grinstead J, Jacobsen JD, Grinstead L, Schantz A, Stenfoss HH, Nielsen SP. Prediction of ovulation. Fertil Steril 52:388–393, 1989.
14. Cahill DJ, Wardle PG, Harlow CR, Hull MGR. Onset of the preovulatory luteinizing hormone surge: Diurnal timing and critical follicular prerequisites. Fertil Steril 70: 56–59, 1998.
15. Leader L, Russell T, Clifford K, Stenning B. The clinical value of ClearPlan home ovulation detection kits in infertility practice. Aust NZ J Obstet Gynaecol 31:142–144, 1991.
16. Behre HM, Kuhlage J, Gassner C, Sonntag B, Schem C, Schneider HPG, Nieschlag E. Prediction of ovulation by urinary hormone measurements with the home use ClearPlan fertility monitor: Comparison with transvaginal ultrasound scans and serum hormone measurements. Hum Reprod 15:2478–2482, 2000.
17. Bonnar J, Flynn A, Freundl G, Royston R, Snowden R. Personal hormone monitoring for contraception. Br J Fam Plan 24:128–134, 1999.
18. Fehring RJ, Schlaff WD. Accuracy of the Ovulon fertility monitor to predict and detect ovulation. J Midwif Women's Health 43:117–120, 1998.
19. Albrecht BH, Fernando RS, Regas J, Betz G. A new method for predicting and confirming ovulation. Fertil Steril 44:200–205, 1985.
20. Fernando RS, Regas J, Betz G. Ovulation prediction and detection with the CUE ovulation predictor. Hum Reprod 3:419–424, 1988.
21. Moreno JE, Khan-Dawood FS, Goldzieher JW. Natural family planning: Suitability of the CUE method for defining the time of ovulation. Contraception 55:233–237, 1997.
22. Freundl G, Bremme M, Frank-Herrmann P, Baur S, Godehardt E, Sottong U. The CUE fertility monitor compared to ultrasound and LH peak measurements for fertile time ovulation detection. Adv Contracep 12:111–121, 1996.
23. Robinson JN, Lockwood GM, Dalton JDE, Franklin PA, Farr MMC. A randomized prospective study to assess the effect of the use of home urinary luteinizing hormone detection on the efficiency of donor insemination. Hum Reprod 7:63–65, 1992.
24. Kossoy L, Hill GA, Herbert CM, Brodie BL, Dalglish CS, Dupont WD, Wentz AC. Therapeutic donor insemination: The impact of insemination timing with the aid of a urinary luteinizing hormone immunoassay. Fertil Steril 49:1026–1029, 1988.
25. Irons DW, Singh M. Evaluation of transvaginal sonography combined with a urinary luteinizing hormone monitor in timing donor insemination. Hum Reprod 9:1859–1862, 1994.
26. Anderson RA, Eccles SM, Irvine DS. Home ovulation testing in a donor insemination service. Hum Reprod 11:1674–1677, 1996.
27. Horne G, Jamaludin A, Critchlow JD, Falconer DA, Newman MC, Oghoetuoma J et al. A 3 year retrospective review of intrauterine insemination, using cryopreserved

donor spermatazoa and cycle monitoring by urinary or serum luteinizing hormone. Hum Reprod 13:3045–3048, 1998.
28. Odem RR, Durso NM, Long CA, Pineda JA, Strickler JA, Gast MJ. Therapeutic donor insemination: A prospective randomized study of scheduling methods. Fertil Steril 55:976–982, 1991.
29. Barratt CLR, Cooke S, Chauhan M, Cooke ID. A prospective randomized controlled trial comparing urinary luteinizing hormone dipsticks and basal body temperature charts with time donor insemination. Fertil Steril 52:394–397, 1989.
30. Brook PF, Barratt CLR, Cooke ID. The more accurate timing of insemination with regard to ovulation does not create a significant improvement in pregnancy rates in a donor insemination program. Fertil Steril 61:308–313, 1994.
31. Wainer R, Merlot F, Ducot B, Bailly M, Tribalat S, Lombrosco R. Prospective randomized comparison of intrauterine and intracervical insemination with donor spermatazoa. Hum Reprod 10:2919–2922, 1995.
32. Corsan GH, Blotner MB, Bohrer MK, Sheldon R, Kemmann E. The utility of a home urinary LH immunoassay in timing the postcoital test. Obstet Gynecol 81: 736–738, 1993.
33. Nulsen J, Wheeler C, Ausmanas M, Blasco L. Cervical mucus changes in relationship to urinary luteinizing hormone. Fertil Steril 48:783–786, 1987.
34. Jeng LL, Moore RM, Kaczmarek RG, Placek PJ, Bright RA. How frequently are home pregnancy tests used? Results from the 1988 national maternal and infant health survey. Birth 18:11–13, 1991.
35. Bastian LA, Nanda K, Hasselblad V, Simel DL. Diagnostic efficiency of home pregnancy test kits: A meta-analysis. Arch Fam Med 7:465–469, 1998.
36. Hicks JM. Home testing: To do or not to do? Clin Chem 39:7–8, 1993.
37. Daviaud J, Fournet D, Ballongue C, Guillem G-P, Leblanc A, Casellas C, Pau B. Reliability and feasibility of pregnancy home-use tests: Laboratory validation and diagnostic evaluation by 638 volunteers. Clin Chem 39:53–59, 1993.
38. Doshi ML. Accuracy of consumer performed in-home tests for early pregnancy detection. Am J Public Health 76:512–514, 1986.
39. Latman NS, Bruot BC. Evaluation of home pregnancy test kits. Biomed Instrum Technol 23:144–149, 1989.
40. O'Conner JF, Ellish N, Kakuma T, Schlatterer J, Kovalevskaya G. Differential urinary gonadotropin profiles in early pregnancy and early pregnancy loss. Prenat Diagn 18:1232–1240, 1998.
41. Kovalevskaya G, Birken S, Kakuma T, O'Conner JF. Early pregnancy human chorionic gonadotropin (hCG) isoforms measured by an immunometric assay for choriocarcinoma-like hCG. J Endocrinol 161:99–106, 1999.
42. Butler SA, Khanlian SA, Cole LA. Utility of home pregnancy test devices for early pregnancy hCG. Clin Chem 47:2131–2136, 2001.
43. Christensen H, Thyssen HH, Schebye O, Berget A. Three highly sensitive "bedside" serum and urine tests for pregnancy compared. Clin Chem 36:1686–1688, 1990.
44. Gelletlie R, Nielsen JB. Evaluation and comparison of commercially available pregnancy tests based on monoclonal antibodies to human choriogonadotropin. Clin Chem 32:2166–2170, 1986.

45. Armbruster DA. Choriogonadotropin and pregnancy testing: Prozone phenomenon defined. Clin Chem 33:742, 1987.
46. Yoo A, Zaccaro J. Falsely low serum hCG level in a patient with hydatidiform mole caused by the "high-dose hook effect." Lab Med 31:431–435, 2000.
47. Stickle DF, Gronowski AM, Olsen GA, Fellows PA, Avery MB. Decreased signal intensity of Sure-Vue serum/urine qualitative hCG test at high [hCG]. Clin Chem 46:A3, 2000.
48. Planet G. False-positive pregnancy test. Clin Chem 36:1522–1523, 1990.
49. Baker LD, Yert LW, Chase MC, Dale E. Evaluation of a "do-it-yourself" pregnancy test. Am J Public Health 66:166–167, 1976.
50. Arends J, Uldall A. The reliability of pregnancy tests performed by trained and untrained persons. Dan Med Bull 24:115–116, 1977.
51. Hicks JM, Iosefsohn M. Reliability of home pregnancy-test kits in the hands of laypersons. N Engl J Med 320:320–321, 1989.

18
Fetal Fibronectin

David G. Grenache and Ann M. Gronowski
Washington University School of Medicine, St. Louis, Missouri, U.S.A.

FETAL FIBRONECTIN

The fibronectin family of proteins is found in the extracellular matrix and plasma. Fibronectins interact with specific adhesion molecules on cell surfaces and have been implicated in the regulation of cell differentiation, proliferation, migration, and apoptosis (1). Fetal fibronectin (fFN) is an immunologically unique fibronectin that contains an epitope referred to as the oncofetal domain that is recognized by the monoclonal antibody FDC-6 (2). During gestation, fFN's location at the choriodecidual interface suggests a role for this protein in anchoring the fetal trophoblast to the maternal decidua (3). Fetal fibronectin is released into cervicovaginal secretions before the onset of labor, and although the mechanism of this release is not clear, it has been suspected to occur by either mechanical or inflammatory mechanisms (4).

Although fFN is detectable in cervicovaginal secretions during the first 24 wk of pregnancy, it typically declines to undetectable concentrations between weeks 24 and 34. Numerous studies have reported that cervicovaginal fFN concentrations ≥50 ng/mL indicate a high risk for preterm delivery in both symptomatic (3,5–9) and asymptomatic women (10 -13). While these and other studies have utilized a microtiter plate ELISA assay for fFN (Adeza Biomedical, Sunnyvale, CA) fewer studies have utilized the rapid fFN assays available from the same manufacturer. The focus of this chapter is the rapid assays for fFN and their utility in predicting preterm delivery. In addition to its use as a marker of preterm delivery, this chapter also addresses the use of rapid fFN in guiding the treatment of preterm labor, its effect on admissions and cost savings, its ability to predict the onset of *term* labor, its use as a selection criterion for labor induction and a predictor of success, and its utility in predicting preterm delivery in twin gestations.

RAPID QUALITATIVE ASSAYS FOR FETAL FIBRONECTIN

Two rapid assays for fFN are currently marketed by Adeza Biomedical that utilize the anti-fFN monoclonal antibody FDC-6. The first assay is a membrane immunogold assay. This assay utilizes an antihuman fibronectin–gold colloid conjugate that binds to fFN present in the specimen. Detection of the fFN–gold colloid complex is accomplished by passing the specimen through a membrane containing a monoclonal antibody specific for fFN that binds the complexes, producing a visible spot within 5 min. Specimens with a fibronectin concentration >50 ng/mL will produce a positive result within a control ring that is interpreted visually. This assay is not available in the United States and its use has been reported in the literature only from countries other than the United States.

The second assay, the Rapid fFN Cassette, is available in the United States and was U.S. Food and Drug Administration (FDA) approved for marketing in 1998. It is also a membrane immunoassay and uses a monoclonal anti-fFN antibody coupled to a blue microsphere and an immobilized polyclonal goat anti-FN antibody. The intensities of the test and control lines on the device are interpreted with the TLi™ analyzer. Specimens with fFN concentrations >50 ng/mL are resulted as positive. Although this assay is the only one exclusively used in the United States to measure fFN, we were unable to identify any published studies of the Rapid fFN Cassette used in conjunction with the TLi analyzer; therefore all of the data presented here represent fFN analyses performed using the immunogold assay.

FETAL FIBRONECTIN AND PREDICTING PRETERM DELIVERY

Preterm delivery of an infant, defined as delivery prior to completion of 37 wk of gestation, occurs in ~11% of all pregnancies and is a significant cause of neonatal morbidity and mortality (14,15). Major causes of preterm birth include premature labor, spontaneous rupture of the membranes, and elective delivery induction for medical intervention (16). While medical standards for diagnosing and treating preterm labor exist, the management of these women is complicated by the fact that many women have no observable risk factors for preterm labor and are not treated until they actually develop cervical dilation, after which point intervention strategies often fail to prevent delivery (4). Additionally, the majority do not go on to deliver preterm infants, making the decision of who to actually hospitalize a difficult one.

Predicting preterm labor has traditionally relied on methods that are neither sensitive nor specific, such as obstetrical history or symptoms and epidemiological risk factors (17). A rapid method to accurately distinguish women who have preterm labor and who are likely to deliver preterm infants from those who have apparent preterm labor and are unlikely to deliver prematurely would prevent unnecessary and potentially risky interventions and could reduce treatment costs. One such method is the detection of fetal fibronectin in the cervicovaginal fluid.

Numerous studies using a microtiter plate ELISA fFN assay have been published on the clinical utility of fFN in predicting preterm delivery. Nearly all of them have produced similar results regarding the accuracy of fFN for both symptomatic and asymptomatic women with preterm labor. While the negative predictive value (NPV) of fFN is excellent, the positive predictive value (PPV) is not nearly as robust. The high number of false positive results encountered with the assay means that all women with preterm labor and a positive fFN test result receive standard treatment for preterm labor, even those women in whom preterm delivery is not likely to occur.

One of the first studies to utilize the rapid detection of fFN as a predictor of early delivery enrolled 36 women with singleton pregnancy between 20 and 34 wk of gestation (18). All patients had a diagnosis of threatened preterm labor with intact membranes and a cervical dilation ≤2 cm. Cervicovaginal fluid was collected and analyzed for fFN and results of the assay were not available to physicians treating the patients. Fetal fibronectin was detected in 11 patients, five of whom delivered infants at <34 wk of gestation and six of whom delivered at ≥34 wk of gestation. A negative fFN result was recorded in 25 patients, none of whom delivered infants before 34 wk of gestation. These data yield a 100% sensitivity, an 81% specificity, a 46% positive predictive value (PPV), and a 100% negative predictive value (NPV) (Table 1, Study 1) (18). There was no significant difference in the weeks of gestation at time of sampling between the positive and negative groups (29.9 and 29.5 wk, respectively) but there was a significant difference in the number of days between sampling and delivery (34.3 days in fFN positive women compared with 60.4 days in fFN negative women, $p < 0.02$) (18). These findings are similar to those reported with the use of a microtiter plate ELISA fFN assay. The high NPV essentially rules out preterm delivery and suggests that it may be possible to delay or avoid unnecessary interventions in women with symptoms of preterm labor and a negative fFN result.

A follow-up study by the same group was conducted to evaluate the rapid fFN assay in routine clinical practice and to determine if knowledge of the fFN would influence patient management (19). This retrospective study examined 70 women with singleton pregnancy at <34 wk of gestation and with symptoms of preterm labor (defined as regular uterine contractions). All patients had intact

Table 1 Summary of Selected Rapid Fetal Fibronectin Studies

Study	Reference	Use of fetal fibronectin	Study type	*n*	Gestational age (wk)	Endpoint	Sensitivity (%)	Specificity (%)	PPV (%)[b]	NPV (%)[c]
1	Parker et al. (18)	Predict preterm birth	Prospective	36	20–34	PTD[a] <34 wk	100	81	46	100
2	Chuileannain et al. (19)	Management of preterm labor	Retrospective	70	<34	PTD <34 wk	90	82	45	98
3	Benattar et al. (20)	Prognosis of preterm labor	Prospective	124	24–36	Delivery w/in 7 days	89	90	42	99
						Delivery w/in 14 days	69	93	57	95
						Delivery w/in 21 days	46	91	58	81
						PTD <32 wk	73	91	55	97
						PTD <37 wk	36	91	50	85
4	Giles et al. (24)	Management of preterm labor	Prospective	151	24–34	PTD <36 wk	63	75	27	93
5	Ahner et al. (25)	Predict onset of term labor	Prospective	100	Date of confinement	Delivery w/in 48 hr	81	91	86	88
6	Ahner et al. (28)	Criterion of labor induction	Prospective	64	≥38	Delivery w/in 24 hr	68	89	93	57
7	Oliveira et al. (21)	Predict preterm delivery in twin gestations	Prospective	52	24–34	PTD <34 wk	80	38	24	89
						PTD <37 wk	89	50	68	80

[a] PTD = preterm delivery.
[b] PPV = positive predictive value.
[c] NPV = negative predictive value.

membranes and had cervical dilation <2 cm. Twenty women were positive for fFN and the remaining 50 were negative. Ten women delivered at <34 wk of gestation, nine of whom were fFN positive (sensitivity 90%) and 60 women delivered at ≥34 wk of gestation, 49 of whom were fFN negative (specificity 82%) (19). The positive and negative predictive values of the fFN assay in identifying women at risk of preterm birth were nearly identical to the previous study at 45% and 98%, respectively (see Table 1, Study 2). Similarly, women with a positive fFN were significantly more likely to deliver prior to 34 wk of gestation compared with those with a negative fFN test ($p = 0.00002$). The study also showed that women with a positive fFN received corticosteroids ($n = 56$) and tocolytic therapy ($n = 70$) more often than those with a negative result (19).

Another study that evaluated the utility of the rapid fFN test in the prediction of preterm delivery reached similar conclusions, although they included women up to 36 wk of gestation (20). One hundred twenty-four women between 24 and 36 wk of gestation and who were diagnosed with preterm labor by regular uterine contractions and cervical changes were entered into the study, including 14 twin pregnancies. All patients had intact membranes and cervical dilation ≤3 cm. The results of fFN testing were not available to the obstetrician and all patients received tocolysis. Nineteen patients tested positive and 105 tested negative for fFN. Preterm delivery occurred in 47% (9 of 19) of the fFN positive patients and in 15% (16 of 105) of fFN negative patients (20). Patients were grouped according to delivery within 7, 14, or 21 days of sampling and before 32 or after 37 wk of gestation. The sensitivity, specificity, NPV, and PPV of fFN were determined for each group (see Table 1, Study 3). The presence of fFN in cervicovaginal secretions had a high sensitivity for delivery within seven days (89%) that decreased, not unexpectedly, to 46% at day 21. The absence of fFN in patients with symptoms of preterm labor was able to rule out preterm delivery within seven days with excellent accuracy (99% NPV). The high NPV continued until day 14, after which it decreased to 81% at day 21. The inclusion of the 14 twin pregnancies in the study was reported to have had no effect on the results, although others have reported a lower NPV for predicting preterm delivery in a population of women with twin gestations (21). Still, this is additional supportive evidence for the use of a rapid fFN test to predict preterm delivery in patients with preterm labor.

FETAL FIBRONECTIN AND TREATMENT OF PRETERM LABOR

The decision to treat a patient presenting with apparent preterm labor is a difficult one, especially if the patient has intact membranes and a closed cervix. The physician must decide whether to provide tocolytic therapy immediately or wait and watch for cervical dilation as a definitive sign of preterm labor. Tocolytic drugs can stop uterine contractions for up to 48 hr and allow time for the administration of corticosteroids in an attempt to decrease the likelihood of neonatal respiratory distress (16). Unfortunately, initiating treatment after cervical dilation frequently fails to prevent preterm birth (4). If treatment is provided to all women with symptoms of preterm labor, then 50–80% of all patients will receive unnecessary tocolytic therapy (22).

The use of fFN in guiding treatment of preterm labor has been reported (22). Women between 25 and 34 wk of gestation and with symptoms of preterm labor were considered eligible for the prospective study if they had intact membranes and a cervix that was <3 cm dilated. Women with vaginal bleeding or a history of sexual intercourse within the past 24 hr were excluded (the latter of which has been associated with the presence of fFN) (23). Sixteen patients were entered into the study and were compared with 32 historical control patients, none of whom had been evaluated for fFN status and had been managed according to standard protocols, including tocolysis. Patients who tested positive for fFN received tocolysis, glucocorticoid, and vitamin K, while fFN negative patients received only glucocorticoid and vitamin K and received tocolysis only if cervical changes occurred. Three of the 16 patients (19%) in the study group tested positive for fFN and received tocolytics compared with 30 patients (94%) in the control group who received tocolysis ($p < 0.0001$) (22). There were no significant differences between the two groups in regard to week of delivery or neonatal outcome. Although the number of patients in the study group was small, the data illustrate that the high NPV of the fFN assay can be utilized to reduce the use of tocolytics in patients who are not likely to benefit from them.

The use of fFN testing has also been shown to reduce maternal transfer to tertiary obstetrical units, resulting in cost savings (24). This is especially important for women with symptoms of preterm labor who first present to rural hospitals with small obstetrical units. Transferring all symptomatic women to tertiary care units generates significant costs to the referring and receiving hospitals and is clearly a disruption for the patients and their families. Clearly, identifying the best patients to transfer would be more beneficial. This prospective study examined the effect of fFN testing on maternal transfer from rural referral hospitals to a tertiary obstetrical unit at a regional medical center. The study enrolled 151 patients admitted to either the primary hospital ($n = 53$) or one of nine referring hospitals ($n = 98$) with a diagnosis of preterm labor with intact membranes and who were between 24 and 34 wk of gestation. Patients who had vaginal bleeding, recent sexual intercourse, or vaginal examination in the preceding 24 hr were excluded. Of 106 patients with a negative fFN test result, 99 (93%) delivered at ≥36 wk of gestation and seven (7%) delivered at <36 wk (one by elective cesarean delivery and five within seven days after the fFN test was performed; three of whom had cervical dilation >3 cm and two of whom had a closed cervix)

(24). Of 45 patients with a positive fFN test result, 11 (24%) delivered within seven days of testing, one (2%) delivered at 34 wk of gestation, and 33 (73%) delivered at ≥36 wk of gestation (24). Seven fFN positive patients had a cervical dilation >3 cm and all delivered within eight days of testing (24). These data produce a sensitivity of 63%, a specificity of 75%, and a positive and negative predictive value of 27% and 93%, respectively, for predicting birth at <36 wk of gestation (see Table 1, Study 4). Notably, inclusion criteria included cervical dilation <5 cm. Cervical dilation >3 cm is usually considered to be a contraindication for performing fFN testing. Of the 98 patients admitted to the referral hospitals, only 11% (7 of 65) with a negative fFN test result were transferred to the tertiary obstetrical unit compared with 88% (29 of 33) with a positive fFN test result (24). The authors indicate that this significant difference resulted in a cost savings of $30,297.47 because road or air ambulance had not been used to transport 81% of the fFN negative patients. Furthermore, an additional savings of $153,120 was realized because 58 patients with a negative fFN were not treated according to their standard protocol (admission for tocolysis and corticosteroid; average 7-day admission). Finally, the average hospital admission for patients transferred with a negative fFN was 7.6 days shorter than for patients with a positive fFN test result, which produced an average savings of $2970 per patient (24). While it is clear that a cost savings was realized by the utilization of fFN testing in women with symptoms of preterm labor, it should be noted that these savings will vary depending on the level and frequency of transport. This particular study was performed at a hospital that services the northern half of the state of New South Wales, Australia, and the nine referral hospitals varied in distance from 9–506 miles.

FETAL FIBRONECTIN AND TERM LABOR

Fetal fibronectin has also been shown to be a useful predictor of the onset of term labor. One prospective study examined 100 women who had reached their date of confinement and who did not have regular uterine contractions or ruptured membranes and who had cervical dilation ≤3 cm (25). Specimens for fFN analysis were collected at a single, routine clinic visit. In addition to fFN analysis, patients had cervical assessment by means of a modified Bishop score* (scale 0–12). Patients were divided into those women delivering within 48 hr and those

* First described in 1964, Bishop (30) developed a scoring system based on factors correlated with uterine ripeness, including cervical dilation, percentage effacement, and others (30). The modified Bishop score was proposed by Burnett (31) to increase its predictability for successful induction and decreased morbidity rates associated with induction. Higher scores are associated with uterine readiness.

delivering >48 hr after fFN testing. Patients who did not deliver vaginally were excluded from the analysis. Forty-one patients delivered within 48 hr of sampling, four of whom did not deliver vaginally. The fFN assay was positive for 30 and negative for seven (81% sensitivity) (25). This population's median Bishop score was 5. Fifty-nine patients delivered >48 hr after sampling, three of whom did not deliver vaginally. The fFN assay was negative for 51 and positive for five (91% specificity) (25). The mean Bishop score of this group was 4. Women who delivered within 48 hr of fFN sampling had a significantly higher frequency of positive fFN compared with those who delivered later than 48 hr after sampling ($p < 0.0001$). In addition, the fFN assay had higher predictive values (88% NPV and 86% PPV) (see Table 1, Study 5) compared with the Bishop score in regard to the onset of spontaneous labor (77 and 55%, respectively) (25).

A separate study comparing the fFN result of 78 women (37–41 wk of gestation) to the modified Bishop score reported similar findings (26). Cervicovaginal specimens were collected from patients at each clinic visit beginning at 38 wk of gestation and through to the onset of labor. All patients entered spontaneous labor and two were delivered by cesarean section. The mean time to delivery in patients who had a positive fFN result at their last clinic visit was 3 ± 1.9 days. This was significantly shorter than the mean time to delivery in those who had a negative fFN result at their last clinic visit, 5.7 ± 3.9 days (26). There was no significant difference between high or low Bishop scores or the mean time to delivery. As in the previous study, the presence of fFN in cervicovaginal secretions indicates that the onset of labor is imminent. These findings are clinically useful in that they may allow better management of women in whom labor induction is being considered.

FETAL FIBRONECTIN AND LABOR INDUCTION

The induction of labor, defined as the initiation of uterine contractions prior to the onset of spontaneous labor, is a common obstetrical practice that has increased in frequency from 90 per 1000 live births in 1989 to 184 per 1000 live births in 1997 (27). In order to avoid complications of labor induction, such as prolonged labor due to the lack of uterine readiness, careful assessment of uterine status is essential and is most commonly determined by the Bishop score (27). The clinical use of the rapid fFN assay in labor induction has recently been described. One study compared the ability of fFN to serve as a more sensitive selection criterion for the induction of labor than the Bishop score (28). Entered into the study were 64 women at ≥38 wk of gestation who were scheduled for labor induction with prostaglandin E_2 and who did not have regular contractions or ruptured membranes and whose cervical diameter was ≤3 cm. Fetal fibronectin was measured with a rapid assay and reconfirmed with a microtiter plate ELISA assay, and only concordant results were included in the statistical analyses. Labor induction was considered successful if vaginal delivery occurred within 24 hr after the application of cervical prostaglandin tablets (cesarean deliveries were not included). Concordance was found in 63 specimens; one specimen produced a quantitative result of 1740 ng/mL but a negative qualitative result (28). A positive fFN result was recorded for 30 women, 27 of whom had vaginal deliveries and three of whom were delivered by cesarean section (28). Twenty-five of these patients were delivered within 24 hr of induction. The median Bishop score of this population was 5. The remaining 33 women had a negative fFN result, with 27 delivering vaginally, five by cesarean section, and one by vacuum extraction. Of the 28 women with spontaneous deliveries, 12 gave birth within 24 hr of induction. The median Bishop score in this population was 4. Ninety-three percent (25 of 27) of fFN positive women gave birth vaginally within 24 hr of induction compared with 43% (12 of 28) of fFN negative women ($p < 0.0001$) (28). Multiple logistic regression identified fFN as a significant predictor of delivery within 24 hr of labor induction ($p = 0.0022$) (28). For predicting delivery within 24 hr of labor induction, the rapid fFN assay had a better specificity (89%), NPV (57%), and PPV (93%) compared with the Bishop score, 67%, 50%, and 81%, respectively (28). The sensitivities were the same at 68% (see Table 1, Study 6). These data suggest that labor induction should not be attempted in women with a negative fFN result, as these patients had more unsuccessful inductions and prolonged deliveries. Labor induction can be considered in women with a positive fFN result, although, as already mentioned, these patients are likely to enter labor spontaneously and in short order.

A second study also investigated the use of the rapid fFN assay as a predictor of successful labor induction in term patients (29). This prospective study enrolled patients under an inclusion criteria of >36 wk of gestation and intact membranes who were determined by a managing obstetrician to require labor induction. The induction protocol was not dictated by the study and was left to the discretion of the clinician. Of 160 patients enrolled in the study, 108 had a positive fFN test, with the remaining 52 testing negative (29). The mean Bishop score was significantly higher in the fFN positive patients (4.3 ± 1.5) compared with the fFN negative patients (3.4 ± 1.4) ($p = 0.0002$) (29). The frequency of cesarean section in fFN negative patients was 27% (14 of 52), which was significantly higher compared with 15% (16 of 108) of fFN positive women ($p = 0.05$) (29). Fetal fibronectin positive women also had shorter intervals from the time of first prostaglandin dose to time of delivery (21.3 hr) compared with fFN negative women (35.8 hr) ($p = 0.0001$). This latter finding remained significant even when patients who delivered by cesarean section were excluded from the analysis. Stepwise logistic regression revealed that, compared with a Bishop score of >5, fFN was a highly significant and independent predictor of delivery between 18 and 24 hr after induction (29). Interestingly, a Bishop score >5 did not improve the predictive ability of a positive fFN result and demonstrated no independent predictive value. With the exception of the frequency of cesarean delivery, these differences remained similar in a subpopulation of 73 nulliparous women with Bishop scores ≤5. This is noteworthy in that the Bishop score was developed as a system for scoring multiparous women and there are limited data on the utility of the Bishop score for predicting successful induction in nulliparous patients (29). The reliability of a low Bishop score for predicting successful induction in nulliparous women is therefore questionable. The data from this study suggest that, regardless of the Bishop score, the presence of fFN in cervicovaginal secretions is a predictor of successful induction in both multiparous and nulliparous patients.

FETAL FIBRONECTIN AND PRETERM DELIVERY IN TWIN GESTATIONS

The incidence of perinatal mortality is significantly higher for twin pregnancy compared with singleton pregnancy, a fact attributed to the increased likelihood of preterm delivery with twin gestations (21). The use of fFN testing to predict preterm delivery at <34 and <37 wk of gestation in asymptomatic women with twin pregnancies has been reported (21). This prospective study collected cervicovaginal specimens for fFN testing every two weeks (24–34 wk of gestation) from 52 asymptomatic patients. All patients began the study with an undilated cervix and a cervical length ≥1 cm. A total of 247 samples were collected and analyzed for fFN. The occurrence of at least one fFN positive specimen was considered to be a positive result, and results were not available to the managing clinicians. Thirty-seven patients had a positive fFN test and 15 were fFN negative. Preterm delivery at <37 wk of gestation occurred in 25 patients with a positive fFN result and in three patients with a negative fFN result (89% sensitivity) (21). Delivery at ≥37 wk of gestation occurred in 12 fFN positive and 12 fFN negative patients (50% specificity) (21). Delivery occurred at <34 wk of gestation in 10 patients, eight of whom had a positive fFN (80% sensitivity) (21). The specificity of fFN at <34 wk gestation was 38% (26 of 42) (see Table 1, Study 7). The use of fFN in asymptomatic twin pregnancies appears to be clinically useful in that it allowed for the early identification of women who were likely to enter preterm labor. However, in contrast to data from singleton pregnancies, the lower specificity at <34 and <37 wk of gestation in this population makes the fFN test a poor screening test for predicting preterm delivery in twin gestations. Additionally, the rapid fFN device available in the United States is only approved for use in predicting preterm delivery in symptomatic, not asymptomatic, women with twin gestations.

CONCLUSIONS

The use of a rapid assay for fFN appears to be an effective clinical tool for predicting preterm delivery. Its value as a discriminator between "true" and "false" preterm labor lies in its high negative predictive value. By effectively identifying symptomatic women who are not likely to deliver preterm infants, fFN testing is able to provide better patient care and management as well as produce significant cost savings. This has been shown repeatedly using both the microtiter plate ELISA assays (data from which were not addressed here) as well as the rapid assay. It also has apparent benefit in predicting the onset of term labor and as a criterion for selecting patients who are most likely to benefit from labor induction. These findings, however, have not been frequently reported and should be investigated more thoroughly.

REFERENCES

1. Magnusson MK, Mosher DF. Fibronectin structure, assembly, and cardiovascular implications. Atheroscler Thromb Vasc Biol 18:1363–1370, 1998.
2. Matsuura H, Takio K, Titani K, Greene T, Levery SB, Salyan ME, Hakomori S. The oncofetal structure of human fibronectin defined by monoclonal antibody FDC-6. Unique structural requirement for the antigenic specificity provided by a glycosylhexapeptide. J Biol Chem 263:3314–3322, 1998.
3. Lockwood CJ, Senyei AEDMR, Casal D, Shah KD, Thung SN, Jones L, et al. Fetal fibronectin in cervical and vaginal secretions as a predictor of preterm delivery. N Engl J Med 325:669–674, 1991.
4. Ascarelli MH, Morrison JC. Use of fetal fibronectin in clinical practice. Obstet Gynecol Surv 52:1S–12S, 1997.
5. Morrison JC, Allbert JR, McLaughlin BN, Whitworth NS, Roberts WE, Martin R. Oncofetal fibronectin in patients with false labor as a predictor of preterm delivery. Am J Obstet Gynecol 168:538–542, 1993.
6. Inglis SR, Jeremias J, Kuno K, Lescale K, Peeper Q, Chervenak FA, Witkin SS. Detection of tumor necrosis factor-alpha, interleukin-6, and fetal fibronectin in the lower genital tract during pregnancy: Relation to outcome. Am J Obstet Gynecol 171:5–10, 1994.
7. Iams JD, Casal D, McGregor JA, Goodwin TM, Kreaden US, Lowensohn R, Lockitch G. Fetal fibronectin improves the accuracy of diagnosis of preterm labor. Am J Obstet Gynecol 173:141–145, 1995.

8. Burrus DR, Ernest JM, Veille JC. Fetal fibronectin, interleukin-6, and C-reactive protein are useful in establishing prognostic subcategories of idiopathic preterm labor. Obstet Gynecol 173:1258–1262, 1995.
9. Bartnicki J, Casal D, Kreaden US, Sailing E, Vetter K. Fetal fibronectin in vaginal specimens predicts preterm delivery and very low birthweight infants. Am J Obstet Gynecol 174:971–974, 1996.
10. Lockwood CJ, Wein R, Lapinski R, Casal D, Berkowitz G, Alvarez M, Berkowitz RL. The presence of cervical and vaginal fetal fibronectin predicts preterm delivery in an inner-city obstetric population. Am J Obstet Gynecol 169:798–804, 1993.
11. Leeson SC, Maresh MJA, Martindale T, Mahmood T, Muotune A, Hawkes N, Baldwin KJ. Detection of fetal fibronectin as a predictor of preterm delivery in high risk asymptomatic pregnancies. Br J Obstet Gynecol 103:48–53, 1996.
12. Goldenberg RL, Mercer BM, Meis PJ, Cooper RL, Das A, McNellis D. The preterm prediction study: Fetal fibronectin testing and spontaneous preterm birth. Obstet Gynecol 87:643–648, 1996.
13. Morrison JC, Naef RW, Botti JJ, Katz M, Belluomini JM, McLaughlin BN. Prediction of spontaneous preterm birth by fetal fibronectin and uterine activity. Obstet Gynecol 87:649–655, 1996.
14. Ventura SJ, Martin JA, Curtin SC, Matthews TJ, Park MM. Births: Final data for 1998. National Vital Statistics Report 48:1–99, 2000.
15. Guyer B, Hoyert DL, Martin JA, Ventura SJ, MacDorman MF, Strobino DM. Annual summary of vital statistics—1998. Pediatrics 104:1229–1246, 1999.
16. Goldenberg RL, Rouse DJ. Prevention of premature birth. N Engl J Med 339:313–320, 1998.
17. Lockwood CJ, Kuczynski E. Markers of risk for preterm delivery. J Perinat Med 27:5–20, 1999.
18. Parker J, Bell R, Brennecke S. Fetal fibronectin in the cervicovaginal fluid of women with threatened preterm labour as a predictor of delivery before 34 weeks' gestation. Aust NZ J Obstet Gynecol 35:257–261, 1995.
19. Chuileannain FN, Bell R, Brennecke S. Cervicovaginal fetal fibronectin testing in threatened preterm labour-translating research findings into clinical practice. Aust NZ J Obstet Gynecol 38:399–402, 1998.
20. Benattar C, Taieb J, Fernandez H, Lindendaum A, Frydman R, Ville Y. Rapid fetal fibronectin swab-test in preterm labor patients treated by betamimetics. Eur J Obstet Gynecol 72:131–135, 1997.
21. Oliveira T, De Souza E, Mariani-Neto C, Camano L. Fetal fibronectin as a predictor of preterm delivery in twin gestations. Int J Gynecol Obstet 62:135–139, 1998.
22. Watson DL, Kim SJ, Humphrey MD. Study of cervicovaginal fetal fibronectin status to guide treatment of threatened preterm labour. Aust NZ J Obstet Gynecol 38:185–187, 1998.
23. Shimoya K, Hashimoto K, Shimizu T, Saji F, Murata Y. Effect of sexual intercourse on fetal fibronectin concentration in cervicovaginal secretions. Am J Obstet Gynecol 179:255–256, 1998.
24. Giles W, Bisits A, Knox MMG, Smith R. The effect of fetal fibronectin testing on admissions to a tertiary maternal-fetal medicine unit and cost savings. Am J Obstet Gynecol 182:439–442, 2000.

25. Ahner R, Kiss H, Egarter C, Zeillinger R, Eppel W, Karas H, Husslein P. Obstetrics: Fetal fibronectin as a marker to predict the onset of term labor. Am J Obstet Gynecol 172:134–137, 1995.
26. Luton D, Guibourdenche J, Sibony O, Braig S, Benzakine Y, Oury J-F, et al. Fetal fibronectin in the cervical secretion predicts accurately the onset of labor at term. Eur J Obstet Gynecol 74:161–164, 1997.
27. Hadi H. Cervical ripening and labor induction: Clinical guidelines. Obst Gynecol 43:524–536, 2000.
28. Ahner R, Egarter C, Kiss H, Heinzl K, Zellinger R, Shatten C, et al. Fetal fibronectin as a selection criterion for induction of labor. Am J Obstet Gynecol 173:1513–1517, 1995.
29. Garite TJ, Casal D, Garcia-Alonso A, Kreaden US, Jimenez G, Ayala J, Reimbold T. Fetus-placenta-newborn: Fetal fibronectin: A new tool for the prediction of successful labor induction. Am J Obstet Gynecol 175:1516–1521, 1996.
30. Bishop E. Pelvic scoring for elective induction. Obstet Gynecol 24:266–268, 1964.
31. Burnett J. Prediction scoring: An objective approach to induction of labor. Obstet Gynecol 28:479–483, 1966.

Index